NUTRITION AND DIET RESEARCH PROGRESS

ALLICIN

THE NATURAL SULFUR COMPOUND FROM GARLIC WITH MANY USES

Nutrition and Diet Research Progress

Additional books and e-books in this series can be found on Nova's website under the Series tab.

NUTRITION AND DIET RESEARCH PROGRESS

ALLICIN

THE NATURAL SULFUR COMPOUND FROM GARLIC WITH MANY USES

DIANA R. CUNDELL
EDITOR

nova
Medicine & Health
New York

Additional color graphics may be available in the e-book version of this book.

Library of Congress Cataloging-in-Publication Data

Library of Congress Cataloging-in-Publication Data

Names: Cundell, Diana R., editor.
Title: Allicin : the natural sulfur compound from garlic with many uses / [edited by] Diana R. Cundell.
Identifiers: LCCN 2020000022 (print) | LCCN 2020000023 (ebook) | ISBN 9781536173390 (hardcover) | ISBN 9781536173406 (adobe pdf)
Subjects: LCSH: Garlic--Therapeutic use.
Classification: LCC RM666.G15 A5753 2020 (print) | LCC RM666.G15 (ebook) | DDC 615.3/2478--dc23
LC record available at https://lccn.loc.gov/2020000022
LC ebook record available at https://lccn.loc.gov/2020000023
ISBN: 978-1-53617-339-0

Published by Nova Science Publishers, Inc. † New York

CONTENTS

PREFACE

Allicin is the major active sulfur-containing moiety that is released when garlic cloves are crushed or damaged. Since its first recorded use in ancient times to ward off snakebites and by the physician Hippocrates to treat pneumonia and heal wounds, allicin has come a long way and its attributes now include antimicrobial and anti-insecticidal activities. Given the rapid appearance of resistant microbes and insects, allicin clearly has merit in these spheres, even more so as resistance does not appear following its usage. More recently allicin has been successfully used as a complementary treatment for chronic inflammatory diseases, which include type II diabetes, cardiovascular disease and even certain tumors. Having a "natural" medicine, which is associated with an absence of side effects, can only be beneficial in conditions requiring long-term usage and it is clear that allicin's potential as an individual or adjunct medicine needs to be evaluated. The gold standard for phase III human studies are double blind randomized placebo controlled trials and allicin's success in this area is just beginning to be realized. Allicin has great potential, and maximizing its bioavailability could be enhanced using computational chemistry methodology combined with the stabilization methods already used for other phytomedicines, such as curcumin. Given the attention it deserves, it is likely that allicin will provide much needed alternative management strategies for decreasing infection and disease over the next decade.

ACKNOWLEDGMENTS

Many individuals are involved in the creation of a book, providing a support system that allows it to grow and develop as an entity. First, my thanks go to my daughter Olivia and husband Michael who were both my anchors to daily life and the effective sounding board for ways to explain the information. My fellow authors proved that the ability to take information from diverse sources and knit it into a homogeneous product was possible. I am forever grateful for their camaraderie and teamwork. Good reviewers are also hard to find but our group of individuals, experts in their fields, challenged the group of writers that produced this book to dig deeper and explain more fully. We all learned a great deal from their supportive critique and their names are listed below. I would also like to thank our illustrator, Dr. Kathryn Mickle, for using her abilities to create figures that are both clear and elegantly constructed. Finally, thank you reader for your interest in the field of herbal medicine and particularly allicin. It is only through the spread of information about this field that it has the chance to continue to develop to its full potential.

Reviewers

Salvatore Agosta, Ph.D., Center for Environmental Studies, Virginia Commonwealth University, Richmond, VA

Anne H. Bower, Ph.D., Professor of Biology, College of Life Sciences, Jefferson University, Philadelphia, PA

Anupriya Chaudhuri, Ph.D., Adjunct Professor of Microbiology, College of Life Sciences, Jefferson University, Philadelphia, PA

William C. Heppenstall, D.O., Philadelphia College of Osteopathic Medicine Internal Medicine Residency
Affiliated Hospitals: Roxborough Memorial and Chestnut Hill, Philadelphia, PA

Lili Fox Velez, Ph.D., Scientific Writer, Baltimore, MD

Karren Jensen, Ph.D., Technical Writer, Stryker Instruments Division, Stryker Corp, Kalamazoo MI

John D. Kelly IV, M.D., Co-Director Sports Medicine Fellowship, Director, Sports Shoulder and Professor of Clinical Orthopedic Surgery, University of Pennsylvania, Philadelphia, PA

Monique E. Maubert, Ph.D., Research Associate, Department of Surgery, Jefferson University, Philadelphia, PA

Genevieve Regan, Ph.D. Assistant Professor of Biology, College of Life Sciences, Jefferson University, Philadelphia, PA

Frank Wilkinson, Ph.D., Associate Professor of Biochemistry, Associate Dean for Undergraduate Programs, College of Life Sciences, Jefferson University, Philadelphia, PA

Illustrator

Kathryn E. Mickle, Ph.D., Associate Professor of Biology and Associate Program Director of Pre-Medical Studies, College of Life Sciences, Jefferson University, Philadelphia, PA

In: Allicin
Editor: Diana R. Cundell
ISBN: 978-1-53617-339-0

Chapter 1

ALLICIN: HISTORY, ETHNOBOTANY AND USES AS TOLD PRIMARILY BY THE GARLIC PLANT

Diana R. Cundell*, PhD
College of Life Sciences, Jefferson University, Philadelphia, PA, US

ABSTRACT

Garlic (*Allium sativum* L.) has been in general use for diverse medicinal purposes, most notably infections, heart disease, snake bites, worms and tumors for at least 5,000 years (3,000 B.C.). Most scholars now attribute these capabilities to the *de novo* synthesis of the organosulfur compound allicin (diallyl-thiosulfinate) when the plant is crushed. Allicin is the major organosulfur compound generated by garlic and protects the plant against predation or attack by insects or microbes. Apart from garlic several wild edible allium species namely *A. ampeloprasum* (Elephant garlic), A. *hirtifolium* (Persian shallot), *A. scorodoprasum* L. (Korean garlic), *A. senescens* (Holub), *A. shoenoprasum* (chives), *A. tricoccum* (Ramp, wild leek), A. *ursifolium* (Ransom/bear garlic) and *A. vineale* (crow garlic) also generate allicin, albeit in lesser amounts. Together these allium species have a geographic distribution that covers much of the Earth's surface and this is reflected by a colorful and srikingly similar historical medicinal past. Historical and ethnobotanical awareness are key to understanding the potential ways a phytochemical can be used. Since the success and spread of medicinal garlic is the story of early allicin use this will be the focus for this chapter. Particular attention will also be given to the other allium species and their uses in indigenous populations. Each of these topics will be discussed in more depth in subsequent chapters.

Keywords: history, diallyl-thiosulfinate, allium

1. INTRODUCTION

The genus *Allium* is believed to consist of between 600 and 750 members [1]. Although all allium generate malodorous organosulfur compounds, which give the plants their name (from

---

* Corresponding Author's Email: Diana.Cundell@jefferson.edu.

the Greek αλεω meaning *to avoid*), those of the methiin/allliin type generate the highly biologically active molecule allicin (diallyl-thiosulfinate) (see Chapter 2 for details) [2, 3]. First discovered in 1944 by Cavallito and Bailey [4, 5], allicin is released via the enzyme allinase when these plants are crushed or attacked by predators such as animals, insects or infectious agents [2, 4]. Allicin (diallyl-thiosulfinate) has been shown to exhibit antimicobial [2, 4], insecticidal [6], immunostimulant [4], antitumor [4] and cardioprotective [4] properties. The individual medicinal qualities of allicin will be the subject of future chapters as they are somewhat extensive, but at this point our journey begins with the source material for this intriguing thiosulfinate.

Allicin is estimated to constitute at least 70% of the organosulfur molecules in freshly, crushed garlic and its activity can be maintained in alcohol for periods of up to 14 days, drying or freezing [4]. When heated or allowed to naturally degrade, allicin generates diallyl disulfide and trisulfide, both of which are still antimicrobial [7, 8]. At least 8 edible allium have been directly shown to generate allicin other than the cultivar garlic (*A. sativum*) [1, 3, 4, 8-13]. Wild varieties generating only 10-50% of the amount of allicin that garlic does [9], although they possess similar organosulfur profiles [3, 9]. Between them, the nine allicin-producing allium species are well distributed geographically (Table 1) and have therefore provided a consistent source of phytomedicines for indigenous peoples around the globe [1, 3, 14, 15, 17]. It is important to note that despite there being allicin in several allium species it is the bulb of *Allium sativum* that remains the best and most reliable source.

Table 1. Cultivated and wild Allium species producing allicin

Allium species	Common name	Native geographical distribution	References
Allum ampeloprasum var ampeloprasum	Elephant garlic	South Europe to West Asia	[10, 14]
Allium hirtifolium	Persian shallot	Central to southwest Asia	[11, 15]
Allium sativum	Garlic	Central Asia mountainous regions	[1, 4]
Allium schoenoprasum	Chives	Europe, Temperate Asia and North America	[3, 16]
Allium scorodoprasum	Korean garlic	Eurasia (dryer areas)	[12, 17]
Allium senenscens	Holub	Central and Submediterranean Europe	[3]
Allium tricoccum	Ramp*	North America	[9, 18]
Allium ursinum	Ransom, bear's garlic*	Europe and Asia	[13]
Allium vineale	Crows garlic*	Europe, northwest Africa, Middle East	[8]

*Species frequently described as "wild garlic" by indigenous peoples.

At this point the reader may be wondering why, given the diversity of medicinal allium species available, it was that the bulbs of *A. sativum* achieved widespread use as a phytomedicine? It is likely that this comes in part at least from both an ease of garlic cultivation and the ability of the bulbs to remain unspoiled following extended periods of storage [1]. The origins of garlic may be from the wild allium species *A. longicuspis* Regel [1]. Botanists believe that the closeness between *A. longicuspis* and *A. sativum* appears to have also allowed them to interbreed, originally producing fertile plants [1].

Harvesting these "wild garlic" plants, ancient people discovered that separating and planting the individual cloves from the bulb rapidly increased their yield! [1] So now traders had a product that was still viable after a long voyage [1] and their customers found that they could not only use but also grow their purchased garlic. Although native to Central Asia, garlic tolerated a wide diversity of climates, especially those of the Mediterranean, thereby allowing its consistent availability for medicinal purposes [1]. In fact, the name "*sativum*" means "cultivated" and again relates back to the continued growth of this particular variant of Allium as well as its continued propagation by asexual cultivation of the garlic bulb cloves [1]. So successful was this practice that the *A. sativum* plant that was created required human interventions to allow its continued propagation; i.e., it is sterile [1].

Historical research can teach us a great deal about the potential medicinal uses of allicin/ garlic and provides a basis for scientific investigations of its efficacy [19-27]. Fortunately for us, investigating the ancient uses of the garlic bulb are possible since these uses were written down in several ancient Egyptian [25, 27], Roman [24, 27] and Greek [23, 25, 28] texts. These ancient sources are not the only ways we can learn about garlic; however, oral histories and folklore about wild garlic species can be confusing [8, 9, 13] and there are also several species involved [13]. Despite this, these accounts do provide possible confirmation of some of allicin's activities and will be referred to throughout this chapter. Since much of early histories and medicinal usages of garlic-allicin are intertwined the reader may assume they are interchangeable in this discussion.

2. History of the Medicinal Usage of Garlic and Other Allium Species

Ancient texts describe the culinary and medicinal use of garlic in many civilizations including Mesopotamia, China, Egypt and Rome [1, 19-28]. Medical practitioners and healers of the time describe elaborate decoctions of the bulb for the treatment of between 20 and 30 prevailing illnesses endemic to the regions [19-28].

But which culture actually began the practice of growing garlic? There is some debate among scholars as to where garlic first began to be deliberately cultivated and used [21, 22, 29, 30]. Some point to the descriptions of medicinally used garlic on excavated 3rd millenium B.C. cuneform Sumarian stone tablets that point to the fertile crescent of Mesopotamia (Fertile Crescent of Tigris and Euphrates Valleys) [21, 22]. In nearby Iran, surviving Zoroastrian writings from the 6th Century B.C. describe medicinal garlic use [19]. Other scholars point to biochemical and molecular evidence of the farming of wild garlic by semi-nomadic Central Asian tribes approximately 10,000 years ago [31]. If we instead take fertile clones as our indicator then garlic was probably first a wild, fertile plant growing in the Central Asian Region of the Tien Shan Mountains [29, 30]. All the "garlic" used historically after this point is the cultivated form, namely *A. sativum* [1].

What ever its origins, garlic's medicinal use was certainly widespread amongst many dfferent ethnographic groups by the early 1900s [1, 19-28]. Historical medicinal "prescriptions" in these populations were varied and involved either chewing cloves of garlic, drinking garlic-infused wine or applying it to a surface lesion freshly crushed as a type of poultice with honey as an "anchor" [21-28] (Table 2).

Table 2. Historical medicinal uses of garlic

Date	Location	Uses	Comments	References
2,600-2,100 B.C.	Euphrates River Valley	Fevers, inflammation, strained muscles, loose bowels and parasites	Information from Sumerian Tablets	[19, 20]
2000 B.C. and earlier	China	Respiration and digestive issues, fatigue, headache, insomnia	Garlic suggested to provide heat and be a "yang" food	[21, 22, 24]
~1500 B.C.	Egypt	Circulatory issues, insect/parasite infection Abnormal growths	Described in Codex Ebers (1550 B.C.)	[24-26]
~1400-1800 B.C.	Greece	Respiratory issues, purging, abdominal growths	Hippocrates incorporated into "therapeutic armamentarium"	[23, 27]
40-100 A.D.	Rome	Infections, arterial "cleansing,' bites, gastrointestinal issues and arthritis	Dioscorides and Pliny the elder provide the roots of pharmacology	[24, 25, 28]
100-300 A.D.	India	Heart disease, arthritis, worm infections and digestive issues	Tibbi, Unarni and Ayurvedic first advocate	[22, 27]
800 A.D.-1500	Europe	Digestive and breathing disorders, plague, animal bites	St. Hildegard von Bingen and Pietro Mattioli define treatments	[26, 27]
1800s	North America	Diuretic, pulmonary diseases of children and adults	John Gunn and Joseph Richards were reference works of the time	[27]

2.1. Ancient Civilizations and Garlic

The ancient Sumerians (2600-2100 BCE) and Chinese (as early as 2700 BCE) were the earliest civilizations to explore garlic's healing qualities [9-14, 24].
Mesopotamia is believed to have been a fairly inhospitable place with marshes and associated disease when first colonized by the ancient Sumerians [20]. Garlic was beneficial in treating the fevers and parasites that were common in that area and may have even helped the civilization to persist [19, 20]. Mesopotamia appears also to be the origin of using garlic to fight demons, possibly because disease and demons were regarded as synonymous at this period of history [20]. Garlic was also extensively employed in Traditional Chinese Medicine (TCM) as a "stimulating" agent effecting improvement in a "depressed" body system and effecting removal of various respiratory and digestive issues that may well have been infectious in nature [24].

Scholars believe that Central Asian traders might have brought their cultivatable garlic west to Sumeria and East to China, Korea and Japan [31]. From Mesopotamia, garlic is also likely to have been exported to India and Egypt after 3,000 B.C. when these markets were first established [31]. India and Egypt appear to have utilized garlic for similar medicinal purposes, namely to correct circulation issues and for the removal of infections and parasites [25-27]. A later Indian manuscript, the *Charaka-Samhita*, probably written in around 300 A.D., also advocates the use of garlic to treat leprosy, although this practice seems not to have been adopted by other cultures of the time [32].

An ancient record of Egyptian medical practices, the *Codex Ebers*, lists over 30 uses for garlic and is remarkable for first prescribing its use to remove abnormal growths [25, 27]. Compiled in around 1550 BCE such "growths" might represent abscesses or tumors or both, but is of particular interest to scholars since allicin has been demonstrated to possess anti-tumor efficacy [4]. Much of the Egyptian medical practices appear to have impressed themselves amongst Jewish slaves living there at the time [27]. These may have also been incorporated into the religious Talmud, believed to have been written in about 200 A.D. which speaks of garlic use for prevention of parasites and other infections [27].

The trade routes that had brought garlic to Egypt are believed to have reached regions of Ancient Greece at the same time (1400-1800 BCE) [33]. Particularly valued by the Greeks, Hippocrates (460-370 BCE) made it part of his *armamentarium*, recommending it as a treatment for many ailments including as a purgative agent, the elimination of abdominal tumors, and to treat parasites such as helminths [24, 27]. He was also the first to suggest its antitoxin effects against snake and animal bites [24]. Greek traditions, including their medical practices, were adopted by Rome as that city-state developed and the Roman use of garlic was first encouraged by the Greek physician Diocorides in his work *De Materia Medica*, which was written somewhere between 50 and 70 AD [25, 28]. Dioscorides used garlic for similar ailments as he had done in Greece but was the first to employ garlic to "clean the arteries " [25, 28]. Further studies on garlic were provided by another Greek physician, Pliny the Elder [25, 27]. In his major work *Historica Naturalis*, written around 77 AD, Pliny listed over twenty garlic uses that included the treatment of poisons and toxins [25, 27]. The works of Pliny the Elder are particularly significant, since they were the first medical texts to be translated, with Arabic allowing their usage far beyond Rome and Greece [34]. Dioscorides *Materia Medica* was also hand copied and translated into mutiple languages, including Arabic, German, French and Spanish; and the ubiquity of this reference work probably fueled the use of medicinal garlic in Medieval Europe [35].

2.2. Middle Ages and the Renaissance

The conquering Romans are believed to have brought garlic with them to the more northern European climes in or around 54 AD [27]. Little is known of how garlic's medicinal use gained ground in these countries, but early knowledge and cultivation of the plant appears to have been through monastery gardens [27]. One major literary work on medicinal plants was authored by Walahfrid Strabo in around AD 840 [36]. *Hortulus* (meaning *little garden*) was a descriptive narrative of the herbs grown in a monastary garden and their various uses [36]. It is to be noted that garlic was suggested as important for many purposes including the treatment of various respiratory and digestive ailments [36].

By the 12th Century AD garlic's medicinal uses were being promoted by the leading medical practitioner of the day, the Abbess St. Hildegard von Bingen [25]. St. Hildegard von Bingen was a great proponent of garlic and made the first suggestions that it only be used raw since cooking destroyed its medicinal qualities [25]. An analysis of European herbal practices in the 13th century by John Grieg [37] suggests that garlic was in common use in gardens between 1323 and 1340. By the 16th Century, the physician Pietro Mattioli began instituting the growth of what were termed "physic gardens" at large Italian Universities [27]. These herbal gardens contained many plant species including garlic [27]. Pietro Mattioli advocated garlic's use for digestive issues, worm infestations and for the first time to help during childbirth [27]. Dr. Mattioli's major work *Discorsi* both interpreted the plant species involved and extended the earlier works of the Greek Dioscorides [38]. Mattioli's writings were translated into French, German, Czech and Latin, which allowed their use across much of Europe [38].

In England, by the 16th and 17th centuries garlic was also in common usage, and typically employed to treat toothache, dropsy, animal bites and the deadly bubonic plague [27]. Paracelsus (1493-1591) appears to have been the major driving force in recommending the use of garlic as a preventative for plaque [39]. Clearly this approach gained widespread acceptance as plague doctors carried cloves of garlic to protect themselves from "the odor" of the disease [27]. Grave diggers who buried the plague dead also drank wine containing crushed garlic cloves [40]. Little was understood of the nature of garlic's curative properties so the bulb was primarily administered during this period in ways that removed its more bitter qualities, namely in honey or wine [27].

2.3. Garlic's Medicinal Uses in 18th, 19th and Early 20th Centuries

Scholars assume that by the 18th century garlic had entered mainstream medicinal use by the majority of the European populace [24]. In 1791 the renowned British physician Dr. William Lewis continued to promote the use of garlic in his *Materia Medica* for the treatment of many conditions including "*To warm and stimulate the solids, attenuate thick humours, and resist putrefaction, seem to be its primary virtues. Hence, in hot bilious constitutions, where there is already a degree of irritation, where the juices are thin and acrimonious, or the viscera or intestines unsound, it is apparently improper, and seldom fails to produce head-aches, flatulencies, thirst, febrile heats, and inflammatory symptoms in various shapes. In cold sluggish phlegmatic habits, on the other hand, it proves a salutary and powerful corroborant, expectorant, diuretic, and, if the patient is kept warm, sudorific.*" [41]. Another British physician Dr. William Woodville in his 1790 work *Medical Botany* also advocated its use as "*an expectorant, a diuretic in dropsies, to remove worms and as an external application to remove tumors*" among others [42]. Later herbalists such as the noted Nicholas Culpepper, who published his *Culpepper's Herbal* in 1858, also echoed similar uses for garlic as a treatment for "*wind colick, obstructions of the kidneys and dropsies*" among others [43].

In contrast, during most of the 17th and 18th centuries early Puritan American settlers initially shunned garlic, choosing instead to use indigenous plants for their medicinal remedies [27, 32, 40]. By 1799, garlic was again in use medicinally; primarily due to its cultivation by the Shaker communities [32, 40]. In the 1800s, in keeping with their relatives back in Europe, most Americans followed the herbal remedies published by Dr. John Gunn in 1830 and revised in 1878 [27, 32, 40]. Alternately called *Gunn's Domestic Medicine* or *The Home Book of Health*, this armamentarium again featured garlic's diverse uses and included it being a diuretic, a treatment for worms, fevers and other infections and as a general tonic [27, 32, 40].

Although the great microbiologist Louis Pasteur observed selective bactericidal activity of crushed garlic in 1858 [24], which should have perpetuated its use, the late 1800s marked the point at which "patent" and "scientific medicines" (often comprised of alcohol and opiates) gained favor amongst the European and American populace [40].

Even as Western medicine became grounded in germ theory and laboratory experimentation, garlic was used to combat or alleviate illnesses [24, 40]. In the early 20th century, garlic was used as a topical treatment for wounded British soldiers in World War 1 [24, 40] and subsequently to treat victims of the 1918-1919 influenza epidemic in the United States [40]. However, the advent of the antimicrobial drugs that began with penicillin in 1928, also turned people towards a more scientific approach to medicine and away from what were perceived as "the old ways" of herbal remedies [40].

2.4. Other Medicinal Allium Species That Have Folklore Significance

Prior to the Rennaisance, the cultivation and use of garlic for both culinary and medicinal purposes was restricted to the ruling class of most European countries [27]. As a result substitutes for its efficacy were sought among wild plants that might be easily gathered [8,13]. The universal distribution of chives (*A. schoenoprasum* L.) meant it was used for many medicinal purposes including antimicrobial activity, and to lower blood pressure [44,45]. Similarly elephant garlic (*A. ampeloprasum*) was consumed medicinally to decrease "inflammation" includin respiratory symptoms of cough and sore throat as well as a digestive calming aid [14]. It is also one of the few other allium species to be included in Dioscorides *Materia Medica* [14]. Indigenous people living in the mountainous areas of central Europe gathered *A. senescens* that they called "Holub" for use in controlling circulatory/ cardiovascular and digestive ailments [3]. Similarly in mountainous areas of Iran, *A. hirtifolium,* called "Mosir" by the local population, was used to "strengthen" the digestive system [46].

Ethnobotanists believe that "garlic" entering much of European folk lore in Medieval and early Rennaisance times and used by manual laborers may have actually been either of two relative "wild garlic" species; *A. ursinum* called "bear's garlic" or "ramson"[13] or *A. vineole,* called "crow's garlic" [8]. "Ramson" had similar uses as traditional garlic, namely the treatment of respiratory disease such as bronchitis and colds, as a detoxifying agent, to treat infections and prevent cardiovascular disease [13, 47]. Widespread as essentially a weed in Europe and Asia *A. ursinum* was used by local people primarily as a detoxifying [13] and cardiovascular agent [47]. *A. vineole* was introduced by settlers as a weed to North America [8]. Although not frequently used medicinally by the Europeans, the Cherokee appear to have used "crow garlic to treat colds [48, 49], as a juice for earache [47] and to relive flatulence [49]. The Iroquois prepared a liquid "tonic," which was drunk to relieve the patient of worms [48] .

North America had its own species of indigenous allium *A. triococcum* commonly called "ramp" [18]. "Ramps" appear to have been prolific throughout North America and were particularly used medicinally in Appalachia [50]. They were typically employed for similar uses as "crow" garlic, namely to treat colds and flu [50] as well as a cure for scurvy [51].

3. Ethnobotany and Ethanopharmacology of Garlic and Other Allium Species

The concept of food as medicine was common in ancient times especially in plants like garlic which were widely available around the world by the Middle Ages [4, 11, 13, 19-24]. Even Hippocrates said "Let food be thy medicine and medicine thy food" [52]. Thus a diet rich with medicinal foods and spices would provide a secondary mechanism to promote wellness. Studies of the *materia medica* used by these ancient peoples demonstrate that the methodologies and practices, especially those advocated by Dioscorides, were continued well into the 1800s [35].

Even today the oral traditions of *materia medica* in developing nations still center around plant-based healing methods [35, 53, 54]. In India and in Nigerian village communities, the garlic bulb is employed not just as a food but also medicinally to treat bacterial infections [53], colds, malaria [54], cardiovascular disease [53] and as a diuretic [54]. Africans, other than the Egyptians, began to use garlic relatively late in the Middle Ages [33], but it is now in common use by the approximately 80% of native people who rely on plant-based medicines [54].

Traditional healing practices are still used in remote parts of Europe such as the Basilica Region of southern Italy [55]. The traditional healer does not refer to texts and knowledge is communicated orally from person to person, with a respected elder maintaining that role until they die [35, 54, 55]. It seems likely that the use of plant-based pharmaceuticals remains strong in these groups based on a combination of poverty, tradition and lack of accces to pharmaceutical medicines [35, 54, 55].

Ethnobotanists have investigated these, and other traditional healing practices, identifying the medicinal plants involved, how they were being used and what illnesses they were involved in treating [35, 52, 56]. For many scientists there were too many coincidences across disparate cultures all doing the same or similar things with particular plants; therefore from ethnobotany the field of ethnopharmacology was born [52, 56]. Ethnopharmacology is a relatively recent field that examines the traditional uses of plants to identify strategies for drug bioprospecting [35, 56, 57]. During the past half century ethnopharmacologic investigations have encouraged the study and development of plant and phytochemical use and several plant-derived products have entered mainstream pharmaceuticals as a result [58, 59].

Plants appear to be the primary source for at least ¼ of all pharmaceuticals and account for widely used medications as those to treat pain (aspirin), cancer (Taxol®), dry eye (pilocarpine), heart disease (Digoxin) and malaria (artemesin) [58, 59]. Despite the obvious successes of drugs derived rom natural products, bioprospecting has not been the main method for identifying new treatments or potential cures [59]. Currently, drug development companies seem to prefer pursuing combinatorial chemstry and high throughput screening, which since the 1980s, has not produced the number of breakthroughts one might expect [59, 60]. Instead, over half the successful new medicines developed in the last twenty years have been either natural products, analogs or their semi-synthetic structural mimics [60]. Given these facts, dismissing plant-derived medicines as "snake oil cures" with their positive results being "mere coincidence" or "placebo" seem shortsighted [61, 62], Another issue muddying the waters is that, like allicin, many phytochemicals are contained in foods and spices [63]. As a result, their use blurs the lines of understanding of how they actually work since each plant contains many different moieties, any of which might act synergistically or be independently responsible for the bioactivity [63]. Once the primary phytochemical is clear and can be consistently separated from the background plant products then bioprospecting research can proceed along classical lines to first identify its effects in isolated target cells, and then on to well-designed preclinical animal models [63].

4. Connecting Allicin with Garlic; Lessons from the Ethnobotanist and Ethnopharmacologist

Garlic owes its bioactive qualities to allicin and traditional preparations would both activate and preserve the activity of this volatile thiosulfinate [4, 21-29, 44-51]. Allicin has been tested in a number of *in vitro* isolated cell/preclinical animal models of disease and appears to shows potential efficacy in treating a number of different diseases (Table 3). Most historical "prescriptions" involved either chewing cloves of garlic, drinking garlic-infused wine, or applying it to a surface lesion freshly crushed as a type of poultice [21-29]. Similarly the other allium species were typically ingested raw or as a "tea" [44-52].

4.1. Effects of Allicin/Garlic on Human Health

Given the traditional antimicrobial uses of garlic, it was not a surprise that the first scientific studies of the juice of crushed cloves observed potent antibacterial and antifungal activity [5, 87]. Cavellito and Bailey also observed that the major antimicrobial properties in the garlic clove were associated with a highly volatile component they called allicin [5, 87]. Since Cavellito and Bailey's discovery of allicin in 1944 the thiosulfinate has been demonstrated to possess broad spectrum antimicrobial activity against bacteria, fungi, protozoa, viruses as well as killing schistosomiasis and roundworms (Table 3). Allicin's antimicrobial mechanism and its spectrum of activity are the subject of future chapters, but it is important for the reader to note that, unlike conventional pharmaceuticals, no resistance to this natural product has ever appeared [67]. Studies also suggest that the antimicrobial activity of allicin may be complementary or synergistic to currently available pharmaceuticals [88, 89]. *Mycobacterium tuberculosis* is killed more efficiently with a combination of chloramphenicol or streptomycin with allicin [89].

Allicin is also effective against antibiotic-resistant "superbugs" such as methicillin-resistant *Staphylococcus aureus* and difficult to treat infections like group B streptococci [90]. MRSA is able to enhance its efficacy through the formation of antibiotic-impenetrable biofilms [91]. Many successful pathogens possess this capability and have been challenging to eliminate from the surfaces they colonize, which include indwellling devices such as cannulae and implants [91]. Biofilms are the root cause of numerous chronic infectious diseases including plaque and gingivitis, kidney stone formation and tuberculosis [91] Allicin is able to kill the bacteria associated with these infections, and decrease the thickness of any biofilms that do form [79, 92, 93].

Table 3. Medicinal uses of allium species correspond with allicin properties

Illness treated	Demonstrated allicin properties	References
Arthritis	Attenuated rheumatoid arthritis (rat model) Reduced in vitro cytokine production by human osteoarthritic chondrocytes	[64] [65]
Bites (animal)	Antimicrobial against several bacteria including normal skin flora (staphylococcal species) likely to be introduced into wounds	[4, 66]
Cardiovascular issues (diuretic, dropsy, heart disease)	Reduced hyperlipidemia, triglycerides, blood pressure and weight (rat model) Vasodilatation of pulmonary blood vessels (rat model) Improvement of cardiac and renal function in rat model of chronic kidney disease	[67, 68] [69] [70]
Gastrointestinal issues (infections, loose bowels)	Antimicrobial against several gastrointestinal infectious agents including the bacteria Escherichia coli, Helicobacter pylori, Enterococci, Shigella species, the protozoa Giardia lamblia and Entamoeba histolytica and cocksackie virus Suppresses colitis in rat and mouse model of irritable bowel disease (IBD)	[4, 66, 71, 72] [73, 74]
Insecticidal and insect repellant	Kills mosquitoes and pests that contaminate stored products such as flour and maize	[6, 75]
Respiratory issues (colds, asthma, tuberculosis)	Antiviral against several respiratory viruses including influenza B and parainfluenza Prevents Mycobacteria tuberculosis from colonizing human monocytes *in vitro* Abrogates airway eosinophilic infiltrate and bronchoalveolar lavage levels of inflammatory cytokines in mouse model of allergic asthma	[72] [76] [77]
Toothache	Allicin-containing garlic extract kills 19 types of oral bacteria, including caries-producing Streptococcus mutans as well as the primary bacterial cause of gingivitis (Porphyromonas gingivalis)	[78, 79]
Tumors (abnormal growths)	Mechanism probably associated with depletion of glutathione levels in cells and/or renewed induction of apoptosis Decreased in vitro proliferation and increased mortality of several malignant cell lines including human breast, cervix, colon, liver, lung, skin and stomach	[4, 80-82] [81-84]
Worm infestations	Allicin as effective as commonly used medication (praziquantel) to kill Schistosomula mansoni in murine model of schistosomiasis Kills roundworm eggs (Ascaridia galli) in infected chickens	[85] [86]

The antifungal activity of allicin has been demonstrated for both human disease and plant pathogens [2] (See Chapter 5). Allicin is able to inhibit the growth of the dimorphic pathogen *Cryptococcus neoformans* and the skin dermatophte *Trichophyton rubrum* [94]. It is also able to inhibit growth and biofilm formation by the yeast *Candida albicans*; an organism which produces millions of infections around the world and is a particular issue in immunocompromised indviduals [94, 95]. When combined with the antifungal drugs fluconazole and itraconazole, allicin also enhanced the killing of the yeast *Candida albicans* [89]. Studies demonstrated that freshly pressed garlic juice, high in allicin levels, was able to kill fungi infecting carrot seeds and also enhance the germination of those seeds [92]. Allicin may constitute a "natural pesticide" since it is able to eliminate a series of important plant pathogens including brassica dark leaf spot (*Alternaria brassicola*), collar rot (*Plectospherella cucumerina)* and rust (*Botrytis cinerea*) [2, 96, 97].

One of the many traditional uses of garlic was as a treatment for "worms" [27], which could have been a general term covering illnesses caused by many separate internal parasited. Indeed, allicin has been shown to kill or remove a variety of these organisms [66]. Allicin is able to kill several important protozoans including *Plasmodium* (malaria)[98], *Leishmania* species [66], *Entamoeba histolytica* [66], *Trypanosoma brucei* [99] and *Giardia lamblia* [66] in addition to roundworms (*Ascaris* species)[85] and liver fluke (*Schistosomula* species)[86]. These parasites cause untold suffering, especially in developing nations where a combination of poor sanitation and access to medical care resulted in a million deaths from parasites in 2013 alone [100]. Studies have suggested that the antibacterial, antifungal and antiparasitic mechanisms of action of allicin occur from its ability to easily penetrate phospholipid membranes and bind to proteins containing thiol groups [66, 86, 99]. Several enzymatic targets have been identified including cysteine proteases [99], alcohol dehydrogenases [101], and the acetyl coA forming system [102] and all are lethal to the microbe if damaged (see Chapters 5-7 for further detail). Allicin is also able to enhance natural killer cell (NK) activity[102]. Since these cells are involved in innate immune protection particularly against intracellular pathogens and tumors [63], this also contributes to the activity of allicin against parasites, fungi and bacteria such as *Mycobacteria.*

Other antiviral effects of allicin involve multiple mechanisms, which vary between the agents involved [73, 74, 79, 103-111]. Discussed further in chapter 8, two notable viruses that allicin may impair are the retroviruses HIV and REV [104]. REV highly oncogenic and associated with development of lymphoma and sarcoma tumors in infected animals [104]. Studies suggest allicin has two other effects to remove the abnormal cells: apoptotic programmed cell death [81] and glutathione depletion [80]. Given that cancer cells fail to undergo normal apoptotic cell death this is an important activity for allicin [104]. Apoptosis is also used by T lymphocytes and NK cells to cause virally-infected cells to release their bioburden [106] providing another potential link between allicin's effectiveness against both viruses and tumors. In chapter 12, we will discuss the activities of allicin and interleukin-2 (IL-2) in more detail, in particular how these appear to act synergisticaly to decrease pancreatic cancer survival in a murine model through priming of both T and NK cells [107]. Allicin has also shown direct *in vitro* activity against a broad spectrum of cancer cell types including human breast, cervical, colon, liver, lung, skin and stomach cancer cells [81-86].

Allicin's immunomodulatory abilities, targeting NF-κB and decreasing proinflammatory cytokine expression, appear to be at the heart of its effectiveness in many other chronic inflammatory diseases (see Chapter 3 for further details). These include cardiovascular illness, type II diabetes [67, 68], asthma [77], arthritis [65], IBD [73, 74], Alzheimer's disease [108, 109] and periodontitis [79] (see Chapters 9-11 for further details). Immune enhancing effects also probably explain the successful use of garlic by the Ancient Egyptians to "fuel" the pyramid builders [25], and in Ancient Greece as a "performance enhancer" [27]. Our modern understanding of "performance enhancing" could well include the activities of allicin that have been associated with improvements in cardiovascular healh including decreased blood pressure [67] and triglycerides [68] together with a reduction in body fat [68]. Discussed in chapter 10 allicin, and its breakdown metabolite ajoene, also inhibits platelet aggregation [110], and therefore has a major impact in maintaining vascular health and preventing artherosclerosis [68-70, 111]. The major metabolite of allicin, ajoene, is also able to impair the cellular formation of nitric oxide (NO) [111]. Human atherosclerotic lesions generate a combination of nitric oxide and high levels of superoxide called peroxynitrite [111]. Peroxynitrite increases platelet aggregation via low density lipoprotein (LDL) and perpetuate the generation of atherosclerotic lesions [4, 111]. Thus, by reducing NO and superoxide synthesis, allicin is able to abrogate these effects [4]. Further, allicin has been shown to reduce insulin and glucose levels in a fructose-induced hyperinsulinemic rat model supporting the use of this organosulfur compound in diabetes treatment [67, 68]. This latter property of allicin will be further discussed in Chapter 9.

Because allicin appears to influence the fundamental pathways of NF-κB activation, cyclooxygenase-2 (COX-2) activation, cytokine and NO expression [65, 79] it could prove useful in conditions that at first seem dissimilar, but are controlled by proteins that alicin can influence. For example, although the initiating stimuli are separate, being bacterial (*P. gingivalis*) infection for periodontitis [79] and cartilage degeneration for osteoarthritis [65], in both cases the effects of these systems is to suppress osteoclastogenesis and decrease levels of healthy bone [65, 79]. Discussed further in chapter 11, allicin is of interest in these conditions since there is currently no effective long term strategy for their treatment other than surgical removal of affected bone 65, 79]. Studies of the efficacy of allicin on IBD, such Crohn's and ulcerative colitis are fewer in the literature but nonetheless suggestive of its utility in managing these conditions [73, 74]. Intriguingly, IBD was known to Ancient Greco-Roman scholars as a "chronic diarrheal" disease [112] and garlic was commonly used as an intervention for it [25, 28]. Two animal models of colitis were abrogated by allicin pre-treatment and suggested further delineation of NF-κB cell expression associated with inhibition of downstream p38 and mitogen-activated protein kinase (MAPK) pathways [73] as well as the signal transducer signal protein (STAT) [74]. Both pathways are important in the maintenance of healthy bone and implicated in the pathophysiology of osteoarthritis [113], demonstrating the need to connect these studies to completely understand the cellular targets of the thiosulfinate.

COX-2 expression has long been associated with chronic inflammatory responses and is known to play a role in both allergies and tumors [63]. Overexpression of this form of cyclooxygenase enzyme has been shown in a number of tumor cell lines including those of the colon, lung, breast and stomach [63]. Specific COX-2 antagonists are currently unavailable pharmaceutically [114], but should allicin provide a selective activity it is clear that the thiosulfinate would have utility in treating a number of chronic inflammatory diseases (see Chapter 3). In terms of asthma, studies are limited but allicin may also possess antihistamine-like activity [115], as well as preventing airway inflamamation by preventing eosinophil migration [77].

What we now term Alzheimer's Disease was considered senility or a "normal" process of aging" by the Ancient Greeks and Romans and therefore not intervened with medically [116]. More recently it has been added to the list of chronic inflammatory disease and studies, particularly in animal models, have begun to clarify how the neurodegeneration occurs in this condition [108, 109]. Alzheimer's risk factors include age, genetic inheritance and also cardiovascular disease (see Chapter 11)[109]. Apart from mitigating atherosclerosis [67, 68] allicin has been shown to alter two biochemical anomalies in animal models of Alzheimer's disease [108, 109]. The first is in ameliorating the decrease in the neurotransmittor acetylcholine (Ach) thereby slowing the samage in cognitive abilities [108]. Even more exciting, research in 2018 demonstrated that allicin could reduc the production of amyloid plaques in a murine model of Alzheimer's disease [109]. This efect was mediated via the c-Jun terminal kinase (JNK) signaling pathway which plays a major role in brain physiology [117].

Current medications for Alzheimer's have focused solely on improving Ach levels and are not without substantial side effects [118]. Finding a medication easily able to cross the blood-brain barrier and that affects multiple pathways in the condition may be another way allicin could be a very useful treatment.

4.2. Additional Uses for Allicin in Agriculture and Food Safety

Added to the direct human benefits allicin is also effective as an insecticidal compound [6] (see Chapter 9) and is therefore able to both prevent infestations by the disease-carrying vectors such as the mosquito [6] and urban house fly (*Musa* domestica) [119] as well as help treat diseases they carry. Insect pests including weevils and borer beetles are responsible for the loss of up to 40% of all grains harvested around the world, particularly in developing nations [120]. These are difficult to control and for some may contaminate more than 50% of stored cereal crops [120]. Allicin has been found to be both repellent and lethal to several storage pests including the mealworm beetle (*Tenebrio mollitor*) [121] and the red flour beetle (*Tribolium castaneum*) [122]. Together these infest grains, flour, pasta and even pet food [121, 122]. Allicin also inhibits the growth and survival of the tobacco cutworm moth *Spodoptera litura* [123], which preferentially attacks soybeans, groundnuts and results in crop losses of at least 20% [124]. Organic farmers and those in developing countries are particularly interested in allicin's antimicrobial use for these and other plant species [96, 97, 125], animal husbandry [126] and even aquaculture [127].

Conclusion and Future Directions

Our journey with allicin has taken us from the historical widespread ethnobotanical uses of the lowly garlic bulb (Table 2), and into its discovery just over seventy years ago as a broad spectrum antimicrobial agent Table 3). During the past decade, allicin has emerged as having the potential to provide a safe, naturally sourced alternative treatment to several common chronic inflammatory conditions including Alzheimer's disease, tumors, and osteodegenerative syndromes (Table 3). Given the diverse properties of allicin, it seems likely to provide many potential interventions for many illnesses that continue to plague mankind. So what are the best future directions for allicin to be used in the future? Identifying the optimal future targets for allicin, as for other natural and pharmaceutical entities, requires an examination of our societal needs; especially important given the upheavals of climate change and the coming world population explosion. Both will be especially felt by the residents of developing nations where resources are already limited.

Discussed in chapter 14, climate change is likely to exacerbate the food insecurities and health issues that are already the bane of developing nations [128]. More aggressive vectors carrying microbes resistant to antimicrobial agents will necessitate the development of new treatments [128]. By 2050, our planet's population will have grown by another two billion people and around one fifth of these people will be over 65 [129]. Most of this population increase will be in developing nations who will also need to address how to manage the significant numbers of individuals suffering from the chronic inflammatory conditions associated with aging including tumors, neurodegenerative and osteodegenerative illnesses [129]. Most developing countries, including India, China and many African nations, still use traditional, plant-based medicines primarily through a lack of access (and sometimes trust) of "modern" pharmaceuticals [129]. Researchers in these countries are already exploring the scientific basis for their traditional medicines and developing modified or stabilized forms that can ensure consistent bioavailability [63]. Given the confidence that already exists in developing nations it is likely that phytomedicines, including allicin, have the potential provide an inexpensive, available therapies for many chronic inflammatory conditions [63, 129]. Developing nations are also adopting the strategies of organic farming and aquaculture as the yield and nutritional benefits of the foods produced far outweigh factory farming methods [130]. Here, as in human healthcare, allicin has the potential to provide a natural, safe method to treat animal and plant-based disease thereby decreasing animal and crop losses and maintaining food security. Just as the lowly garlic bulb provided both food and medicinal uses to human societies of the past, allicin may in turn be able to do the same for our world and its uncertain future.

References

[1] Block, Eric 2010. "Chapter 1 *Allium* botany and cultivation, ancient and modern." In: *Garlic and other alliums: The Lore and the Science*. Royal Society of Chemistry, www.rsc.org.

[2] Borlinghaus, Jan, Frank Albrecht, Martin C. H. Grulke, Ifeanyi D. Nwachukwu, and Alan J. Slusarenko 2014. "Allicin: Chemistry and biological properties." *Molecules* 19(8): 12591-12618.

[3] Vlase, Laurian, Marcel Parvu, Elena Alina Parvu, and Anca Toju 2013. "Chemical constituents of three *Allium* species from Romania." *Molecules* 18: 114-127. Accessed September, 1 2018. https://doi.org/10.3390/molecules18010114.

[4] Rahman, Mohammad S. 2007. "Allicin and other functional active components in garlic: health benefits and bioavailability." *Int J Food Properties* 10: 245-268.

[5] Cavallito, Chester J., and John H. Bailey 1944. "Allicin, the antibacterial principle of *Allium sativum*. I. Isolation, physical properties and antibacterial action." *J. Am Chem. Soc.* 66:1950-1951.

[6] Revay, Edita E., Yosef Schlein, Onie Tsabari, Vasily Kravchenko, Whitney Qualls, Rui De-Xue, John C. Beier, Sekou F. Traore, Seydou Doumbia, Axel Hausman and Günter C. Müller 2015. "Formulation of attractive toxic sugar bait (ATSB) with safe EPA-exempt substance significantly diminishes the *Anopheles sergentii* population in a desert oasis." *Acta Tropica, 150*, 29–34. Accessed September 10, 2018. http://doi.org/10.1016/j.actatropica.2015.06.018.

[7] Tsao, Shyh-Ming, and Mei-Chin Yin 2001. "In vitro activity of four diallyl suphides occurring naturally in garlic and Chinese leek oils." *J. Med Microbiol.* 50: 646-649.

[8] Satyal, Prabodh, Jonathan D. Craft, Noura S. Dosoky, and William N. Setzer 2017. "The chemical compositions of the volatile oils of garlic (*Allium sativum*) and wild garlic (*Allium vineale*)." *Foods,* 6(8): 63. Accessed September 10, 2018. doi: 10.3390/foods6080063.

[9] Calvey, Elizabeth M., Kevin D. White, Jean E. Matusik, Deyou Sha, and Eric Block 1998. "Allium chemistry: identification of organosulfur compounds in ramp (Alliu tricoccum) homogenates." *Phytochemistry* 49(2): 359-364.

[10] Tchórzewska, Dorota, Jan Bocianowski, Agnieszka Najda, Agnieszka Dąbrowska, and Krystyna Winiarczyk 2017. "Effect of environment fluctuations on biomass and allicin level in *Allium sativum* (cv. Harnas, Arkus) and *Allium ampeloprasum* var. *ampeloprasum* (GHL)." *J Applied Botany Food Quality* 90: 106—114.

[11] Mikaili, Peyman, Surush Maadirad, Milad Moloudizargari, Shahin Aghajanshakeri, and Shadi Sarahroodi 2013. "Therapeutic uses and pharmacological properties of garlic, shallot and their biologically active compounds." *Iranian J. Basic Med. Sci.* 16: 1031-1048.

[12] Tasci, Bahtinur, Halil Kutuk H., and Ilkay Koca 2016. "Determination of alliin and allicin in the plant of *Allium scorodoprasum* L. subsp. *rotundum* by using the infrared spectroscopy technique." *Acta Hortic.* 1143: 133-138.

[13] Sobolewska, Danuta, Irma Podolak, and Justyna Makowska-Wąs 2015. "*Allium ursinum:* botanical, phytochemical and pharmacological overview." *Phytochem Rev.*, 14: 81-97.

[14] Dey. Purnima, and Kazi Layla Khaled 2015. "An extensive review on *Allium ampeloprasum*." *Int J. Sci. Res.* 4(7): 371-377. ISSN Online 2309-7614.

[15] Gimdil, Reza, Hassan Shahgoli, Absalt R. Ajiorloo, and Morad Shaban 2013. "Study on phenology stages of cultivated Persian shallot (Allium hirtifolium) in Mashad region." *Int. J. Farming Allied Sci.* 2(s): 1223-1225.

[16] Courteau, Jacqueline. *"Allium schoenoprasum: Wild Chives."* Accessed September 10, 2018. http://eol.org/pages/1084938/overview.

[17] Tasci, Bahtinur, and Ilkay Koca I 2016. "Use of *Allium scorodoprasum* L. subsp. *rotundum* as food." *Acta Hort.* 1143: 153-158.

[18] Nault, Andree, and Daniel Gagnon 1993. "Ramet demography of Allium tricoccum, a spring ephemeral, perennial forest herb." *J. Ecology* 81. 101-119.

[19] Bayan, Leila, Peir H. Koulivand, and Ali Gorji. 2014. "Garlic: a review of potential therapeutic effects." *Avicenna Journal of Phytomedicine* 4(1): 1-14.

[20] Heinerman, John. 1993. "*The healing benefits of garlic: from pharoahs to pharmacists.*" New Caanan, CT: Keats Publishers.

[21] Bellamy, David J., and Andrea Pfister. 1992. "*World medicine: plants, patients and people.*" Oxford, UK: Blackwell Publishers.

[22] Woodward Penny. 1996. "*Garlic and friends: The history, growth and use of edible Alliums*" pp 2-22. Melbourne Australia: Hyland House.

[23] Totelin, Laurence 2014. "When foods became remedies in Ancient Greece: The curious case of garlic and other substances." *J. Ethnopharmacol.* 167:30-37. http://doi.org/10.1016/j.jep.2014.08.018.

[24] Petrovska, Biljana B., and Svetlana Cekovska 2010. "Extracts from the history and medical properties of garlic." *Pharmacogn. Rev.*, 4(7): 106-110.

[25] Bergner, Paul. 1996. "*The healing power of garlic.*" Pp 3-26. Rocklin, CA: Prima Publishing,

[26] Lawson, Larry D. 1998. "Garlic: a review of its medicinal effects and indicated active compounds." In: *Phytomedicines of Europe. Chemistry and Biological ACS Symposium*

Series 691 (Lawson L. D. & Bauer R eds.), pp 176-209. American Chemical Society, Washington D.C.

[27] Moyers, Susan. 1996. "*Garlic in health, history and world cuisine.*" pp 1-36. St. Petersberg, FL: Suncoast Press.

[28] Riddle, John M. 1996. "The medicines of Greco-Roman antiquity as a source for medicines today." In: *Prospecting for drugs in ancient and medieval European texts: A scientific approach* (Holland B. K. ed), pp 7-17, Amsterdam, The Netherlands: Harwood Academic Publishers.

[29] Hong, Chong-Jian, and Takeomi Etoh T 1996. "Fertile clones of garlic (*Allium sativum* L.) abundant around the Tien Shan mountains." *Breeding Science* 46: 349-353.

[30] Shah N. C. 2014. "*Allium Sativum* (Garlic): The folk and modern uses- Part 1." *The SciTech Journal* 1(5) ISSN 2347-7318. Accessed September 10, 2018. http://thescitech.com/admin/includes/abstractpdf/2014-9-05536cdd2c1d2a2.pdf.

[31] Kamanetsky, Rina, Furkat Khassanov, Haim D. Rabinowitch, Jacques Auger, and Christopher Kik 2007. Garlic Diversity and Genetic Resources. *Medicinal and Aromatic Plant Sciences and Biotechnology* 1(1): 1-5.

[32] Rivlin, Richard S. 2001. "Historical perspectiive on the use of garlic. *J. Nutrition*, 131(3): 951S-954S."

[33] Etoh Takeomi, and Philip W. Simon. 2002. "Diversity, fertility and seed production of garlic." In Rabinowitch H. D., Currah eds. *Alllium crop science recent advances* pp 101-117. CAB International, Wallingford, UK: CAB International.

[34] Saad, Bashar, Hassan Azaizeh, and Omar Said 2005. "Tradition and persectives of Arab herbal medicine: A review." *Evid. Based Complement. Alternat. Med.* 2(4): 475-479.

[35] De Vos, Paula 2010. "European Materia Medica in historical texts: Longevity of a tradition and implications for future use." *J. Ethnopharmacol.* 132(1): 28-47.

[36] Strabo, Walahfrid. 840 AD. "Hortulus." Translated by Raef Payne, commentary by Wilfrid Blunt. *The Hunt Botanical Library*, Pittsburgh, PA, 1966. Accessed on November 5, 2019 http://www.huntbotanical.org/admin/uploads/hibd-hortulus-facsimile.pdf.

[37] Grieg, John. 1995 for 1996. "Archeobotanical and historical records compared – a new look at the taphonomy of edible and other useful plants from the 11th to the 18th century." *Circea* 12:211-247. Accessed on November 5, 2019. http://www.envarch.net/publications/circaea/12.2/12-2-whole.pdf#page=53.

[38] Daxecker, Franz 2005. "The botanist and doctor Pietro Andrea Matthioli." *Klin Monbl. Augenheilkd.*, 222(6): 516-517. [Article in German].

[39] Hahn, G. 1996. "History, folk medicine and legendary uses of garlic." In*: Garlic: The Science and Therapeutic Appreciation of Allium sativum L. and related species,* pp 1-24, (eds H. P. Koch and L. D. Lawson), 2nd Edition, Baltimore, MD: Williams and Wilkins.

[40] Cherry, Robin. 2014. "*Garlic an edible biography. The history, politics, and mythology behind the world's most pungent food with over 100 recipes.*" 1st Edition Boston: Roost Books. ISBN 978-1-61180-160-6. Accessed on November 5, 2019. https://en.calameo.com/read/000039257d3fc86f63e66.

[41] Lewis, William. 1791. "*An Experimental History of the Materia Medica.*" J. Johnson, London, England. Accessed on November 5, 2019. https://chestofbooks.com/health/materia-medica-drugs/Experimental-History-Materia-Medica/index.html.

[42] Woodville, William, and James Philips. 1790. "*Medical botany: containing systematic and general descriptions wth plates, of all the medicinal plants, indigenous and exotic, comprehend in the catalog of the materia medica.*" Printed and sold for the author by James Philips, London, England 1790-1793.

[43] Culpepper, Nicholas. 1858. "*Culpepper's Herbal: A comprehensive description of nearly all herbs.*" Published by W. Foulsham and Company Ltd., London, England. Accessed on November 5, 2019. https://archive.org/details/culpeperscomplet00culpuoft/page/n4.

[44] Leporatti, Maria L., and Stephanie Ivancheva 2003. "Preliminary comparative analysis of medicinal plants used in the traditional medicine of Bulgaria and Italy." *J Ethnopharmacol.*, 87: 123-142.

[45] Stajner, Dubravka, Jasna Canadanovic-Brunet, and Aleksey Pavlovich 2004. "*Allium schoenprasum* L., as a natural antioxidant." *Phytother. Res.*, 18: 522-524.

[46] Aleebrahim-Dehkordy, Elahe, Abdollah Ghasemi-Pirbalouti, and Mahmoud Mirhosein M 2016. "A comprehensive review of *Allium hirtifolium* Boiss as a medicinal and edible plant." *Der Pharmacia Lettre*, 8(1): 188-196.

[47] Bombicz, Mariann., Daniel Priksz., Balazs Varga., Rudolf Gesztelyi, Attila Kertesz, Peter Lengyel, Peter Balogh, Dezso Csupor, Judit Hohmann, Harjit P. Bhattoa, David D. Haines, and Bela Juhasz 2016. "Anti-Atherogenic Properties of *Allium ursinum* Liophylisate: Impact on Lipoprotein Homeostasis and Cardiac Biomarkers in Hypercholesterolemic Rabbits." *International Journal of Molecular Sciences*, 17(8), 1284. Accessed September 10, 2018. http://doi.org/10.3390/ijms17081284.

[48] Moerman Daniel E. 1998. "*Native American Ethnobotany.*" Portland OR: Timber Press.

[49] Hamel, Paul B., and Mary U. Chiltoskey. 1975. "*Cherokee Plants and their uses – A 400 year history.*" Herald Publishing Company, NC, USA.

[50] Cavender, Anthony 2006. "Folk medical uses of plant foods in Southern Appalachia, United States." *J Ethnopharmacol.*, 108: 74-84.

[51] Chapman, Sasha 2005. "Quantum Lccks." *Toronto Life* 39(4): 85-86.

[52] Yeung, Andy W. K., Michael Heinrich, and Atanas G. Atanasov 2018. "Ethnopharmacology – A bibliometric analysis of research meandering between medicine and food science." *Frontiers in Pharmacology*, volume 9, article 215 doi:10.3389/phar.2018.00215.

[53] Tahseen, Moh A., and Garima Mishra 2013. "Ethnobotany and diuretic activity of some selected Indian medicinal plants: A scientific review." *The Pharma Journal*, 2(3): 109-121.

[54] Mesfin, Kalayu, Gebru Tekle, and Teklemichael Tefshay 2013. "Ethnobotanical study of traditional medicinal plants used by indigenous people of Gemad district Northern Ethiopia." *J. Medicinal Plants Studies* 1(4): 32-37.

[55] Montesano, Vincenzo, Donatella Negro, Giurlio Sarli, Antonino De Lisi, Gaetano Laghetti, and Karl Hammer 2012. "Notes about the uses of plants by one of the last healers in the Basilicata Region (Southern Italy)." *J. Ethnobiol. Ethnomedicine*, 2012, 8:15. Accessed September 10, 2018. http://www.ethnobiomed.com/content/8/1/15.

[56] Heinrich, Michael 2000. Ethnobotany and its role in drug development. *Phytother. Res.* 14: 479-488.

[57] Adams, Michael, Caroline Berset C., Michael Kessler, and Matthias Hamburger 2009. "Medicinal herbs for the treatment of rheumatic disorders: A survey of European herbals form the 16th and 17th century." *J. Ethnopharmacol.* 121(2): 343-359.
[58] Buenz, Eric J., David J. Schnepple, Brent A. Bauer, Peter L. Elkin, John M. Riddle, and Motley Timothy J. 2004. "Techniques: Bioprospecting historical herbal texts by hunting for new leads in old tomes." *Trends in Pharmacological Sciences*, 25(9): 494-498.
[59] Dias, Daniel A., Sylvia Urban, and Ute Roessner 2012. "A historical overview of natural products in drug discovery." *Metabolites* 2:303-336.
[60] Newman, David J., and Morgan M. Cragg 2007. "Natural products as sources of new drugs over the last 25 years." *J. Nat. Prod.,* 70: 461-477.
[61] Shapiro, Arthur K. 1959. "The placebo efffect in the history of medical treatment: Implications for psychiatry." *American J. of Psychiatry* 116:298-304.
[62] Sneader Walter. 2005 "*Drug Discovery: A History.*" Hoboken, NJ: Wiley.
[63] Cundell, Diana R. 2014. Herbal phytochemicals as immunomodulators *Current Immunology Reviews 2014*, Volume 10 Issue 2 ISSN:1875-631X(Online), ISSN:1573-3955(Print) Accessed September 10, 2018. http://benthamscience.com/journal/index.php?journalID=cir.
[64] Jayanthi M. K., Sushima Naidu, V. Pramod, and Sunil 2015. "Antioxidant and antiarthritic activity of allicin in animal models." *IJPSR* 6(3): 1150-1155. Accessed September 10, 2018. http://ijpsr.com/bft-article/antioxidant-and-antiarthritic-activity-of-allicin-in-animal-models/?view=fulltext.
[65] Wang Lin, Hai-Tao Pan., Bing Wang, Yang Liu, Kai Fei, and Wei-Feng Han W. F. 2016. "Allicin reduces IL-1β-induced inflammatory cytokines via attenuating the NF-κβ and MMP-3 activation in human osteoarthritis chondrocyte model." *Int. J. Clin. Exp. Pathol.,* 9(10): 10320-10326.
[66] Ankri, Serge, and David Mirelman 1999. "Antimicrobial properties of allicin from garlic." *Microbes and Infection* 2:125-129.
[67] Elkayam, Amitai., David Mirelman, Edna Peleg., Meir Wilchek, Talia Miron, Aharon Rabinkov, Sigal Sadetzki, and Talma Rosenthal 2000. "Comparison of the effects of allicin and Enalapril on blood pressure, insulin and triglycerides levels in fructose-induced hyperinsulinemic-hyperlipidemic hypertensive rats." *American Journal of Hypertension* 14: 377-381.
[68] Elkayam, Amitai., David Mirelman, Edna Peleg, Meir Wilchek, Talia Miron T., Aharon Rabinkov, Mor Oron-Herman, and Talma Rostenthal 2003. "The effects of allicin on weight in fructose-induced hyperinsulinemic-hyperlipidemic hypertensive rats." *American Journal of Hypertension* 16: 1053-1056.
[69] Kaye Alan D., Bracken J. de Witt, Muhammad Anwar, Donald E. Smith, Chang J. Feng, Philip J. Kadowitz, and Bobby D. Nossaman 2000. "Analysis of responses of garlic derivatives in the pulmonary vascular bed of the rat." *J. Appl. Physiol.* 89: 353-358.
[70] García-Trejo Ehécatl M. A., Abraham S. Arellano-Buendía, Raúl Argüella-García, María I. Loredo-Mendoza, Fernando E. García-Arroyo, Mónica G. Arellana-Mendoza, María C. Castillo-Hernández, Gustavo Guevara-Balcázar, Edilia Tapie, Laura G. Sánchez-Lozada, and Horacio Osorio-Alonso 2016. "Effects of allicin on hypertension and cardiac function in chronic kidney disease." *Oxidative Medicine and Cellular Longevity* 2016, ArticleID 3850402. Accessed September 10, 2018. http://dx.doi.org/10.1155/2016/3850402.

[71] Jonkers, Daisy, Judith Sluimer, and Ellen Stobberingh 1999. "Effect of garlic on vancomycin-resistant enterococci." *Antimicrob. Agents Chemother.* 43(12): 3045. Accessed September 10, 2018 https://www.ncbi.nlm.nih.gov/pmc/articles/PMC89616/.

[72] Tsai, Yen, Linda L. Cole., Larry E. Davis, Steven J. Lockwood, Victoria Simmons, and Gaynor C. Wild 1985. "Antiviral properties of garlic: invitro effects on influenza B, Herpes simplex and cocksackie viruses." *Planta Med.*, 5: 460-461.

[73] Li, Chen, Wei Lun., Xinmei Zhao, Shan Lei, Yandong Guo, Jiayi Ma, and Facho Zhi 2015. "Allicin Alleviates Inflammation of Trinitrobenzenesulfonic Acid-Induced Rats." *Inflammation, 2015* 434692. Accessed September 10, 2018. http://doi.org/10.1155/2015/434692.

[74] Pandurangan, Ashok. K., Salmiah Ismail, Zeinab Saadatdoust, and Norhaisan M. Esa 2015. "Allicin Alleviates Dextran Sodium Sulfate- (DSS-) Induced Ulcerative Colitis in BALB/c Mice." *Oxidative Medicine and Cellular Longevity 2015* 605208. Accessed September 10, 2018 http://doi.org/10.1155/2015/605208.

[75] Rahman, G. K. M. Mustafizur, and Naoki Motoyama N. 2000. "Repellant effect of garlic against stored product pests. *Journal of Pesticide Science* 25(3): 247-252." Accessed September 10, 2018. https://doi.org/10.1584/jpestics.25.247.

[76] Hasan, Nazarul, Nabiha Yusuf, Zahra Toossi, and Najmul Islam 2006. "Suppression of *Mycobacterium tuberculosis* induced reactive oxygen species (ROS) and TNF-α mRNA expression in human monocytes by allicin." *FEBS Letters*, 580(10): 2517-2522.

[77] Zare Ahad, Parvaneh Farzaneh, Zahra Pourpak, Fatemeh Zahedi, Mostafa Moin, Shahram Shahabi, and Zuhair M. Hassan 2008. "Purified aged garlic extract modulates allergic airway inflammation in Balb/c mice." *Iranian Journal of Allergy, Asthma and Immunology*, 7(3):133–141.

[78] Bakri, Issam M., and C. W. Ian Douglas 2005. "Inhibitory effect of garlic extract on oral bacteria." *Archives of Oral Biology* 50: 645-651.

[79] Guan, Xiaoxu, Yi Zhou, Hui Chen, Chaowei Wang, and Huiming Wang 2018. Antibacterial, anti-inflammatory, and anti-osteoclastogenesis roles of allicin in periodontitis. *Int. J. Clin. Med.*, 11(7): 6721-6730.

[80] Hirsch, Keren, Michael Danilenko, Judith Giat J, Talia Miron, Aharon Rabinko, Meir Wilcheck, David Mirelman, Joseph Levy, and Yoav Sharoni 2000." Effect of purified allicin, the major ingredient of freshly crushed garlic on cancer cell proliferation." *Nutrition and Cancer* 38(2): 245-254.

[81] Ooommen, Suby, Ruby J. Anto, Gopal Srinivas, and Devarajan Karunagaran 2004. "Allicin (from garlic) induces caspase-mediated apoptosis in cancer cells." *Eur. J. Pharmacol.* 485: 97-103.

[82] Park, Sook-Yooung, Seong-Jun Cho, Hak-chul Kwon, Kang-Ro Lee, Dong-Kwon Rhee, and Suhkneung Pyo 2005. "Caspase-independent cell death by allicin in human epithelial carcinoma cells: Involvement of PKA." *Cancer Letters* 224: 123-132.

[83] Gruhlke, Martin C. H., Carole Nicco, Frederic Batteux, and Alan J. Slusarenko 2017. "The Effects of Allicin, a Reactive Sulfur Species from Garlic, on a Selection of Mammalian Cell Lines." *Antioxidants*, 6(1). Accessed September 10, 2018. http://doi.org/10.3390/antiox6010001.

[84] Chu, Yun-Lin, Chi-Tang Ho, Jing-Gung Chung, Raghu Rajasekaran, and Lee-Yan Sheen 2012. "Allicin induces p53-mediated autophagy in Hep G2 human liver cancer

cells." *J. Agric. Food Chem.*, Aug 29; 60(34):8363-71. Accessed September 10, 2018. doi: 10.1021/jf301298y. Epub 2012 Aug 15.

[85] Metwally, Dina M, Ebtesam M. Al-Olayan, Mohammad Alanazi, Sanaa B. Alzahrany, and Abdelelhabib Semlali 2018. "Antichistosomal and anti inflammatory activity of garlic and allicin compared with that of praziquantel in vivo." *BMC Complementary and Alternative Medicine* 18:135 Accessed September 10, 2018. https://doi.org/10.1186/s12906-018-2191-z.

[86] Hossain, Md. Shakhayet, Anita R. Dey, Nurjahan Begum, and Md. Abdul Alim 2015. "*In vitro* efficacy of medicinal plant material on the inhibition of development of egg of *Ascaridia galli." The Journal of Advances in Parasitology*, 2(1): 5-10. Accesssed September 12, 2018. doi: http://dx.doi.org/10.14737/journal.jap/2015/2.1.5.10.

[87] Block Eric, 1985. "The chemistry of onions and garlic." *Sc. Am.*, 252:94-99.

[88] Gupta, K. C. Sen, and Ren Viswanathan 1955. "Combined action of streptomycin and chloramphenicol with plant antibiotics against tubercle bacilli. I Streptomycin and chloramphenicol with cepharanthine. II. Streptomycin and allicin." *Antibiot. Chemother.* 5:24-27.

[89] Li, Guoliang, Xudong Ma, Lisha Deng, Xixi Zhao, Yuejiao Wei, Zhongyang Gao, Jing Jia, Jiru Xu, and Chaofeng Sun 2015. "Fresh garlic extract enhances the antimicrobial activities of antibiotics on resistant strains *in vitro." Jundishapur Journal of Microbiology* 8.5 (2015): e14814. *PMC*. Web. Accessed September 12, 2018. doi: 10. 5812/jjm.14814.

[90] Cutler, Ronald R., Michel Odent, Hussein Hajj-Ahmad, Sunil Maharajan, Norman J. Bennett, Peter D. Josling, Vanessa Ball, Paulette Hatton, and Martino Dall'Antonia 2009. "*In vitro* activity of an aqueous allicin extract and a novel allicin topical gel on Lancefield group B positive streptococci." *Journal of Antimicrobial Chemotherapy* 63(1): 151–154. https://doi.org/10.1093/jac/dkn457.

[91] Cundell, Diana R., and Frank Wilkinson 2017. "Chapter 3 Plant Factors inhibitory to Biofilm Formation," pages 59-120. In eBook *Biofilms: Characterization, Applications and Recent Advances* ISBN 978-1-53610-138-6.

[92] Mohsenipour, Zeinab, and Mehdi Hassanshahian 2015. "The Effects of *Allium sativum* Extracts on Biofilm Formation and Activities of Six Pathogenic Bacteria." *Jundishapur Journal of Microbiology*, *8*(8), e18971. Accessed September 12, 2018. http://doi.org/10.5812/jjm.18971v2.

[93] Ranjbar-Omid, Mahsa, Mohsen Arzanlou, Mojtaba Amani Seyyedeh K. S., Al-Hashem., Nour A. Mozafari, and Hadi P. Doghaleh 2015. "Allicin from garlic inhibits the biofilm formation and urease activity of *Proteus mirabilis in vitro." FEMS Letts.,* May;362(9). pii: fnv049 Epub 2015 Apr 2. Accessed September 12, 2018. https://doi.org/10.1093/femsle/fnv049.

[94] Kim, Young-Sun, Kyung S. Kim, Ihn Han, Mi-Hyun Kim, Min H. Jung, and Hun-Kuk Park 2012. "Quantitative and Qualitative Analysis of the Antifungal Activity of Allicin Alone and in Combination with Antifungal Drugs." *PLoSONE* 7(6), e38242. Accessed September 12, 2018. http://doi.org/10.1371/journal.pone.0038242.

[95] Khodavandi, Alireza, Fahimeh Alizadeh, Nabil S. Harmal, Shiran M. Sidik, Fauziah Othman, Zamberi Sekawi, Mohammad A. F. Jahromi, Kee-Peng Ng, and Pei-Pei Chong 2011.Comparison between efficacy of allicin and fluconazole against *Candida albicans*

in a mous model. *FEMS Microbiology Letts.* 315(2): 87-93. Accessed September 12, 2018. https://doi.org/10.1111/j.1574-6968.2010.02170.x.

[96] Perelló, Analia, Martin C. H. Gruhlke, and Alan J. Slusarenko 2013." Effect of garlic extract on seed germination, seedling health, and vigour of pathogen-infested wheat." *J. Plant Prot. Res.* 53: 317-323.

[97] Carlucci, A., M. L. Raimondo, J. Santos and A. J. L. Phillips 2012. "*Plectosphaerella* species associated with root and collar rots of horticultural crops in southern Italy." *Persoonia: Molecular Phylogeny and Evolution of Fungi* 28: 34-38. Accessed September 14, 2018 http://doi.org/10.3767/003158512X638251.

[98] Feng, Yonghui, Xiaotong Zhu, Quinhui Wang, Yongjun Jiang, Hong Shiang, Liwang Cui, and Yaing Cao 2012. "Allicin enhances host pro-inflammatory responses and protects against acute murine malaria infection." *Malaria J.* 11: 268. Accessed on September 14, 2018. doi: 10.1186/1475-2875-11-268.

[99] Waag, Thilo, Christoph Gelhaus, Jennifer Rath, August Stitch, Matthias Leippe, and Tanja Schirmeister 2010. "Allicin and its derivatives are cysteine protease inhibitors with antiparasitic activity." *Bioorg., Med. Chem. Lett.* 20(18): 5541-5543.

[100] Hotez, Peter, and Jennifer Herricks 2015." One million deaths from parasites." *PLoS Blogs* Posted January 16th, 2015. Accessed September 13, 2018. https://blogs.plos.org/speakingofmedicine/2015/01/16/one-million-deaths-parasites/.

[101] Ankri, Serge, Talia Miron, Aharon Rabinkov, Meir Wilchek, and David Mirelman 1997. "Allicin from garlic strongly inhibits cysteine proteases and cytopathic effects of Entamoeba histolytica." *Antimicrob. Agents Chemother.* 10: 2286-2288.

[102] Focke, Manfred, Andrea Feld, and Hartmut K. Lichtenthaler 1990. "Allicin a naturally occurring antibiotic from garlic, specifically inhibits acetyl-CoA synthase." *FEBS Letts.* 261:106-108.

[103] Walder R., Z. Kalvatchev, D. Garzaro, M. Barrios, and R. Apitz-Castro 1997. "In vitro suppression of HIV replication by ajoene [(e)-(z)-4,5,9-trithiadodeca-1,6,11-triene-9-oxide]."*Biomedicine and Biopharmacother.* 51(1): 397-403. Accessed on September 20, 2018. http://www.academia.edu/8123663/In_vitro_suppression_of_HIV1_ replication_ by_ajoene_e_-_z_-4_5_9-trithiadodeca-1_6_11-triene-9_oxide.

[104] Wang, Liyuang, Hongchao Jiao, Jinpeng Zhao, Xiaojuan Wang, Shuhon Sun, and Hai Lin 2017. "Allicin alleviates reticuloendotheliosis virus-induced immunosuppression via ERK/mitogen-activated protein kinase pathway in pathogen-free chickens" *Frontiers in Immunology*, 8:1856. Accessed September 14, 2018. doi: 10.3389/fimmu. 2017.01856.

[105] Prasad, Kailash, Victor A. Laxdal, Ming Yu, and Barbara L. Raney 1995. "Antioxidant activity of allicin, an active principle in garlic." *Mol. Cell. Biochem.* 148: 183-189.

[106] Simon Marcus M., Paul Waring, Mario Lobigs, Ahmed Nil, Thao Tran, Ron T. Hla, Seo Chin, and Arno Müllbacher 2000. "Cytotoxic T cells specifically induce Fas on target cells, thereby facilitating exocytosis-independent induction of apoptosis." *J. Immunol.* 165(7): 3663-3672.

[107] Wang, Con-Jun, Chao Wang, Jiang Han, Yong-Kun Wang, Lin Tang, Dong-Wei Shen, Yi Zhao, Rong-Hua Xu, and Hui Zhang 2013. "Effect of combined treatment with interleukin 2 and allicin on pancreatic cancer." *Mol. Biol. Rep.* 40: 6579-6585.

[108] Kumar, Suresh 2015. "Dual inhibition of acetylcholinesterase and butyrylcholinesterase enzymes by allicin." *Indian Journal of Pharmacology 47*(4), 444–446. http://doi.org/10.4103/0253-7613.161274.

[109] Zhang, Hao, Ping Wang, Yixue Xue, Libo Liu., Zhen Li, and Yunhui Liu 2018. "Allicin ameliorates cognitive impairment in APP/PS1 mice via suppressing oxidative stress by blocking JNK signaling pathways." *Tissue and Cell*, 50:89-95.

[110] Apitz-Castro, Rafael, Juan J. Badimon, and Lina Badimon 1992. "The effect of ajoene, the major antiplatelet compound from garlic, on platelet thrombus formation." *Thrombosis Res.* 68(2): 145-155.

[111] Dirsch, Verena M., Alexandra K. Kiemer, Hildebert Wagner, and Angelika M. Vollmar 1998. "Effect of allicin and ajoene, 2 compounds of garlic, on inducible nitric-oxide synthase." *Atherosclerosis* 139: 333-339.

[112] Mulder, Daniel J., Angela J. Noble, Christopher J. Justinich, and Jaclyn M. Duffin 2014. "A tale of two diseases: the history of inflammatory bowel disease." *J. Crohns Colitis*, 8(5): 1341-1348.

[113] Cundell, Diana R., and Kathryn E. Mickle 2018. "Osteoarthritis: potential for herbal medicines as therapies in the management of chronic inflammatory damage." *Current Immunology Reviews,* 14:1-13. E Pub ahead of print link. Accessed on September 14, 2018. http://www.eurekaselect.com/node/162555/article/osteoarthritis-potential-for-herbal-medicines-as-therapies-in-the-management-of-chronic-inflammatory-damage.

[114] Wilkinson, Frank, and Diana R. Cundell 2014. "From test tube to clinical trial; promising herbs with NF-κB and COX-2 activity." *Current Immunology Reviews 2014*, Volume 10 Issue 2 ISSN: 1875-631X (Online), ISSN: 1573-3955(Print). Accessed September 14, 2018 http://benthamscience.com/journal/index.php?journalID=cir.

[115] Kyo, Eikai., Naoto Uda, Shigeo, Kasuga, and Yoichi Itakura 2001. "Immunomodulatory effects of aged garlic extract." *J. Nutr.* 13(3s):1075s-1079s.

[116] Smith, Martin, Alison Atkin, and Clare Cutler 2017. "An age old problem ? Estimating the impact of dementia on past human populations." *Journal of Aging and Health* 29(1): 68-98.

[117] Coffey, Eleanor T. 2014. "Nuclear and cytosolic JNK signalling in neurons." *Nat Rev Neurosci.* 15:285–299. doi: 10.1038/nrn3729.

[118] Inglis, Fiona 2002. "The tolerability and safety of cholinesterase inhibitors in the treatment of dementia." *Int J Clin Pract Supp*l. 127:45–63.

[119] Bell, Howard A., Andrew G. Cuthbertson, and Neil Audsley 2016." The potential use of allicin as a biopesticide for the control of the housefly *Musa domestica* L." *Int. J. Pest Management*, 62(2): 111-118.

[120] Kumar, Deepak, and Prasanta Kalita 2017. "Reducing postharvest losses during storage of grain crops to strengthen food security in developing countries." *Foods* 6(1) 8. Accessed September 16, 2018. http://doi.org/10.3390/foods6010008.

[121] Plata-Rueda, Anglelica, Luis C. Martínez., Marcello H. D. Santos, Flávio L. Fernandes, Carlos F. Wilcken, Marcus A. Soares, José E. Serrão, and José C. Zanuncio 2017. "Insecticidal activity of garlic essential oil and their constituents against the mealworm beetle, *Tenebrio molitor* Linnaeus (Coleoptera: Tenebrionidae)." *Scientific Reports* 7 46406. Accessed on September 15, 2018. http://doi.org/10.1038/srep46406.

[122] Huang, Yan, Shao X. Chen, and Shuit H. Ho 2000. "Bioactivities of methyl allyl disulfide and diallyl trisulfide from essential oil of garlic to two species of stored-product pests, Sitophilus zeamais (Coleoptera: Curculionidae) and Tribolium castaneum (Coleoptera: Tenebrionidae)." *Journal of Economic Entomology* 93(2): 537–543. Accessed on September 20, 2018 https://doi.org/10.1603/0022-0493-93.2.537.

[123] Meriga, Balaji, Ramgopal Mopuri, and T. MuraliKrishna 2012. "Insecticidal, antimicrobial and antioxidant activities of *Allium sativum* bulb." *Asian J. Tropical Med.* 5(5): 391-395.

[124] Fand, Babasaheb B. N., Nitin T. Sul, Santanu K. Bal, and P. S. Minhas 2015. "Temperature Impacts the Development and Survival of Common Cutworm (*Spodoptera litura*): Simulation and Visualization of Potential Population Growth in India under Warmer Temperatures through Life Cycle Modelling and Spatial Mapping." *PLoS ONE*, *10*(4), e0124682. Accessed September 20, 2018. http://doi.org/10.1371/journal.pone.0124682.

[125] Anwar, Awais, Emma Gould, Ryan Tinson, Murree Groom, and Chris J. Hamilton 2017. "Think Yellow and Keep Green—Role of Sulfanes from Garlic in Agriculture." *Antioxidants*, *6*(1), 3. Accessed September 20, 2018. http://doi.org/10.3390/antiox6010003.

[126] Mayer, Maria, Christian R. Vogl, Michele Amorena, and Matthias Hamburger 2014. "Treatment of organic livestock with medicinal plants: A systematic review of European ethnoveterinary research." *Forsch Komplementmed.*, 21: 375-386. Accessed September 20, 2018. https://doi.org/10.1159/000370216.

[127] Erguig, Marwane, Mohamed Yahyaoui, and Mohammed Fekhaoui 2015. "The use of garlic in aquaculture." *Eur. J. Biotech. Bioscience*, 3: 28-33. Accessed September 20, 2018. http://www.biosciencejournals.com/vol3/issue8/pdf/15.1.pdf.

[128] Luber, George, & Natasha Prudent. 2009. "Climate change and human health." *Transactions of the American Clinical and Climatological Association* 120: 113-7.

[129] Lutz, Wolfgang, and Samir KC. 2010. "Dimensions of global population projections: what do we know about future population trends and structures?" *Philosophical Transactions of the Royal Society of London. Series B, Biological Xciences*, *365*(1554), 2779-91. doi: 10.1098/rstb.2010.0133.

[130] Schoonbeek, Sanne, Hossein Azadi, Hossein Mahmoudi, Ben Derudder, Philippe De Maeyer, and Frank Witlox. 2013. "Organic agriculture and undernourishment in developing countries: Main potentials and challenges." *Critical Reviews in Food Sciences and Nutrition* 53(9): 917-928. doi: 10.1080/10408398.2011.573886.

In: Allicin
Editor: Diana R. Cundell
ISBN: 978-1-53617-339-0

Chapter 2

CHEMISTRY AND BIOCHEMISTRY OF ALLICIN

***Gwendolyn Moise**, PhD**
and Mary Ann Wagner-Graham, PhD
College of Life Sciences, Department of Biological and Chemical Sciences,
Jefferson University, Philadelphia, PA, US

ABSTRACT

Allicin, a phytochemical produced by members of the *Allium* genus, contains a unique thiosulfinate (-SS(O)-) functional group which conveys the chemical properties and activities of allicin. The primary chemical actions of allicin include scavenging of free radical species, oxidation of reduced thiols, and participation in disulfide exchange reactions. In biological systems, allicin inactivates proteins and enzymes with critically important cysteine residues or disulfide bonds, and depletes levels of common cellular reductants like cysteine and glutathione. *In vitro*, allicin is made from diallyl disulfide, with a performic acid catalyst to promote formation of allyl sulfenic acid, which then condenses to form allicin. *In vivo*, allicin is produced by alliinase (E.C. 4.4.1.4), a pyridoxyl-5'-phosphate-dependent C-S lyase, from alliin (S-allyl-L-cysteine sulfoxide) substrate. Alliin and alliinase are held in separate compartments of garlic bulb cells and mixed only when plant tissue is crushed or cut. The greatest production of allicin is achieved by *A. sativum* plants. Due to inherent instability of allicin, many commercial and pharmaceutical products contain alliin and alliinase for *in situ* production of allicin. Alliinase is well-characterized regarding substrate specificity, inhibitor compounds, and structure. There are many protocols for purification of alliinase from garlic plants and garlic powder. Recombinant and matrix-immobilized forms of alliinase have been developed for improved manufacture of allicin on demand.

* Corresponding Author's Email: Gwendolyn.Moise@Jefferson.edu.

Keywords: allicin, diallyl thiosulfinate, allylthiosulfinate, diallyl disulfide-oxide, 539-86-6, garlic

INTRODUCTION

Allium satavum L. more commonly known as garlic, can be found all around the world. Because of its uniquely pungent odor, garlic has been used in many different ways for centuries. Some of the more notable ways include as a spice for cooking, as a vampire repellent, and as a medicinal herb. It has been used in traditional medicine from around the globe. References to its medicinal properties have been found in ancient China, India, Egypt and PreRomanic Germany [1]. While some of the famous properties of garlic, such as the smells warding off evil spirts, can't be tested, the medicinal properties have been heavily studied. The most biologically active compound found in garlic comes from a small sulfur compound called allicin. In the PubChem database allicin has over 69 different depositor-supplied names listed, and the most common IUPAC name is 3-prop-2-enylsulfinyl-sulfanylprop-1-ene. One of the most interesting properties of garlic is that the intense and distinctive smell is almost nonexistent until the garlic has been crushed or cut. Allicin and its degradation products cause the distinctive smell, so therefore are not made until the precursor alliin and the enzyme alliinase are combined when the cells are cut or crushed. Allicin is not only pungent, but also highly bioactive, which means that it is unstable and ephemeral. On the other hand, the precursor alliin, S-allyl-L-cysteine sulfoxide, is relatively stable and is the limiting factor on the amount of allicin produced by garlic. Alliin, because of its stability, is being used in pharmaceutical compounds.

Allicin is a small organic molecule with a molecular mass of 162.3 g/mol and contains both sulfur and oxygen atoms and is classified as a reactive sulfur species (RSS). RSS have been defined as "redox-active sulfur-containing molecules that are able, under physiological conditions, to either oxidize or reduce biomolecules" [2]. The structure of allicin is shown in Figure 1 and the nature of the unique –S–S=O– functional group has been extensively studied. The original view of the bond was that of a highly polar sigma bond between one of the sulfurs and the oxygen atom as seen in Figure 1, part C, but on further inspection it was reclassified as a dative bond and shown with an arrow (Figure 1, part B). This arrow shows that the two electrons forming the bond both come from the sulfur atom and are not equally shared. This dative bond is most commonly seen in metal coordinate complexes where the ligand is electron rich and the bond is formed by a ligand-suppling the pair of electrons. In organic chemistry, dative bonds are seen mostly in Lewis acid acid-base pairs. The arrow depiction of the dative bond indicates electrons shared by the oxygen atom are supplied by the sulfur atom, so there are six electrons forming three free electron pairs around the oxygen atom making it highly nucleophilic and unstable. This form of representation has also fallen out of favor for the more common sulfur-oxygen double bond as seen in Figure 1, part A. This "S=O" representation implies two electrons are supplied by both sulfur and oxygen. While the double bond representation is more conventional, it does not adequately convey the inherent instability of the dative bond or polar bond models, and so the older representations (S→O and S–O) are still often used.

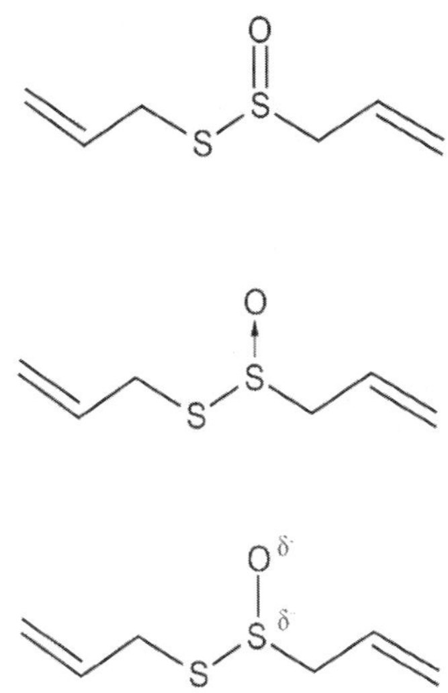

Legend: Part A shows the structure of allicin with the conventional sulfur-oxygen double bond. While not as accurate, it shows that both sulfer and oxygen contribute two electrons in the bond. Part B shows the structure of allicin as a dative bond, where the arrow points from the sulfur to the oxygen atom showing that two electrons from sulfur contribute to the bond and no electrons from oxygen are used to make the bond. Part C shows the structure of allicin with a highly polar bond between the sulfur and oxygen representing unequal sharing of electrons not usually observed in a sigma bond between sulfur and oxygen.

Figure 1. Chemical structure of allicin.

1. Chemical Properties

1.1. Inherent Instability

Allicin is a highly reactive molecule and therefore inherently unstable, but measures of instability are highly varied. Some extracts of allicin can last months without loss of activity, while others last only an hour before noticeable loss of acivity. The ability of a 1% (w/v) aqueous extract of garlic powder to fully kill *E. coli* O-157 bacteria was retained after boiling at 100°C for 20 min [3], and pure allicin added to HCl solutions pH 1-5 had no loss of allicin for 2 hours [4]. Later studies [5] found that the half life of allicin in aqueous solution was 30-40 days at 23 °C. Another study [6] found that the half life of allicin in aqueous solution is 6.5 days at 23°C, but about 1 year at 4°C, showing that the decomposition of allicin in an aqueous solution is heavally dependant on the temperature of that solution. Now why are there differences in these studies? All of these studies are done with natural extracts of garlic, so some of the variability comes with the diffent strains of garlic while others come from the difference in pH, buffers, and concentrations used, not all of which are reported. In 2010 these results were confirmed by a study [7] finding that allicin in aqueous garlic extract, Iranian garlic strain, using just distilled water, no buffers or added chemicals, at 4°C the half life was >150 days and at 22°C the half life was about 20 days. Aqueous extract concentration is 1.2 mg/mL was determined by HPLC. So while boiling the solution for 20 mins, or dropping the pH to 1, seemed to not affect overall activily of an extract because there was enough allicin left after boiling to kill the *E. coli* even at the lowered concentration. The decomposition of allicin is highly temperature dependent and the rate of decomposition increases as the solution is heated. No loss of antimicrobial activity of aqueous garlic extract (10 g bulb/10 mL distilled water) was seen after storage at 4°C for 1 week or at -80°C for 6 months [8]. So, while allicin is not stored in the garlic it can readly be made by crushing garlic and can be stored in diluted aqueous in a -80 °C freezer for months at a time.

The stability of allicin can be increased. Plant-derived porous silicon extracted from bamboo nodal joints preserved the antibacterial activity of garlic etract from decomposition with UV light, affording retention of 95% of antibacterial activity as compared to a control of garlic extract alone [9].

Allicin is inherently unstable because it is highly reactive. The –S–S=O– functional group can reduce any free thiol group or participating in disulfide bond reactions. Allicin primarily acts as an oxidation agent and oxidizes any accessible reduced thiol group –SH. In the blood there are many small molecules and proteins with exposed reduced thiol groups for allicin to react with. A study looking into the reactivity of allicin in the stomach and in the blood found that allicin is highly reactive in blood samples, 83% of allicin was lost during mixing with methanol-denatured heparinized blood, and no allicin could be detected after 5 minutes with heparinized blood. Inversely at gastric pH of 1.2 allicin is very unreactive, after 1 day of incubation in water at pH 1.2, 80% remained [10]. Allicin reactivity is based in electron rich oxygen atom and once it is protonated at low pHs the reactivity is dramatically reduced [10]. In protein tyrosine phosphatases (PTP), a reduced thiol at the active site is required for activity, so any oxidation of it nullifies activity [11]. The addition of new disulfide bonds in proteins changes the 3D structure of a protein and therefore can alter is catalytic ability. Additionally, allicin scavenges hydroxyl radicals in biological tissues. These mechanisms are those by which allicin is bioactive.

1.2. Purification and Preparation of Allicin

Allicin can be extracted from garlic using just distilled water and crushed garlic bulbs, though more commonly a neutral phosphate buffer (60 mM, pH 7.00, 1% NaCl) with 10% sucrose for stability is used for extraction [12]. Chemical composition of the extract varies according to the type of solvent employed. In one study common bioacitve componds such as alliin and allicin were not present in the water-based extract, but were detected in the butanolic garlic extract [13]. Allicin can also be extracted with dichlorormethane or acetonitrile [12]. Allicin is soluble in water, which is easily obtained and non-toxic, but more soluble in polar organic solvents. Therefore water is the most common solvent used to extract allicin and its precursur alliin, although not the most efficient. For more details on different extraction techniques see references [14-19]. While allicin is the main bioactive compound, alliin is more stable and therefore can be a more desired extract. Alliin is more soluble in water than allicin and therefore can also be extracted from garlic with distilled water. Garlic bulbs contain 0.62-1.78% alliin by weight, as determined by using both HPLC and an alliinase-based biosensor monitoring rate of ammonia production [20].

Allicin can be synthesized in lab via the radical addition of oxygen to diallyl disulfide (DADS). To synthesise allicin, DADS is mixed with aqueous hydrogen peroxide in the presence of performic acid as a catalyst Figure 2. Other acids can be used but performic acid gave the highest yields [21]. The reaction is run at 0°C and purifed via a sillica gel column chromatography. Prior to addition of diallyldisulfide, performic acid is generated in a 100 min reaction at room temperature by combination of formic acid and hydrogen peroxide [21]. This approach using performic acid proceeds more quickly, yields greater amount of allicin, and concommitant with a lesser amount of undesired byproducts than the same reaction performed with peracetic acid at 20 °C [21].

The rate limiting step is the formation of the hydroxyl radical, so to speed up the reaction, formic acid and peroxide can be mixed together on ice before the DADS is added. The mechanism for the formation of allicin was proposed using the oxidative cleavage of the disulfide bond in DADS by hydroxyl-radicals generated when peroxide is mixed with formic acid [21]. This leaves allyl sulfonic acid and allyl radical. Another hydroxyl-radical can then convert the allyl radical into a second allyl sulfonic acid. The two allyl sulfonic acid molecules can then combine in a dehydration reaction to form allicin (Figure 2).

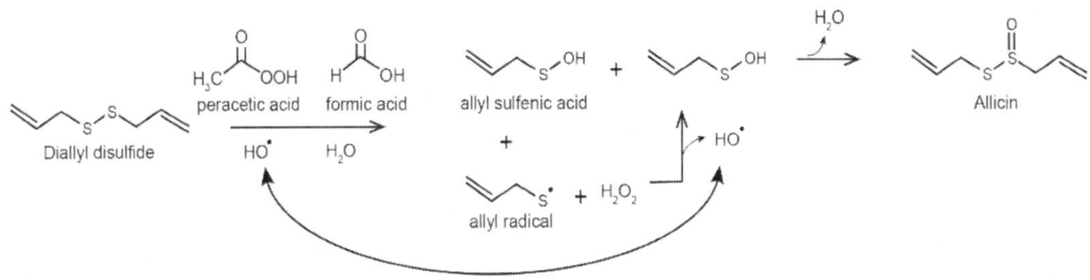

Legend: Oxidative cleavage of the S–S bond in DADS by hydroxyl-radicals forms two units of allyl sulfonic acid, which then condense to form allicin.

Figure 2. Synthesis of allicin from diallyl disulfide DADS.

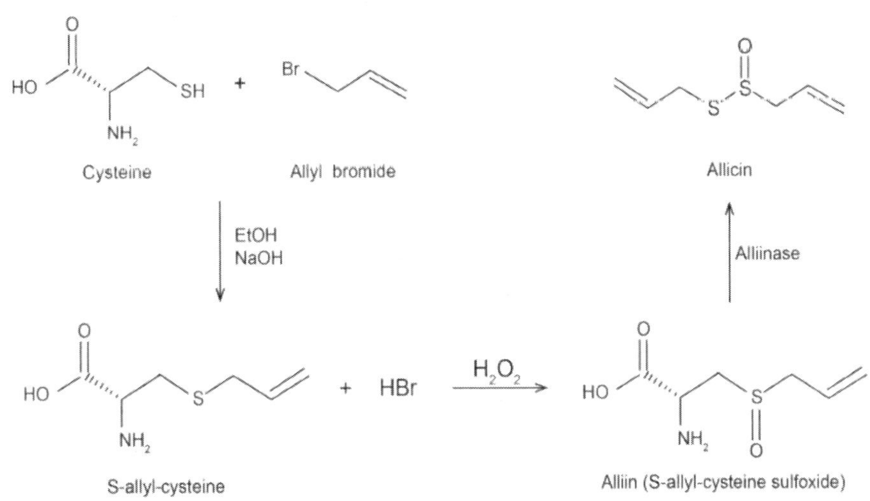

Legend: S-cysteine and allyl bromide are mixed in solvent ethanol with sodium hydroxide. The sulfur does a nucleophilic substitution of the bromide and forms S-allyl-cysteine. Then the direct oxidation of the sulfur atom is achieved by hydroxyl-radicals to form alliin. Alliin can then be converted to allicin using the enzyme alliinase.

Figure 3. Synthetic pathway of the formation of alliin.

While allicin is the main bioactive compound in garlic, its precurser alliin is much more stable and can be stored dried at room temperature for years. Alliin is converted to allicin by the enzyme alliinase (Figure 3). A more thorough summary of alliinase structure and mechanism is provided later in this chapter. Alliinase is found in many different *Allium* species in addition to garlic, and is a very promiscuous enzyme, having many different substrates and roles. Garlic is the only species to make allicin because it is the only species to make alliin in any quantity. Alliin can be synthesised starting with L-cysteine and allyl bromide. The sulfur in L-cysteine is deprotinated with sodium hydroxide and does a nucleophilic substitution of bromide to form S-allyl-cysteine. The sulfur in S-allyl-cysteine can then be oxidized by hydrogen peroxide to form S-allyl-cysteine sulfoxide, alliin [1]. Alliin can then be converted to allicin using the enzyme alliinase, or stored and used as an active pharmaceutical ingredient. When alliin is mixed with alliinase, allicin can be made *in vivo*.

1.3. Structural Analogues and Synthetic Derivatives

Early studies with synthetic branched-chain derivatives of alkyl thiosulfonates showed that the minimal inhibitory concentration for complete shutdown of microbial growth increased with the degree of branching of the alkyl side chains bookending the –S–S=O– functional group [22]. The authors of that study suggested bulkier molecules are restricted from permeating the cell membrane. We know many of allicin's biological actions depend upon its passage into the cell's interior. The passage of allicin into the cell is limited by diffusion [12], so the better is it at slipping through the cell wall, the more biological activity it has. The rigid, flat allyl side groups provide just enough hydrophobic character to ease passage of allicin through the cell membrane, without adding bulk to hinder its slippage between closely packed membrane phospholipids. Therefore, no increases to the sidechain have found an increase in biological activity. Alkyl thiosulfinates can be employed in a variety of synthetic reactions, as described [23].

2. Biochemical Properties of Alliinase

2.1. Natural Synthesis of Allicin by Alliinase

Allicin is a natural, highly-reactive sulfhydryl modifying agent produced in response to attack of plant tissues by pests or animals, and a focus on enzymatic formation of allicin *in vivo* is warranted. The enzyme responsible for allicin formation was named alliinase by Stoll and Seebeck [24], the research team who solved the structure of allicin in 1948. Alliinase (E.C. 4.4.1.4) is alternatively known as alliin lyase, cysteine sulfoxide C-S lyase, and L-cysteine sulfoxide lyase. Of nine *Allium* species assessed for alliinase activity, crude extract of *Allium sativum* contained the highest specific activity for alliinase at 178 umol min^{-1} mg^{-1} [12]. To state that alliinase produces allicin is technically incorrect since alliinase does not make allicin directly, but produces allyl sulfenic acid, and two molecules of allyl sulfenic acid nonenzymatically combine to form one molecule of allicin [24]. Figure 4 shows an overview of the reaction performed by alliinase. In the process, pyruvate and ammonia are liberated, and the activity of alliinase is measured by either discontinuous (endpoint measurement of total product formed) or continuous (rate of product formation) assay; Table 2 summarizes popular assay methods and conditions.

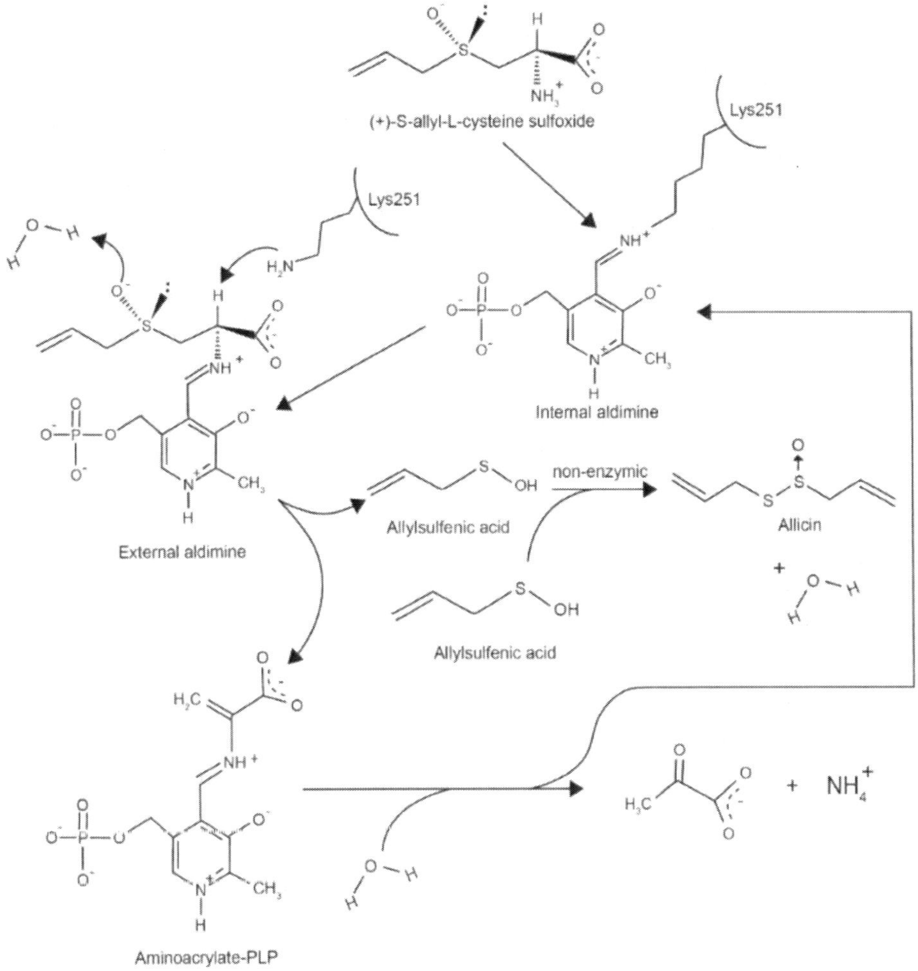

Legend: In one catalytic cycle, alliin is converted to allyl sulfenic acid, pyruvate, and ammonia. Two molecules of allyl sulfenic acid nonenzymically condense to yield one molecule of allicin, thus two catalytic cycles of alliinase are required to produce one molecule of allicin. Here, the resting state of the enzyme is shown with an internal aldimine formed between the pyridoxal-5'-phosphate cofactor and the ε-amino group of Lys251, as seen in structure 1LK9 [25]. The active site of structure 2HOX contained an aminoacrylate-PLP intermediate [26]. Further details regarding catalytic mechanism are presented in the text, under the section 2.5, "Substrate specificity, inhibitor compounds, modifying agents, and mechanism".

Reference sources for figure: [25, 26, 27, 28].

Figure 4. The reaction performed by alliinase.

Alliinase protein is abundant in garlic bulb tissue, estimated 12% [14, 29] by weight of soluble bulb proteins. Alliinase accounts for one of two prominent protein bands observed on SDS-PAGE of garlic bulb homogenate [30]. Western-blotting with anti-allinase antibodies shows alliinase is most accumulated in bulbs, less so in leaves, and absent in roots, but nearly twice the amount of alliinase activity was present in roots as comparted to bulbs, suggesting a variant and highly active isoform of alliinase is present in roots [31]. A root-specific isoform was isolated and characterized in *A. cepa* [32], but the same has not yet been described for *A. sativum*.

Tight control of allicin production limits damage to the plant, and the biochemical synthesis of allicin is a beautiful example of compartmentalized metabolism. Alliinase is sequestered inside membrane-bound vacuoles [33, 34] while alliin substrate, (+)-S-allyl-L-cysteine sulfoxide, is in the cytoplasm. In the garlic bulb, alliinase is exclusive to bundle sheath cells, as determined by intrinsic pyridoxyl-5'-phosphate fluorescence, activity staining with alliin and nitroblue tetrazolium (NBT), and immunohistochemical staining of sliced bulb tissue with anti-alliinase antibodies using an alkaline phosphatase/NBT/5-bromo-4-chloro-3-indoyl phosphate (BCIP) detection system [34].This finding was confirmed by immunohistochemical localization of alliinase on tissue prints of sectioned bulbs using peroxidase-labeled anti-alliinase polyclonal antibodies [35]. Both alliinase and cysteine synthase, an enzyme required to make alliin substrate, are localized to bundle sheath cells, as determined with FITC-labeled goat anti-rabbit IgG detection of polyclonal rabbit anti-alliinase and anti-cysteine synthase antibodies [36]. Northen blotting suggests alliinase is constituitvely expressed [37].

Alliinase is catalyticly active against multiple forms of S-alkylated-L-cysteine sulfoxides, but the specific substrate needed to produce allicin is alliin, (+)-S-allyl-L-cysteine sulfoxide. The amount of S-alkyl/alkenyl-L-cysteine sulfoxides present in 17 different *Allium* species was quantitated, and although 10 of the species screened produced detectable amounts of (+)-S-allyl-L-cysteine sulfoxide, only *A. sativum* preferentially made this allicin precursor in large quantities, as approximately 75% of all cysteine sulfoxides produced by *A. sativum* [12]. Another source determined alliin constituted 87% of the cysteine sulfoxides and γ-glutamylcysteines in bulbs of mature plants, but only 25% if harvested 7 weeks early [5]. Thus, although alliinase enzyme is present in other plants and also some bacteria [28, 32, 38 - 43], ability to produce allicin is restricted to those species which also contian a completed metabolic pathway to generate (+)-S-allyl-L-cysteine sulfoxide, *i.e.*, alliin. Evidence suggests alliin is synthesized in leaves and transferred to bulbs upon maturity of the plant [44]. The highest concentration of alliin was found in leaves, and alliin accumulation increased with supplementation of calcium sulfate [45]. Cysteine synthase is obligate for manufacture of cysteine, including that built into either serine or glutathione, and both the cytosol and chloroplast isoforms of cysteine synthase are most highly transcribed in leaves of young plants before appearance of the second leaf [46].

Both serine and glutathione have been proposed as possible precursors of the amino acid backbone of alliin [47]. The definitive donor of the allyl group is not yet identified, and it seems formation of the allyl group's carbon-carbon double bond is the step unique to formation of alliin. Garlic bulb callus cells grown in culture did not manufacture alliin when fed solely glutathione or serine [48], but did make alliin when fed either S-allyl-cysteine or allyl thiol [49], although at a lesser yield when fed allyl thiol [48]. Even cultured onion cells, which do not make alliin in large quantities, were able to do so when fed allyl cysteine [48]. Addition of ^{14}C-labeled valine lead to accumulation of both radiolabeled S-2-carboxypropyl cysteine and S-2-carboxypropyl-glutathione [47, 50], which seems to suggest methylacrylyl-CoA derived from valine provides the allyl group, and notably this path is present in the MetaCyc database [51] pathway for alliin metabolism. However, the ^{14}C-label from valine, although incorporated into isoalliin in both garlic and onion, was not present in alliin [47].

Recent work [52] described three γ-glutamyl transpeptidases (AsGGT1, AsGGT2, AsGGT3) from *A. sativum*, which when expressed in *S. cerevisiase*, permit generation of S-allyl-L-cysteine from exogenously supplied glycylglycine and γ-glutamyl-S-allyl-L-cysteine, but not γ-glutamyl-S-allyl-L-cysteine sulfoxide. GFP-fusion constructs of AsGGT1 and AsGGT3 are cystol-bound when expressed in *A. cepa* cells, but AsGGT2 translocates to the vacuole [52]. After removal of the glytamyl residue, the sulfur atom of S-allyl-L-cysteine is oxidized by a novel FAD and NADPH dependent flavin monooxygenase (AsFMO1), creating (+)-S-allyl-L-cysteine sulfoxide [53]. More work is required to clarify the sulfur and allyl group donors and the in the alliin synthesis pathway.

2.2. Purification and Isolation of Alliinase

Purification of alliinase from homogenized garlic cloves is relatively straightforward, and similar methods permit isolation of active alliinase also from garlic powder. An overview (Table 1) of purification strategies and reports is provided, although not exhaustive. Commonly, purification schemes begin with ammonium sulfate or polyethelene glycol fractionation of proteins from homogenized cell lysates. Pelleted proteins are collected and resuspended before further purification by column chromatography. Since alliinase is a glycolsyated protein, Concanavalin A Sepharose affinity chromatrography facilitates purification. Approaches using ConA-Sepahrose affinity matrix recover alliinase from the resin with α-D-mannoside. Supplementation with 20 – 25 μM pyridoxal-5'-phosphate (PLP) helps to avoid loss of PLP cofactor. While inclusion of glycerol (10%) or sucrose (10%) assists in preserving activity, addition of at least 1% sodium choride to storage buffer is critical for preservation of alliinase activity; buffer without NaCl offered no stabilizing effect, even when sucrose, glycerol, or PLP was present alone or in combination [19]. A chloride binding loop plays a key role in alliinase structure [25, 26]. Some purification protocols include β-mercaptoethanol, as this was seen to preserve activity of *A. cepa* alliinase [14, 29].

Alliinase purified from garlic powder yielded different size bands on SDS-PAGE (53 and 54 kDa), suggesting alliinase is modified during the clove dehydration process, as alliinase from fresh cloves yielded a single band [54]. The specific activity of alliinase from garlic powder (252 U/mg) was less than that from fresh cloves (332 U/mg), and the K_m values for (+)- and (-)-S-allyl-L-cysteine sulfoxide were slightly higher those for the alliinase from garlic powder [54].

2.3. Physical Characteristics of Alliinase

The coding sequences for alliinase in *Allium sativum*, *A. cepa*, and *A. ascalonicum*, were identified through hybridization of a degenerate radiolabeled DNA probe, reflecting the N-terminal sequence (residues 1-7) of allinase enzyme, to a library of cDNA molecules isolated from bulb tissue and cloned into the pT_7T_3 18 U phagemid at the *EcoRI* site and hosted in *E. coli* XL1 Blue [30]. The coding sequence for alliinase was isolated also from both λgt11 and λZAPII cDNA libraries of *A. sativum* [31].

Table 1. Overview of alliinase purification methods

Summary of Approach[a] [Referenced work]	Homogenization buffer	SA (U/mg)[b]
Fresh garlic from Davis, CA; 1% protamine sulfate precipitation followed by 35% $(NH_4)_2SO_4$ cut; resuspended pellet applied to Sephadex G200; authors comment that ion-exchange chromatography (CM- or DEAE-Sephadex) provided no additional purification [55].	20 mM sodium phosphate, pH 7.5; 10% glycerol	37.6
Garlic from Davis, CA; 35% $(NH_4)_2SO_4$ cut; resuspended pellet applied to hydroxylapatite column, followed by ConA Sepharose chromatography [55].	20 mM sodium potassium phosphate, pH 7.0; 10% glycerol; 5% NaCl; 5% polyvinylpolypyrrolidone (PVPP); 0.05% β-mercaptoethanol; 1 mM PMSF	214
Garlic from a local market in Davis, CA; approach is as in [14, 29].	20 mM sodium potassium phosphate, pH 7.0; 0.05% β-mercaptoethanol; 10% glycerol; 1 mM PMSF; 5 mM EDTA	109
Spanish garlic; complicated purification scheme without use of Con-A Sepharose; Three $(NH_4)_2SO_4$ fractionations; nine different buffer compositions, ranging from 20 mM potassium phosphate pH 7.0 to Tris-HCl to 25 mM histidine-HCl, pH 5.25, but all containing 10% glycerol, and all but two buffers including 20 μM PLP; only a 3.7% recovery of alliinase activity [18].	20 mM potassium phosphate, pH 7.0; 5% NaCl; 5% PVPP; 10 mM EDTA; 0.05% β-mercaptoethanol; 10% glycerol; 20 μM PLP; 1 mL Wacker "SE2" silicone oil per 100 mL	390
Source of garlic not specified; 25% PEG-8000 fractionation; pellet resuspended and applied to hydroxylapatite; 50% $(NH_4)_2SO_4$ fractionation; resuspended pellet applied to Ultrapac TSK Phenyl 5PW (hydrophobic interaction) HPLC column [31].	20 mM sodium phosphate, pH 7.2; 10% glycerol; 1 mM PMSF; 20 μM PLP	260
Source of garlic not specified; initial 25% PEG-8000 precipitation; resuspended pellet applied to ConA Sepharose; no other chromatography used [17].	50 mM HEPES, pH 7.2; 10% glycerol; 1 mM PMSF; 1 mM $CaCl_2$; 20 μM PLP	115.4
Starting material was garlic powder, 100 g; 45% $(NH_4)_2SO_4$ cut; applied resuspended pellet to Sephadex S 200 HR, then proceeded to ConA Sepharose [19].	60 mM phosphate pH 7.0; 10% glycerol; 5% NaCl; 0.5% PVP; 0.05% β-mercaptoethanol; 5 mM EDTA; 1 mM PMSF; note dialysis buffer contains 60 mM phosphate pH 7.0; 1% NaCl; 10% sucrose; 25 μM PLP; 0.02% NaN_3	20
Purification schema as in [19], above; starting material is either 2.5 g fresh *A. sativum* var. *pekinense* cloves or 100 g garlic powder from "Cangshan" garlic [54].	60 mM phosphate, pH 7.0; 10% glycerol; 5% NaCl; 0.5% PVP; 0.05% β-mercaptoethanol; 5 mM EDTA; 1 mM PMSF	252 (powder) 332 (fresh)
Egyptian garlic; purification approach as in [17], but with HiLoad 20/60 Superdex 200 after ConA Sepharose column [16].	50 mM HEPES, pH 7.2; 10% glycerol; 1 mM Pefabloc; 1 mM $CaCl_2$; 1 mM $MgCl_2$; $MnCl_2$; 3 mM NaN_3; 20 μM PLP	660

a – For detailed information, see reference paper.

b – Specific activity as reported in the original work. As a variety of enzyme assays were used, these values cannot be easily compared from one laboratory to another.

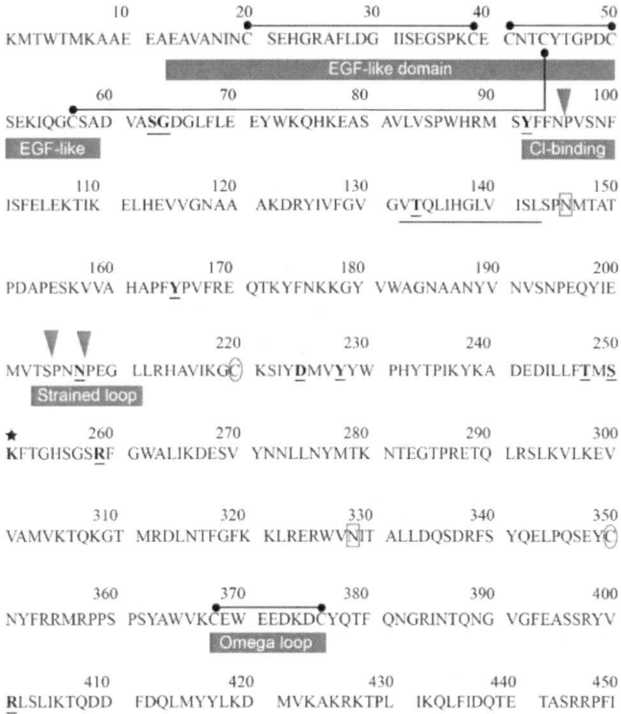

Legend: Features of alliianse are mapped onto primary sequence from UniProtKB/SwissProt record Q01594.1 [30]. For simplicity, only sequence of the mature protein is shown, and signal peptide is omitted. Cys-cys bridges are indicated by bar/circle connectors. Free cys residues are circled. Residues involved in noncovalent substrate or cofactor binding are bolded and underlined; Tyr165 stabilizes specifically PLP. Helix 132-143 is underlined by a solid bar. Covalent PLP attachment site, Lys251, is starred. Glycosylated Asn residues are boxed. Cis-peptide bonds are indicated by filled triangles. Notable tertiary features are labeled with text boxes below sequence.

References used to construct figure: [16, 25, 26, 30, and 56].

Figure 5. Map of alliinase primary sequence.

Analysis of the cDNA sequence suggests alliinase is translated as an inactive 486-aa preproprotein, with posttranslational cleavage predicted to occur between amino acids 30 and 31 [30]. However, cleavage at this position does not account for presence of a lysine at the N-terminus, as determined by N-terminal amino acid sequencing of the enzyme purified from garlic cloves [30]. Based on the cDNA sequence, the mature protein has 448 amino acid residues, active as a homodimer of 51.5 kDa subunits [31]. Figure 5 presents a composite map of the primary sequence of alliinase.

Alliinase belongs to the fold type I group of PLP-dependent enzymes [57]. Multiple sequence alignment analysis suggested alliinase contains an N-terminal epidermal growth factor (EGF) like domain, from Glu13 to Ala59, the first example noted for a plant-derived enzyme [16]. This was confirmed by crystallographic data revealing the structure of alliinase (1LK9) at 1.53 Å resolution [25], generated from alliinase crystallized with with S-ethyl-L-cysteine [16]. Subsequently, two well-resolved structures of alliianse were presented [26]: 2HOX shows the holo-enzyme co-crystallized with (+)-S-allyl-L-cysteine at 1.40 Å resolution, and 2HOR shows the apo form at 1.61 Å. Interestingly, the PLP cofactor was in complex with an aminoacrylate intermediate in the holoenzyme; the donor of the aminoacrylate group could be either S-ethyl-L-cysteine included in the crystallization buffer or alliin present in the garlic bulb [26]. The models of both groups [25, 26] show alliinase as a homodimer with active sites at the dimer interface, monomeric subunits containing PLP cofactors, and many of the same binding interactions between the protein and cofactor and/or substrate mimic. The structures differ in that 1LK9 [25] resolved to show an equal mixture of PLP participating either in an internal aldimine with Lys251 or in external aldimine with aminoacrylate intermediate, while 2HOX [26] shows only the external aldimine.

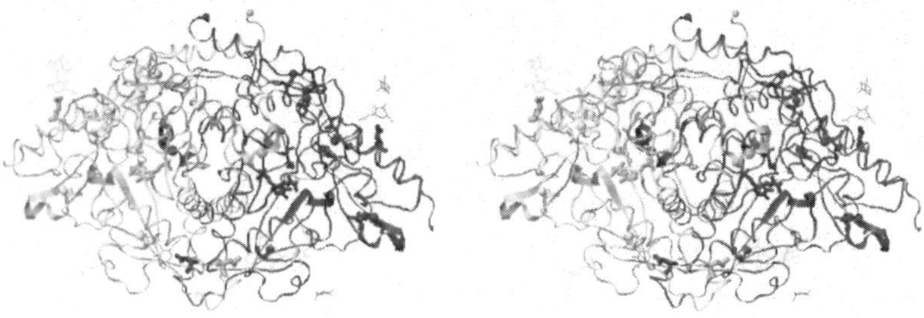

Legend: Stereoscopic overview of alliinase structure 2HOX [26]. Subunit A (light gray) and subunit B (dark gray) constitute the active homodimer. N-termini at top are marked by filled spheres. The aminoacrylate-PLP intermediates at the dimeric interfaces are embraced by the chloride-binding loop (chloride atom shown) and strained loop, both shown as broad ribbons. The omega loops are indicated as broad ribbons. Carbohydrate residues (wireframe) of Asn146 are at bottom of image; those of Asn328 are at top of image; Asn anchors displated in bold wireframe. Cysteinyl sulfur atoms shown as large spacefill.
Figure generated using *Jmol* 14.20.4.

Figure 6. Overview of alliinase quaternary structure.

Alliinase activity is dependent upon pyridoxal-5'-phosphate (PLP) cofactor, and PLP-modifying reagents hydroxylamine and sodium cyanide promoted loss ofalliinase activity [55]. Penicillamine also strongly inhibits alliinase [58]. The pyridoxal-5'-phosphate cofactor conveys a yellow color to the enzyme, with an absorbance maximum of the enzyme at 415 nm [18, 55], or 430 nm [14] which is suppressed upon addition of 3 mM L-cysteine, which forms a thiazolidine complex with PLP that absorbs at 330 nm [14, 29, 55]. Sodium borohydride reduction shifts the PLP peak to 325 nm, and subsequent lysylendopeptidase digestion of sodium borohydride treated and denatured alliinase from *A. cepa* identified Lys285 was as the PLP binding site, which aligns to Lys251 in the garlic enzyme [59]. Site-directed mutagenesis of the corresponding lysine residue in the *A. tuberosum* alliinase revealed recombinant K280A and K280R enzymes expressed in yeast lacked alliinase activity, although they were still recognized by anti-alliinase antibodies [28]. And, ultimately, crystal structure analysis confirms Lys251 as the covalent PLP binding site [25, 26].

The fluorescence profile of PLP-bound alliinase is as follows: λ_{ex} = 430 nm, λ_{em} = 519 nm; λ_{ex} = 390 nm, λ_{em} max = 511 nm, λ_{em} min = 460 nm; λ_{ex} = 330 nm, λ_{em} = 391 nm [16]; λ_{ex} = 290 nm, λ_{em} = 340 nm; λ_{ex} = 640 nm, λ_{em} = 420-435 nm (with shoulder) [18]. Alliinase has an extinction coefficient of ε_{280}=7.9 x 10^4 M^{-1} cm^{-1}, both by calculation and experimental comparison with ovalbumin [31]. Estimation of alliinase can be achieved by means of absorbance of the PLP cofactor, using ε_{410}=2.92 mM^{-1} cm^{-1} [14].

Alliinase is estimated to be 5.5% carbohydrate by weight [14], with the following alditol acetate-derivatized sugars detected by gas liquid chromatography, as percent of total carbohydrate: mannose, 43%; glucose, 34%; arabinose, 9%; galactose, 8%; xylose, 5% [29]. The mature alliinase protein has four asparagine residues which may be glycosylated: Asn19, Asn146, Asn191, Asn328 [30]. Sequencing of cyanogen bromide and chymotryptic fragments of alliinase define Asn146 as a glycosylation site [17]. Alliinase may exist in various glycosylation states in solution, as this may account for different crystal and unit cell geometries obtained under different crystallization conditions [16]. X-ray crystallography indicates only Asn146 and Asn328 are glycoslyated, with the carbohydrate moiety of Asn146 located at the dimeric interface, while that of Asn328 is surface accessible [25, 26]. Structure data shows Asn191 at the protein surface may be glycosylated in the enzyme without PLP, although quality of refraction data was insufficient to identify definitively any carbohydrates present [26]. The 2HOX structure [26] shows six carbohydrate residues at Asn146: the main chain consists of mannose $\alpha(1\rightarrow3)$ mannose $\beta(1\rightarrow4)$ N-acetylglucosamine $\beta(1\rightarrow4)$ N-acetylglucosamine, N-linked to Asn146, with xylose $\beta(1\rightarrow2)$ linked to the proximal mannose, and fucose $\alpha(1\rightarrow3)$ linked to the proximal N-acetylglucosamine. The same proximal four residues are observed also in 1LK9 [25]. Carbohydrate residues discernable at Asn328 include two N-acetylglucosame residues and a terminal mannose [26].

The glycosylated nature of alliinase permits interaction with lectins, such as the heterodimeric mannose-binding lectin ubiquitously present in the garlic bulb [60]. Both alliinase and lectin co-eluted from Concanavalin-A Sepharose washed with α-D-mannoside, as determined by western-blotting using polyclonal rabbit anti-alliinase-IgG and anti-lectin-IgG, and visualized with alkaline phosphatase-labeled goat anti-rabbit IgG [17]. N-terminal sequencing confirmed the lectin as *Allium sativum* agglutinin I (ASAI), a heterodimer of 11.5 and 12.5 kDa subunits [17]. Additionally, alliinase (although only 5% of total activity in garlic bulb crude extract) co-immobilized on a mannose-Sepharose 4B column with ASAI, with identity of ASAI again confirmed by observation of 11.5 and 12.5 kDa bands on SDS-PAGE and N-terminal sequencing [35]. The alliinase:ASAI complex produces allicin [35, 61]. Incidentally, the extent of glycosylation of alliinase increases from 5.4% to 8.5% upon complexation with ASAI [35].

2.4. Measuring Alliinase Activity

The most popular method for measuring alliinase activity is via continuous monitoring of pyruvate formation as alliin is converted to allyl sulfenic acid; absorbance at 340 nm decreases as lactate dehydrogenase depletes NADH during the reduction of pyruvate to lactate [38]. Perhaps a note of caution is warranted, as 500 μM allicin reduces activity of rat muscle lactate dehydrogenase [62]. Table 2 contains references of kinetic studies and indicates popularity of this assay approach. Alternatively, total pyruvate is measured in a discontinuous assay, after denaturation of alliinase, by complexation of pyruvate with 2,4-dinitrophenylhydrazine under basic conditions yielding a thiosemicarbazone [24] which absorbs at 520 nm [28]. Additionally, alliinase activity can be monitored directly and continuously by measuring the rate of fast, nonenyzmatic reaction of allicin with 4-mercaptopyridine (4-MP) ($\varepsilon_{324\ nm}$ = 19, 800 M^{-1} cm^{-1}) to form 4-allomercapto-thiopyridine, which does not appreciably absorb at 324 nm [63].

Similarly, allicin rapidly combines with 2-nitro-5-thiobenzoate (NTB) ($\varepsilon_{412\ nm}$ = 28, 300 M^{-1} cm^{-1}), bleaching absorbance of NTB as S-allylmercapto-NTB is formed [58]. When measuring alliinase activity as rate of allicin production, keep in mind production of one allicin molecule requires two alliin molecules and two alliinase cycles; for convenience of calculation, the extinction coefficients for 4-MP and NTB may be halved. The production of ammonia can be measured by various colorimetric methods [24], or by means of an ammonia electrode.

Slightly different assay conditions across various research groups make it difficult to compare kinetic data of alliinase extracted from different *A. sativum* varietals or using different purification techniques. In some reports, criticial information such as temperature of the assay mixutre is not provided. In almost no case is a linear working range of the assay referenced.

The paper most commonly referenced for measurement of alliinase activity [38] focused on alliinase from *A. cepa*, which prefers (+)-S-ethyl-L-cysteine sulfoxide as substrate, and that paper presents two methods of determining alliinase activity – the discontinuous colorimetric measurement of pyruvate and the continuous monitoring of pyruvate formation using LDH. Thus, care must be taken to differentiate which assay was used to assess alliinase activity in works referencing this source. The temperature of the discontinuous assay is specified as 37°C, but the temperature of the continuous assay is not stated explicitly. Most commonly, one unit of alliinase activity is the amount of enzyme needed to produce 1 μmole of pyruvate per min at 23°C [55].

Reported pH optima range from 5 to 7.0 [12, 18, 19, 24, 31, 55, 64], with the most commonly reported optima 6.5 and 7.0. Interestingly, the pI of alliinase is near its pH optimum, with reports as 6.35 [31] and 7.0 [29]. The earliest reported pI was 4.0 [24]. Although the temperature optimum for alliinase is 31 - 40ºC [12, 18, 24, 54, 64], activity is also seen at 0ºC [24].

2.5. Substrate Specificity, Inhibitor Compounds, Modifying Agents, and Mechanism

Alliinase from garlic is specific for only the L-cysteine form of (±)-S-allyl-D,L-cysteine sulfoxide [24, 62]. However, alliinase is tolerant to both the identity of the S-alkyl/alkenyl group and the absolute configuration of groups around the sulfur atom, although the naturally-occurring dextrorotatory form is preferred [12, 24, 54]. Activity of alliinase decreases through this series: (+)-S-allyl-, (±)-S-allyl-, (±)-S-ethyl-, (-)-S-allyl-, (±)-S-methyl-, (±)-S-butyl-, (±)-S-propyl-L-cysteine sulfoxide [12, 18, 54]. These substrate specificities extend to alliinases in other members of the *Allium* genus beyond *A. sativum*, including *A. sphaerocephalon*, *A. victorialis*, *A. hymenorrhizum*, *A. saxatile*, *A. obliquum*, *A. subhirsutum*, *A. jesdianum*, and *A. stipulatum* [12]. Thus, the factor which limits other members of the Alliaciae from making allicin is the availability of the completed metabolic pathway for making alliin substrate. Although the activity of alliinase with (±)-S-propyl-L-cysteine sulfoxide as substrate is poor, the K_m for this substrate is similar to the K_m for racemic alliin (Table 2), possibly because the 2-propenyl group constrains geometry of alliin and minimizes conformations unfavorable to substrate docking or catalysis, and also because allylsulfenate is a better leaving group than propanesulfenate. No alliinase activity was seen with the S-allyl, S-propyl, or S-ethyl substituted thioether (non-sulfoxide) forms of S-alkyl-L-cysteine [18]. Rather, S-allyl [58], S-propyl, S-ethyl, and S-methyl [55] substituted L-cysteines act as competitive inhibitors. Interestingly, alliinase co-crystallized with S-ethyl-L-cysteine [16] suggests S-ethyl-L-cysteine may be a slow-substrate of alliinase, as S-ethyl-L-cysteine was seen in a external aldimine with the PLP cofactor [25].

Table 2. Reported K_m and K_i values for alliin and alliin analogues

Substrate*	K_m (mM)	Comment and Referenced Citation of Assay	Reference
(+)-S-allyl-L-cysteine sulfoxide	0.5	Unknown, as in [14]	[65]
	1.1	Continuous monitoring of pyruvate [38]; temperature not specified	[31]
	1.28	Continuous monitoring of pyruvate [31, 38] at 23°C	[58]
	1.45	Continuous monitoring of allicin [58] at 23°C	[58]
	1.11	Continuous monitoring of pyruvate [38] at 25°C. For alliinase from garlic powder, Km = 1.56 [54]	[54]
	1.25	Continuous monitoring of pyruvate [38] at 25°C, in a minimally purified preparation	[12]
	1.90	Continuous monitoring of allicin at 23°C [58]	[63]
	1.93	Continuous monitoring of allicin at 23°C [63]	[63]
(±)-S-allyl-L-cysteine sulfoxide	2.9	Continuous monitoring of pyruvate at room temperature [31, 38]	[16]
	6	Discontinuous monitoring of pyruvate [55] at 23°C	[55]
	2.2	Continuous monitoring of pyruvate [38] at 35°C	[18]
	3.3	Continuous monitoring of pyruvate [38] at room temperature	[14]
(-)-S-allyl-L-cysteine sulfoxide	2.28	Continuous monitoring of pyruvate [38] at 25°C. For alliinase from garlic powder, K_m = 2.80 [54]	[54]
(±)-S-butyl-L-cysteine sulfoxide	5	Discontinuous monitoring of pyruvate [55] at 23°C	[55]
(±)-S-propyl-L-cysteine sulfoxide	3	Discontinuous monitoring of pyruvate [55] at 23°C	[55]
	1.1	Continuous monitoring of pyruvate [38] at 35°C	[18]
(±)-S-ethyl-L-cysteine sulfoxide	4.9	Continuous monitoring of pyruvate [38] at 35°C	[18]
	5.7	Continuous monitoring of pyruvate [38] at room temperature	[14, 29]
	6	Discontinuous monitoring of pyruvate [55] at 23°C	[55]
(±)-S-methyl-L-cysteine sulfoxide	15	Discontinuous monitoring of pyruvate [55] at 23°C	[55]
Inhibitor: S-allyl-L-cysteine	2.32 (K_i)	Continuous monitoring of allicin [58] at 23°C, with (+)-S-allyl-L-cysteine sulfoxide substrate	[58]
Inhibitor: S-propyl-L-cysteine	5 (K_i)	Discontinuous monitoring of pyruvate [55] at 23°C, with (±)-S-ethyl-L-cysteine sulfoxide substrate	[55]
Inhibitor: S-ethyl-L-cysteine	18 (K_i)	Discontinuous monitoring of pyruvate [55] at 23°C, with (±)-S-methyl-L-cysteine sulfoxide substrate	[55]
	8 (K_i)	Discontinuous monitoring of pyruvate [55] at 23°C, with (±)-S-ethyl-L-cysteine sulfoxide substrate	[55]
Inhibitor:S-methyl-L-cysteine	33 (K_i)	Discontinuous monitoring of pyruvate [55] at 23°C, with (±)-S-ethyl-L-cysteine sulfoxide substrate	[55]

* - See Figure 7 for structures; inhibitor compounds, with K_i values in units of mM, are indicated.

Summary of assay conditions as described in works referenced in Table 2:

[38]: 33.3 mM Tris, pH 7.3; 16.7 μM PLP; 66.7 μM NADH; 50 uL of a 1:10 dilution of LDH stock; 3 mL reaction volume; temperature not indicated, but presumed to be 37°C, which was temperature of the discontinuous assay

[55]: 200 mM sodium potassium phosphate, pH 6.5; 25 μM PLP; 2 mL reaction volume; 23°C; 5-10 min reaction; terminate with 10% TCA; colorimetric detection of pyruvate as in [66]

[14, 29]: as in [38], but with sodium potassium phosphate pH 6.5 as buffer

[18]: 100 mM potassium phosphate pH 6.5; 20 μM PLP; 167 μM NADH; 3 mL reaction volume; 35°C

[31]: 100 mM sodium phosphate, pH 6.5; 200 μM NADH; 25 μM PLP; 10 U LDH; 1 mL reaction volume; temp not specified, but references [38], which uses 37°C

[58]: 50 mM sodium phosphate, pH 6.5; 1 mM EDTA; 20 uM PLP; 0.1 mM NTB; 1 mL reaction volume; 23°C

[12, 54]: 60 mM phosphate, pH 7.0; 400 μM NADH; 18 U LDH; 1 mL reaction volume; 25°C

[16]: 100 mM sodium phosphate, pH 6.5; 20 μM PLP; 200 μM NADH; 3 U LDH; 300 μL reaction volume; room temp

[63]:50 mM sodium phosphate, pH 7.2; 2 mM EDTA; 20 μM PLP; 0.1 mM 4-MP

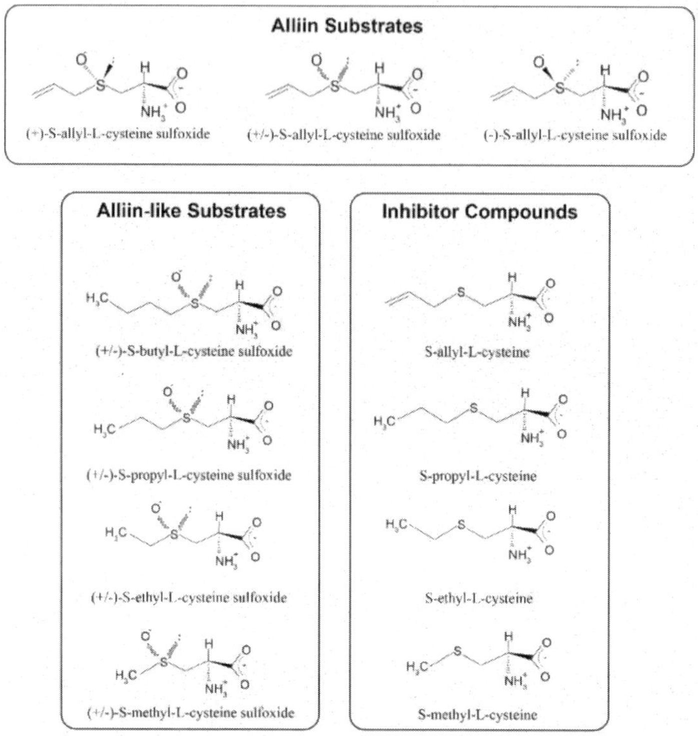

Legend: Compounds mentioned in Table 2 are presented in three groups: alliin substrates, alliin-like substrates, and inhibitor compounds. Note the different possible stereochemistries of the chiral sulfur atom in alliin; wavy lines indicate configurations present in racemic mixtures. Sulfur atoms of the inhibitor compounds each possess two non-bonding electron pairs, which are not expressly shown.

Figure 7. Structures of alliin and alliin-like compounds referenced in Table 2.

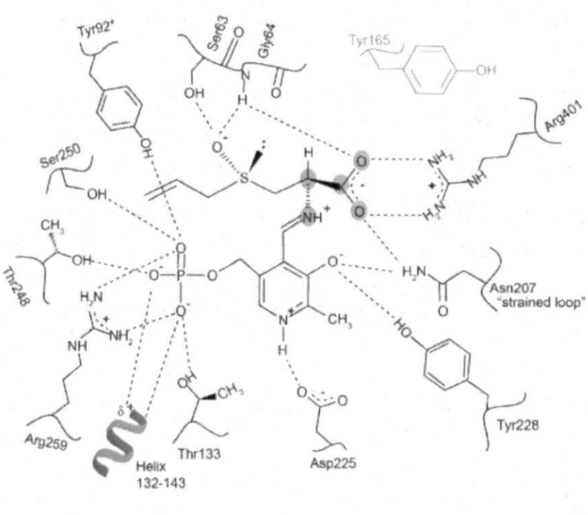

Legend: Residues of alliinase involved in substrate and co-factor binding. Alliin substrate modeled in [25]. Important residues and features as indicated in [25, 26]. Water molecules are not shown. The 2-propenyl group of alliin is located near the phenol ring of Tyr92*, which is provided by the complementary monomer [25]. Tyr165 stabilizes pyridine ring of PLP through π-π stacking. The positions of shaded atoms were fixed when modeling alliin substrate in place of S-ethyl-L-cysteine present in 1LK9 [25].

Figure 8. Substrate and cofactor binding.

Substrate binding occurs at the interface between the subunits of homodimeric alliinase enzyme [25]. (+)-S-allyl-L-cysteine sulfoxide was modelled at the active site, by fixing positions of the alliin α-carbon, carboxylate carbon, caboxylate oxygens, and the amino nitrogen to the positions of the corresponding atoms in the pyridoxal phosphate-aminoacrylate external aldimine seen in the crystal structure [25] (Figure 8).Preference of alliinase for the (+)-S forms of the substrate is explained by molecular modeling using crystal structure data, which shows substrate binding is stabilized by hydrogen bonding between the oxygen of the (+)-S substrate sulfoxide and the protonated hydroxyl of Ser63, and between the sulfoxide oxygen and the peptide backbone nitrogen of Gly64 [25]. These interactions are unavailable for (-)-S substrates, so the binding of the (-)-S substrates is weaker [25]. Different S-allkyl substitions are tolerated since these project away from the binding pocket toward solvent.

Alliinase activity is moderated by a variety of metal ions and small molecules. S-propyl-L-cysteine is a more potent competitive inhibitor (K_i = 5 mM) than S-methyl-L-cysteine (K_i = 33 mM), with S-ethyl-L-cysteine sulfoxide as substrate [55]. Divalent cations at 2.5 mM in the reaction yielded mixed results, with iron, magnesium, manganese, and cobalt enhancing alliinase activity by 27-35%, while nickel and copper reduced alliinase activity by 33 and 52%, respectively; alliinase was blind to calcium and cadmium [55]. However, one group saw no effects of metal ions or EDTA on alliinase activity [18]. Rabbit anti-alliinase antibodies inactivate alliinase [31].

Allicin inactives enzymes by modifying free sulfhydryl groups important in catalysis. Some reports state allicin inactivates alliinase, but no experimental plan or data is shown [31, 67]. Eight of ten cysteine residues in each alliinase monomer are bound up in intra-chain disulfide linkags [25, 26, 56], and the remaining two surface-exposed cysteines (Cys 220 and Cys350) can be chemically modified to immobilize alliinase on solid support without noticeable loss of activity [56]. No sulfhydryl group is necessary for catalysis. Thus, if alliinase activity fades over the course of the reaction, it is not likely due to chemical modification of a sulfhydryl residue by alliicin, and more likely due to simple product inhibition. Further experiementation is needed to clarify this point.

A panel of chemical modification agents was used to identify catalytically important amino acid residues in alliinase [68]. No appreciable loss of activity was seen upon incubation of 10 μM alliinase with 10 mM of any of the following agents: dithiothreitol (DTT), 1-ethyl-3-(3-dimethylaminopropyl)carbodiimide (EDC), 1-cyclohexyl-3-(2-morpholinoethyl)carbodiimide (CMC), diethylpyrocarbonate (DEPC), iodoacetate, maleic anhydryde, or 5 mM phenylmethylsulfonyl fluoride (PMSF) [68]. While extended N-bromosuccinimide (NBS) modification of alliinase modified six tryptophan residues, only a brief (8 sec) exposure to NBS caused full loss of activity; Edman degradation of tryptic peptides of alliinase exposed to NBS for 8 sec identified Trp182 as obligatory for alliinase activity [68]. Structures 2HOX and 2HOR [26] show the indole side chain of Trp182 is surface-accessible, although the indole residue is sandwiched between Helix 165-175 and the beta strand containing Trp182 [25, 26]. NBS-modification of Trp182 likely causes loss of activity through perturbation of tertiary structure. Since 20 mM N-acetylimidazole caused 50% loss of activity, a tyrosine residue was deemed important for activity of the enzyme [68]. The phenol ring of Tyr165 at the N-terminus of Helix 165-175 stabilizes the pyridine ring of the pyridoxal phosphate cofactor through π-π stacking interactions [25, 26].

During the reaction, the bond between PLP and Lys251 is broken [25]; refer to Figure 4. In one proposed mechanism [26], the internal aldimine between Lys251 and the C4' carbonyl carbon of PLP is replaced by an external aldimine when the amino group nitrogen of alliin displaces that of the ε-amino group by nucleophilic attack. This explains the observation [24] that alliin analogues with substituted alpha-amino groups were not substrates of alliinase. Further, aminooxyacetic acid (210 mM) covalently modifies the aldehyde of PLP, forming a stable oxime and causing complete loss of alliinase activity [69, 70], presumably by preventing formation of the external aldimine between PLP and substrate. Modification of alliinase with 2 mM succinic anhydride caused 60% loss of activity, suggesting that a lysine residue is critically important for catalysis [68]. Lys251 may act as a general base catalyst to accept a hydrogen from the alliin α-carbon, leading to collapse of the external aldimine, cleavage of the bond between the alliin sulfur and the β-carbon, release of allylsulfenic acid, generation of an aminoacrylate intermediate, and reformation of the internal aldimine [26]. In subsequent non-enyzmatic reactions, the aminoacrylate intermediate is hydrolyzed to pyruvate and ammonia, while two molecules of allylsulfenic acid condense to form alliicin [24, 71]; water molecules in the active site may facilitate these reactions by rapid hydrolysis of the aminoacrylate [26].

Not all have agreed, however, that allicin is formed via non-enzymatic condensation of two molecules of allylsulfenic acid. Lawson and Hughes [72] suggested condensation of allylsulfenic acid may be enzymic in nature, since the half-life of allylsulfenic acid – if comparable to that of methylsulfenic acid - is greater than the rate of alliinase-catalyzed formation of allicin, and also cite an observation [73] that allicin formed in garlic extract is optically active, while synthetically prepared is not.

Alliinase moonlights as a poor lyase of cystine (K_m for cystine = 2.65 mM; pH optimum 7.5; temp optimum 44°C), acting about 1000 times slower than when using alliin as substrate, and forming thiocysteine which enters back onto allinase to be enzymatically converted to disulphine which rapidly decomposes to hydrogen sulfide and elemental sufur [74]. With each successive β-elimination, pyruvate and ammonia are liberated, yielding two molecules of pyruvate and ammonia for each cystine degraded. Formation of polysulfides occurs when disulfine combines with allylsulfenic acid or with allicin directly [74].

3. Enzymes Targeted by Allicin

Enzymes with catalytically important cysteine residues are ubiquitous in nature [75], and those with a solvent-accessible thiol are potential targets for allicin. A comprehensive review describes small-molecule, pharmaceutical drug inhibition of a broad range of cysteine-dependent proteases, such as cathepsins, caspases, and proteases associated with infectious diseases - all associated with disease conditions and each a potential therapeutic target [76]. In theory, allicin could modify and inhibit any of these.

Allicin covalently modifies cysteine to S-allylmercaptocysteine, confirmed via NMR and mass spectrometry [77]. Additionally, covalent modification by allicin of proteins, including non-enzymic proteins, is global in nature [78]. Reducing agents can restore some enzymic activity [62], based upon the chemical microenvironment of the allicin-modified cysteine.

Table 3. Enzymes inhibited by allicin

Enzyme	Notes	Reference
Acetyl-CoA synthetase	Allicin (100 μM) causes 85% loss of activity of acetyl-CoA synthetase from yeast. Inhibition could be reversed upon gel-filtration, suggesting a non-covalent mode of inhibition. Dithioerythritol did not rescue the enzyme.	[81]
Alcohol dehydrogenase	ADH from *Thermoanaerobium brockii* was protected from modification by $NADP^+$, and the presumed target was Cys203. Activity could be 75% restored by 1 mM DTT, but not by glutathione.	[77]
	Inactivation of horse liver ADH was enhanced by NAD^+, and while the cysteine target could not be identified, Cys46 and Cys174 were excluded. β-mercaptoethanol (5 mM), but not glutathione or dithiothreitol, restored 50% of ADH activity.	[77]
	ADH from both yeast and liver (source unspecified) inhibitited by 500 μM allicin.	[62]
Alkaline phosphatase	Allicin (500 μM) inhibits the enzyme from ox or rabbit serum.	[62]
Bacterioferritin comigratory protein (BCP) peroxiredoxin from *B. cenocepacia* J2315	Recombinant (His tag) protein expressed in *E. coli* (strain not specified). Cys44 and Cys98 modified by allicin, confirmed by mass spectrometry. Similar result observed with aqueous garlic extract. Modification can be reversed with TCEP (tris (2-carboxyethyl) phosphine).	[8]
DNA-polymerase	Allicin (200 μM) promoted 20% loss of activity of DNA-directed-DNA-polymerase β from rat, and 15% activity loss in the human DNA-directed-DNA-polymerase λ. Note that diallyldisulfide, diallyltrisulfide and alliin at the same concentration provide greater inhibition than allicin.	[86]
Lactate dehydrogenase	500 μM allicin inhibits lactate dehydrogenase activity in 5% ($^{w}/_{v}$) extract of rabbit muscle.	[62]
Papain	Inhibited by 500 μM allicin.	[62]
	Complete inhibition achieved with 60 μM allicin. Likely target is surface-accessible Cys25. Glutathione (5 mM) restores activity.	[77]
Protease activity in *P. gingivalis* extracts	*P. gingivalis* contains multiple cysteine-proteases. 2 h incubation with garlic extract (55 μg/mL allicin) destroyed 95% activity against azocoll (1 mg/mL; meaurses general protease activity) and 93% activity against benzoyl-arginine naphthylamide (BANA; 440 μg/mL; measures trypsin-protease activity), while co-incubation with 2 mM DTT reduced inhibition by 20%.	[87]
Succinic dehydrogenase	Actvitiy in 10% ($^{w}/_{v}$) rat liver homogenate was 90% inhibited by 333 μM allicin; diluted aqueous garlic extract completely inhibits.	[62]
Succinic oxidase	Only 8% activity remained after 14 min incubation with 250 μM allicin, and inhibition was attributed to effects of allicin on succinic dehydrogenase activit. Cysteine at 1 mM protected against modification by 140 μM allicin.	[62]
Triose phosphate dehydrogenase	Allicin (100 μM) offered 100% inhibition of activity from muscle acetone powder [88].	[62]
Tyrosinase	Allicin (1 mM) provides 45% inhibition. Details about the source of the enzyme and assay conditions are lacking.	[62]
Urease	Diluted aqueous garlic extract caused 67% loss of activity (67%), with greater inhibition at alkaline pH. Cysteine, GSH and BAL (2:3-dimercaptopropanol) protects activity. Urease source not specified.	[62]
	Within 30 min, 7 μg allicin fully destroyed urease activity in *P. mirabilis* lysate. DTT (5 mM) rescued the enzyme. Cys319 is a crucial residue for urease activity [90]	[89]
Xanthine oxidase	200 μM allicin caused 95% inhibition of xanthine oxidase from milk. 16.7 mM methylene blue afforded 100% protection from modification by 100 μM allicin, while 100 μM methylene blue partly protected activity. Inihibition by allicin was pH dependent, and greater inhibition was seen at lower pH.	[62]
	Complete inhibition of the rat liver enzyme was accomplished with 250 μM allicin.	[62]

For example, the activity of allicin-modified *Thermoanaerobium brockii* alcohol dehydrogenase (TBAD) could be rescued by β-mercaptoethanol and dithiothreitol, but allicin-treated horse liver alcohol dehydrogenase could be restored only by β-mercaptothanol; glutathione could restore activity of papain but not TBAD [77]. Allicin destroys the pool of reduced glutathione in the cytoplasm [78 - 80], reducing ability of the cell to rescue these thiol-modified enzymes. As a final note, not all enzymes inhibited by allicin contain a catalytically important sulfhydryl group, however, and acetyl-CoA synthetase serves as an example [81].

In addition to the enzymes listed in Table 3, allicin at 500 μM inhibited also the following enzymes: adenosine triphosphatase from rat skeletal or cardiac muscle extract, cholinesterase, and glyoxylase [62]. The same landmark paper [62] found that allicin (500 μM) did not inhibit lipase, rennin, pepsin, trypsin, invertase, alpha-amylase, esterase (serum), D-amino acid oxidase, ascorbic acid oxidase, catalase, or carbonic anhydrase. Surprisingly, carboxylase, adenosine triphosphatase, and beta-amylase, all sulfhydryl-dependent enzymes, were not affected by 500 μM allicin [62].

Both extracellular and intracellular proteins are potential targets of allicin. Allicin is freely permeable through biological membranes, with a permeability coefficient of ~ 0.2 cm s^{-1}, determined using the value of 1.77 ± 0.31 for a partition coefficient (K_p) for a hexane/water system [79]. The second-order rate constant for oxidation of GSH in 100 mM sodium chloride, 10 mM sodium phosphate, pH 7.0, is 48.66 ± 2.45 M^{-1} s^{-1}, at 24°C [79].

Rat muscle lactate dehydrogenase (LDH) was inhibited by 500 μM allicin [62], and inactivation of rat muscle LDH with p-mercuribenzoate [82] suggested a thiol was catalytically important. Ethyl methanethiosulphonate modification of pig heart LDH [83] confirmed presence of a critical Cys165, which when thioethylated, increased the K_m for pyruvate nearly 300 fold over that for the native enzyme and caused an 85% reduction in maximum rate, most likely due to structural perturbation, as no cysteine plays a direct role in catalysis. Cys 165 maps to Cys 163 in LDH from rat muscle [84].

At the time of Wills's work [62], the mechanism of xanthine oxidase was not known, but since allicin inhibited xanthine oxidase, it was proposed that xanthine oxidase contained a critical sulfhydryl group. Xanthine oxidase contains a molybdenum(IV) atom and an Fe-S center, and a molybdenum(IV)-sulfhydryl species is formed as a proton is removed from C-8 of xanthine [85].

4. Biochemical Fate of Allicin

The concentration of GSH in whole human blood varies widely across the population and depends upon factors such as health status and age, but the average value is 1 mM [91]. In blood, allicin can react rapidly with GSH, forming S-allylmercaptoglutathione (GSSA) and sulfenic acid; allicin also reacts with cysteine to form S-allylmercaptocysteine (CSSA) [77, 92]. Thus, GSH and other free thiols in blood, such as free cysteine or cysteine residues of blood proteins, would have potential to reduce the effects of allicin. Serum protected succinic dehydrogenase and urease from allicin-induced loss of activity [62]. The combination of GSH and allicin form GSSA and sulfenic acid, which have multiple fates as recently summarized [1]: GSSA can combine with a second molecule of GSH to form oxidized glutathione and allylmercaptan, and two molecules of allylmercaptan can combine to form diallyldisulfide.

Allylsulfenic acid has potential to oxidize another thiol group, either on reduced GSH or on a free or protein-bound cysteine, as well as combining with a second sulfenic acid to form allicin [1, 92].

Glutathione reductase replenishes intracellular GSH by reduction of oxidized glutathione. Studies in *E. coli* suggest allicin shifts the ratio of GSH:GSSG in the cell, possibly because GSSA is not acted upon by glutathione reductase [78]. A recent report suggests that GSSA may be a poor substrate for yeast glutathione reductase, with the rate of oxidation of 0.3 mM NADPH by glutathione reductase using 0.125 mM GSSA as substrate was exceptionally slow - total loss of $A_{340\ nm}$ was just less than 0.09 after 50 min [93]. NADPH is known to decompose at a very slow rate in buffers less than pH 7.5, and rate of decomposition is accelerated by phosphate and is dependent upon ionic strength [94]; the rate of NADPH degradation [93] is similar to the nonenzymic decomposition rate [94].

Products of allicin combination with GSH and cysteine thiols are biologically active. Both GSSA and CSSA are reactive disulfides and can inhibit thiol-containing enzymes alcohol dehydrogenase from *Thermoanaerobium brockii* and also papain [95, 96]. Both allicin and allylsulfenic acid can combine with reduced cyeteine thiols, forming CSSA, an activated disulfide, which has potential to participate in disulfide exchange reactions and form inter-and intra-disulfide bonds [1, 96]. Allicin promoted aggregation of proteins in *E. coli* [78], perhaps through formation of interprotein disulfide linkages. Paradoxically, allicin did not promote formation of the disulfide bond required for activity of cytosol-bound, secretion-signal deficient alkaline phosphatase [78].

Allicin also acts to scavenge free oxygen radicals. Allicin from a commercial preparation (Garlicin) inhibited combination of ·OH with lipids to form malondialdehyde in a dose-depdendent mannor in rabbit liver homogenates [97].

Beyond targeted inhibition of enzymes, allicin can promote global metabolic changes within the cell. Allicin (250 μM) inhibits respiration in yeast by 43% and respiration in rat muscle or rat liver by 50% [62]. This observation can possibly be explained by the ability of allicin to deplete levels of GSH in rat hepatocytes [80], which in turn affects the level of S-glutathionylation of proteins that control the rate of oxidative phosphorylation in the cell [98]. A comprehensive overview of how allicin acts to disrupt intracellular signaling pathways is presented in Chapter 3.

5. Development of Alliinase for Commercial and Pharmaceutial Use

Due to the highly unstable nature of allicin, a common approach is to generate allicin immediately prior to use through the action of alliianse on alliin. Many commercial garlic supplements contain alliin and alliinase rather than allicin. Therefore, presentation of the considerations for making alliinase attractive for commercial applications is warranted.

5.1. Stability

Alliinase, like any protein, is subject to denaturation and loss of activity, and a range of stabilities is reported in the literature The variation is attributed to differences in alliinase source, purification method, composition of storage buffer, storage temperature, and whether or not buffer was supplemented with stabilizing agents like glycerol, sucrose, sodium chloride, and/or PLP. Inclusion of 10% glycerol in purification buffers is a common technique for preserving alliinase activity [18, 31, 55, 56]. A combination of sodium chloride (1%), 25 μM PLP, and 10% sucrose preserved alliinase activity for at least 500 days, when stored at -20 °C [19].

Complete loss of alliinase activity was seen after 14 days at 3 °C, although the storage buffer is not listed [24]. Inclusion of 10% glycerol in the isolation steps preserved alliinase activity for 30 days when stored at -10 °C, and provided protection even upon multiple freeze-thaw cycles [55]. Alliinase experienced no appreciable difference in pH or temperature profiles or optima when stored freeze-dried or in solution, although more alliinase activity was lost in aqueous preparations, as compared to lyophylized preparations, when both were stored at 4 °C for 35 days [64]. As expected, alliinase irreversibly loses all activity in synthetic gastric juice [18, 72]. Encouragingly, no appreciable loss of alliinase activity, as judged by yield of allicin, was observed in garlic powder (50 mg/mL) in simulated pancreatic fluid containing protease [72].

Higher temperature is also deleterious to alliinase, with greater than 80% loss of activity after 10 min at 50 °C in 250 mM Tris-HCl, pH 7.5, even with inclusion of 10% glycerol and 20 uM PLP [18]. Alliinase is stabilized against thermal denaturation at 57 °C by polyols that raise osmotic potential of solution, with 1 M glycerol preserving alliinase activity better than either 1 M sorbitol or 1 M glucose [61].

The stability of alliinase decreases with increasing purity of preparation [19]. Perhaps highly purified alliinase is stripped away from ASAI, which provides a stabilizing effect [35]. Alliinase-ASAI complexes retained alliinase activity after multiple freeze-thaw cycles, and even up to 2 years when stored in 50 mM sodium acetate, 200 mM sodium chloride buffer, pH 6.5 buffer at 0-2 °C [35]. Complexation of alliinase with ASAI also protected against thermal denaturation and preserved activity, but simple addition of glycerol to the solution was more effective at temperatures above 30 °C [61]. It seems concanavalin A can play a similar stabilizing role as ASAI, as alliinase is stable for up to one year at 4 °C when stored bound to ConA Sepharose [54]. Interestingly, ultrasound waves (40 kHz, 0.5 W cm^{-1}) increased specific activity of purified alliinase preparation from 597 to 878 nmol of pyruvate formed from S-allyl-L-cysteine per minute per milliliter of enzyme preparation, but oddly, added PLP (up to 0.5 mM) inhibited enzyme activity while added L-cysteine (up to 10 mM), usually an inhibitor compound, activated the enzyme [99].

5.2. Recombinant Expression Systems

Recombinant expression of alliianse is attractive because the manufacture of functional protein is controlled and not dependent on growth condition or variety of the plant. Recombinant alliinase was expressed in *Xenopus oocytes* after microinjection of alliinase mRNA manufactured *in vitro* from the cloned cDNA sequence, and although a protein band of expected size was observed on SDS-PAGE, no information regarding functionality of the recombinant protein was provided [31]. Functional recombinant alliinase was obtained through amplification by polymerase chain reaction of cDNA for alliinase from *A. sativum*, with subsequent cloning and expression in *E. coli* BL21(DE3) (pET3b vector), *S. cerevisiae* (pPT2bL2 vector), and *P. pastoris* (pHIL-D2 and pPIC9 vectors) [100]. Alliinase was obtained in all hosts as non-functional inclusion bodies, and activity was restored in refolding buffer [100]. Functional recombinant alliinase from *A. tuberosum*, which has 64.3% amino acid sequence identity with that from *A. sativum*, was expressed in both *E. coli* BL21 (DE3) with a pET15b vector, and *Saccharomyces cerevisiae* INVSc1 using a pYES2 system [28]. Recombinant alliinase from *A. cepa* expressed in bacterial, yeast, insect, or mammalian cell expression systems, is available for purchase [101]. Production of recombinant alliinase is described in an international patent document [102].

5.3. Commercial Dietary Supplements

Although liquid formulations of allicin stabilized by proprietary methods are available, most garlic supplements contain alliin and alliinase, and produce allicin upon dissolution. Of 24 commercially available dietary supplements, 83% tested according to U.S. Pharmacopeia Method 742A standard yielded less than 15% of the allicin generated when tablets/capsules were ground and dissolved in room temperature water at 50 g/mL, with sampling for allicin content at 30 min incubation [70]. USP Method 742A standard simulates transit through stomach to test the efficacy of enteric-coated drugs, and entails incubation of the tablet or capsule in 0.1 M HCl followed by 45 min in 200 mM sodium phosphate buffer, pH 6.8, before sampling for active compound(s). Low production of allicin was attributed to loss of alliinase activity, rather than destruction of alliin, since addition of exogenous alliinase lead to production of the full amount of allicin formed under optimal conditions [70].

Encapsulation of pure alliinase in alginate particles afforded retention of 50-60% activity after 30 min at pH 2.0, followed by 240 min at pH 7.4, simulating the pH changes similar to those found in the digestive tract, and suggested that alginate encapsulation may allow oral adminstration of an alliin and alliinase combination without loss of activity in the acid environment of the stomach [103].

The method used to process garlic bulbs to make garlic powder incorporated into dietary supplements greatly affected the amount of allicin generated, with lyophilization (0% loss of alliin; 22% loss of alliinase) superior to drying at 55 °C (16% loss of alliin; 48% loss of alliinase) [70]. Cycling the temperature used to dry sliced garlic bulbs from 40 C to 60 °C for 20 min cycles, for a total of 100 min, yielded dried material with alliinase activity notably higher than drying at a constant temperature at either 40 or 60 °C [104].

5.4. Use of Alliinase in High-Capacity Allicin Bioreactors

Purified alliinase was coupled directly and covalently *via* amino groups (ε-amino groups of lysine residues) to para-nitrophenyl- or cyanogen bromide- activated cellulose or sepharose in the prescence of added PLP to protect Lys251, producing a column matrix which not only stabilizes alliinase but enhances its specific activity [105]. Gram-quantities of allicin were produced from alliin (4 mg/mL in 50 mM phosphate buffer, pH 6.5, with 20 μM PLP; flow rate 7 ml/h) for two weeks continuously, at room temperature, and alliinase activity of the column was stable for up to one year at 4 ºC with "periodic" use [105]. Similarly, glutaraldehyde was used to cross-link amino groups of alliinase to amino groups on N-succinyl-chitosan matrix, again with inclusion of PLP to protect Lys251 [106]. Alliinase coupled to N-succinyl-chitosan retained activity for at least five uses of the matrix, and cross-linked alliinase had a more basic pH optimum (pH 7.0, coupled; pH 6.0, free), higher temperature optimum (40 °C coupled; 30 ºC free), and greater thermal stability (60% loss of activity after 3 h at 45 °C for coupled alliinase) than free alliinase (94% loss of activity) in the same system [106]. Alliinase biotinylated at surface-accessible free –SH groups (Cys 220 and Cys 350), and imobilized on streptavidin-coated plates showed similar activity to native alliinase [56]. An additional benefit of production of allicin in this manner is that alliinase is not subject to product inhibition. A method for production of allicin by use of alliinase mechanically released from a natural source is covered by a US Patent [107], and immobilization of alliinase on synthetic or naturally-derived supports is also patented [108]. The use of antibody-coupled alliinase for *in-situ*, cell-level targeting of allicin production to treat cancers or infections is also described in a US Patent [109].

Besides production of allicin, immobilized alliinase can be used to quantitate alliin in plant preparations. Alliinase coupled to ConA-agarose was used to measure alliin content in garlic bulb extracts, with a linear range of 10 uM – 1 mM alliin, when ammonia production was measured by ammonia electrode [20]. Alliinase coupled to chitosan microspheres via glutaraldehyde cross-linking was incorporated into an analytical microinjection tool could measure alliin content in plant tissue; this system also had a linear range of 10 μM – 1 mM alliin, and measured rate of alliinase activity with an ammonia electrode [110].

6. Future Directions and Summary

6.1. Allicin as a Starting Material for Other Bioactive Compounds

A recent review of redox active sulfur species [111] summarizes structures and biological functions of the many currently known sulfur species and classifies allicin as a "reactive sulfur secondary metabolite". Allicin in solution decomposes and recombines to form polysulfide (also known as "polysulfane") species, such as diallylsulfide, diallyldisulfide, diallyltrisulfide, and others, which have enhanced and expanded functionalities beyond those of allicin [112]. Along these lines, the polysulfides formed by allicin decomposition can further decompose to release hydrogen sulfide, with important biological activities of its own [113].

6.2. Variations on a Thiosulfinate Theme

Selenium sits just below sulfur in group 6 of the periodic table, and therefore may substitute for sulfur in organic molecules. As presented in a recent review [114], incorporation of selenium into common reducing agents like glutathione, cysteine, and mercaptoethanol, alters their redox potential, increasing their ability to act as reductants. Selenium-substituted allicin (and/or selenium-substituted forms of its breakdown products allyl sulfenic acid and allyl mercaptan) would have modified redox properties compared to the native forms and may be useful in augmenting or restricting reactions of these compounds *in vivo*.

Allicin is a model for development of novel bioactive compounds based upon the thiosulfinate functional group. Polyethylene glycol-based ointment containing a synthetic allicin-inspired compound (4-aminobenzenthiosulfoacid S-alkyl ester), was active against *Bacillus mesentericus*, *Escherichia coli*, *Aspergillus niger*, and *Candida lipolytica*, and was, in most cases, more effective than commercially available antimicrobials [115]. Multiple variations of 4-acylaminobenzenethiosulfoacid S-esters also showed antimicrobial activity [116].

Varacin B and varacin C are naturally occuring compounds having an allicin-like thiosulfinate group in the context of a cyclic trisulfide present on a five-member ring; similar varacin A contains only the trisulfide *sans* the oxygen atom [117]. Varacin A, B, and C were isolated from a *Polycitor* sp. harvested from the Sea of Japan just off the East Coast of the Lazovsky Nature Reserve in Russia, and these compounds are antimicrobial toward *Staphylococcus aureus*, *Bacillus subtilis*, and *Saccharomyces cerevisiase* [117], possibly due to the reactive trisulfide and trisulfide-S-oxide (R-SSS(O)-R) groups. Leinamycin, produced by *Streptomyces atroolivaceus* S-140 contains a thiosulfinate group essential for antitumor activity via alkylation of DNA [118].

6.3. Other Applications of Allicin

The unique chemistry of allicin fits this molecule for multiple applications. As of this writing, a search of the database of US Patents filed since 1976 [119] returns 552 hits for keyword "allicin". Applications are wide-ranging in nature, with allicin incorporated as a key active ingredient or as a potential additive. Selected patent examples include use of allicin as a preservative for blood products [120], as a component of an insect and deer repellent [121], as a component of packaging for smokeless tobacco [122], as an active ingredient in a patch applied to the skin over an insect bite [123]. Allicin can be combined with azetidine and proline derivative angiotensin-converting enzyme (ACE) inhibitors to improve efficiency of these drugs for lowering blood pressure [96].

Garlic extract was used for "green" synthesis of silver nanoparticles in mild temperatures (25-60°C), and garlic extract concentration influenced the size of silver nanoparticles [124]. Developers of the method suggested that sugars in the garlic extract act as reducing agents while allicin and other sulfur compounds protect the silver nanoparticles from oxygen radicals, and found the particles to be stable for at least nine months [124]. Silver nanoparticles prepared in this way were not toxic to vascular smooth muscle cells in culture when applied at 25 μg/mL, but silver nanoparticles appliced at a concentration of 50 μg/mL caused about 30% loss of cell viability, an amount similar to that observed with an equivalent amount of garlic extract alone [124]. This is only one example of the use of garlic extract (and allicin) in greener, more earth-friendly chemical synthesis.

Given the variation in allicin content across different varietals of *A. sativum*, which is magnified further by varied growth conditions, there is a great opportunity for biotechnologists to engineer a system for controlled production of alliin, alliinase, and allicin. An early review discusses then-current developments toward use of genetically modified garlic and onion species for increased production of allicin [125]. An ideal system may consist of a bacterial two-strain approach, in which one bacterial strain contains all genes for *de novo* synthesis of alliin, and a second strain produces highly active, thermostable recombinant alliinase. Full allicin production is achieved "on demand" as manufactured alliin and alliinase are combined. An international intellectual property filing [102] describes the preparation and application of recombinant alliinase. A novel and clevel method for allicin production was recently described. An engineered heavy-chain-only camel antibody with PLP-dependent alliinase activity (nanobody VHH C10) was expressed in *E. coli* BL21(DE3), and has K_m (1.32 mM) and V_{max} (0.453 min^{-1}) similar to those of purified *A. sativum* alliinase enzyme (K_m = 1.49 mM; V_{max} = 0.888 min^{-1}), as measured by production of pyruvate [126]. Excitingly, VHH C10 nanobody was able to inhibit growth of mouse melanoma B16 F10 cells in vitro, when provided with alliin substrate [126].

In summary, allicin is a small but highly reactive molecule with a range of applictions limited only by its own inherent instability and the human imagination. Advances in biotechnology are aiding development of stable alliinase enzyme for on-demand production of allicin from alliin. Novel chemicals, modelled upon or incorporating allicin, are being developed as pharmaceutical therapies.

REFERENCES

[1] Borlinghaus, Jan, Frank Albrecht, Martin C.H. Grulke, Ifeanyi D. Nwachukwu, and Alan J. Slusarenko. 2014. "Allicin : Chemistry and biological properties". *Molecules* 19(8) : 12591-12618.

[2] Gruhlke, Martin C.H., and Slusarenko, Alan J. 2012. "The Biology of Reactive Sulfur Species (RSS)." *Plant Physiology and Biochemistry* 59 (October): 98–107. doi:10.1016/j.plaphy.2012.03.016.

[3] Sasaki, Jin-ichi, Takeshi Kita, Kunio Ishita, Hidemitsu Uchisawa, and Hajime Matsue. 1999. "Antibacterial activity of garlic powder against *Escherichia coli* O-157." *Journal of Nutritional Science and Vitaminology*, 45(6), 785–790. doi:10.3177/jnsv.45.785.

[4] Lawson, Larry D., Steven G. Wood, and Bronwyn G. Hughes. 1991. "HPLC analysis of allicin and other thiosulfinates in garlic clove homogenates." *Planta medica* 57(3):263-270.

[5] Lawson, L.D. 1996. "The composition and chemistry of garlic cloves and processed garlic. In *Garlic: the Science and Therapeutic Application of Allium sativum and Related Species,* 2nd edn. pp. 37-107. Edited by H.P. Kock L.D. Lawson Baltimore MD: Williams Wilkins.

[6] Fujisawa, Hiroyuki, Kaoru Suma, Kana Origuchi, Hitomi Kumagai, Taiichiro Seki, and Toyohiko Ariga. 2008. "Biological and chemical stability of garlic-derived allicin." *Journal of Agricultural and Food Chemistry* 56 (11): 4229-4235.

[7] Arzanlou, Mohsen, and Shahab Bohlooli. 2010. "Inhibition of streptolysin O by allicin – an active component of garlic." *Journal of Medical Microbiology.* 59:1044-1049. doi: 10.1099/jmm.0.019539-0.

[8] Wallock-Richards, Daynea, Catherine J. Doherty, Lynsey Doherty, David J. Clarke, Marc Place, John R.W. Govan, and Dominic J. Campopiano. 2014. "Garlic revisited: antimicrobial activity of allicin-containing garlic extracts against *Burkholderia cepacia* complex." *PloS One* 9 (12): e112726. doi:10.1371/journal.pone.0112726.

[9] Le, Nguyen T, Kalluri, Jhansi R, Loni, Armando, Canham, Leigh T, and Coffer, Jeffery L. 2017. "Biogenic Nanostructured Porous Silicon as a Carrier for Stabilization and Delivery of Natural Therapeutic Species." *Molecular Pharmaceutics* 14 (12): 4509-14. doi:10.1021/acs.molpharmaceut.7b00638.

[10] Freeman, Fillmore and Yukihiro Kodera. 1995. "Garlic chemistry: stability of S-(2-propenyl)-2-propene-1-sulfinothioate (allicin) in blood, solvents, and simulated physiological fluids." *Journal of Agricultural and Food Chemistry* 43(9): 2332-2338.

[11] Peters, Günther H, Branner, Sven, Møller, Karin B, Andersen, Jannik N, and Møller, Niels Peter H. 2003. "Enzyme Kinetic Characterization of Protein Tyrosine Phosphatases." *Biochimie* 85 (5): 527–34. doi: 10.1016/S0300-9084(03)00036-1.

[12] Krest, I., J. Glodek, and M. Keusgen. 2000. "Cysteine sulfoxides and alliinase activity of some *Allium* species." *Journal of Agricultural and Food Chemistry* 48 (8): 3753-3760. doi: 10.1021/jf990521.

[13] Rajinder Kaur, Atul Tiwari, Manish Manish, Indresh K Maurya, Rakesh Bhatnagar, and Samer Singh. 2017. "Common garlic (*Allium sativum* L.) has potent anti-*Bacillus anthracis* activity." *bioRxiv* 162214; doi: https://doi.org/10.1101/162214.

[14] Nock, Linda P. and Mendel Mazelis. 1986. "The C-S lyases of higher plants: preparation and properties of homogeneous alliin lyase from garlic (*Allium sativum*)." *Archives of Biochemistry and Biophysics* 249 (1): 27-33.

[15] Feldberg, R.S., S.C. Chang, A.N. Kotik, M. Nadler, Z. Neuwirth, D.C. Sundstrom, and N.H. Thompson. 1988. "*In vitro* mechanism of inhibition of bacterial cell growth by allicin." *Antimicrobial Agents and Chemotherapy* 32 (12): 1763-1768.

[16] Kuettner, Bartholomeus E., Rolf Hilgenfeld, and Manfred S. Weiss. 2002. "Purification, characterization, and crystallization of alliinase from garlic." *Archives of Biochemistry and Biophysics* 402 (2): 192-200.

[17] Rabinkov, Aaron, Wilchek, Meir, and Mirelman, David. 1995. "Alliinase (alliin Lyase) from Garlic (*Alliium sativum*) Is Glycosylated at ASN 146 and Forms a Complex with a Garlic Mannose-Specific Lectin." *Glycoconjugate Journal* 12 (5): 690–98. https://doi.org/10.1007/BF00731266.

[18] Jansen, Herwig, Bernd Müller, and Karl Knobloch. 1989. "Characterization of an alliin lyase preparation from garlic (*Allium sativum*)." *Planta Medica* 55 (5): 434-439.

[19] Krest, I. and M. Keusgen. 1999. "Stabilization and pharmaceutical use of alliinase." *Die Pharmazie* 54 (4): 289-293.

[20] Keusgen, Michael, Martina Jünger, Ingo Krest, and Michael J. Schöning. 2003. "Development of a biosensor specific for cysteine sulfoxides." *Biosensors and Bioelectronics* 18 (5): 805-812.

[21] Albrecht, Frank, Roman Leontiev, Claus Jacob, and Alan J. Slusarenko. 2017. "An Optimized Facile Procedure to Synthesize and Purify Allicin." *Molecules (Basel, Switzerland)* 22 (5): 770.

[22] Small, L.A., Bailey, J.H. and Cavallito, C.J. 1947. "Alkyl thiosulphinates." *Journal of the American Chemical Society* 69, 1710–1713.

[23] Block, Eric and John O'Connor. 1974. "Chemistry of alkyl thiosulfinate esters. VII. Mechanistic studies and synthetic applications." *Journal of the American Chemical Society* 96 (12): 3929-3944.

[24] Stoll, A. and E. Seebeck. 1951. "Chemical Investigations on Alliin, the Specific Principle of Garlic." *Advances in Enzymology and Related Subjects of Biochemistry* 11: 377-400.

[25] Kuettner, E. Bartholomeus, Rolf Hilgenfeld, and Manfred S. Weiss. 2002. "The active principle of garlic at atomic resolution." *Journal of Biological Chemistry* 277 (48): 46402-46407.

[26] Shimon, L.J., Rabinkov, A., Shin, I., Miron, T., Mirelman, D., Wilchek, M., Frolow, F. 2007. "Two structures of alliinase from *Alliium sativum* L.: apo form and ternary complex with aminoacrylate reaction intermediate covalently bound to the PLP cofactor." *J. Mol. Biol.* 366(2): 611-625. doi: 10.1016/j.jmb.2006.11.041

[27] Block, Eric. 1985. "The Chemistry of Garlic and Onions." *Scientific American*. 252(3):114-9.

[28] Manabe, T., A. Hasumi, M. Sugiyama, M. Yamazaki, and K. Saito. 1998. "Alliinase [S-alk(en)yl-L-cysteine sulfoxide lyase] from *Allium tuberosum* (Chinese chive) - purification, localization, cDNA cloning and heterologous functional expression." *European Journal of Biochemistry* 257 (1): 21-30.

[29] Nock, L.P., and Mazelis, M. 1987. "The C-S Lyases of Higher Plants: Direct Comparison of the Physical Properties of Homogenous Alliin Lyase of Garlic (*Allium sativum*) and Onion (*Allium cepa*)." *Plant Physiology*, 85(4): 1079-1083.

[30] Damme, Els J.M., Smeets, Koen, Torrekens, Sophie, Leuven, Fred, Goldstein, Irwin J., and Peumans, Willy J. 1992. "The Closely Related Homomeric and Heterodimeric Mannose-binding Lectins from Garlic Are Encoded by One-domain and Two-domain Lectin Genes, Respectively." *European Journal of Biochemistry* 206 (2): 413–20. doi:10.1111/j.1432-1033.1992.tb16941.x.

[31] Rabinkov, A., X.Z. Zhu, G. Grafi, G. Galili, and D. Mirelman. 1994. "Alliin lyase (alliinase) from garlic (*Allium sativum*). Biochemical characterization and cDNA cloning." *Applied Biochemistry and Biotechnology* 48 (3): 149-171. doi:10.1007/bf02788739.

[32] Lancaster, Jane E., Martin L. Shaw, Meeghan D. Pither Joyce, John A. McCallum, and Michael T. McManus. 2000. "A novel alliinase from onion roots. Biochemical characterization and cDNA cloning." *Plant Physiology* 122 (4): 1269-1279.

[33] Lancaster, Jane E. and H.A. Collin. 1981. "Presence of alliinase in isolated vacuoles and of alkyl cysteine sulphoxides in the cytoplasm of bulbs of onion (*Allium cepa*)." *Plant Science Letters* 22 (2): 169-176.

[34] Ellmore, George S., Ross S. Feldberg. 1994. "Alliin lyase localization in bundle sheaths of the garlic clove (*Allium sativum*)". *American Journal of Botany*. 81(1): 89-94. doi:10.1002/j.1537-2197.1994.tb15413.x.

[35] Smeets, Koen, Els J.M. Van Damme, Fred Van Leuven, and Willy J. Peumans. 1997. "Isolation and Characterization of Lectins and Lectin-Alliinase Complexes from Bulbs of Garlic (Allium Sativum) and Ramsons (Allium Ursinum)." *Glycoconjugate Journal* 14 (3): 331-343.

[36] Yamazaki, Mami, Mitsuyo Sugiyama, and Kazuki Saito. 2002. "Intercellular localization of cysteine synthase and alliinase in bundle sheaths of *Allium* plants." *Plant Biotechnology* 19 (1): 7-10.

[37] Smeets, Koen, Els J.M. Van Damme, and Willy J. Peumans. 1997. "Developmental Regulation of Lectin and Alliinase Synthesis in Garlic Bulbs and Leaves." *Plant Physiology* 113 (3): 765-771.

[38] Schwimmer, Sigmund, and Mendel Mazelis. 1963. "Characterization of alliinase of *Allium cepa* (onion)." *Archives of Biochemistry and Biophysics* 100 (1): 66-73. doi: 10.1016/0003-9861(63)90035-3.

[39] Lohmüller, Eva-Maria, J. Landshuter, and K. Knobloch. 1994. "On the isolation and characterization of a C-S-lyase preparation from leek, *Allium porrum*." *Planta Medica* 60 (4): 337-342.

[40] Mazelis, M., and R.K. Creveling. 1975. Purification and properties of S-alkyl-L-cysteine lyase from seedlings of acacia farnesiana willd. *The Biochemical Journal* 147 (3): 485-91.

[41] Hamamoto, Arlene, and Mendel Mazelis. 1986. "The C-S lyases of higher Plants 1: isolation and properties of homogeneous cystine lyase from broccoli." *Plant Physiology* 80 (3): 702-706.

[42] Kamitani H, Esaki N, Tanaka H, Imahara H, Soda K. 1990. Purification and characterization of S-alkylcysteine α, β-lyase from pseudomonas putida. *Journal of Nutritional Science and Vitaminology* 36 (4-SupplementI): 339-47.

[43] Chhabria, Sagar and Krutika Desai. 2018. "Purification and characterisation of alliinase produced by *Cupriavidus necator* and its application for generation of cytotoxic agent: allicin." *Saudi Journal of Biological Sciences* 25 (7): 1429-1438.

[44] Jones, Meriel G., H.A. Collin, A. Tregova, L. Trueman, L. Brown, R. Cosstick, J. Hughes, J. Milne, M.C. Wilkinson, A.B. Tomsett, and B. Thomas. 2007. "The Biochemical and Physiological Genesis of Alliin in Garlic". *Medicinal and Aromatic Plant Science and Biotechnology* 1(1):21-24.

[45] Nasim, Sekh Abdul, Bhupinder Dhir, Rashmi Kapoor, Samar Fatima, Mahmooduzzafar, and Abdul Mujib. 2010. "Alliin Production in various Tissues and Organs of Allium Sativum Grown Under Normal and Sulphur-Supplemented in Vitro Conditions." *Plant Cell, Tissue and Organ Culture (PCTOC)* 101 (1): 59-63.

[46] Mitrová, Katarina, Svoboda, Pavel, Milella, Luigi, and Ovesná, Jaroslava. 2018. "Alliinase and Cysteine Synthase Transcription in Developing Garlic (*Allium sativum* L.) over Time." *Food Chemistry* 251(2018): 103–9. doi:10.1016/j.foodchem.2017.12.090.

[47] Granroth, B. Biosynthesis and decomposition of cysteine derivatives in onion and other Allium species. *Annales Academiae Scientiarum Fennicae* A 154: 4-71. In Jones, Meriel G., Hughes, Jill, Tregova, Angela, Milne, Jonothan, Tomsett, A. Brian, and Collin, Hamish A. 2004. "Biosynthesis of the Flavour Precursors of Onion and Garlic." 2004. *Journal of Experimental Botany* 55(404): 1903-1918. doi:10.1093/jxb/erh138.

[48] Hughes, J., A. Tregova, A.B. Tomsett, M.G. Jones, R. Cosstick, and H.A. Collin. 2005. "Synthesis of the flavour precursor, alliin, in garlic tissue cultures." *Phytochemistry* 66 (2): 187-194.

[49] Ohsumi, Chieko, Takahisa Hayashi, and Konosuke Sano. 1993. "Formation of alliin in the culture tissues of *Allium sativum*. Oxidation of S-allyl-L-cysteine." *Phytochemistry* 33 (1): 107-111.

[50] Suzuki T, Sugii M, and Kakimoto T. 1962. "Metabolic incorporation of L-valine-C^{14} into S-(2-carboxypropyl) glutathione and S-(2-carboxypropyl) cysteine in garlic." *Chemical and Pharmaceutical Bulletin (Tokyo)* 10 (4): 328-331. In Jones, Meriel G., Hughes, Jill, Tregova, Angela, Milne, Jonothan, Tomsett, A. Brian, and Collin, Hamish A. 2004. "Biosynthesis of the Flavour Precursors of Onion and Garlic." 2004. *Journal of Experimental Botany* 55(404): 1903-1918. Doi:10.1093/jxb/erh138.

[51] Caspi, Ron, Richard Billington, Carol A. Fulcher, Ingrid M. Keseler, Anamika Kothari, Markus Krummenacker, Mario Latendresse, Peter E. Midford, Quang Ong, Wait Kit Ong, Suzanne Paley, Pallavi Subhraveti, and Peter D. Carp. 2018. "The MetaCyc Database of metabolic pathways and enzymes." *Nucleic Acids Research* 46 (D1): D633-D639.

[52] Yoshimoto, Naoko, Ayami Yabe, Yuka Sugino, Soichiro Murakami, Niti Sai-Ngam, Shin-Ichiro Sumi, Tadamitsu Tsuneyoshi, and Kazuki Saito. 2015a. "Garlic γ-glutamyl transpeptidases that catalyze deglutamylation of biosynthetic Intermediate of Alliin." *Frontiers in Plant Science* 5: 758.

[53] Yoshimoto, Naoko, Misato Onuma, Shinya Mizuno, Yuka Sugino, Ryo Nakabayashi, Shinsuke Imai, Tadamitsu Tsuneyoshi, Shin-ichiro Sumi, and Kazuki Saito. 2015b. "Identification of a flavin-containing S-oxygenating monooxygenase involved in alliin biosynthesis in garlic." *The Plant Journal* 83 (6): 941-951.

[54] Krest, I. and M. Keusgen. 1999. "Quality of Herbal Remedies from Allium Sativum: Differences between Alliinase from Garlic Powder and Fresh Garlic." *Planta Medica* 65 (2): 139-143.

[55] Mazelis, M. and L. Crews. 1968. "Purification of the Alliin Lyase of Garlic, Allium Sativum L." *The Biochemical Journal* 108 (5): 725-730.

[56] Weiner, Lev, Irina Shin, Linda J.W. Shimon, Talia Miron, Meir Wilchek, David Mirelman, Felix Frolow, and Aharon Rabinkov. 2009. "Thiol-disulfide organization in alliin lyase (alliinase) from garlic (*Allium sativum*)." *Protein Science : A Publication of the Protein Society* 18 (1): 196-205. doi: 10.1002/pro.10.

[57] Schneider, G, Kack, H, and Lindqvist, Y. 2000. "The Manifold of Vitamin B6 Dependent Enzymes." *Structure* 8 (1): R1–R6. doi:10.1016/S0969-2126(00)00085-X.

[58] Miron, Talia, Aharon Rabinkov, David Mirelman, Lev Weiner, and Meir Wilchek. 1998. "A spectrophotometric assay for allicin and alliinase (alliin lyase) activity: reaction of 2-nitro-5-thiobenzoate with thiosulfinates." *Analytical Biochemistry* 265 (2): 317-325.

[59] Kitamura, Nobuko, Naoya Shimomura, Junji Iseki, Mamoru Honma, Seiya Chiba, Satoshi Tahara, and Junya Mizutani. 1997. "Cysteine-S-conjugate β-lyase activity and pyridoxal phosphate binding site of onion alliin lyase." *Bioscience, Biotechnology, and Biochemistry* 61 (8): 1327-1330. doi: 10.1271/bbb.61.1327.

[60] van Damme, E.J., K. Smeets, S. Torrekens, F. van Leuven, I.J. Goldstein, and W.J. Peumans. 1992. "The closely related homomeric and heterodimeric mannose-binding lectins from garlic are encoded by one-domain and two-Domain lectin genes, respectively." *European Journal of Biochemistry* 206 (2): 413-420.

[61] Shin, Irina, David Mirelman, Lev Weiner, Enrique Villar, Valery L. Shnyrov, and Aharon Rabinkov. 2018. "Stabilization of Alliinase from Garlic by Osmolytes and the

Mannose-Specific Lectin ASAI." *Journal of Pharmacy and Pharmacology* 6 (5) 437-447. doi:10.17265/2328-2150/2018.05.001.

[62] Wills, E.D. 1956. "Enzyme Inhibition by Allicin, the Active Principle of Garlic." *The Biochemical Journal* 63 (3): 514-520.

[63] Miron, Talia, Irina Shin, Guy Feigenblat, Lev Weiner, David Mirelman, Meir Wilchek, and Aharon Rabinkov. 2002. "A spectrophotometric assay for allicin, alliin, and alliinase (alliin lyase) with a chromogenic thiol: reaction of 4-mercaptopyridine with thiosulfinates." *Analytical Biochemistry* 307 (1): 76-83.

[64] Mallika, Thapa, Elshareif Omer, Zhang Lianfu, and State Key. 2014. "Separation and purification of alliinase and alliin from garlic (*Allium sativum*)." *Journal of Academia and Industrial Research (JAIR)*. 2(11): 599 – 605.

[65] Kazaryan Goryachenkova 1978. *Biochemistry* 43: 1502-1508. In Nock, Linda P. and Mendel Mazelis. 1986. "The C-S lyases of higher plants: preparation and properties of homogeneous alliin lyase from garlic (*Allium sativum*)." *Archives of Biochemistry and Biophysics* 249 (1): 27-33.

[66] Friedemann, T.E, and G.E. Haugen. 1943. "Pyruvic acid II. The determination of keto acids in blood and urine." *Journal of Biological Chemistry* 147: 415-42.

[67] Ankri, Serge, and David Mirelman. 1999. "Antimicrobial Properties of Allicin from Garlic." *Microbes and Infection* 2: 125–29. doi:10.1016/S1286-4579(99)80003-3.

[68] Jin, Young Nam, Youngsok Choi, Changyuan Yang. 2001. "Identification of an essential tryptophan residue in alliinase from garlic (*Allium sativum*) by chemical modification. *Bull. Korean Chem. Soc.* 22(1):68-76.

[69] Müller, B. 1990. "Garlic (*Allium sativum*): Quantitative analysis of the tracer substances alliin and allicin." *Planta Medica* 56 (6): 589–90. https://doi.org/10.1055/s-2006-961198.

[70] Lawson, Larry D. and Z.J. Wang. 2001. "Low Allicin Release from Garlic Supplements: A Major Problem due to the Sensitivities of Alliinase Activity." *Journal of Agricultural and Food Chemistry* 49 (5): 2592-2599.

[71] Block, E. 1992. "The organosulfur chemistry of the genus *Allium* – Implications for the organic chemistry of sulfur." *Angew. Chem. Int. Ed. Engl.*, 31: 1135-1178. doi:10.1002/anie.199211351.

[72] Lawson, Larry D. and Bronwyn G. Hughes. 1992. "Characterization of the formation of allicin and other thiosulfinates from garlic." *Planta Medica* 58(4): 345-350.

[73] Müller BH, *Beitrag zur Charakterisierung und Analytik von Alliin und Allicin in Knoblauch und seinen Zubereitungen [Characterization and analysis of alliin and allicin in garlic and its preparations]*, Dissertation Universitat Erlangen Nurnberg 1991.

[74] Keusgen, Michael. 2008. "Unusual cystine lyase activity of the enzyme alliinase: direct formation of polysulphides." *Planta Medica* 74 (1): 73-79.

[75] Nagahara, Noriyuki. "Catalytic Site Cysteines of Thiol Enzyme: Sulfurtransferases," *Journal of Amino Acids,* vol. 2011, Article ID 709404, 7 pages, 2011. doi:10.4061/2011/709404.

[76] Leung-Toung, Regis, Wanren Li, Tim Tam, and Khashayar Kaarimian. 2002. "Thiol-Dependent Enzymes and their Inhibitors: A Review." *Current Medicinal Chemistry* 9 (9): 979-1002.

[77] Rabinkov, Aharon, Talia Miron, Leonid Konstantinovski, Meir Wilchek, David Mirelman, and Lev Weiner. 1998. "The mode of action of allicin: trapping of radicals

and interaction with thiol containing proteins." *Biochimica et Biophysica Acta.* 1379: 233-244.

[78] Müller, Alexandra, Jakob Eller, Frank Albrecht, Pascal Prochnow, Katja Kuhlmann, Julia Elisabeth Bandow, Alan John Slusarenko, and Lars Ingo Ole Leichert. 2016. "Allicin induces thiol stress in bacteria through S-allylmercapto modification of protein cysteines" *J. Biol. Chem.* 291(22): 11477-11490. doi:10.1074/jbc.M115.702308.

[79] Miron, Talia, Aharon Rabinkov, David Mirelman, Meir Wilchek, and Lev Weiner. 2000. "The mode of action of allicin: its ready permeability through phospholipid membranes may contribute to its biological activity." *BBA - Biomembranes* 1463 (1): 20-30. doi: 10.1016/S0005-2736(99)00174-1.

[80] Wu, Chih-Chung, Yung-Lin Chu, and Lee-Yan Sheen. 2012. "Allicin modulates the antioxidation and detoxification capabilities of primary rat hepatocytes." *Journal of Traditional and Complementary Medicine* 2 (4): 323-330.

[81] Focke, Manfred, Andrea Feld, and Hartmut K. Lichtenthaler. 1990. "Allicin, a naturally occurring antibiotic from garlic, specifically inhibits acetyl-CoA synthetase." *FEBS Letters* 261 (1): 106-108.

[82] Dube, S.K., O. Ronholt, and D. Pressman. 1963. "The chemical nature of the enzyme site of rabbit muscle lctic acid dehydrogenase". *The Journal of Biological Chemistry.* 238(2): 613-617.

[83] Bloxham, David P., Ram P. Sharma, and David C. Wilton. 1979. "A detailed investigation of the properties of lactate dehydrogenase in which the 'essential' cysteine-165 is modified by thioalkylation." *Biochem. J.* 177:769-780.

[84] Tsuji, Soichi, Masood A. Qureshi, Esther W. Hou, Walter M. Fitch, and Steven S. -L Li. 1994. "Evolutionary relationships of lactate dehydrogenases (LDHs) from mammals, birds, an amphibian, fish, barley, and bacteria: LDH cDNA sequences from *Xenopus*, pig, and rat." *Proceedings of the National Academy of Sciences of the United States of America* 91 (20): 9392-9396.

[85] Stockert, Amy L., Sujata S. Shinde, Robert F. Anderson, and Russ Hille. 2002. "The reaction mechanism of xanthine oxidase: evidence for two-electron chemistry rather than sequential one-electron steps." *Journal of the American Chemical Society* 124 (49): 14554-14555.

[86] Nishida, Masayuki, Takahiko Hada, Kouji Kuramochi, Hiromi Yoshida, Hideki Yoshida, Yuko Yonezawa, Isoko Kuriyama, Fumio Sugawara, and Yoshiyuki Mizushina. 2008. "Diallyl Sulfides: Selective Inhibitors of Family X DNA Polymerases from Garlic (Allium Sativum L.)." *Food Chemistry* 108 (2): 551-560.

[87] Bakri, I.M. and C.W.I. Douglas. 2005. "Inhibitory effect of garlic extract on oral bacteria." *Archives of Oral Biology* 50 (7): 645-651.

[88] Mackworth, Jane F. 1948. "The inhibition of thiol enzymes by lachrymators." *Biochemical journal.* 42:82-90.

[89] Ranjbar-Omid, Mahsa, Mohsen Arzanlou, Mojtaba Amani, Seyyedeh Khadijeh Shokri Al-Hashem, Nour Amir Mozafari, and Hadi Peeri Doghaheh. 2015. "Allicin from garlic inhibits the biofilm formation and urease activity of *Proteus mirabilis in vitro.*" *FEMS Microbiology Letters* 362 (9). doi: 10/1093/femsle/fnv049.

[90] Todd, M.J., and R.P. Hausinger. 1991. "Identification of the essential cysteine residue in *Klebsiella aerogenes* urease." *Journal of Biological Chemistry* 266 (36): 24327-24331.

[91] Richie, JP, Jr, L. Skowronski, P. Abraham, and Y. Leutzinger. 1996. "Blood glutathione concentrations in a large-scale human study." *Clinical Chemistry* 42 (1): 64-70.

[92] Miron, Talia, Irving Listowsky, and Meir Wilchek. 2010. "Reaction mechanisms of allicin and allyl-mixed disulfides with proteins and small thiol molecules." *European Journal of Medicinal Chemistry* 45 (5): 1912-1918.

[93] Horn, Tobias, Wolfgang Bettray, Alan J. Slusarenko, and Martin C.H. Gruhlke. 2018. "S-Allylmercaptoglutathione is a substrate for glutathione reductase (E.C. 1.8.1.7) from yeast (*Saccharomyces cerevisiae*)." *Antioxidants (Basel, Switzerland)* 7 (7): 86.

[94] Wu, JT, LH Wu, and JA Knight. 1986. "Stability of NADPH: Effect of various factors on the kinetics of degradation [Published Erratum Appears in Clin Chem 1987 may;33(5):724]." *Clinical Chemistry* 32 (2): 314-319.

[95] Rabinkov, Aharon, Talia Miron, David Mirelman, Meir Wilchek, Sabina Glozman, Ephraim Yavin, and Lev Weiner. 2000. "S-Allylmercaptoglutathione: The reaction product of allicin with glutathione possesses SH-modifying and antioxidant properties." *BBA - Molecular Cell Research* 1499 (1): 144-153.

[96] Miron, Talia, Aharon, Rabinkov, David Mirelman, and Meir Wilchek. 2002. *"Allylmercaptocaptopril compounds and uses thereof."* US Patent Number 7,241,902, filed May 30, 2002, and issued July 10, 2007.

[97] Prasad, Kailash, Victor A. Laxdal, Ming Yu, and Barbara L. Raney. 1995. "Antioxidant activity of allicin, an active principle in garlic." *Molecular and Cellular Biochemistry.* 148: 183-89. doi:10.1007/BF00928155.

[98] Mailloux, Ryan J., and Jason R. Treberg. 2016. "Protein S-glutathionlyation links energy metabolism to redox signaling in mitochondria." *Redox Biology* 8 (C): 110-118.

[99] Wang, Jing, Chengtao Wang, Yanping Cao, Baoguo Sun, and Yingjie Mo. 2011. "Effect of ultrasound on the activity of alliinase from fresh garlic." *Ultrasonics - Sonochemistry* 18 (2): 534-540.

[100] Weik, Robert, Andrej Francky, Gerald Striedner, Peter Raspor, Karl Bayer, and Diethard Mattanovich. 1998. Recombinant expression of alliin lyase from garlic (*Allium sativum*) in bacteria and yeasts. *Planta Medica* 64 (4): 387-8.

[101] *MyBioSource.com.* "Alliinase recombinant protein". 2019. https://www.mybiosource.com/alliinase-recombinant-protein/alliin-lyasc/1007620.

[102] Mirelman, David, Aharon Rabinkov, Gad Galili, Gideon Grafi, Xiao-Zhu Zhu, and Meir Wilchek. 1994. *"Recombinant alliinase, its preparation and pharmaceutical compositions comprising it."* World Intellectual Property Organization Application Number WO1993US09785, filed October 7, 1993, and published April 28, 1994.

[103] Ko, J.A., Y.L. Lee, H.J. Jeong, and H.J. Park. 2012. "Preparation of encapsulated alliinase in alginate microparticles." *Biotechnology Letters* 34 (3): 515-518. doi: 10.1007/s10529-011-0791-5.

[104] Méndez Lagunas, Lilia L. and François Castaigne. 2008. "Effect of Temperature Cycling on Allinase Activity in Garlic." *Food Chemistry* 111 (1): 56-60.

[105] Miron, T., H. SivaRaman, A. Rabinkov, D. Mirelman, and M. Wilchek. 2006. "A method for continuous production of allicin using immobilized alliinase." *Analytical Biochemistry* 351 (1): 152-154. doi: 10.1016/j.ab.2006.01.030.

[106] Zhou, Jianqin. 2009. "Immobilization of alliinase and its application: Flowinjection enzymatic analysis for alliin." *African Journal of Biotechnology*. 8(7): 1337-1342.

[107] Williams, David Michael, and Chandra Mohan Pant. 2002. *"Process for production of allicin."* US Patent Number 7,179,632, filed July 4, 2002, and issued February 20, 2007.

[108] Mirelman, David, Meir Wilchek, Talia Miron, Aharon Rabinkov, Hephzibah Sivaraman. 1997. *"Garlic alliinase covalently bound to carrier for continuous production of allicin."* US Patent Number 6,689,588 B1, filed April 14, 1997, and issued February 10, 2004.

[109] Rabinkov, Aharon, Talia Miron, David Mirelman, Meir Wilchek. 2003. *"Site-specific in situ generation of allicin using a targeted alliinase delivery system for the treatment of cancers, tumors, infectious diseases and other allicin-sensitive diseases."* US Patent Number 7,445,802, filed December 31, 2003, and issued November 4, 2008.

[110] Zhou, Jian Qin and Jian Wen Wang. 2009. "Immobilization of alliinase with a water soluble–insoluble reversible N-succinyl-chitosan for allicin production." *Enzyme and Microbial Technology* 45 (4): 299-304. doi:10.1016/j.enzmictec.2009.07.007.

[111] Giles, Gregory I, Nasim, Muhammad Jawad, Ali, Wesam, and Jacob, Claus. 2017. "The Reactive Sulfur Species Concept: 15 Years On." *Antioxidants (Basel, Switzerland)* 6(2). doi:10.3390/antiox6020038.

[112] Anwar, Awais, Emma Gould, Ryan Tinson, Javaid Iqbal, and Chris Hamilton. 2018. "Redox Modulation at Work: Natural Phytoprotective Polysulfanes from Alliums Based on Redox-Active Sulfur." *Current Pharmacology Reports* 4 (5): 397-407.

[113] Pluth, Michael D., T. Spencer Bailey, Matthew D. Hammers, Matthew D. Hartle, Hillary A. Henthorn, and Andrea K. Steiger. 2015. "Natural Products Containing Hydrogen Sulfide Releasing Moieties." *Synlett* 26 (19): 2633-2643.

[114] Toohey, John I., and Arthur J.L. Cooper. 2014. "Thiosulfoxide (Sulfane) Sulfur: New Chemistry and New Regulatory Roles in Biology." *Molecules (Basel, Switzerland)* 19 (8): 12789-12813.

[115] Lubenets, Vira, Olena Karpenko, Mykola Ponomarenko, Gleb Zahoriy, Aelita Krychkovska, Volodymyr Novikov, Kyiv JSC "Darnytsia" Ukraine, et al. 2013. "Development of New Antimicrobial Compositions of Thiosulfonate Structure." *Chemistry Chemical Technology* 7 (2): 119-124.

[116] Lubenets, Vira, Sofiya Vasylyuk, Nataliya Monka, Khrystyna Bolibrukh, Olena Komarovska-Porokhnyavets, Diana Baranovych, Rostyslav Musyanovych, et al. 2017. "Synthesis and antimicrobial properties of 4-acylaminobenzenethiosulfoacid S-esters." *Saudi Pharmaceutical Journal* 25 (2): 266-274. doi: 10.1016/j.jsps.2016.06.007.

[117] Makarieva, Tatyana N., Valentin A. Stonik, Andrei S. Dmitrenok, Boris B. Grebnev, Vladimir V. Isakov, Nikolai M. Rebachyk, and Yakov W. Rashkes. 1995. "Varacin and Three New Marine Antimicrobial Polysulfides from the Far-Eastern Ascidian Polycitorsp." *Journal of Natural Products* 58 (2): 254-258.

[118] Pan, Guohui, Zhengren Xu, Zhikai Guo, Hindra, Ming Ma, Dong Yang, Hao Zhou, Yannick Gansemans, Ziangcheng Zhu, Yong Huang, Li-Xing Zhao, Yi Jiang, Juanhua Cheng, Filip van Neuwerburgh, Joo-Won Suh, Yanwen Duan, and Ben Shen. 2017. "Discovery of the Leinamycin Family of Natural Products by Mining Actinobacterial Genomes." *Proceedings of the National Academy of Sciences of the United States of America* 114 (52): E11131-E11140.

[119] United States Patent and Trademark Office. *"USPTO patent full-text and image database."* August 6, 2019. http://patft.uspto.gov/netahtml/PTO/search-bool.html.

[120] Goodrich, Laura L. 2003. *"Antimicrobial blood treatment using allicin and related compounds."* US Patent Number US 2003/0077264 A1, filed September 18, 2002, and published April 24, 2003.

[121] Numata, Richard, and Ryan Willey. 2018. "*Grease-like gel for repelling insects and preventing undesirable behavior in hoofed animals.*" US Patent Number 10,212,93, filed January 19, 2018, and issued February 26, 2019.

[122] Adams, John M., and Tommy C. Holland. 2015. *"Coal packaging for smokeless tobacco."* US Patent Number 9,888,716, filed March 26, 2015, and issued February 13, 2016.

[123] Daeef, Salha, F.H. *"Kit containing patches and omposition for insect bite treatment."* US Patent Number 9,517,213, filed March 10, 2015, and issued December 13, 2016.

[124] Von White, Gregory, Kerscher, Petra, Brown, Ryan M, Morella, Jacob D, Mcallister, William, Dean, Delphine, and Christopher L Kitchens. 2012. "Green Synthesis of Robust, Biocompatible Silver Nanoparticles Using Garlic Extract." *Journal of Nanomaterials* 2012 (January). Article ID 730746. Doi:10.1155/2012/730746.

[125] Bhagyalakshmi, N., R. Thimmaraju, L. Venkatachalam, K.N. Chidambara Murthy, and R.V. Sreedhar. 2005. "Nutraceutical Applications of Garlic and the Intervention of Biotechnology." *Critical Reviews in Food Science and Nutrition* 45 (7-8): 607-621.

[126] Li, Jiang-Wei, Xia, Lijie, Su, Youhong, Liu, Hongchun, Xia, Xueqing, Lu, Qinxia, Yang, Chunjin, and Reheman, Kalbinur. 2012. "Molecular Imprint of Enzyme Active Site by Camel Nanobodies: Rapid and Efficient Approach to Produce Abzymes with Alliinase Activity." *The Journal of Biological Chemistry* 287 (17): 13713-13721.

In: Allicin
Editor: Diana R. Cundell
ISBN: 978-1-53617-339-0

Chapter 3

General Biochemical Pathways of Inflammation and Allicin

Diana R. Cundell*, PhD[*]
College of Life Sciences, Jefferson University, Philadelphia, PA

Abstract

Allicin is the major biologically active thiosulfinate produced when garlic is damaged. Since its discovery in 1944, allicin has been shown to have primarily anti-inflammatory effects mediated through several important biochemical pathways including the glutathione (GSH) redox, NF-E2, p45related factor (Nrf2), nuclear factor kappa beta (NF-κβ), phosphoinositide-3-phosphate/protein kinase B (P13K/Akt), nitric oxide synthases (NOS) and all three mitogen activated kinase pathways (MAPKs). One landmark study in 1956, reported that allicin was able to inhibit fourteen of twenty eight enzymes tested and that all contained an accessible thiol group. So how does allicin produce these effects? Allicin pentrates cell membranes easily, oxidizes the thiol group of GSH and raises the overall cellular redox potential. Oxidized GSH reduces cellular stress by "mopping up" or preventing the formation of excessive reactive oxygen species (ROS) as well as preventing apoptosis. Elevations of ROS in healthy cells triggers the activation of the Nrf2 pathway and results in upregulation of antioxidant enzymes including catalase and superoxide dismutase (SOD). Activation of Nrf2 also suppresses NF-κβ expression, in turn affecting MAPK and overall cellular activation. To date, allicin has been demonstrated to affect at least one of these pathways in over fifty *in vitro* or *in vivo* models of acute or chronic infammatory disease. Acute inflammatory models include those generated by infectious agents as well as damage to the central nervous system (ischemic stroke, subarachnoid hemorrhage and traumatic brain injury). Chronic inflammatory models in which allicin has reported effects on underlying biochemical pathways include Alzheimer's, cardiovascular disease, osteoarthritis, osteoporosis as well as renal and hepatotoxic syndromes. This chapter will first explore the studies of allicin's effects on the biochemical pathways of acute and chronic inflammation. The intersection of these biochemical targets will then be discussed in order to provide a greater understanding of how allicin may prove useful in both acute and chronic inflammatory diseases.

---

[*] Corresponding Author's Email: Diana.Cundell@jefferson.edu.

Keywords: ERK, iNOS, JNK, MAPK, NF-κB, Nrf2, NO, P13K/Akt, and ROS

INTRODUCTION

Allicin's first cellular effects were described in 1944, when it was identified as the major thiosulfinate of garlic cloves that was antibacterial [Cavallito 1944]. Cavallito [2] later classified the bactericidal activity of allicin as one that attacks all enzymes possessing sulfhydryl groups, especially those containing cysteine and cysteine peptides. A landmark paper in 1956, by Wills [3], examined the ability of allicin to impair the activity of enzymes in eukaryotic cells. Using freshly generated allicin, Wills demonstrated that the thiosulfinate was able to impair the activity of an impressive fourteen enzymes of the twenty eight he tested. Wills [3] reported that all the majority of enzymes allicin impaired contained sulfhydryl groups but also some that did not contain these groups, for example glyceraldehyde 3-phosphate dehydrogenase (GADPH). At that point analysis of how allicin functioned on eukaryotic enzymes underwent a hiatus of over forty years, until biochemists again began to examine its effects. The literature now contains nearly fifty more papers on the ability of allicin to either upregulate or impair six major and central pathways central to maintenance of health and prevention of apoptosis in healthy eukaryotic *in vitro* and *in vivo* models of disease [4-56]. Temporary changes in the functioning of all six are required for a eukaryotic cell to rid itself of an infection and during the healing that follows [57-67]. This is particularly true for the central pathway of nuclear factor kappa beta (NF-κB), which in turn feeds into and controls the regulation of the the mitogen-activated protein kinases (MAPK), nitric oxide synthases (NOS), the generation of rective oxygen species (ROS) and the NF-E2, p45-related factor 2 (Nrf2) signaling pathways [57-68].

If the stimulus is not removed then chronic inflammation ensues with a sustained alteration to these cellular pathways, resulting in accelerated cell death due to a shift in the redox cell environment and consequent activation of mitochondrial-based caspase and non-caspase based systems [64-66]. Allicin's ability to affect sulfhydryl groups also affects the major redox controlling systems in eukaryotic cells namely glutathione (GSH)[69]. By binding to this group allicin is able to create an oxidative state in the cell, which results in its preservation i.e., lack of apoptosis from the damaging stimuli of ROS [69]. The biochemistry of allicin was last fully evaluated by Jan Borlinghaus in 2014 [69] and considered by him to possess two major effects on healthy cells. Borlinghaus considered the primary anti-inflammatory property of allicin to be the positive effects of the thiosulfinate on GSH as well as levels of ROS-metabolizing enzymes including superoxide dismutase (SOD) and catalase [69]. Allicin's effects on redox pathways in acute and chronic inflammation has been researched in over twenty studies [4-26]. These include *in vitro* [4-9] and *in vivo* [10-26] models of acute infection [5, 6, 23] and central nervous system inflamation [9-13, 17, 18, 25, 26] as well as chronic inflammatory conditions affecting the brain [9-12], heart [4, 14], kidneys [9-21], liver [15, 26], cartilage and bone [8, 24].

Borlinghaus identified allicin's secondary major property as its ability to directly switch on the Nrf2 signaling pathway [5, 10, 11, 15, 20, 21, 27-29]. As will be discussed later in the chapter, allicin, like other phytochemicals, is able to attach directly to the Kelch ECH associating protein-1 system (Keap-1) subunit of this enzyme [11, 69]. Nrf2 both switches off

ROS production as well as engaging in cross talk with NF-κB to reduce the overall inflammatory levels in the cell [11, 69, 70]. Allicin has been able to inhibit NF-κB in fourteen either *in vitro* [5, 30-34] or *in vivo* animal studies [15, 16, 22, 29, 35-38] in keeping with this capacity. Since the central work of Borlinghaus [69], over thirty further studies have appeared on allicin that have begun to identify its important cellular targets [4, 5, 8, 9, 11, 14-27, 29-33, 35, 37, 38, 42, 44, 45, 47-49, 55, 56].

Dissecting how allicin actually works in healthy cells becomes more complex at this point since these pathways begin to intersect and cross talk with each other [57-68]. For example Keap 1 also regulates the phosphoinositide-3-phosphate/protein kinase B (P13K/Akt) pathway [71] and suppression of NF-κB impacts the MAPK pathways and NOS synthesis [65, 67, 68]. Allicin has been reported to modify either P13K/Akt or NOS enzymes in over twenty *in vitro* or *in vivo* studies [4, 7, 8, 14, 19, 21, 22, 29, 31, 32, 36, 39-47] and to influence MAPK in a further ten [8, 12, 18, 36, 44, 47-49, 51, 52].

Setting aside the complexities of cellular biochemistry until the end of the chapter, it is first necessary to first examine each of the pathways allicin impacts as individual entities. An analysis of the studies performed on each pathway will be combined with an explanation of the underlying mechanism allicin uses to achieve these effects. Finally, in "putting it together" the target mechanisms elucidated for allicin in healthy cells undergoing inflammation will be discussed. Several studies have examine the effects of allicin or garlic extract on cholesterol and the enzymes involved in its synthesis [53-56]. These will be discussed further in Chapter 10 and their analysis will not appear here. Many investigators have also examined the influence of allicin on tumor cell integrity, biochemical pathways and apoptosis and analysis of these abnormal cells will appear in "Chapter 13 Tumoricidal activities of allicin".

1. Biochemical Pathways Modulating Inflammation – The Basics

Inflammation is typically initiated through interaction of foreign antigen or cell surface molecules with pattern recognition receptors (PRR) which include the Toll-like receptor group (TLR) [57]. PRR stimulation initiates a signaling complex which in turn activates the TGFβ-activated MAP 3 kinase 1 (TAK-1) [57]. TAK-1 can directly activate NF-κB as well as two MAPK kinase pathways, namely Jun amino-terminal kinases (JNK) and p38 [58]. By initiating the expression of MAP 3 tumor progression locus 2 protein (TPL2) it is also able to switch on a third MAPK pathway called extracellular-initiated kinase or ERK [58]. Activation of PRR/TLR on immune response cells, particularly macrophages in this manner also produces a convergence of the NF-κB and p38 MAPK pathway to allow iNOS transcription via the Janus-kinase signal transductors/activators of transcription (JAK-STAT) pathway producing nitric oxide (NO) [59]. Activation of the JAK-STAT pathway, which in turn results in the expression of signal transduction and activator of transcription 3 (STAT3) [60]. Alongside these powerful pathways inflammation also involves activation of the P13K/Akt pathway and its variable interaction with NF-κB, ERK and TLR signaling i.e., the pathway can either be switched on or off [61].

Both NO and reactive oxygen species (ROS) can either enhance or suppress the activities of other pathways and, in doing so are central to effective control of inflammatory responses or persistence into chronic inflammation [62-64]. ROS and NF-κB are considered to participate in what is termed "crosstalk" [65]. Several genes upregulating ROS are produced by NF-κB during periods of inflammation/oxidative cell stress and then switched off to allow cell survival [65]. Oxidative stress and the ROS produced can also activate the NrF2 signaling pathway which both switches off ROS through generation of antioxidative enzymes [65] and inhibits NF-κB activity [66]. NF-κB expression may also be influenced by p38 and ERK MAPK pathways [67, 68]. MAPK p38 inhibits NF-κB through interfering with its coactivating molecules [67]. Different organ systems may also depend on these biochemical pathways [68]. Discussed later, a prime example is the inverse relationship between NF-κB and ERK in controlling survival and maturation of osteoclasts in bone [68]. A summary of how these pathways intersect is shown in Figure 1.

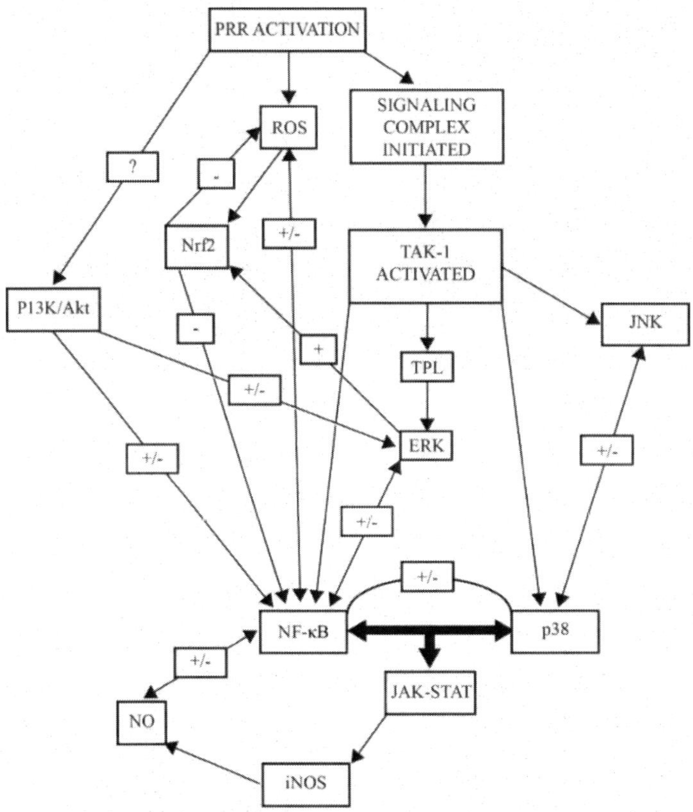

Legend: Crosstalk is common among biochemical pathways and indicated as negative reinforcement (-), positive (+) or variable (+/-).

Abbreviations: ERK (extracellular-initiated kinase) iNOS (inducible nitric oxide synthase), JAK-STAT (Janus-kinase signal transductors/ activators of transcription), JNK (Jun amino-terminal kinases), NF-κB (nuclear factor kappa beta), NO (nitric oxide), Nrf2 (NF-E2, p45-related factor 2), Abbreviations: ERK (extracellular-initiated kinase) iNOS (inducible nitric oxide synthase), JAK-STAT (Janus-kinase signal transductors/activators of transcription), JNK (Jun amino-terminal kinases), NF-κB (nuclear factor kappa beta), NO (nitric oxide), Nrf2 (NF-E2, p45-related factor 2), P13K/Akt (phosphoinositide-3 phosphate/protein kinase B), PRR (pattern recognition) ROS (reactive oxygen species), TAK-1 (TGFβ-activated MAP 3 kinase) and TPL2 (tumor progression locus 2 protein).

References used to construct diagram: [57-67].

Figure 1. Biochemical pathways of inflammation.

2. ALLICIN AND THE REDOX ENVIRONMENT OF CELLS

Twenty-three studies have appeared in the literature to suggest that allicin has efficacy in ameliorating the redox environment of *in vitro* or *in vivo* models of acute and chronic inflammatory conditions [4-26]. A description of the experimental design and results of these studies is shown in Table 1.

The six *in vitro* models of allicin [4-9] and seventeen *in vivo* [10-26] all demonstrated changes in the redox environment involving upregulation of primarily GSH and the enzymes involved in its creation, namely glutathione peroxidase (GpX), glutathione reductase (GR) and glutathione transferase (GST) [5, 6, 9-11, 13, 15-17, 19, 20, 22, 24-26]. Thioredoxin levels were also increased in a single *in vitro* study of allicin's (10, 30 or 100 µg/ml for 24 h) effects on murine osteoblasts [8]. Thioredoxin, provides a second buffer system to control cellular ROS levels and can directly modulate several biochemical pathways simultaneously including NF-κB and P13K/Akt [72]

Table 1. Allicin studies reporting significant increase in redox enzymes #

***In vitro* studies**	**Experimental design**	**Reference**
Cardiac ischemia	H9c2 cells pre-treated with allicin (0.2, 0.5 or 1 µM 1 h) and exposed to hypoxic stress (5% CO_2, 95% N_2) for 12 h; ↑ SOD	[4]
Infection	HUVECs treated with allicin (40 µg/ml) and LPS (1 µg/ml) for 24 h: allicin ↑ CAT, GpX, GST and SOD compared with LPS alone	[5]
	PBMC from patients with vaginitis treated with allicin (0-500 ng/ml); allicin allicin ↑ GpX compared with cells from healthy patients	[6]
Inflammation	HUVEC incubated with TNF-α (5 ng/ml) in the presence or absence of allicin (500 µg/ml) for 20 h; ↓ release of H_2O_2 (CAT activated)	[7]
OP	Murine osteoblast-like line MC3-T3-E1 cells treated with hydrogen peroxide (200 µM) for 6 h then allicin (10, 30 or 100 µg/ml) for 24 h; ↑ thioredoxin activity	[8]
PkD	*In vitro* assay rat PC12 cells incubated with allicin (50 µM) for 2 h then exposed to 6-OHDA for 24 h; ↑ GPx, GSH levels	[9]
AD	20-month old male C57BL/6 mice (n =16 per group) received allicin (180 mg/kg/day, oral) for 8 weeks. Compared with 3-month old and 20-month old; ↑ GPx, GSH levels and total antioxidant capacity in hippocampus	[10]
	Sprague Dawley rats (n = 12, 4 groups) treated with allicin (180 mg/kg oral) or sulforaphane (12 mg/kg oral) for 16 weeks then injected into lateral ventricle with tunicamycin (TM) (5 µl); Both allicin and sulforaphane ↑ GpX and GSH activity	[11]
	Kunming mice (n =20) AD model (Aβ injected into brains); allicin (180 mg/kg/ day for 14 days injected i.p.) and compared with PBS; ↑SOD	[12]
Animal models	**Experimental design**	**Reference**
ASCI	Male New Zealand white rabbits (n = 8 per group) pretreated with allicin (1, 10 or 50 mg/kg oral) for 14 days then given aortic occlusion spinal injury. Changes evaluated 4 and 24 h after reperfusion; ↑ oxidative enzymes (SOD, catalase, GpX and GST) ↓ ROS	[13]
Exhaustive cardiac stress	Sprague-Dawley rats (n = 8 per group) underwent exhaustive swimming training for 7 weeks and supplemented with allicin (4.2, 6.3 or 12.6 mg/kg i.p.); ↑ SOD in cardiac tissue	[14]
Hepatotoxicity (arsenic-induced)	Wistar rats (n = 24) administered allicin (30 mg/kg by i.p. injection) 1 h before arsenic oxide (3 mg/kg) given by gavage for 7 days; ↑ SOD and GpX in hepatic tissues	[15]
IBD	Balb/c mice (n = 6) given 2.5% DSS in drinking water with or without allicin (10 mg/kg) for 7 days; ↑ oxidative enzymes (SOD, GpX and GR)	[16]

Table 1. (Continued)

Animal models	Experimental design	Reference
IS	C57BL/6 mice (n =15) pretreated with allicin (50 mg/kg oral) for 14 days and middle cerebral artery occluded. Changes evaluated after 1 and 24 h; ↑ oxidative enzymes (SOD, GpX and GST)	[17]
	Mongolian Gerbils (n = 9) and bilateral common carotid arteries occluded (7 minutes) and administered allicin (20, 40 or 80 mg/kg, intragastric) for 7 days; ↑ SOD	[18]
Kidney toxicity (ConA)	Concanavalin A (15 mg/kg injected subcutaneously) administered to Sprague Dawley rats (n = 6) with or without allicin (50 mg/kg/day via gavage) for 28 days; renal tissue from animals treated with allicin demonstrated ↑ GSH and SOD	[19]
Chronic kidney disease	Wistar rats (n = 6) model created by kidney ablation and administered allicin (40 mg/kg orally) for 6 weeks then cardiac tissue with and without allicin compared; allicin ↑ CAT, SOD and GpX compared with CKD animals that had not received allicin	[20]
Chronic kidney disease	Wistar rats (n = 12 per group) model created by kidney ablation and administered allicin (40 mg/kg orally), losartan alone (20 mg/kg/day) or allicin plus losartan for 6 weeks then kidney tissue for three treatments compared with controls; renal cortex ↑ SOD similar for both allicin and losartan although losartan was better at restoring CAT than allicin	[21]
LPS-induced stress	Sprague Dawley rats (n = 20) given 80 mg/kg allicin by IV tail injection for 8 days after being given LPS (5 mg/kg) by injection; ↑ GpX and SOD in bronchoalveolar lung tissue	[22]
Bacterial infection	New Zealand rabbits (n =50, 5 groups), four groups infected with *Pasteurella multocida* (2 x 10^5 infected RBC i.n.); control, untreated, allicin (50 mg/kg/day, orally), norfloxacin (100 mg/kg/day, orally) or allicin and norfloxacin combined; allicin and allicin-norfloxacin groups showed ↑ SOD	[23]
OA	Albino rats (n =6) given 100 mg/kg of allicin or piroxicam by gavage. OA provoked by 0.01 ml turpentine oil injected into knee joint and changes assessed after 6 h; allicin believed to exert anti-inflammatory effects by ↓ROS through ↑ GpX and CAT	[24]
SAH	Sprague Dawley rats (n = 15) treated with allicin (70 mg/kg i.p.) 30 minutes after injection of blood into pre-chiasmatic cistern; ↑ oxidative enzymes (SOD, GSH)	[25]
Toxicity of glycidamide (brain, liver)	Balb/c mice (n = 5 per group) administered glycidamide (50 mg/kg by i.p. injection) for 7 days then allicin (5, 10 or 20 mg/kg intragastrically) plus glycidamide for 7 more days; ↑ in GpX, GSH and SOD following allicin (20 mg/kg) treatment with tissue responsiveness of liver > kidney > brain > lung	[26]

redox enzymes include CAT (catalase), GpX (glutathione peroxidase), GR (glutathione reductase), GSH (glutathione), GST (glutathione transferase), SOD (superoxide dismutase) and thioredoxin

Abbreviations used in the table: AD (Alzheimer's disease), ASCI (acute spinal cord injury), h (hour), HUVEC (human vein endothelial cells), IBD (inflammatory bowel disease), i.n. (intranasal), i.p. (intraparenterally), IS (ischemic stroke), LPS (lipopolysaccharide), OA (osteoarthritis), OP (osteoporosis), PkD (Parkinson's disease), ROS (reactive oxygen species), SAH (subarachnoid hemorrhage)

Dosages of allicin used for the six *in vitro* studies are in the micromolar range and similar to each other, allowing for realistic comparisons to be made [4-9]. The sixteen *in vivo* studies varied between 20 and 180 mg/kg allicin given for as little as thirty minutes [25], to more than one month [10, 11, 14, 19-21, 26] after the experimental condition was established. Route of administration for the animal models was via the oral route for ten studies [10, 11, 13, 16-18, 20, 21, 23, 24] and injection for the remaining seven [12, 14, 15, 19, 22, 25, 26]. The dosages are realistic given that an achievable physiological concentration of allicin, would be of the order of 37 mg/g, which is comparable to levels in freshly chopped cloves [73]. Several of the animal studies have reproducibly focused on allicin's effects on acute or chronic changes in redox levels in three major organ systems, namely the kidney [19-21, 26], liver [15, 26] and brain [10-13, 17, 18, 25, 26]. Allicin's effects on promoting antioxidant enzymes has been studied the most frequently using acute (acute spinal cord injury, ischemic stroke, subarachnoid hemorrhage) and chronic (Alzheimer's; AD) models of neurodegenerative disease [10-13, 17, 18, 25, 26]. Both short-term [25] and long term [10-13, 17, 18, 26] neuroprotection was also seen in these models (see Chapter 12 for more details). In all seven *in vivo* studies allicin (20-180 mg/kg/ day) administration was associated with an increase in antioxidant enzyme expression in the *ex vivo* brain tissues, and also corroborated by a single *in vitro* study [9].

Interestingly, one study in which allicin was injected identified that different tissues varied in their responsiveness to allicin administration with the liver, kidneys and brain being most responsive and the lung least responsive [26]. This may represent the primary clearance of allicin through the liver, when it is introduced directly into the circulation [26]. Injected allicin (30 mg/kg) was effective at reducing arsenic-induced damage in a rat model of toxicity [15] and at lower levels (4.2-12.6 mg/kg/day) reduced the damage to cardiac myocytes in a rodent model of exhaustive stress [14]. Allicin given orally (15 or 40 mg/kg) was also able to elevate antioxidant enzymes in three separate studies of chronic kidney disease [19-21].

So why have researchers examined inflammatory models of these particular organ systems with respect to allicin's effects on antioxidant enzymes? Mammalian liver, brain, kidney and heart have the highest metabolic activity of the body, with brain and liver being the most active [74]. This elevated metabolism also correlates with more ROS and have developed responsive antioxidant systems as a result, particularly in the liver [75] and brain [76]. It also means that during acute or chronic inflammation when infiltrating neutrophils and macrophages generate additional ROS [63] the balance may be difficult to maintain in these organs [75, 76]. Chronic production of ROS (often referred to as oxidative stress) is associated with various inflammatory syndromes, especially in these organs, including atherosclerosis [64], cirrhosis [75] and neurodegenerative conditions [76]. Although not mirrored by any human trials, the biochemical effects of allicin on the redox environment clearly warrant further study, particularly in those conditions for which effective strategies are not currently available.

3. Allicin and Nrf2

Nine studies have appeared in the literature to suggest that allicin has efficacy in ameliorating the redox environment in acute and chronic inflammatory conditions by upregulating the expression of Nrf2 [5, 10, 11, 15, 20, 21, 27-29]. A description of the experimental design and results of these studies is shown in Table 2.

Only a single *in vitro* study was performed on the effects of allicin (40 μg/ml) on an inflammation model in human endothelial cells [5]. The eight *in vivo* studies varied between 20 and 250 mg/kg allicin given for as little as one week [15], to more than one month [10, 11, 20, 21, 27-29] after the experimental condition was established. Route of administration for the animal models was via the oral route for seven studies [10, 11, 15, 20, 21, 28, 29] and injection for the remaining investigation [26]. The dosages are realistic given that an achievable physiological concentration of allicin [73]. Several of the animal studies have reproducibly focused on allicin's effects on acute or chronic changes in Nrf2 levels in four major organ systems, namely the kidney [20, 21], liver [15], brain [10, 11, 27] and heart [28, 29]. Five of these eight studies demonstrated allicin increased both antioxidant enzyme levels as well as

Nrf2 levels in animal models of AD [10, 11], chronic kidney disease [20, 21], arsenic-induced liver damage [15].

Table 2. Allicin studies reporting significant increase in Nrf2 expression

In vitro model	Experimental design	Reference
Infection	HUVECs treated with allicin (40 μg/ml) and LPS (1 μg/ml) for 24 h: allicin ↑ Nrf2 expression	[5]
AD	20-month old male C57BL/6 mice (n =16 per group) received allicin (180 mg/kg/day, oral) for 8 weeks. Compared with 3-month old and 20-month old C57BL/6 mice; ↑ Nrf2 activity and of downstream targets NQ01 and γ-GCS	[10]
	Sprague Dawley rats (n = 12, 4 groups) treated with allicin (180 mg/kg oral) or sulforaphane (12 mg/kg oral) for 16 weeks then injected into lateral ventricle with tunicamycin (TM) (5 μl); Both allicin and sulforaphane ↑ Nrf2 activity and of downstream targets NQ01 and γ-GCS	[11]
ASCI	Sprague Dawley rats (n = 18, 3 groups) treated with allicin (2, 10 or 50 mg/kg i.p.) immediately after undergoing laminectomy and having rod-damage spinal cord. Changes assessed at 7, 14, and 21 days post trauma. ↑ expression of Nrf2 (astrocyte and neuronal); blocking Nrf2 with specific inhibitors ↓ allicin protection	[27]
Cardiac Hypertrophy	Sprague Dawley rats (n=9) infused with angiotensin (250 mg/kg via osmotic pump) for 14 days and fed allicin (180 mg/kg) for 8 weeks; ↑ Nrf2 in cardiac tissue compared with control animals without angiotensin	[28]
Chronic kidney disease	Wistar rats (n = 6 per group) model created by kidney ablation and administered allicin (40 mg/kg orally) for 6 weeks then cardiac tissue with and without allicin compared; allicin ↓ serum BUN and creatinine indicating renal improvement and ↓ angiotensin 1 receptor expression in the heart and ↑ Nrf2 and ↓Keap compared with CKD animals that had not received allicin	[20]
Chronic kidney disease	Wistar rats (n = 12 per group) model created by kidney ablation and administered allicin (40 mg/kg orally), losartan alone (20 mg/kg/day) or allicin plus losartan for 6 weeks then kidney tissue for three treatments compared with controls; renal cortex ↑ Nrf2 and ↓ Keap expression was similar for allicin and losartan	[21]
Diabetes	Fructose fed (65% of feed) Sprague Dawley rats (n = 7) also supplemented 250 mg/ kg/day fresh garlic homogenate for 8 weeks; ↑ Nrf2 in cardiac tissue compared with control animals without fructose	[29]
Hepatotoxicity (arsenic-induced)	Wistar rats (n = 24) administered allicin (30 mg/kg by i.p. injection) 1 h before arsenic oxide (3 mg/kg) given by gavage for 7 days; ↑ Nrf2 in liver tissue using a KLF9 mechanism and associated with ↓ AST and ALT enzymes in blood and hepatic tissues	[15]

Abbreviations used in the table: AD (Alzheimer's disease), ALT (alanine transferase), ASCI (acute spinal cord injury), AST (aspartame transferase), BUN (blood urea nitrogen), γ-GCS (gamma glutamyl cysteine synthase), h (hour), HUVEC (human vein endothelial cells), i.p. (intraparenterally), Keap (Kelch ECH associating protein-1 system), KLF9 (Krueppel-like factor 9), NQO1 (NADPH quinone dehydrogenase 1), Nrf2 (NF-E2, p45-related factor 2)

Further studies of allicin's mechanism upregulation of Nrf2 has come from five animal studies [10, 11, 15, 20, 21]. Two rodent models of AD [10, 11] documented that long term administration of allicin (180 mg/ kg/day) for eight or sixteen weeks increased hippocampal expression of Nrf2 together with downstream targets gamma glutamyl cysteine synthase (γ-GCS) and and NADPH quinone dehydrogenase 1 (NQO1). NQO1 expression is also induced by Nrf2 and protects cells against oxidative stress by acting on endogenous cellular quinones, preventing apoptosis [77]. γ-GCS is the first enzyme in the synthetic cascade that results in GSH, so this may be the primary target for allicin in this pathway [78]. One animal study of arsenic-induced hepatotoxicity [15] demonstrated allicin (30 mg/kg i.p.) increased expression of SOD and GpX as well as Nrf2 and its downstream target Krueppel-like factor 9 (KLF9). KLF9 is another important independent responder to cellular oxidative stress and modulates cell death and oxidative injury [15]. Activation of Nrf2 by allicin, which results in upregulation of NQ01, γ-GCS and KFL9, provides a negative feedback for NF-κB activity [66]. Through inhibiting NF-κB, Nrf2 also inhibits expression of cyclooxygenase 2 (COX-2) genes, whose products are implicated in chronic inflammation [66]. Nrf2 also suppresses vascular endothelial adhesion molecules (VCAM-1 and ICAM-1), as well as blood vessel inducing (angiogenesis) factors that include metalloproteinases (MMP) [66]. This cenral effect of allicin on Nrf2 thereby has widespread effects on controlling the inflammatory process.

4. Allicin and NF-κB

Fourteen studies, six *in vitro* and eight *in vivo*, have appeared in the literature to suggest that allicin has efficacy in reducing NF-κB expression environment in inflammatory conditions [5, 15, 16, 22, 29-38]. A description of the experimental design and results of these studies is shown in Table 3.

The eight *in vivo* studies varied between 20 and 250 mg/kg allicin given for as little as one week [15, 16, 22, 36, 38], to more than one month [29, 35, 37] after the experimental condition was established. Route of administration for the animal models was via the oral route for five of the eight studies [16, 29, 35-37] and injection for the remaining investigations [15, 22, 38]. The dosages are realistic given that an achievable physiological concentration of allicin [73].

The studies investigating the effects of allicin on NF-κB expression focused primarily on four areas, namely models of infection [5, 22, 33, 34, 37], diabetes [29, 30, 35], cartilage and bone damage [31, 32, 38] and toxic or cirrhotic liver [15, 36]. Three of the *in vitro* studies [5, 33, 34] and two *in vivo* studies [22, 37] investigated allicin's effects on NF-κB in models of infection. Allicin has been investigated both *in vitro* (40 μg/ml and 100 μM) and *in vivo* (80 mg/kg) in bacterial models of toxic shock i.e., using lipopolysaccharide (LPS)[5, 22, 34]. In all three models, NF-κB expression was significantly reduced [5, 22, 34] and for the *in vivo* model this correlated with a decrease in bronchial swelling [34]. Although a much higher dosage was ultilized for the vesicular stomatitis virus (VSV)(10-50 mg/ml) [33], this is also one of the earliest antiviral studies on allicin. More recent antiviral *in vivo* studies have seen biochemical effects on NF-κB in the μg or μM range [37]. The large study of the effects of allicin (300 or 600 mg/kg) on the highly fatal reticuloendotheliosis virus (REV), demonstrated that a reduction in the expression of NF-κB, together with inflammatory cytokines was seen in the bird's thymus and speen [37]. Discussed further in Chapter 8, REV kills by inducing a shutdown of the immune system by producing a chronic inflammatory cascade [37]. Ultimately the immune system shrinkage or tumors that result from REV infection kill the animals and no preventative strategy exists [37].

Three models of diabetes, one *in vitro* [30] and two *in vivo* [29, 35] reported decreases in NF-κB expression in aortic cells [30], cardiac [29] and renal tissue [30]. Both *in vivo* studies gave allicin (50 or 250 mg/kg) to the diabetes-induced rats for either five [29] or eight [30] weeks before examining the animals' tissues. NF-κB was significantly decreased ($p<0.05$) in both studies [29, 35]. Induced rodent hepatic damage through arsenic (3 mg/kg)[15] or concanavalin A (15 mg/kg) [36] was associated with elevated NF-κB expression and this was significantly decreased by one week of allicin treatment (21 mg/kg or 30 mg/kg)[15, 36]. Whether this was a direct effect on NF-κB or due to Nrf2 increase (seen in two studies)[15, 29] is unclear however. Another mechanism of action for allicin was suggested by a single study on a murine model of inflammatory bowel disease (IBD) [16]. One week of allicin (10 mg/kg) treatment decreased the expression of STAT-3 [16]. As previously stated, STAT-3 is typically co-expressed with NF-κB and its activation is associated with synthesis of NO [58, 59]. As will be discussed in the next section, the findings of several studies that allicin is able to impair inflammatory expression of NO [7, 31, 36, 39] may support this as a mechanism.

Table 3. Allicin studies reporting significant change in NF-κB/RANKL

***In vitro* models**	**Experimental design**	**Reference**
Diabetes	Murine aortic cell line (high glucose, ↓ oxygen) with allicin (10 μg/ml) for 24 h; ↓ NF-κB	[30]
OA	Murine chondrocytes pretreated with allicin (5 and 10 μM) for 2 h and stimulated with IL-1β for 24 h; ↓ NF-κB	[31]
	Human chondrocytes pretreated with allicin (2.5, 5 and 10 μM) for 1 h then stimulated with IL-1β for 30 minutes; ↓ NF-κB	[32]
Infection	Human monocyte (THP), rat fibroblast (MT-1) and human cervical (WISH) cells pretreated with allicin (10, 25 and 50 mg/ml) then inoculated with VSV; ↓ NF-κB effects seen in all three cell lines	[33]
	HUVECs treated with allicin (40 μg/ml) and LPS (1 μg/ml) for 24 h; ↓ NF-κB	[5]
	Human isolated white blood cells incubated with allicin (100 μM/L) and LPS (10 μg/ml) for 20 h ↓ NF-κB	[34]
Animal models	**Experimental design**	**Reference**
Diabetes	Fructose fed (65% of feed) Sprague Dawley rats (n = 7) also supplemented 250 mg/kg/day fresh garlic homogenate for 8 weeks; ↓ NF-κB seen in cardiac tissue	[29]
	Streptozotocin (50 mg/kg/ i.p.) in Wistar rats (n=6) after 30 days given allicin (16 mg/kg/day gavage) for another 4 weeks; ↓ NF-κB seen in renal cortex	[35]
Hepatic damage	Concanavalin A (15 mg/kg injected into tail vein) administered to Balb/c mice 7 days (n =10) prior to allicin (21 mg/kg/day via gavage); ↓ NF-κB seen in liver as early as 2 h after allicin administration	[36]
	Wistar rats (n = 24) administered allicin (30 mg/kg by I.P. injection) 1 h before arsenic oxide (3 mg/kg) given by gavage for 7 days; ↓ NF-κB seen in hepatic tissues	[15]
IBD	Balb/c mice (n= 6) given 2.5% DSS in drinking water with or without allicin (10 mg/kg) for 7 days; ↓ STAT-3 activation indicative of ↓ colonic NF-κB	[16]
***In vitro* models**	**Experimental design**	**Reference**
Infection	REV-infected white Leghorn chickens (two groups of n=40) treated with 300 mg/kg or 600 mg/kg allicin for 5 weeks; ↓ NF-κB seen in thymus and spleen	[37]
	Sprague Dawley rats (n=20) given 80 mg/kg allicin by IV tail injection for 8 days after receiving LPS (5 mg/kg) by injection; ↓ NF-κB seen in bronchoalveolar lung tissue	[22]
PD	Sprague Dawley rats (n =) for 7 days given allicin (4 or 8 mg/L injection); ↓ NF-κB gingivomucosal tissue, RANKL ↓ in osteoclast activity from rodent tibia	[38]

Abbreviations used in the table: h (hour), HUVEC (human vein endothelial cells), IL-1β (interleukin 1 beta), IV (intravenous), LPS (lipopolysaccharide), NF-κB (nuclear factor kappa beta), OA (osteoarthritis), PD (periodontal disease), RANKL (receptor activator for nuclear factor kappa beta ligand), REV (reticuloendotheliosis virus), STAT-3 (signal transducer and activator of transcription 3), VSV (vesicular stomatitis virus)

Two of the *in vitro* studies examined the effects of allicin on *in vitro* models of osteoarthritis (OA) [31, 32]. In both cases, low doses of allicin (2.5-10 μM) significantly ($p < 0.05$) decreased the chondrocyte expression of NF-κB [31, 32]. Chondrocyte damage, associated with upregulation of NF-κB and consequent reduction of cartilage components, is a hallmark of OA [79]. Discussed further in chapter 11, cartilage damage stimulates bone-destroying osteoclasts in underlying bone [79]. Bone destruction through activated osteoclasts is associated with several osteodegenerative conditions apart from OA including osteoporosis

(OP) and periodontal disease (PD) (see Chapter 11 for details). Interestingly, one very recent study described the ability of injected allicin (4 or 8 mg/L) to decrease the osteoclast expression of receptor activator for nuclear factor kappa beta ligand (RANKL) in a PD model of disease [38]. Taken together, these three studies suggest a direct effect of allicin on NF-κB and RANKL expression in this tissue.

5. Allicin and NO/NOS

Fourteen studies, nine *in vitro* and five *in vivo*, have appeared in the literature to suggest that allicin can affect nitric oxide synthase or NO expression in inflammatory conditions [4, 7, 19, 21, 31, 32, 36, 39-45]. A description of the experimental design and results of these studies is shown in Table 4.

The five *in vivo* studies varied between 10 and 50 mg/kg allicin given for as little as two days week [43], to more than one month [19, 21] after the experimental condition was established. Route of administration for the animal models was via the oral route for one of the studies [21] and injection for the remaining four investigations [19, 36, 43, 45]. The dosages are comparable with an achievable physiological concentration of allicin [73].

The studies investigating the effects of allicin on NOS or NO expression focused primarily on four areas, namely models of cardiac damage or circulatory damage [4, 7, 39-41], brain injury [42, 44, 45], hepatic or kidney damage [19, 21, 36] and OA [31, 32]. NO plays a particularly important role in both the cardiovascular system and brain [80, 81]. Three *in vitro* studies reported that allicin (0.2-500 μg/ml) increased the generation of NO from endothelial derived nitric oxide synthase (eNOS)[4, 40, 41]. One *in vitro* study reported that nitric oxide synthase (iNOS) was reduced in isolated cardiac myocytes [39] by allicin treatment (10-200 μM). A final *in vitro* study also reported a decrease in NO by allicin treatment (500 μg/ml) of activated HUVEC [7], although which NOS was affected was not described. A change in the source of NO levels is associated with the development and persistence of chronic cardiovascular disease [80]. In the healthy environment high NO from constitutional eNOS prevents the deposition of arterial plaques and iNOS is only observed following inflammation [80].

Of the three studies of allicin and NOS in neuronal tissues, two were performed on models of traumatic injury (TBI) [44, 45] and one using an *in vitro* model of spinal cord damage [42]. The two *in vitro* models observed that allicin (1-100 μM) pre-treatment either decreased iNOS but had no effects on neuronal NOS (nNOS) [42] or increased eNOS [44]. The effect of allicin on eNOS expression was confirmed by a rodent craniotomy model of TBI in which intraparenteral injection (10 or 50 mg/kg) was reported to increase phosphorylation of Enos [45]. In the brain there are three variants of NOS [81]. eNOS-derived NO plays a similar role as the general vasculature, namely maintaining the circulation and preventing inflammation [81]. iNOS is produced by central nervous system microglia and other glial cells only following inflammatory events [81]. nNOS is involved in neurotransmitter regulation as well as pain signals and is unique to this tissue [81]. Discussed further in Chapter 12, the potential ability of allicin to increase eNOS derived NO and decrease inflammatory or iNOS-derived NO would be expected to be neuroprotective.

Table 4. Allicin studies reporting significant effects on NO/NOS

In vitro models	Experimental design	Reference
Cardiac ischemia	H9c2 cells pre-treated with allicin (0.2, 0.5 and 1 μM 1 h) and exposed to hypoxic stress (5% CO_2, 95% N_2) for 12 h; ↑ eNOS-derived NO	[4]
	HUVEC incubated with TNF-α (5 ng/ml) in the presence or absence of allicin (500 μg/ml) for 20 h; ↓ NO release	[7]
	Myocytes from neonatal Wistar rats stimulated with LPS (10 μg/ml) in presence or absence of allicin (10, 40, 50 or 200 μM) for 24 hours; ↓ iNOS at higher concentrations (200 μM) by decreasing CAT-2 expression and ↑ at lower concentrations (50 μM)	[39]
Congestive heart failure	Wistar rats (n = 8-10 per treatment) were fed with raw garlic extract (1 g orally) for 3 weeks or 1 days before treatment with monocrotaline (60 mg/kg i.p.), euthanized 3 weeks later and coronary arteries isolated and contracted by raising intraluminal pressure (40 mm Hg); raw garlic preserved the ability of the right coronary arteries to respond to acetylcholine via eNOS derived NO. Boiled or aged garlic (which don't contain allicin) had no such effects.	[40]
Pulmonary artery disease	Rat isolated intralobular pulmonary arteries stimulated with indomethacin (5 mol/) and pre-contracted with phenylephrine (0.1-0.3 mol/L) in presence of allicin (garlic extract 0-500 μg/ml) for up to 10 minutes; allicin relaxed arteries within 3 minutes with an ED_{50} of ~100 μg/ml and ↑ eNOS-derived NO	[41]
OA	Isolated murine chondrocytes activated by incubation with IL-1β (10 ng/ml) in presence or absence of allicin (5 or 10 μM) for 24 h; ↓ IL-1β-induced iNOS activation	[31]
	Isolated human knee OA chondrocytes activated by incubation with IL-1β and incubated in presence or absence of allicin (2.5, 5 and 10 μM) for 24 h; ↓ IL-1β-induced iNOS activation	[32]
Spinal cord neuron damage	Rat spinal cord neurons pretreated with allicin (5 μM 30 minutes) and then activated with glutamate (5 mM) for 24 h; ↓iNOS but had no effects on nNOS	[42]
TBI	Isolated embryonic rat cortical neurons pretreated with allicin (1, 10, 50, 100 or 200 μM) 1 h before injury and assessed for 6-48 h after; ↑ phosphorylated eNOS but not iNOS	[44]
Animal models	**Experimental design**	**Reference**
Hepatic damage	Concanavalin A (15 mg/kg injected into tail vein) administered to Balb/c mice 7 days (n =10) prior to allicin (21 mg/kg/day by gavage); ↓ iNOS seen on liver as early as 2 h after allicin administration	[36]
Kidney damage	Cyclosporine (15 mg/kg injected subcutaneously) administered to Sprague Dawley rats (n = 6) with or without allicin (50 mg/kg/day via gavage) for 28 days; renal tissue from animals treated with allicin demonstrated ↑ nitric oxide activity (eNOS as renoprotective?)	[19]
Kidney damage	Wistar rats (n = 12 per group) model created by kidney ablation and administered allicin (40 mg/kg orally), losartan alone (20 mg/kg/day) or allicin plus losartan for 6 weeks then kidney tissue for three treatments compared with controls; renal cortex ↑ eNOS with allicin being more effective than losartan	[21]
Malaria infection	Balb/c mice (n = 9) infected with *Plasmodium yoelii* (1 x 10^6 infected RBC i.p.), given allicin (3 or 9 mg/kg/day) for 2 days post infection and splenocytes examined; allicin restored acute inflammatory response to parasitemia by elevating levels of macrophage-derived NO (iNOS)	[43]
TBI	Rats (two groups of 18) treated with allicin (10 or 50 mg/kg i.p.) immediately after craniotomy and up to 8 h after. Changes assessed for 7 days; ↑ phosphorylation of eNOS	[45]

Abbreviations used in the table: CO_2 (carbon dioxide), eNOS (endothelial nitric oxide synthase), h (hour), HUVEC (human vein endothelial cells), IL-1β (interleukin 1 beta), iNOS (inducible nitric oxide synthase), i.p. (intraparenteral), nNOS (neuronal nitric oxide synthase), N_2 (nitrogen), NO (nitric oxide), OA (osteoarthritis), TBI (traumatic brain injury), TNF-α (tumor necrosis factor alpha)

Chronic inflammation in liver and kidney disease is associated with upregulation of iNOS indirectly through cellular exposure to pro-inflammatory cytokines or directly by NF-κB activation [82, 83]. In the liver the macrophage-like Kupffer cells are primarily responsible for iNOS synthesis although NO can be secreted through this pathway by all hepatic cells [82]. A single *in vivo* study of a murine model of hepatic damage reported that allicin (21 mg/kg orally) decreased iNOS expression as rapidly as two hours after concanavalin A was injected [36]. Healthy kidney function appears to require a balance between constitutive eNOS expression and induced iNOS and is highly sensitive to redox stress [83]. Studies using targeted inhibitors have shown that either upregulation of eNOS and or downregulation of iNOS during chronic kidney inflammation can prevent renal failure [82]. Two *in vivo* studies of allicin (20 or 50 mg/kg/day) documented a reduction in kidney damage associated with increased expression of eNOS activity [19, 21]. Both were recently performed by the same research group and the second reported that allicin (40 mg/kg/day) was more effective than the angiotensin inhibitor losartan (20 mg/kg/day) [21]. Dysregulation of NO synthesis through inflammatory upregulation of iNOS production by chondrocytes in the articulating cartilage has also been implicated in the etiology of OA [84]. Two recent *in vitro* studies have reported the ability of allicin (2.5-10 μM) to impair iNOS secretion by a cytokine-actvated human chondrocyte model of OA [31, 32].

Finally, allicin (3 or 9 mg/kg/day) was reported in a single *in vivo* study to increase macrophage iNOS secretion in an acute murine malarial infection [43]. Although at first glance this is a confusing effect, this suggests allicin is an adaptogen like many other phytochemicals [57] and thus restores balance rather than impairing or increasing NOS pathways.

6. ALLICIN AND P13K/AKT

Eight studies, five *in vitro* and three *in vivo*, have appeared in the literature to suggest that allicin can affect P13K/Akt expression in inflammatory conditions [8, 14, 22, 29, 31, 44, 46, 47]. A description of the experimental design and results of these studies is shown in Table 5.

Five *in vitro* studies have investigated the effect of allicin (1-100 μM) on separate models of inflammation [8, 31, 44, 46, 47] and excepting the TBI [44] allicin significantly decreased P13K/Akt expression in all these models. Two of the three animal models of chronic inflammation also documented a decrease in P13kAkt expression after allicin (80 or 250 mg/kg/ day) was administered for at least eight days [22, 29]. Administration of lower dose allicin (4-12 mg/kg/day) was reported as ameliorating the exhaustive cardiac stress of rodents through a FOXO3a activation of Akt and sirtuin pathway [14]. Suppression of the P13K/ Akt pathway is easy to explain as it would be associated with a consequent decrease in inflammation, cell demise and would be cytoprotective [62]. So why the differential responses of P13K/Akt in the two cardiac studies [14, 47]? Interestingly, activation of P13K/Akt and upregulation of the forkhead protein FOXO3a is cardioprotective [85]. Thus, the ability of allicin to activate this pathway both *in vitro* [47] and *in vivo* [14] would suggest that this is an additional anti-inflammatory activity for the thiosulfinate.

Table 5. Allicin studies reporting significant alteration in P13K/Akt

***In vitro* models**	**Experimental design**	**Reference**
Angiogenesis	BAEC grown to monolayers (48 h) and treated with allicin (0.2, 0.5, 2 and 4 μM) ↓ phosphorylation of Akt	[46]
Cardiac Hypertrophy	Neonatal rat cardiomyocytes (Wistar rats) incubated with angiotensin (100 nM) for 48 hours then treated with either allicin (25, 50 or 100 μM) or control for a further 48 h; Allicin ↑ phosphorylation of Akt and P13K (50 μM) Effects of 50 μM allicin were reversed by rapamycin (1 μM) indicating these effects are mediated through the P13K/Akt/MTOR pathway	[47]
OA	Murine chondrocytes pretreated with allicin (5 and 10 μM) for 2 h and stimulated with IL-1β for 24 h; ↓ Akt	[31]
OP	Murine osteoblast-like line MC3-T3-E1 cells treated with hydrogen peroxide (200 μM) for 6 h then allicin (10, 30 or 100 μg/ml) for 24 h; ↓ Akt	[8]
TBI	Isolated embryonic rat cortical neurons pretreated with allicin (1, 10, 50, 100 or 200 μM) 1 h before injury and assessed for 6-48 h after; Allicin ↑ phosphorylation of Akt	[44]
Diabetes	Fructose fed (65% of feed) Sprague Dawley rats (n = 7) also supplemented 250 mg/ kg/day fresh garlic homogenate for 8 weeks; ↓ P13K/Akt in cardiac tissue compared with control animals	[29]
Animal models	**Experimental design**	**Reference**
Exhaustive cardiac stress	Sprague-Dawley rats (n= 8 per group) underwent exhaustive swimming training for 7 weeks and supplemented with allicin (4.2, 6.3 or 12.6 mg/kg i.p.); ↑ FOXO3a activation of Akt and sirtuin pathway protecting cardiac tissue	[14]
Infection (LPS-induced stress)	Sprague Dawley rats (n=20) given 80 mg/kg allicin by IV tail injection for 8 days after being given LPS (5 mg/kg) by injection; ↓ P13K/Akt in bronchoalveolar lung tissue compared with control animals	[22]

Abbreviations used in the table: i.p. (intraparenteral), IV (intravenous), BAEC (bovine aortic endothelial cells), FOXO3a (foxhead protein), h (hour), LPS (lipopolysaccharide), OA (osteoarthritis), OP (osteoporosis), P13K/Akt (phosphoinositide-3-phosphate/ protein kinase B), TBI (traumatic brain injury)

7. Allicin and MAPK

Ten studies, seven *in vitro* and three *in vivo*, have appeared in the literature to suggest that allicin can affect one or more of the MAPK pathways during inflammatory conditions [8, 12, 18, 37, 44, 47-49, 51, 52]. A description of the experimental design and results of these studies is shown in Table 5.

Four of the MAPK studies on inflammatory models were performed on the central nervous system [12, 18, 44, 52]. Three of the studies, one *in vitro* [44], and two *in vivo* [12, 52] reported suppression of the MAPK, ERK [44], JNK [52] or p38 [12]. Brain inflammation, especially AD, appears to involve sequential activation of all three MAPK pathways with JNK and p38 particularly being involved in the generation of neurofibrillary tangles [86]. Allicin's abiliy to impair this activation in models of AD [12, 52] and TBI [44] decreased neuronal apoptosis in these models. The final *in vivo* study of ischemic stroke reported ERK as being suppressed by the animals' carotid arteries being occluded and returned to normal unoperated levels by allicin (20-80 mg/kg/day) treatment [18]. Given that this latter study reported a simultaneous activation of SOD [18], and that ERK are activated by growth factors or mitogens [87], allicin may be involved in the immediate healing process occurring in the animals following neuronal damage. Elevated ERK was also observed following allicin treatment in three other studies;

Table 6. Allicin studies reporting significant effects on MAPK#

Models	Experimental design	Results	Reference
In vitro: TBI	Embryonic rat cortical neurons pretreated with allicin (1, 10, 50, 100 or 200 μM) 1 h before injury and assessed for 6-48 h after	↓ERK expression but not total protein levels. Inhibitor studies determined allicin directly affected Akt and ERK pathways	[44]
In vitro: PBMC	Human healthy PBMC incubated for 2 h, stimulated with PHA (20 μg/ml) in the presence or absence of allicin (10 μg/ml)	Allicin ↑ ERK expression through modification of $p21^{ras}$ protein	[51]
In vivo; AD	Kunming mice (n =20) AD model (Aβ injected into brains); allicin (180 mg/kg/ day for 14 days injected i.p.) and compared with PBS	↓p38 levels (preventing neuronal apoptosis)	[12]
In vivo; AD	APP/PS1 4-month old Mice (n = 6); allicin (10 mg/kg/day by gavage) or corn oil for 3 months	↓JNK levels (preventing neuronal apoptosis)	[52]
In vivo IS	Mongolian Gerbils (n = 9) carotid arteries occluded (7 minutes) and administered allicin (20, 40 or 80 mg/kg, intragastric) for 7 days	↑ depressed ERK 1/2 (80 mg/kg allicin) ↑ neurological function all doses.	[18]
In vitro: Cardiac Hypertrophy	Neonatal rat cardiomyocytes (Wistar rats) incubated with angiotensin (100 nM, 48 h) then treated with either allicin (25, 50 or 100 μM) or control for a further 48 h	p-ERK ↑ following allicin treatment compared with that in Ang II-treated cardiomyocytes ($p < 0.01$)	[47]
In vitro and *in vivo:* Obesity	*In vitro*: Murine 3T3-L1 adipocytes exposed to allicin (0-100 ng/ml) for 7 days *In vivo*: C57BL/6J mice (n = 5, per group) fed high fat diet for 8 weeks with or without allicin (1mg/kg every 2 days)	Allicin treatment ↑ERK preventing the change of the adipocytes from white to brown (i.e., bad to good or easy mobilized adipose)	[48]
In vitro: OP	Murine osteoblast-like line MC3-T3-E1 cells treated with hydrogen peroxide (200 μM) for 6 h then allicin (10, 30 or 100 μg/ml) for 24 h	ERK ↑ following treatment with all concentrations of allicin	[8]
In vitro: tuberculosis infection	Peritoneal macrophages derived from C57BL/6 mice infected with *TB* and treated with allicin (30 μg/ml, 1 h)	↑ JNK, ↓ p38 No change in non-phosphorylated levels of SAP/JNK/ p38	[49]
In vivo: REV Infection	REV-infected white Leghorn chickens (two groups of n=40) treated with 300 mg/kg or 600 mg/kg allicin for 14 days	↓elevated ERK, JNK and p38 expression induced by REV in thymus spleen and bursa of animals.	[37]

ERK (extracellular initated kinase), JNK (Jun amino-terminal kinases)
Additional abbreviations used in table: AD (Alzheimer's disease), Ang-II (angiotensin), h (hour), IS (ischemic stroke), OP (osteoporosis), PBMC (peripheral blood mononuclear cells), PHA (phytohemagglutinin), REV (reticuloendotheliosis virus), SAP (stress activated protein kinases), TB (*Mycobacterium tuberculosis*).

three *in vitro* (0-200 nM allicin) [8, 47, 48] and an *in vivo* study (1 mg/kg) [48]. In each of these studies allicin treatment and ERK elevation was associated with either decreased cell death [8, 47] or prevention of terminal differentiation [48] i.e., the pathway was growth related. Allicin's effects on ERK may also relate to its effects on a specific ERK pathway protein, $p21^{ras}$, according to a study published by Patya and colleagues [51]. Healthy peripheral blood mononuclear cells (PBMC) were found to exhibit elevated ERK levels tbetween ten and fifteen minutes after allicin (10 μg/ml) incubation that returned to unstimulated, control levels after thiry minutes [51]. Using T cell leukemia (Jurkat cells) and their mutants, Patya and colleagues [51] also pointed towards allicin's effect on ERK as involving the $p21^{ras}$ protein. The $p21^{ras}$ contains six cysteine residued and is known to be activated following thiol modulation as well as the cellular redox environment [88]. Allicin's redox activities and those on ERK may represent two separate activities, although they clearly impact each other.

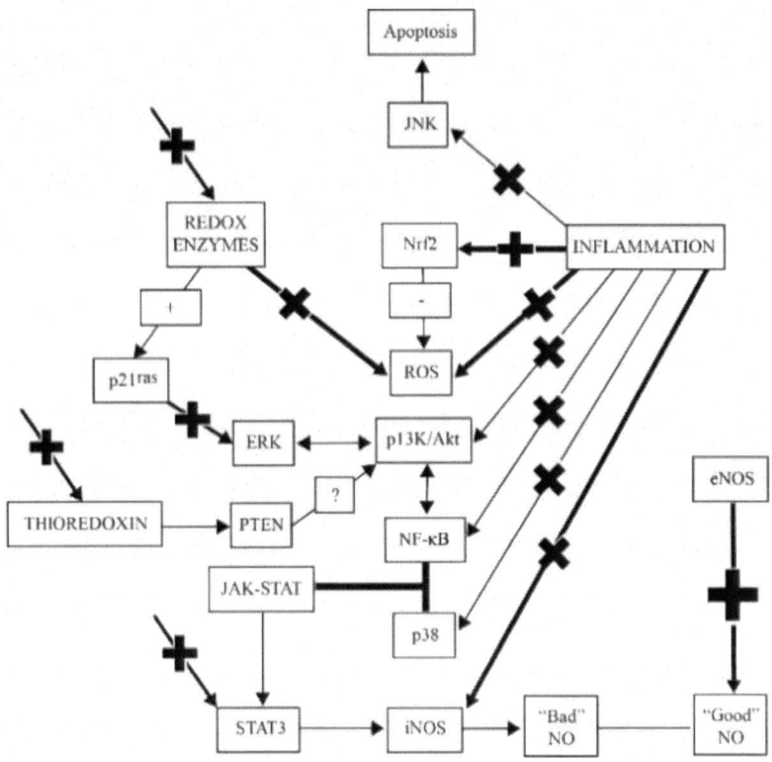

✖ = allicin inhibition ✚ = allicin enhances

Legend: Several pathways are involved in cellular inflammation including NF-κB, Nrf2, P13K/Akt and the three MAPK pathways JNK, ERK and p38. Infllammation also requires tipping the balance of NO synthesis away from between "healthy" eNOS and towards iNOS-derived NO. Allicin decreases inflammation of healthy cells primarily by balancing the redox enzymes resulting in a decrease of ROS and stimulation of Nrf2. Resetting of the eNOS:iNOS-derived NO balance is also a major target for allicin. Thioredoxin may also be a target of allicin and in turn affect regulation of Akt phosphrorylation through PTEN. These four major interventional targets are shown by heavy arrows. Secondary sites of intervention are through interaction with the Akt component of P13K/Akt. These pathways are shown by lighter arrows and in turn downregulate the central "hub" of NF-κB activation and allow cell survival and return to health.

Abbreviations: Bax (apoptosis regulator Bax), Bcl-2 (B-cell lymphoma 2) ERK (extracellular-initiated kinase), iNOS (inducible nitric oxide synthase), JAK-STAT(Janus-kinase signal transductors/activators of transcription), JNK (Jun amino-terminal kinases), NF-κB (nuclear factor kappa beta), NO (nitric oxide), Nrf2 (NF-E2, p45-related factor 2), P13K/Akt (phosphoinositide-3 phosphate/protein kinase B), PTEN (phosphatase and tensin homolog), ROS (reactive oxygen species), STAT3 (signal transducer and activator of transcription 3).

References used to construct diagram: [4-68, 90].

Figure 2. Allicin inhibition points of biochemical pathways of inflammation.

Allicin was reported to variably affect JNK and decrease p38 in two models of chronically-carried infections, namely tuberculosis [49] and REV [37]. Most microbes inactivate JNK as this allows their surivival within a host but some also inactivate p38 by tampering with a protein upstream of both [89]. A good example of this is *Mycobacterium tuberculosis*, which proliferates within macrophages and shuts down both the JNK and p38 pathways of those cells [89]. The ability of allicin (30 μg/ml for 1 hour) to remediate the JNK suppression in *ex vivo* tuberculosis-infected macrophages would allow their removal [49]. This latter fact was further reported by the authors who stated that allicin treatment *"promoted a strong Th1 response leading to a drastic reduction in the mycobacterial burden"* [49]. In contrast, intracellular microbes, like viruses, instead promote co-activation of JNK and NF-κB by mimicking TNF receptors and therefore allow cell survival [61]. Suppression of JNK produced by allicin (300 or 600 mg/kg) in the *in vivo* model of REV would thereby decrease viral survival [37].

8. Putting It All Together; Biochemical Targets for Allicin

Allicin's effects on biochemical pathways have been researched in over fifty studies during the past forty years [3-56]. Strongest evidence exists for this thiosulfinate producing its effect by affecting the redox environment of the cell by targeting either GSH or thioredoxin enzymes [4-26] or binding to the Keap-1 subunit of Nrf2 [15, 20, 21]. Downregulation of Nrf2 and upregulating redox enzymes would downregulate NF-κB [66] and may therefore be an indirect biochemical effect of allicin. This may be an indirect anti-inflammatory mechanism for allicin fourteen studies of allicin and NF-κB [5, 15, 16, 22, 29-38]. Depression of NF-κB by allicin would in turn decrease p38 expression, as was seen in three studies [12, 37, 49]. In contrast, ERK expression is upregulated by allicin, putatively by directly modifiying the thiol groups or redox environment of the downstream $p21^{ras}$ protein or [51]. Since the last major review of allicin [68], evidence has also also emerged for an independent direct on the Akt component of the PI3K/Akt pathway [14, 46]. Interestingly, thioredoxin regulates the activity the of phosphatase and tensin homolog (PTEN), which in turn affects the phosphorylation of Akt and JNK [90]. Allicin's effects may therefore be directly against Akt and JNK or the relative activation of PTEN. A possible mechanistic approach for allicin is shown in Figure 2.

Currently the biochemical studies performed on allicin, whilst promising haven't extended past animal models, which are open to bias. Semi-synthetic, stable forms of allicin exist [91, 92] and double-blind randomized placebo-controlled trials (DBRPCT) could determine whether these biochemical effects translate into effective strategies for the management of human disease. Oxidative stress alone is now known to be a component of many aspects of acute and chronic inflammatory damage, especially that occurring in the brain and cardiovascular system [93]. Specific agonists, for example to Nrf2, are already under development especially from plant-derived products [93] and are expected to find multiple uses in chronic conditions including cardiovascular disease, neurodegenerative illnesses and tumors. Allicin may find a role here.

In addition, allicin possesses unique activities, including its ability to act as an agonist of FOXO3a [14], inhibit RANKL [38], and improve the balance of eNOS versus iNOS-derived NO [4, 39-41]. These effects would correlate with cardioprotective, osteoprotective activities, and neuroprotective activities respectively. Current medications for these conditions are less than selective and no such targeted therapies exist (see Chapters 10 and 11 for details). In addition, many patients with cardiovascular disease, osteoarthritis and neurodegeneration suffer from at least two of these conditions simultaneously [94]. Multiple medications prescribed for these patients (polypharmacy) as a result frequently lead to adverse events and the call for combined therapies [95]. Allicin's activities against at least three (and possibly six) biochemical pathways may provide the potential to provide a therapy, either alone or in combination with other classic or phytomedicines, for many chronic illnesses.

REFERENCES

[1] Cavallito, Chester J. & John, H. Bailey (1944). "Allicin, the Antibacterial Principle of Allium sativum. I. Isolation, Physical Properties and Antibacterial Action." *J. Am. Chem. Soc.*, *66*, 1950-1951. https://pubs.acs.org/doi/abs/10.1021/ja01239a048.

[2] Cavallito, Chester J. (1946). "Relationship of thiol structures to reaction with antibiotics." *J. Biol. Chem.*, *164*, 29-34.

[3] Wills, E. D. (1956). "*Enzyme inhibition by allicin, the active principle of garlic.*," *63*(3), 514-520. doi: 10.1042/bj0630514.

[4] Lina, Ma., Shangke, Chen., Shaochun, Li., Lijuan, Deng., Yikui, Li. & Hao, Li. (2018). "Effect of Allicin against Ischemia/Hypoxia-Induced H9c2 Myoblast Apoptosis via eNOS/NO Pathway-Mediated Antioxidant Activity." *Evidence-Based Complementary and Alternative Medicine*, Article ID 3207973. https://doi.org/10.1155/2018/3207973.

[5] Zhang, Min., Huichao, Pan., Yinjie, Xu., Xueting, Wang., Zhaohui, Qiu. & Li, Jiang. (2017). "Allicin decreases lipopolysaccharide-induced oxidative stress in human vein endothelial cells through suppression of mitochondrial dysfunction and activation of Nrf2." *Cellular Physiology and Biochemistry*, *41*, 2255-2267. https://www.karger.com/Article/FullText/475640

[6] Islam, Najmul., Iqbal, Jawed., Hasan, Nazarul., Fatima, Zeeshan., Thakur, Hamida., Hasan, Nazia, Mahdi., Abbas Ali, Khan., Tamkin, Bano Farzana. & Ansari, Irfan Ahmad. (2008). "Allicin from garlic suppresses TNF-α and augments IFN-γ expressions in monocyte cultures from patients with Vaginitis." Available from *Nature Precedings.* http://dx.doi.org/10.1038/npre.2008.1560.1.

[7] Mo, Sung-Ji., Eun-Wha, Son., Dongquan, Rhee. & Sukhneung, Pyo. (2003). "Modulation of TNF-alpha induced ICAM-1 expression, NO and H_2O_2 production by alginate, allicin, and ascorbic acid in human endothelial cells." *Arch Pharm Res*, *26*, 244-251. https://doi.org/10.1007/BF02976837.

[8] Ding, Guoling., Jinguan, Zhao. & Dianming, Jiang. (2016). "Allicin inhibits oxidative stress-induced mitochondrial dysfunction and apoptosis by promoting P13K/Akt and CREB/ERK signaling in osteoblast cells." *Experimental and Therapeutic Medicine*, *11*, 2553-2560. Doi:10.3892/etm.2016.3179.

[9] Liu, Hao., Ping, Mao., Jia, Wang., Tuo, Wang. & Chang-Hou, Xie. (2015). "Allicin protects PC12 cells against 6-OHDA-induced oxidative stress and mitochondrial dysfunction via regulating mitochondrial dynamics." *Cellular Physiology and*

Biochemistry, *36*, 966-979. Accessed on October 25, 2018. https://www.karger.com/Article/PDF/430271.

[10] Li, Xian-Hui., Chun-Yan, Li., Jiang-Ming, Lu., Rong-Bo, Tian. & Jia, Wei. (2012). "Allicin ameliorates cognitive deficits ageing-induced memory and learning deficits through enhancing of Nrf2 antioxidant signaling pathways." *Neuroscience Letters*, *514*, 46-50. doi: 10.1016/j.neulet.2012.02.054.

[11] Zhu, Yao-Feng., Xian-Hui, Li., Zhi-Peng, Yuan., Chun-Yan, Li., Rong-Bo, Tian., Wei, Jia. & Zhu-Ping, Zhao. (2015). "Allicin improves endoplasmic reticulum related stress-related cognitive deficits via PERK/Nrf2 antioxidative signaling pathway." *Eur. J. Pharmacol.*, *762*, 239-246. https://doi.org/10.1016/j.ejphar.2015.06.002.

[12] Li, Xian-Hui., Chun-Yan, Li., Zhi-Gang, Xiang., Fei, Chong., Zheng-Ying, Chen. & Jiang-Ming, Lu. (2010). "Allicin can reduce neuronal death and ameliorate the spatial memory impairment in Alzheimer's disease models." *Neurosciences (Riyadh)*, *15*(4), 237-243. Accessed on March 13, 2019. http://www.nsj.org.sa/PDFFILES/Oct10/Allicin20100060.pdf.

[13] Zhu, Jin-Wen., Tao, Chen., Jianzhong, Guan., Wen-bo, Liu. & Jian, Liu. (2012). "Neuroprotective effect of allicin on spinal cord ischemia-reperfusion injury via improvement of mitochondrial function in rabbits." *Neurochemistry International*, *61*(5), 640-648. https://doi.org/10.1016/j.neuint.2012.06.021.

[14] Fan, Yongyang., Ran, Zhang., Yang, Li., Caiyi, Lu., Feng, Xu., Chao, Zhu., Yutang, Wang. & Qiao, Xue. (2018). "Allicin prevents rat cardiomyocytes from oxidative injury and apoptosis during repeated exhaustive exercise via Akt and sirtuin 1 pathways." *Int. J. Clin. Exp. Med*, *11*(8), 7885-7895. http://ijcem.com/files/ijcem0068357.pdf.

[15] Yang, Daqian., Zhanjun, Lv., Haili, Zhang., Biying, Liu., Huijie, Jiang., Jingling, Lu., Ruiqi, Baiyun. & Zhigang, Zhang. (2017). "Activation of the Nrf2 signaling pathway involving KLF9 plays a critical role in allicin resisting against arsenic trioxide-induced hepatotoxicity in rats." *Biol Trace Elem Res*, *176*, 192-200. https://doi.org/10.1007/s12011-016-0821-1.

[16] Pandurangan, Ashok K., Salmiah, Ismail., Zeinab, Saadatdoust. & Norhaizan, Mohd. Esa. (2015). "Allicin Alleviates Dextran Sodium Sulfate- (DSS-) Induced Ulcerative Colitis in BALB/c Mice." *Oxidative Medicine and Cellular Longevity*: Article ID 605208. https://doi.org/10.1155/2015/605208.

[17] Kong, Xiangyi., Shun, Gong., Lijuan, Su., Chen, Li. & Yanguo, Kong. (2017). "Neuroprotective effects of allicin on ischemia-reperfusion brain injury." *Oncotarget*, *8*(61), 104492–104507. doi:10.18632/oncotarget.22355.

[18] Yu, Juan., Ru-Xia, Lu., Pen, Yang., Yong-Gan, Cao., Qian-Long, Zhang., Hui, Qiao, Qian Luo., Shu-Zhi, Li., Chang-Lin, Jiang. & Li-Hui, Qu. (2016). "Allicin attenuates global cerebral ischemia/reperfusion injury in gerbils via anti-oxidative and apoptotic pathway." *Int J. Clin. Exp. Med.*, *9*(2), 2375-2382. http://www.ijcem.com/files/ijcem0017226.pdf.

[19] El-Khashef, D. H., El-Kenawi, A. E., Suddek, G. M. & Salem, H. A. (2015). "Allicin ameliorates kidney function and urinary bladder sensitivity in cyclosporine A treated rats." *Human and Experimental Toxicology*, *36*(7), 681-691. doi: 10.1177/0960327116660864.

[20] García-Trejo, Ehécatl M. A., Abraham, S. Arellano-Buendía., Raúl, Argüello-García., María, L. Loredo-Menzoza., Fernando, E. García-Orroya., Moníca, G. Arrelano-

Mendoza., María, C. Castillio-Hernández., Gustavo, Guevara-Balcázar., Edilia, Tapia., Laura, G. Sánchez-Lozada. & Horacio, Osorio-Alonso. (2016). “Effects of Allicin on Hypertension and Cardiac Function in Chronic Kidney Disease.” *Oxidative Medicine and Cellular Longevity*, Article ID 3850402. https://doi.org/10.1155/2016/3850402.

[21] García-Trejo, Ehécatl M. A., Abraham, S. Arellano-Buendía., Omegar, Sanchez-Reyes., Fernando, E. García-Orroya., Raúl, Argüello-García., María, L. Loredo-Menzoza., Edilia, Tapia., Laura, G. Sánchez-Lozada. & Horacio, Osorio-Alonso. (2017). “The beneficial effects of allicin in chronic kidney disease are comparable to Losartan.” *International Journal of Molecular Sciences*, *18*, 1980. doi:10.3390/ijms18091980.

[22] Wang, Xudong., Xiao, Chang., Chao, Chen., Yi, Guo., Xiaoyang, Meng. & Chen, Kan. (2018). “Allicin attenuates lipopolysaccharide-induced acute lung injury in neonatal rats via the P13K/Akt pathway.” *Molecular Medicine Reports*, *17*(5), 6777-6783. https://doi.org/10.3892/mmr.2018.869.

[23] Alam, Rasha T. M., Elshaima, M. Fawzi., Maha, I. Alkhalf., Wafa, S. Alansari., Lotfi, Aleya. & Mohamed, M. Abdel-Daim. (2018). “Anti-Inflammatory, Immunomodulatory, and Antioxidant Activities of Allicin, Norfloxacin, or Their Combination against Pasteurella multocida Infection in Male New Zealand Rabbits,” Oxidative Medicine and Cellular Longevity, vol. 2018, Article ID 1780956, 10 pages, https://doi.org/10.1155/2018/1780956.

[24] Jayanthi, K., Naidu, Sushma., Pramod, V. & Sunil. (2017). “Antioxidant and antiarthritic activity of allicin in animal models.” *International Journal of Pharmaceutical Sciences and Research*, *26*, 1150-1155. Accessed on October 25, 2018. http://ijpsr.com/bft-article/antioxidant-and-antiarthritic-activity-of-allicin-in-animal-models/?view=fulltext.

[25] Shao, Jing., Qi, Wu., Sheng-yin, Lv., Xiao-ming, Zhou., Xiang-sheng, Zhang., Li-li, Wen., Xin, Xue. & Xin, Zhang. (2019). “Allicin attenuates early brain injury after experimental subarachnoid hemorrhage in rats.” *J. Clin. Neurosci.*, *63*, 202-208. https://www.sciencedirect.com/science/article/pii/S0967586818314103.

[26] Wang, En-Ting., Dong-yan, Chen., Huang-you, Liu., Hai-Yang, Yan. & Yuan, Yuan. (2015). “Protective effect of allicin against glycidamide toxicity in male and female mice.” *Gen. Physiol. Biophys.*, *34*, 177-187. doi: 10.4149/gpb_2014038.

[27] Lv, Runxiao., Ningfang, Mao., Jinhui, Wu., Chunwen, Lu., Muchen, Ding. & Xiaochuan, Gu. (2015). “Neuroprotective effect of allicin in a rat model of acute spinal cord injury.” *Life Sciences*, *143*, 114-123. http://dx.doi.org/10.016/j.lfs.2015.11.001.

[28] Li, Xian-Hui., Chun-Yan, Li., Zhi-Gang, Xiang., Jian-Jun, Hu., Jiang-Min, Lu., Rong-Bo, Tiang. & Wei, Jia. (2012). “Allicin ameliorates cardiac hypertrophy and fibrosis through enhancing of Nrf2 signaling pathways.” *Cardiovascular Drugs and Therapy*, *26*(6), 457-465. https://link.springer.com/article/10.1007%2Fs10557-012-6415-z.

[29] Padiya, Raju., Debrabrata, Chowdhury., Roshan, Borkar., Srinivas, R., Manika, P. Bhadra. & Sanjay, K. Banerjee. (2014). “Garlic Attenuates Cardiac Oxidative Stress via Activation of PI3K/AKT/Nrf2-Keap1 Pathway in Fructose-Fed Diabetic Rat.” *PLOS ONE*, *9*(5), e94228. https://doi.org/10.1371/journal.pone.0094228.

[30] Wang, Shu-Li., D-Shan, Liu., Er-Shun, Liang., Yan-Hua, Gao., Ying, Cui., Yu-Zhao, Liu. & Wei, Gao. (2015). Protective effect of allicin on high glucose/hypoxia-induced aortic endothelial cells via reduction of oxidative stress. *Experimental and Therapeutic Medicine*, *10*(4), 1394-1400. doi: 10.3892/etm.2015.2708.

[31] Qian, Yu-Qin., Zhen-Hua, Feng., Xiao-Bin, Li., Zhi-Chao, Hu., Jiang-Wei, Xuan., Xiang-Yang, Wang., Hai-Chao, Xu. & Jiao-Xiang, Chen. (2018). "Downregulating P13/Akt/NF-κB signaling with allicin for ameliorating the progression of osteoarthritis". *Food Funct.*, *19*, 9(9), 4865-4875. doi: 10.1039/c8fo01095a.

[32] Wang, Lin., Hai-Tao, Pan., Bing, Wang., Yang, Liu., Kai, Fei. & Wei-Feng, Han. (2016). "Allicin reduces IL-1β-induced inflammatory cytokines via attenuating the NF-κβ and MMP-3 activation in human osteoarthritis chondrocyte model". *Int. J. Clin. Exp. Pathol.*, *9*(10), 10320-10326. Accessed March 21, 2019. http://www.ijcep.com/files/ijcep0034372.pdf.

[33] Shou, Chunchui., Nanchuan, Weng., Xichun, Chang., Lei, Feng., Hangping, Yao. & Nanping, Wu. (2015). "Effect of allicin on THP-1, MT-2 and WISH cell apoptosis induced by vesicular stomatitis virus (VSV) and the molecular mechanism involved." *African Journal of Biotechnology*, *10*(36), 7040-7047. doi: 10.5897/AJB11.184.

[34] Keiss Hans-Peter., Verena, M. Dirsch., Thomas, Hartung., Thomas, Haffner., Laurence, Trueman., Jacques, Auger., Remi, Kehane. & Angelique, M. Vollmar. (2003). "Garlic (*Allium sativum* L.) modulates cytokine expression in lipopolysaccharide-activated human blood thereby inhibiting NF-κB activity. " *Journal of Nutrition, 133* (7), 2171–2175. https://academic.oup.com/jn/article/133/7/2171/4688391.

[35] Arellano, Buendía., Abraham, S., Montserrat, Tostado González., Omegar, Sánchez Reyes., Fernando, E. García Arroyo., Raúl, Argüello García., Edilia, Tapia., Laura, G. Sánchez Lozada. & Horatio, Osario Alonso. (2018). "Immunomodulatory Effects of the Nutraceutical Garlic Derivative Allicin in the Progression of Diabetic Nephropathy." *International Journal of Molecular Sciences*, *19*(10), 3107. doi:10.3390/ijms19103107 https://www.ncbi.nlm.nih.gov/pmc/articles/PMC6212798/.

[36] Bruck, Rafael., Hussein, Aeed., Eli, Brazovsky., Talia, Noor. & Rami, Hershkoviz. (2005). "Allicin, the active component of garlic, prevents immune-mediated, concanavalin A-induced hepatic injury in mice." *Liver International*, *25*(3), 613-621. doi: 10.1111/j.1478-3231.2005.01050.x.

[37] Wang, Liyuang., Hongchao, Jiao., Jinpeng, Zhao., Xiaojuan, Wang., Shuhon, Sun. & Hai, Lin. (2017). "Allicin alleviates reticuloendotheliosis virus-induced immunosuppression via ERK/mitogen-activated protein kinase pathway in pathogen-free chickens" *Frontiers in Immunology*, *8*, 1856. Accessed November 16, 2018. doi: 10.3389/fimmu.2017.01856.

[38] Guan, Xiaoxu., Yi, Zhou., Hui, Chen., Chaowei, Wang. & Huiming, Wang. (2018). "Antibacterial, anti-inflammatory, and anti-osteoclastogenesis roles of allicin in periodontitis." *Int. J. Clin. Med.*, *11*(7), 6721-6730. Accessed on March 13, 2019 http://www.ijcem.com/files/ijcem0066740.pdf.

[39] Schwartz, Idit F., Rami, Hershkvitz., Adrian, Iana., Ehud, Gnessin., Yoram, Wollman., Tamara, Chernichowski., Miriam, Blum., Yoram, Levo. & Doran, Schwartz. (2002). "Garlic attenuates nitric oxide production in rat cardiac myocytes through inhibition of nitric oxide synthase and the arginine transporter CAT-2 (cationic arginine transporter-2)." *Clinical Science*, *102*(5), 487-493. doi: 10.1042/cs1020487.

[40] Ku, David D., Tarek, Abdel-Razek., Jarel, Dai., Sangae, Kim-Park., Michael, B. Fallon. & Gary, A. Abrams. (2002). "Garlic And Its Active Metabolite Allicin Produce Endothelium- And Nitric Oxide-Dependent Relaxation In Rat Pulmonary Arteries." *Clinical and Experimental Pharmacology and Physiology*, *29*, 84-91. doi:10.1046/j.1440-1681.2002.03596.x.

[41] Sun, Xiaowei. & David, D. Ku. (2006). "Allicin in garlic protects against coronary endothelial dysfunction and right heart hypertrophy in pulmonary hypertensive rats." *American Journal of Physiology-Heart and Circulatory Physiology*, *291*, 5, H2431-H2438. https://doi.org/10.1152/ajpheart.00384.2006.

[42] Liu, Shu-Guang., Peng-Yu, Ren., Guo-Yu, Wang., Shu-Xin, Yao. & Xi-Jing, He. (2015). "Allicin protects spinal cord neurons from glutamate-induced oxidative stress through regulating the heat shock protein 70/inducible nitric oxide synthase pathway." *Food Function*, *6*, 320-329. doi: 10.1039/C4FO00761A.

[43] Feng, Yonghui., Xiaotong, Zhu., Quinhui, Wang., Yongjun, Jiang., Hong, Shiang, Liwang, Cui. & Yaing, Cao. (2012). "Allicin enhances host pro-inflammatory responses and protects against acute murine malaria infection". *Malaria J.*, *11*, 268. Accessed on May 6, 2019. doi: 10.1186/1475-2875-11-268.

[44] Zhou, Yui-fei., Wen-tao, Li., Hong-chen, Han., Da-kuan, Guo., Xiao-sheng, He., Liang, Li., Jin-ning, Song. & Zhou, Fei. (2014). "Allicin protects rat cortical neurons against mechanical trauma injury by regulating nitric oxide synthase pathways." *Brain Research Bulletin*, *100*, 14-21. http://dx.doi.org/10.016/j.brainresbull.2013.10.013.

[45] Chen, Wei., Jun, Qi., Feng, Feng., Mao-de, Wang., Gang, Bao., Tuo, Wang., Mu, Xiang. & Wang-fu, Xie. (2014). "Neuroprotective effect of allicin against traumatic brain injury via Akt/endothelial nitric oxide synthase pathway-mediated anti-inflammatory and anti-oxidative mechanisms." *Neurochemistry International*, *68*, 28-37. http://dx/doi.org/10.016/j.neurint.2014.01.015.

[46] Sela, Uri., Alexander, Brill., Vyacheslav, Kalchenko., Olga, Dashevsky. & Rami, Hershkovitz. (2008). "Allicin inhibits blood vessel growth and downregulates Akt phosphorylation and actin polymerization." *Nutrition and Cancer*, *60*(3), 412-420. http://www.encognitive.com/files/Allicin%20Inhibits%20Blood%20Vessel%20Growth%20and%20Downregulates%20Akt%20Phosphorylation%20and%20Actin%20Polymerization.pdf.

[47] Ba, Lina., Jingquan, Gao., Yunping, Chen., Hanping, Qi., Chonghui, Dong., Hao, Pan., Qianhui, Zhang., Pilong, Shi., Chao, Song., Xueying, Guan., Yonggang, Cao. & Hongli, Sun. (2019). "Allicin attenuates pathological cardiac hypertrophy by inhibiting autophagy via activation of PI3K/Akt/mTOR and MAPK/ERK/mTOR signaling pathways." *Phytomedicine*, *58*, 152765. https://doi.org/10.1016/j.phymed.2018.11.025.

[48] Lee, Chung G., Dong Kwon, Rhee., Byung, Oh Kim., Sung, Hee Um. & Suhkneung, Pyo. (2019). "Allicin induces beige-like adipocytes via KLF15 signal cascade. " *The Journal of Nutritional Biochemistry*, *64*, 13-24. https://doi.org/10.1016/j.jnutbio.2018.09.014.

[49] Dwivedi, Ved P., Debapriya, Bhattacharya., Mona, Singh., Ashima, Bhaskar., Santosh, Kumar., Parveen, Sobia., Luc, Van Kaer. & Gobardhan, Das. (2018). Allicin enhances antimicrobial activity of macrophages during Mycobacterium tuberculosis infection. *Journal of Ethnopharmacology*. https://doi.org/10.1016/j.jep.2018.12.008.

[50] Mayeux, P. R., Agrawal, K. C., Jen-Sie, H. Tou., Barry, King., Lipton, H. N., Hyman, A. L., Kadowitz, J. L. & MacNamara, F. D. B. (1989). "The pharmacological effects of allicin, a constituent of garlic oil." *Agents Actions*, *25*(1-2), 182-190. doi: 10.1007/BF01969110.

[51] Patya, Miriam., Muayad, A. Zahalka., Alexey, Vanichkin., Aharon, Rabinkov., Talia, Miron., David, Mirelman., Meir, Wilchek., Harry, M. Lander. & Abraham,

Novogrodsky. (2003). "Allicin stimulates lymphocytes and elicits an antitumor effect: a possible role of p21^ras." *International Immunology, 16*(2), 275-281.

[52] Zhang, Hao., Ping, Wang., Yixue, Xue., Libo, Liu., Zhen, Li. & Yunhui, Liu. (2018). "Allicin ameliorates cognitive impairment in APP/PS1 mice via suppressing oxidative stress by blocking JNK signaling pathways." *Tissue and Cell, 50*, 89-95. doi:10.3389/fnana.2015.00032.

[53] Gupta, Nisha. & Todd, D. Porter. (2001). "Garlic and garlic-derived compounds inhibit human squalene monooxygenase". *J. Nutr., 131*, 1662–1667.

[54] Focke, Manfred, Andrea, Feld. & Harmut, K. Lichtenthaler. (1990). "Allicin, a naturally occurring antibiotic from garlic, specifically inhibits acetyl-CoA synthetase". *FEBS Lett., 261*, 106–108.

[55] Oi, Yuriko., Mika, Imafuku., Chiaki, Shishido., Yutaka, Kominato., Syoji, Nishimura. & Kazuo, Iwai. (2001). "Garlic Supplementation Increases Testicular Testosterone and Decreases Plasma Corticosterone in Rats Fed a High Protein Diet." *The Journal of Nutrition, 131*(8), 2150–2156, https://doi.org/10.1093/jn/131.8.2150.

[56] Yin, Lu., He, Zhuojin., Shen Xiuying, Shen., Xiaolu, Xu., Jie, Fan., Shaohu, Wu. & Deyong, Zhang. (2012). "Cholesterol-Lowering Effect of Allicin on Hypercholesterolemic ICR Mice." *Oxidative Medicine and Cellular Longevity*: Article ID 489690 https://doi.org/10.1155/2012/489690.

[57] Cundell, Diana R. (2014). Herbal phytochemicals as immunomodulators Current Immunology Reviews 2014, Volume 10 Issue 2 ISSN:1875-631X(Online), ISSN:1573-3955(Print) Accessed September 10, 2018. http://benthamscience.com/journal/index.php?journalID=cir.

[58] Arthur, J. C. Simon. & Steven, C. Ley. (2013). "Mitogen-activated protein kinases in innate immunity". *Nature Reviews Immunology, 13*, 679–692.

[59] Lowenstein, Charles J. & Elizabeth, Padalko. (2004). "iNOS (NOS2) at a glance". *Journal of Cell Science, 117*, 2865-2867. doi: 10.1242/jcs.01186.

[60] Forbes, Lisa R., Josh, Milner. & Elie, Haddad. (2016). "STAT3: A year in Review". *Current Opinion in Hematology, 23*(1), 23–27. http://doi.org/10.1097/MOH.0000000000000206.

[61] Hawkins, P. T. & Stevens, L. R. (2015). P13K signaling and inflammation. *Biochem. Biophys. Acta, 1851*, 882-897. https://doi.org/10.1016/j.bbalip.2014.12.006.

[62] Kutz, Helmut., Gilbert, Reisbach., Ute, Shultheiss. & Arnd, Keiser. (2008). "The c-Jun N-terminal kinase pathway is essential for cell transformation by the latent membrane protein 1 of Epstein-Barr virus". *Virology, 371*(2), 246-256. Accessed September 26, 2018. https://www.clinicalkey.com/#!/content/playContent/1-s2.0-S0042682207006368?returnurl=https:%2F%2Flinkinghub.elsevier.com%2Fretrieve%2Fpii%2FS0042682207006368%3Fshowall%3Dtrue&referrer=https:%2F%2Fwww.ncbi.nlm.nih.gov%2F.

[63] Ibiza, S. & Serrador, J. M. (2008). "The role of nitric oxide in the regulation of adaptive immune responses". *Immunología, 27*(3), 103-117.

[64] Mittal, Manish., Mohammed, R. Siddiqui., Khiem, Tran., Sekhar, P. Reddy. & Asrar, B. Malik. (2014). "Reactive Oxygen Species in Inflammation and Tissue Injury". *Antioxidants & Redox Signaling, 20*(7), 1126–1167. http://doi.org/10.1089/ars.2012.5149.

[65] Morgan, Michael J. & Zheng-gang, Liu. (2011). "Crosstalk of reactive oxygen species and NF-κB signaling". *Cell Research*, *21*(1), 103–115. http://doi.org/10.1038/cr.2010.178.

[66] Ahmed, S .M. U., Lin, Luo., Akhileshwar, Namani., Xiu, Jan Wang. & Xiuwen, Tang. (2016). "Nrf2 signaling pathway: Pivotal roles in inflammation". *Biochmimica et Biophysica Acta*, *1863*, 585-597. http://dx.doi.org/10.1016/j.badis.2016.11.005.

[67] Saha, Ramendra N., Malabendu, Jana. & Kallipada, Pahan. (2007). "MAPK p38 regulates NF-κB activity in primary human astrocytes by acteylation of p65". *The Journal of Immunology*, *179*(10), 7101-7109. doi: https://doi.org/10.4049/jimmunol.179.10.7101.

[68] Miyazaki, Tsuyoshi., Hideki, Katagiri., Yumi, Kanegae., Hiroshi, Takayanagi., Yasuhiro, Sawada., Alichiro, Yamamoto., Mattew, P. Pando., Tomoichiro, Asano., Inder, M. Verma., Hiromi, Oda., Kozo, Nakamura. & Sakae, Tanaka. (2000). "Reciprocal Role of ERK and Nf-κb Pathways in Survival and Activation of Osteoclasts". *The Journal of Cell Biology*, *148*(2), 333–342.

[69] Borlinghaus, Jan., Frank, Albrecht., Martin, C. H. Grulke., Ifeanyi, D. Nwachukwu. & Alan, J. Slusarenko. (2014). "Allicin: Chemistry and biological properties". *Molecules*, 19(8), 12591-12618.

[70] Abed, Dhulfigar A., Melanie, Goldstein., Haifa, Albanyan., Huijuan, Jin. & Longgin, Hu. (2015). "Discovery of direct inhibitors of Keap1-Nrf2 protein-protein interaction as potential therapeutic and preventive agents." *Acta Pharmaceutica Sinica. B*, *5*(4), 285–299. doi:10.1016/j.apsb.2015.05.008.

[71] Si Qin, Si. & De-Xing, Hou. (2017). The Biofunctions of Phytochemicals and Their Applications in Farm Animals: The Nrf2/Keap1 System as a Target. *Engineering*, *3*(5), 738-752. https://doi.org/10.1016/J.ENG.2017.03.011.

[72] Cross, Janet V. & Dennis, J. Templeton. (2006). "Regulation of cysteine transduction through protein cysteine oxidation." *Antioxidants & Redox Signaling* http://doi.org/10.1089/ars.2006.8.1819.

[73] Rahman, Mohammad S. (2007). "Allicin and other functional active components in garlic : health benefits and bioavailability". *Int J Food Properties*, *10*, 245-268.

[74] Wang, Zhimiang., Zhiliang, Ying., Anja, Bosy-Westphal., Junyi, Zhang., Britta, Schautz., Wiebke, Later., Steven, B. Heymsfield. & Manfred, J. Müller. (2010). "Specific metabolic rates of major organs and tissues across adulthood: evaluation by mechanistic model of resting energy expenditure." *Am J Clin Nutr.*, *92*(6), 1369-77. doi: 10.3945/ajcn.2010.29885.

[75] Li, Sha., Hor-Yue, Tan., Ning, Wang., Zhang-Jin, Zhang., Lixing, Lao., Chiwoon, Wong. & Yibin, Feng. (2015). "The Role of Oxidative Stress and Antioxidants in Liver Diseases." *Int J Mol Sci.*, *16*(11), 26087-124. doi: 10.3390/ijms161125942.

[76] Angelova, Plamina R. & Andrey, Y. Abramov. (2018). "Role of mitochondrial ROS in the brain: from physiology to neurodegeneration. *FEBS Letters*, *582*, 692-702. Accessed April 2, 2019. https://febs.onlinelibrary.wiley.com/doi/pdf/10.1002/1873-3468.12964.

[77] Atia, Ahmed., Nadia, Alrawaiq. & Azman, Abdullah. (2014). "A review of NAD (P)H:quinoneoxidoreductase 1 (NQO1): A multifunctional antioxidant enzyme." *J. Applied Pharm. Sci.*, *4*(12), 118-122. Accessed on May 24, 2019 https://www.japsonline.com/admin/php/uploads/1401_pdf.pdf.

[78] Lu, Shelley C. (2009). "Regulation of glutathione synthesis." *Mol Aspects Med.*, *30*(1-2), 42-59. doi: 10.1016/j.mam.2008.05.005.

[79] Cundell, Diana R. & Kathryn, E. Mickle. (2018). "Osteoarthritis: potential for herbal medicines as therapies in the management of chronic inflammatory damage". *Current Immunology Reviews*, *14*, 1-13. E Pub ahead of print link. Accessed on September 25, 2018 http://www.eurekaselect.com/node/162555/article/osteoarthritis-potential-for-herbal-medicines-as-therapies-in-the-management-of-chronic-inflammatory-damage.

[80] Kawashima, Seinosuke. & Mitsuhiro, Yokoyama. (2004). "Dysfunction of endothelial nitric oxide synthase and atherosclerosis". *Atherosclerosis, Thrombosis and Vascular Biology*, *24*, 998-1005.

[81] Garry, P. S., Ezra, M., Rowland, M. J., Westbrook, J. & Pattinson, K. T. S. (2015). "The role of the nitric oxide pathway in brain injury and its treatment — From bench to bedside." *Experimental Neurology*, *263*, 235-243. https://doi.org/10.1016/j.expneurol.2014.10.017.

[82] Iwakiri, Yasuko. (2015). "Nitric oxide in liver fibrosis: The role of inducible nitric oxide synthase." *Clinical and Molecular Hepatology*, *21*(4), 319–325. doi: 10.3350/cmh.2015.21.4.319.

[83] Goligorsky, Michael S., Sergey, V. Brodsky. & Eisei, Noiri. (2002). "Nitric oxide in acute renal failure: NOS versus NOS." *Kidney International*, *81*(3), 855-861. doi: https://doi.org/10.1046/j.1523-1755.2002.00233.x.

[84] Vuolteenaho, K., Moilanen, T., Knowles, R. G. & Moilanene, E. (2007). "The role of nitric oxide in osteoarthritis." *Scand. J. Rheumatol.*, *36*(4), 247-258. https://www.tandfonline.com/doi/full/10.1080/03009740701483014.

[85] Aoyagi, Toshinori. & Takashi, Matsui. (2011). Phosphoinositide-3 kinase signaling in cardiac hypertrophy and heart failure. *Current Pharmaceutical Design*, *17*(18), 1818–1824. Accessed on May 27, 2019. https://www.ncbi.nlm.nih.gov/pmc/articles/PMC3337715/.

[86] Kaminska, Bozina., Agata, Gozdz., Malgorzata, Zawadzka., Alecsandra, Ellert-Miklaszewska. & Maciej, Lipko. (2009). MAPK "Signal Transduction Underlying Brain Inflammation and Gliosis as Therapeutic Target." *Anat Rec*, *292*, 1902-1913. doi:10.1002/ar.21047.

[87] Morrison, Deborah H. (2012). "MAP kinase pathways". *Cold Spring Harbor Perspectives in Biology* doi: 10.1101/cshperspect.a011254. Accessed on September 25, 2018. http://cshperspectives.cshlp.org/content/4/11/a011254.

[88] Sethuraman, Mahadevan., Nicolas, Clavreul., Hua, Huang., Mahadeva, E. McComb., Catherine, E. Costello. & Richard, A. Cohen. (2007). "Quantification of oxidative posttranslational modifications of cysteine thiols of p21ras associated with redox modulation of activity using isotope-coded affinity tags and mass spectrometry." *Free Radical Biology and Medicine*, *42*(6), 823–829. doi:10.1016/j.freeradbiomed.2006.12.012.

[89] Kim, Kyoung H., Doo, R. An., Jinsu, Song., Ji, Y. Yoon., Hyoun, S. Kim., Hye, J. Yoon., Ha, N. Im., Jieun, Kim., Sang, J. Lee., Ki-Hye, Kim., Hye-Mi, Lee., Hie-Joon, Kim., Eun-Kyeong, Jo., Jae, Y. Lee. & Se, W. Suh. (2012). "*Mycobacterium tumerculosis* Eis protein initiates suppression of host immune responses by acetylation of DUSP16/MK7". *PNAS*, *109*(20), 7729-7734. Accessed on September 25, 2018.

[90] Lee, Samuel., Soo, M. Kim. & Richard, T. (2013). "Thioredoxin and thioredoxin target proteins: from molecular mechanisms to functional significance." *Antioxidants & Redox Signaling*, *18*(10), 1165–1207. doi:10.1089/ars.2011.4322.

[91] Leontiev, Roman., Nils, Hohaus., Jacob, Claus., Martin, C. H. Gruhlke. & Alan, J. Slusarenko, (2018). "Comparison of the Antibacterial and Antifungal Activities of Thiosulfinate Analogues of Allicin." *Scientific Reports*, *6763*, 8(1). Accessed on February 22, 2019 https://www.nature.com/articles/s41598-018-25154-9.

[92] Lubenets, Vira., Sofiya, Vasylyuk., Nataliya, Monka., Khrystina, Bolibrukh., Olena, Komarovska-Porokhnyavets., Diana, Baranovych., Rostyslav, Musyanovych., Ewa, Zaczynska., Anna, Czarny., Urszula, Nawrot. & Volodymyr, Novikov. (2016). "Synthesis and antimicrobial properties of 4-acylaminobenzenethiosulfoacid S-esters." *Saudi Pharmaceutical Journal: SPJ: The Official publication of the Saudi Pharmaceutical Society*, *25*(2), 266-274. doi: 10.1016/j.jsps.2016.06.007.

[93] Hybertson, Brooks M., Bifeng, Gao., Swapan, K. Bose. & Joe, M. McCord. (2011). "Oxidative stress in health and disease: The therapeutic potential of Nrf2 activation." *Molecular Aspects of Medicine*, *32* (4–6), 234-246. https://doi.org/10.1016/j.mam.2011.10.006.

[94] Weber, Adrian., Shin, H. Mak., Francis, Berenbaum., Jérémie, Sellam., Yong-Ping, Zheng., Yifan, Han. & Chunyi, Wen. (2019). "Association between osteoarthritis and increased risk of dementia: A systemic review and meta-analysis." *Medicine (Baltimore).*, *98*(10), e14355. doi: 10.1097/MD.0000000000014355. Epub 2019 Mar 8.

[95] Maher, Robert L., Joseph, T. Hanlon. & Emily, R. Hajjar. (2014). "Clinical consequences of polypharmacy in elderly." *Expert Opin Drug Saf.*, *13*(1), 57-65. doi: 10.1517/14740338.2013.827660.

In: Allicin
Editor: Diana R. Cundell
ISBN: 978-1-53617-339-0

Chapter 4

IMMUNE SYSTEM EFFECTS OF ALLICIN

Diana R. Cundell*[*], *PhD
College of Life Sciences, Jefferson University, Philadelphia, PA, US

ABSTRACT

The immune system effects of allicin from garlic were first described nearly fifty years after its initial discovery. Like many other phytochemicals, initial studies determined that this thiosulfinate affected primarily innate immune system cells, namely neutrophils and macrophages. Studies of its efficacy in this respect are complicated by the frequent use of *in vivo* models of infectious disease, making it difficult to distinguish between antimicrobial versus immunomodulatory activities. Chronic inflammatory disease models suggest allicin elicits effects primarily on T helper (Th) cells and may shift the balance between Th1 and Th2 subpopulations, as well as influence the expression and trafficking of Th17 and Treg populations. Alllicin produces a dose response curve of efficacy, demonstrating a pro-inflammatory profile at low concentrations and anti-inflammatory effects at elevated concentration levels. This discrepancy makes it very different from current pharmacuticals, and thus has been the issue for general understanding of its mechanism(s) of action and acceptance of its clinical importance. This chapter will review the studies performed on allicin/garlic extract's effects on innate and adaptive immunity, as well as interpret the relevance for the immune system cells involved in acute and chronic inflammatory disease states.

Keywords: B-lymphocyte, interleukin, macrophage, neutrophil, T-helper cell

INTRODUCTION

First discovered in 1944 as the potent antibacterial metabolite from garlic, allicin's effects on the immune system were not investigated until nearly fifty years later [1]. Since this date, twenty-two studies have been performed to evaluate either allicin directly [2-12], garlic oil containing allicin [13-15], or raw garlic/extract [16-28] on immune system activity. Most of

[*] Corresponding Author's Email: Diana.Cundell@jefferson.edu.

these studies have been performed within the last decade [2, 5, 7-9, 11, 13-15, 17, 20, 22, 23, 26-28]. Phytomedicines that are both immunomodulatory and antimicrobial include both allicin [1] and numerous flavonoids [29, 30]. Botanists believe these types of metabolites act as plant sensors, signaling and regulating the levels of microbial growth on the plant surface and activating the immune system cells when needed [29, 30]. However, clearance of a plant-specific microbe by an entity like allicin is not sufficient to prove it has an effect on the mammalian immune system. This chapter will therefore include those studies reporting direct changes to both mammalian and non-mammalian immune system cells, represented by cytokine shifts, phagocytosis, antibody production, or differential expression of lymphocyte subpopulations.

Analysis of the biochemistry of the garlic bulb has revealed a diverse series of chemical entities including the dominant thiosulfinate allicin, as well as other metabolites that have also been reported to be immunoregulatory, such as alliin, ajoene, and S-allyl-L-cysteine (SAC) [31]. Allicin constitutes the major active moiety in freshly crushed garlic or garlic oil preparations, whereas ajoene is the dominant entity in aged garlic (AGE) [31]. In this chapter, focus will therefore be made only on those preparations in which either pure allicin has been utilized or in which the effectiveness can be realistically attributed to its presence i.e., fresh garlic, garlic oil, or commercial formulations such as Allimed®.

Finally, it is important to determine how allicin or allicin-enriched preparations are affecting immune system cell function. Immunomodulating phytomedicines can be classified as adjuvants, immunostimulants, immunomodulators, or adaptogens [29]. Adjuvants are phytochemicals like saponins from *Panax ginseng* [29] that boost T cell system function without actively participating with the cells [32]. Immunostimulants include the well-described *Echinacea purpurea* [33] which improves removal of infections and tumors by typically potentiating innate immune system activity [29]. Immunomodulators, which "balance immune function" i.e., suppress overactive chronic inflammation and improve poorly functioning responses, include the Ayurvedic plant *Nycanthes arbor tristis* (night flowering jasmine) [34]. Finally, there are adaptogens, which include *Panax ginseng*, and function by improving the body's resistance to cellular stress and thereby reduce infections [29]. In order to understand the efficacy of allicin and allicin-enriched garlic preparations on the immune system it will be necessary to first review the mechanisms involved in both the innate and adaptive immune systems.

1. Basics of Immunology: The Innate and Adaptive Immune System

The immune system is a complex but fortunately plastic system which, through sequential activation of non-specific (innate) and specific (adaptive) mechanisms, is able to affect elimination of most pathogens, as well as early malignant cells [35]. Although described as two separate systems, immunologists now consider that adaptive immunity cannot be initiated without first activation of innate immune system cells [35].

1.1. Innate Immunity: Neutrophils, Macrophages and Natural Killer Cells

Innate immunity involves mobilization of neutrophils, macrophages, and natural killer (NK) cells [24, 35, 36-40]. Neutrophils are the "first responders" and accumulate at sites of infection (primarily bacterial) and injury [35, 37]. Their role at this point appears to be immunomodulatory in that they recruit macrophages and NK cells, and under normal conditions act to resolve acute inflammation through phagocytosis of debris and microbes [37]. To perform these functions, neutrophils produce a variety of toxic reactive oxygen species (ROS) including hydrogen peroxide (H_2O_2), hydroxyl radicals, and superoxide [37]. By combining these substances with their endogenous myeloperoxidase (MPO) [37], neutrophils can also produce hypochlorous acid i.e., the active ingredient in household bleach! Release of these products directly onto an internalized microbe typically results in certain death and their release to the external environment initiates oxidative stress which, as has been discussed previously, is the hallmark for induction of acute inflammation (see Chapter 3). Other antimicrobial factors released from neutrophil granules include proteins that sequester iron (lactoferrin), or are directly bacteriocidal (M-ficolin and peptidoglycan recognition protein) [37]. Neutrophils also contain a diverse repertoire of proteases with various activities, including the important antibacterial lysozyme (which disrupts bacterial peptidoglycan), as well as metalloprotease-9 (MMP-9), and neutrophil elastases (which permit new blood vessel growth, as well as remodeling of existing scaffolding following damage) [37].

Macrophages and monocytes are mobilized shortly after neutrophils and appear to constitute the second most common cell type involved in acute inflammatory responses [35, 39]. These cells do most of their killing through the generation of nitric oxide (NO) which decreases pathogen load [39]. ROS are also generated by macrophages and released internally to help eliminate phagocytosed pathogens [39]. NO and ROS are highly toxic to microbes through several mechanisms [39]. Independently, NO can diffuse across microbial membranes and impair DNA repair enzymes, thus inducing microbiostasis [39]. ROS bind to a variety of microbial targets including sulfhydryl groups, iron-sulfur clusters, and cysteine residues and ultimately result in demise [39]. When combined, NO and ROS can also produce the toxic peroxynitrite [39].

Finally, NK cells may also play a role in viral-based or early anti-tumor responses [38]. Activation of NK cells occurs primarily through their interaction with local dendritic cells or macrophages and consequent interaction with interleukin-15 (IL-15) or IL-18 [38]. Without this early cellular promotion they appear not to be fully potent in their activities [38]. Neutrophils also interact with NK cells both in the bone marrow and later in lymphatic tissues where they appear to allow full maturation of the cells to occur as evidenced by the ability of NK cells to secrete pro-inflammatory cytokines following contact with neutrophils [40]. Once a NK cell has detected and attached to its target, killing occurs through the release of toxic molecules stored in intracellular granules [42]; these are identical to those found in T cytotoxic cells and include granzymes and perforin [42]. In addition, NK cells also express tumor necrosis factor alpha (TNFα)-receptor ligands which can activate the Fas pathway in cells to induce apoptosis [42].

Interestingly, unlike other cells active in innate immunity, NK cells appear to possess memory for both tumors and certain viruses [41, 42]. Although this may only represent a month or two of memory [41, 42], unlike the years attributable to adaptive immunity [35], the finding is still a striking one.

All three cell types appear to be "plastic" in nature (i.e., under healthy circumstances they are able to control inflammation such that they neutralize and control the threat to the host) [35, 37, 39, 43]. Should the microenvironment shift, neutrophils and macrophages are able to perpetuate chronic inflammation, by polarizing into subtypes and through the generation of immunosuppressive cytokines [24, 35, 37]. Activated macrophages are considered to be the most important in this regard in that they can secrete cytokines, which may be either pro- or anti-inflammatory depending on their micro-environment [35].

Classic or M1 macrophages, which participate in acute inflammation, secrete large amounts of TNFα, interferon gamma (IFNγ), and IL-6 and -12 [39]. Some of these cytokines (e.g., IL-12 and IL-6) are particularly important for another role of the macrophage: that of presenting antigen [39]. Like neutrophils, macrophages bridge the innate and adaptive immune systems and can present digested bacterial proteins to classic Th ($CD4^+$) cells and induce B-lymphocyte driven antibody responses [39]. In contrast, M2 macrophages are anti-inflammatory, secreting IL-4, IL-10 and IL-13 [39]. Although M2 macrophages play a central role in terminating acute inflammatory responses, their appearance is often associated with chronic illnesses including allergies, the development of type II diabetes, and colitis [39]. Neutrophils are considered to be the cells that terminate acute inflammation through release of the immunosuppressive IL-10 cytokine, as well as by polarizing macrophages to the immunosuppressive M2 phenotype after ingesting apoptotic particles from demised neutrophils (from the neutrophil extracellular trap or NET) [40]. The generation of M2 is beneficial at this point as a termination of inflammation, underlining the importance of the balance of these types of responses. A "reverse migration" of the remaining living neutrophils back to the circulation can also occur at this point, signaling the end of the acute inflammatory response [37].

Like macrophages and neutrophils, NK cells are able to secrete both pro- and anti-inflammatory cytokines [38]. Once fully activated, they can secrete a variety of these communication molecules including TNFα, IL-10, and IL-8 [38]. Several studies suggest that, unlike macrophages and neutrophils, NK cells appear to respond to the environment they are already in rather than influencing it [44, 45]. Finally, activation of NK cells paves the way for involvement of T cytotoxic cells possibly by generating apoptotic debris from lysed, virally-infected, or transformed host cells [38].

1.2. Adaptive Immunity

T lymphocytes (T cells), so called because they are educated and sorted into suptypes in the thymus, play a central role in regulating the initiation and termination of all adaptive responses [35]. From acting as second signal generators to B lymphocytes (B cells) and stimulating their antibody producing abilities, to regulating the activities of T cytotoxic ($CD8^+$) cells, T lymphocyte helper ($CD4^+$) and regulator cells ($CD4^+CD25^+FOXP3$), the T lymphocyte system is also the route which can lead to chronic inflammatory disease [35]. Dendritic cells (DC) play a major role in the maturation of T lymphocytes, which in turn regulate the activities of the mature DC and its role in antigen presentation for immune cell-driven adaptive responses [46]. Mature DC prime Th cells into subpopulations, which are typically balanced in the healthy response to pathogens [45]. Lymphoid-derived DC secrete

IL-12 and promote the conversion of $CD11C^+$ T cells into Th1 cells; whereas the absence of IL-12 results in $CD11C^-$ T cells developing into Th2 cells [46]. DC can also prime naïve T cytotoxic $CD8^+$ cells without Th assistance and also stimulate the proliferation of these cells [47]. Mature DC also maintain survival of naïve T cells [48] and promote the development of T cell memory [49].

DC can also regulate B lymphocyte functions and are able to activate both unstimulated B cells and memory B lymphocytes [46]. In the mucosa, DC promote the induction of immunoglobulin A (IgA) expression on B lymphocytes, through exposing them to transforming growth factor beta (TGFβ) [50].

Finally, like other cells, DC are also plastic to the environment in which they are found [46]. Normally, they release IL-12 and produce a Th1 driven response, but if anti-inflammatory cytokines (e.g., IL-10) or steroids are present they will drive a Th2 response [51]. "Successful" adaptive immunity, therefore, involves polarization of Th cells into either Th1 cells (through interaction with IL-12 from either lymphoid-derived DC, macrophages, or NK cells) [35, 46, 52], or Th2 cells (through interaction with IL-4 from NK, other T cells, mast cells or basophils) [35, 52]. Th1 cells are characterized by their production of pro-inflammatory cytokines including IFNγ and IL-2, which support cell-mediated responses protecting the body against intracellular pathogens including viruses, protozoa, and fungi [35, 52]. Th1 cells regulate the activities of $CD8^+$ T cytotoxic cells [53] through a three-way interaction between $CD8^+$, antigen-presenting cells (macrophage or DC; APC), and cytokines secreted by the Th1 cell which perpetuate the response [53]. Although levels of stimulation required by Th1 cells vary, they appear to be needed if the APC are immature [53]. Once primed, specific $CD8^+$ cells undergo rapid increase in numbers (clonal expansion) [53]. The cellular army created is then specific for its target, which it interacts with through a combination of antigen- and self-recognition molecules (i.e., major histocompatability class 1; MHC I) [53]. Death of the target is then triggered using direct cell-cell contact or the shedding of pre-formed granzyme and perforin granules onto the target cell, resulting in an apoptotic cascade [53].

Some helper cells evolve into Th17 cells through interaction with TGFβ or IL-6 [35, 54]. Th17 are so named because of their unique production of IL-17 and appear to be induced early in adaptive responses against bacteria and help control neutrophil responses through the induction of pro-inflammatory cytokines including TNFα [54]. Like other leukocytes, the activity of Th17 is upregulated by classically proinflammatory cytokines (including TNFα and IL-1β) and downregulated by IL-4, IFNγ, and IL-12 [53]. Th17 cells are plastic to the environment they inhabit—this means they can either be effective participants in healthy host immune responses or contributors to perpetuating chronic inflammatory diseases including autoimmune diseases such as rheumatoid arthritis and allergic conditions [54].

A subgroup of $CD4^+$ cells play a role as immunosuppressors, known as T regulator cells (Tregs) [35]. Tregs are traditionally characterized in the literature to express a combination of CD4, CD25, and the transcription factor forkhead box protein-3 (FOXP3), denoted as $CD4^+CD25^+FOXP3+$ [35]. These cells secrete immunosuppressive IL-10 and TGFβ and are able to prevent autoimmunity [54]. In addition, a subset of Tregs have been described that appear to be induced in the circulation through differentiation of $CD4^+$ cells due to presence of IL-10 and may or may not express FOXP3 [35, 55]. In addition to self-tolerance, Tregs have two additional effects [55]: 1. they can prevent naïve T cell proliferation, thereby preventing over-stimulation of the immune system and also converting those cells into additional Tregs [55]; in this context, Tregs can exert their effects either indirectly through cytokine secretion or by direct cell:cell contact [56]. 2. Tregs are also able to downregulate DC and prevent their acting as antigen presenting cells [56]; in turn, this prevents B cell activation and antibody production [55]. By preventing activation of B lymphocytes responding to autologous antigens this also allows Tregs to prevent the initiation of autoimmune disease [55].

Effective generation of antibody by most activated B cells requires their cooperation with Th2 cells through both antigen- and self-recognition via MHC class 2 (MHC II) [56]. If appropriate, this results in a "go forward" signal through a combination of secretion of cytokines (including IL-4 and IFNγ) and co-stimulatory molecules (that include CD40 and its corresponding ligand) [56]. The B cells selected as suitable for their "best fit" with antigen next undergo clonal expansion and evolution into antibody-secreting plasma cells [56]. Supported by the DC signals previously mentioned [50], Th2 cells also allow for the class switching of antibody molecules from their initial immunoglobulin, M (IgM), to one of three other classes [35, 56].

Specifically, generation of IL-10 by Th2 cells results in the secretion of IgG, which has the ability to remove bacteria and their toxins through activation of the Complement System, as well as activating innate immune cells to remove the targets through lysis [35, 56]. In contrast, Th2 generation of IL-4 and IL-13 results in the allergic antibody IgE, while secretion of TGFβ results in manufacture of IgA [35, 56]. Antibodies of the IgA, IgE, and IgM classes are present on both mucosal tissues and in the circulation; in contrast, IgG is only found in the circulation [56]. IgG has the longest half-life of any of the immunoglobulins and also appears to be the pervading auto-antibody associated with autoimmune conditions [56].

1.3. Allicin, Acute Inflammation and Innate Immune Cells

Allicin's effects on neutrophil, macrophage, and NK function have been investigated in seventeen studies and their findings are summarized in Table 1 below.

1.4. Allicin/Garlic and Innate Immune Cells: General Observations

Review of the literature on allicin/garlic's effects on the innate immune system cells appear to provide confliciting data, with some of the *in vitro* studies suggesting anti-inflammatory activity [2, 4, 13, 16, 18, 19] but other *in vitro* studies reveal activation of these same cells, implying pro-inflammatory activity, and demonstrate rapid clearance of infections [3, 7, 8, 17, 21] and tumors [4]. Use of different preparations of garlic, namely pure allicin [2-9] versus garlic oil [13], fresh garlic [16, 21, 22], or garlic extracts [17-20, 23] also provide an added layer of variability in observed outcomes. As a caveat, garlic extracts (versus fresh garlic) and garlic oil consist of a wide variety of constituents including diallyl sulfides (DADs) and trisulphides (DATS), as well as variable amounts of allicin, thus making it difficult to ascertain the exact contributions of each of these moieties in the reviewed studies [57].

Table 1. Allicin literature studies on innate immune system cells

Neutrophils	Experimental Design	Reference
In vitro	HUVECs treated with fresh garlic extract (1, 10 or 100 ng/ml) for 24 h showed ↓ neutrophil attachment and transmigration in response to FMLP (1 x 10^7 mol/L) in an isolated cell system	[16]
	HUVECs treated with allicin (0-40 μg/ml) and LPS (1 μg/ml) for 24 h; allicin ↓ NF-κB activation in the HUVECs and binding of neutrophils to the activated HUVECs i.e., ↓ inflammation	[2]
	Neutrophil-like cells from HL-60 line incubated with garlic oil (1-10 μg/ml, 60 min); ↓ chemotaxis induced by IL-8 believed to involve cytoskeleton assembly	[13]
In vivo	New Zealand rabbits (n =50, 5 groups), four groups infected with *Pasteurella multocida* (2 x 10^5 infected RBC i.n.); control, untreated, allicin (50 mg/kg/day orally), norfloxacin (100 mg/kg/day orally) or allicin and norfloxacin combined for 5 days; allicin and allicin-norfloxacin groups showed ↑ neutrophil counts (but not macrophages or other leukocytes) and this was also associated with a more rapid clearance of the bacterium in these animals	[3]
	Albino rats (n = 10) fed garlic extract (1 ml/day) and challenged with *Salmonella typhi* (1 x 10^3 oral, single dose) for 7 weeks; ↓ total white cell count but ↑ neutrophil numbers compared with untreated animals	[17]
	Nile tilapia (*Oreochromis niloticus*) fed 3% garlic for 3 months in summer; ↑ neutrophil adherence	[21]
Macrophage/ Monocytes	Experimental Design	Reference
In vitro	HCAECs incubated with garlic extract (0.25-4.0 mg/ml) and IL-1α (10 ng/ml) for 24 h; extract significantly ↓ ($p < 0.05$) adhesion of human monocytes	[18]
	Murine (CD-1) peritoneal macrophages (elicited by 3 ml thioglycolate injection) treated with allicin (1-100 ng/ml) for 20 h; ↑ NO and TNFα, doubling of tumoricidal activity but no effect on phagocytosis when co-incubated with B16 melanoma cells	[4]
	Human healthy PBMC incubated for 2 h, stimulated with PHA (20 μg/ml) in the presence or absence of allicin (10 μg/ml); ↑ ERK levels between ten and fifteen minutes after allicin incubation that returned to unstimulated, control levels after 30 min	[5]
	Human healthy PBMC incubated for 1 h with methylprednisolone (10^{-7}M) or a combination with garlic extract (10 μg/ml). Monocyte stimulation was evaluated by adding LPS (1 μg/ml) for 24 h; Significant ($p < 0.05$) ↓ of production of IL-6, IL-8 and IL-12 and ↑ IL-10	[19]
	Murine macrophage cell line (Raw 264.7), allicin (1-1000 μM) ↑ ROS and ↓ iNOS	[6]
In vivo	BALB/c mice (8-12 weeks) peritoneal macrophages (elicited by 3 ml thioglycolate injection) treated with garlic extract (0-2,000 μg/ml) for 18 h; ↑ chemiluminescence peaking at 150 μg/ml	[20]
	Albino rats (n = 10) fed garlic extract (1 ml/day) and challenged with *Salmonella typhi* (1 x 10^3 oral, single dose) for 7 weeks; ↓ total white cell count but ↑ of monocyte numbers compared with untreated animals	[17]

Table 1. (Continued)

Macrophage/Monocytes	Experimental Design	Reference
In vivo	BALB/c mice (n = 9) infected with *Plasmodium yoelii* (1×10^6 infected RBC i.p.), given allicin (3 or 9 mg/kg/day orally by gavage) for 2 days post infection and splenocytes examined; allicin restored acute inflammatory response to parasitemia by elevating levels of macrophage-derived NO (iNOS) ↑ IFNγ, which feeds back to an increase in macrophage-derived NO Splenic macrophage load was also triple that of untreated animals	[7]
	Rainbow trout (*Onchorhyncus mykiss)* fed allicin from Allimed® (0.5 or 1.0 ml of a 1000 mg/ml Allimed/ 100 g of feed) and challenged with 1×10^5 *Aeromonas hydrophila* for 14 days; ↑ red cells, monocytes, phagocytic index and respiratory burst	[8]
NK Cells	Experimental Design	Reference
In vitro	Human healthy PBMC incubated for 2 h, stimulated with PHA (20 μg/ml) in the presence or absence of allicin (10 μg/ml); ↑ ERK levels between ten and fifteen minutes after allicin incubation that returned to unstimulated, control levels after thirty minutes	[6]
In vivo	C57BL/6 nude mice given a human pancreatic xenograft (n = 60, 15 per group), control, recombinant-IL-2 (20 μg i.v.), allicin (10 mg/kg i.v.) or allicin + recombinant-IL2 for 28 days; after 10 days significant ($p<0.001$) ↑NK cells using either allicin alone or in combination with IL-2 (additive effect)	[9]
	Human volunteers consumed raw garlic (0.5 g/kg) daily for 21 days demonstrated an over 150% increase in tumor killing NK cells compared with those not taking garlic	[22]
Immune Defense Proteins	Experimental Design	Reference
In vivo	Kuruma black tiger shrimp fed garlic paste (10g per 1 kg feed) for 28 days; ↑ expression of innate system genes for hemocyte lysozyme and penaeidins as well as crustins	[23]

Abbreviations used in the table: ERK (extracellular regulated kinase), FMLP (N-formyl l-methionyl leucyl phelylalanine), h (hour), HCAEC (human coronary artery endothelial cells), HUVEC (human vein endothelial cells), IFNγ (interferon gamma), IL (interleukin), iNOS (inducible nitric oxide synthase), i.v. (intravenous), LPS (lipopolysaccharide), NF-κB (nuclear factor kappa beta), NK (natural killer cells), NO (nitric oxide), PBMC (peripheral blood mononuclear cells; typically a mixture of monocytes natural killer cells and lymphocytes), PHA (phytohemagglutinin), ROS (reactive oxygen species), TNFα (tumor necrosis factor alpha)

However, there are two primary differences comparing the *in vivo* and *in vitro* studies, which may explain this apparent contradiction. First, the duration of exposure *in vitro* is less than one day [2, 3, 16] compared with either five [3], forty-nine [17], or eighty-four days [21] for the *in vivo* studies. Second, allicin/garlic was administered orally in the *in vivo* studies, which means that there is likely to have been a breakdown into metabolic derivatives following digestion, including ajoene, and also likely reducing the concentration of allicin [1]. Finally, as will be discussed later, some studies have pointed towards allicin displaying a bell-shaped curve of activity, being pro-inflammatory at lower concentrations but exhibiting anti-inflammatory activity at higher ones [6, 14, 25].

1.5. Neutrophils

Six studies have been performed on the effects of allicin or garlic extracts on neutrophils, three being *in vitro* [2, 13, 16] and three *in vivo* [3, 17, 21]. The only direct studies on the interaction of human neutrophils and resting human vein endothelial cells (HUVECs) suggest garlic extract decreases their attachment and transmigration in an isolated cell system [16]. A second study, which examined allicin's effects against LPS-stimulated HUVECs, also demonstrated a lack of neutrophil adhesion to these cells but did not evaluate the effects of allicin on neutrophil functionality (i.e., ROS generation or cytokine secretion) [2]. Given that allicin is an anti-oxidant this would appear to suggest that its effects are anti-inflammatory. Finally, neutrophil-like cells (HL-60) demonstrated impaired cytoskeleton assembly when exposed to garlic oil [13]. Interestingly, as will be discussed later, purified allicin (100 ng/ml) was directly able to impair actin polymerization of T lymphocytes [10], which would prevent optimal chemotaxis and adhesion. In contrast, the three *in vivo* studies all demonstrated that allicin [3] or garlic [17, 21] increased neutrophil numbers [3, 17, 21], adherence [21], and removal of bacterial infections [3, 17].

1.6. Macrophage/Monocytes

Nine studies have been performed on the effects of allicin or garlic extracts on monocytes, five being *in vitro* [4-6, 18, 19], one *ex vivo* [20], and two *in vivo* [7,8, 17]. Two *in vitro* studies reported garlic extract [19] or garlic oil [18] were anti-inflammatory and suppressed the activities of the monocytes. One study observed that garlic impaired the secretion of pro-inflammatory cytokines from peripheral blood mononuclear cells (PBMC) and increased expression of IL-10 [19]. A second reported that garlic oil impaired attachment of monocytes to IL-1α-activated HUVECs [18]. In contrast, an *ex vivo* study using murine peritoneal macrophages demonstrated enhanced activation of these cells (in the form of a chemiluminescence reporter) that peaked at 150 μg/ml of a garlic extract [20]. A second study demonstrated that oral garlic extract (1 ml/day) resulted in an increase in monocyte counts and accelerated removal of bacteria in mice infected with *Salmonella typhi* [17].

Five studies, all using allicin or the stabilized commercial form Allimed®, demonstrated enhancement of macrophage activation [4-8]. Human PBMC demonstrated a transient increase in extracellular regulated kinase (ERK) activity following exposure to allicin (10 μg/ml) for up to thirty minutes *in vitro* [5]. As previously discussed in Chapter 3, elevation in ERK results in cell survival, primarily through activation of the p21^{ras} pathway [5]. Allicin pre-treatment of isolated murine peritoneal macrophages that were then exposed to B16 melanoma cells resulted in increased expression of TNFα and NO but no effects on ROS [4]. This was also seen in an *in vivo* study on malaria infection of BALB/c mice whereby consumed allicin (given by gavage, 3 or 9 mg/kg/day) increased murine peritoneal macrophage activation, as demonstrated by elevated levels of iNOS [7]. In the latter study, the splenic macrophage load was triple that of the untreated animals [7]. Interestingly, a fifth study on the *in vitro* effects of allicin (0-1000 μM) on the Raw 264.7 murine macrophage cell line reported that iNOS was suppressed but that ROS generation was increased [6]. This apparent discrepancy may be either an issue with the assay itself or with the cell line used; however, this is currently unable to be determined as the experiment has not been repeated. In rainbow trout, Allimed® (0.5 or 1.0 ml of 1000 mg/ml Allimed®/100 g of feed) treatment increased both the monocyte count and level of activation (as assessed by phagocytic ability and respiratory burst) [8]. This elevated monocyte activity also increased the survival of the fish from an aritificially induced *Aeromonas hydrophila* bacterial infection [8].

So why is garlic sometimes pro-inflammatory and at other times anti-inflammatory for macrophages? As stated earlier, the answer may lie in the amount of allicin present in the mixture of agents present in garlic or garlic oil [57]. But what of the mixed response seen when Raw 264.7 cells were exposed to allicin? [6] Raw 264.7 macrophages are a good model for the human cells except in one respect; lipopolysaccharide (LPS) activation of these cells triggers IL-1β secretion in humans but not mice [58]. Some studies suggest that Raw 264.7 resemble stem or precursor macrophages, which would not have all the full attributes of mature cells [59]. As a result, their activation might produce the data seen in the study of the Raw 264.7 macrophages (i.e., suppression of iNOS but elevation of ROS) [6].

1.7. Natural Killer Cells

Three studies have been performed on the effects of allicin or garlic extracts on NK cells, one being *in vitro* [6] and two *in vivo* [9, 22]. The combined studies all reported that either allicin [6, 9] or raw garlic [22], elevated both activation and numbers of NK cells. Of note, PBMC would be expected to contain variable numbers of NK cells but the effects of raw garlic/allicin on this population are much more consistent [9, 22]. Animals from a murine model of pancreatic cancer that were treated with either a combination of allicin and IL-2 or IL-2 alone, demonstrated increases in NK cell numbers and IFNγ [9]. These changes were associated with a concomitant decrease in tumor size in the animals which were enhanced when the two agents were combined [9]. A human study in which volunteers consumed raw garlic (which would possess allicin) demonstrated an over 150% increase in tumor killing NK cells compared with those not taking garlic [22].

1.8. Allicin/Garlic and the Innate Immune System: Putting It Together

When combined, these studies suggest that allicin is pro-inflammatory for certain cell types (monocytes and NK cells) with effects on neutrophils being dependent on the pervading environment (i.e., whether it is an acute inflammatory or chronic inflammatory milieu; Figure 1). Dosage of allicin being used is also an important consideration, with lower concentrations demonstrating a pro-inflammatory profile, but higher concentrations resulting in inhibition of inflammation [6]. Allicin/garlic's effects also appear to be cell-specific, as previously stated. This variability makes allicin unlike any currently described pharmaceutical compound capable of affecting immune system function, as it functions as an immunomodulator rather than an on/off switch.

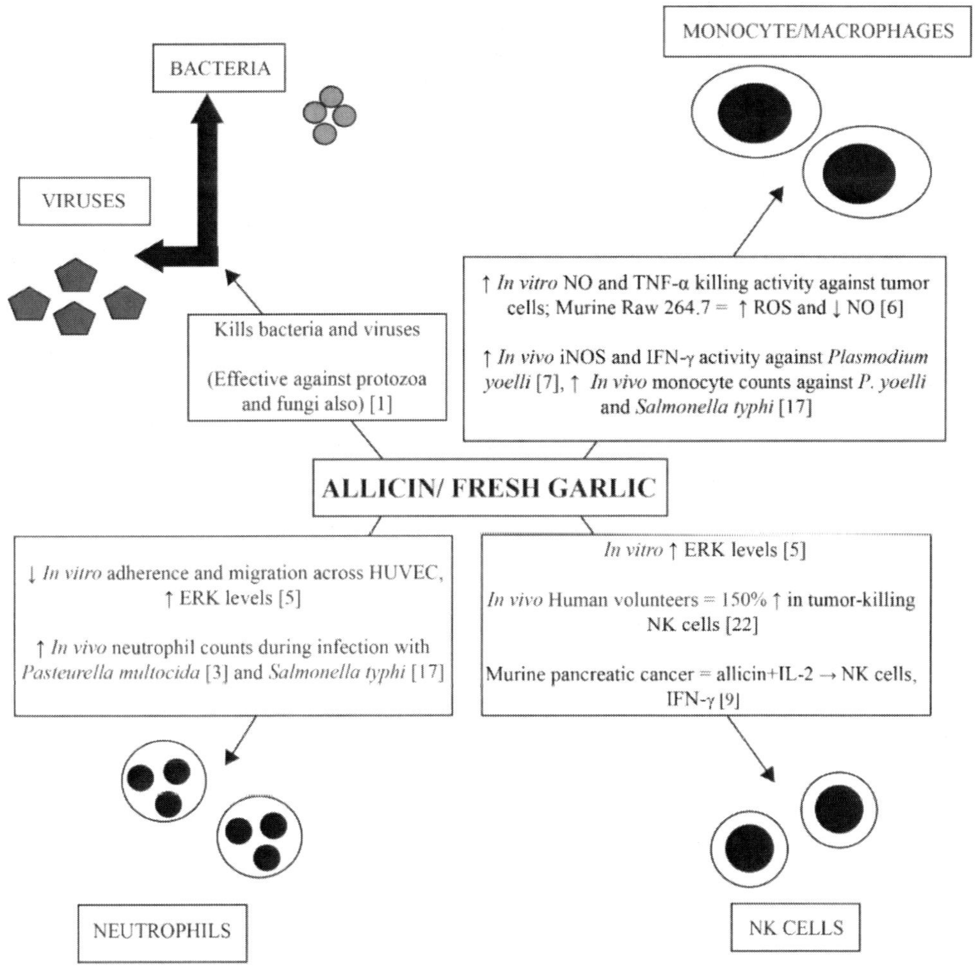

Legend: Allicin and fresh garlic produce reproducible and pro-inflammatory effects in both *in vitro* and *in vivo* studies of monocyte/macrophages and natural killer cells. In contrast, *in vitro* studies of neutrophils have suggested a more anti-inflammatory activity for allicin and fresh garlic whereas *in vivo* the cells become activated. This latter conflict may represent a response to the metabolite of allicin, ajoene, or differential doses being used in the two types of studies.

Abbreviations: ERK (extracellular regulated kinase), HUVEC (human vein endothelial cells), IFNγ (interferon gamma), IL-2 (interleukin 2), NK (natural killer), PBMC (peripheral blood mononuclear cells), and ROS (reactive oxygen species).

References used to construct diagram: [2, 3, 6-9, 16. 17, 21, 22].

Figure 1. Allicin or fresh garlic effects on innate immune system.

Allicin in fresh garlic paste may also upregulate immune system genes coding for antimicrobial proteins according to one *in vivo* study [23]. Kuruma black tiger shrimp fed garlic paste (10g per 1 kg feed) for 28 days were reported to increase the expression of genes for hemocyte lysozyme, penaeidins, and crustins [23]. All three exhibit particularly effective antimicrobial activity against marine gram-positive bacterial strains [60], and hemocytes are very similar to circulating monocytes in other animals, including humans [61]. Allicin was also found to be effective against infection by the gram-negative fish pathogen *Aeromonas hydrophila* in one *in vivo* study [8]. Taken together, this further supports the ability of allicin to activate monocyte-like cells across many animal species [7, 8, 17].

A final component to allicin's contribution to innate immunity is that it is also a strong and broad-spectrum antibacterial agent shown to affect the growth of at least 12 different gram-positive and gram-negative bacterial species [1] (see Chapter 5). Allicin has been demonstrated to have direct antibacterial activity against *Aeromonas hydrophila* [21], *Pasteurella multocida* [3] and *Salmonella typhi* [1]. In at least three of the *in vivo* models of infection, some of the resulting activity of allicin may be due to direct antibacterial activity, in addition to activating neutrophils [3, 17] and monocytes [8, 17]. Only a single human study has appeared in the literature with respect to allicin or garlic's effects on innate immune system cells [22]. This study was both unblinded and appeared only in abstract form, however it did demonstrate a dramatic increase in NK cell number following raw garlic consumption [22]. Clearly, additional human double-blind, randomized, placebo-controlled trials (DBRPCT) are needed to effectively evaluate allicin's activities with respect to human innate immune system cells.

2. Allicin and Adaptive Immunity

Allicin's effects on B and T lymphocytes have been investigated in sixteen studies and their findings are summarized in Table 2 below.

2.1. B Lymphocytes

Two *in vivo* studies were performed on B lymphocytes and both reported that allicin at a dose of 50 mg or 100 mg/kg/day [3] or 10 g/kg/day of garlic extract [24] increased activation and secretion of immunoglobulins. In a recent rabbit model of *P. multocida* infection, allicin was found to be additive with the antibiotic norfloxacin (100 mg/kg/day) and increased secretion of both serum IgG and IgM in these animals [3]. The second study reported that an extract of garlic (naturally containing allicin) was able to promote antibody formation following vaccination of chickens with the infectious agents of Newcastle Disease virus and the bacterium *Brucella abortus* [24]. In this study, interestingly, higher levels of garlic extract (30 mg/kg/day) were found to be ineffective [24]. These findings of increased IgG and IgM antibodies production are also suggestive of allicin/garlic in promoting a Th2-based response in these animals.

Table 2. Allicin literature studies on B and T lymphocyte function

B lymphocytes	Experimental design	Reference
In vivo	New Zealand rabbits (n = 50, 5 groups), four groups infected with *Pasteurella multocida* (2×10^5 infected RBC i.n.); control, untreated, allicin (50 mg/kg/day), norfloxacin (100 mg/kg/day) or allicin and norfloxacin combined; serum IgG and IgM levels showed significant decreases ($p < 0.05$) in infected animals, while allicin alone or in combination with norfloxacin demonstrated significant increases ($p < 0.05$), compared to infected rabbits.	[3]
	White Leghorn chickens fed *Allium sativum* or *Allium cepa* a (10 g/kg orally), immunized with Newcastle Disease Virus (NDV), Sheep red blood cells (SRBC), and *Brucella abortus* (BA); chickens showed enhanced anti-NDV, anti-SRBC, and anti-BA antibody production. The authors concluded that enhanced T cell proliferation with dietary garlic might directly/indirectly enhanced B-cell proliferation and differentiation.	[24]
T lymphocytes	**Experimental design**	**Reference**
In vitro	BALB/c mice (8-12 weeks) treated with garlic extract (0-2,000 μg/ml) for 18 h; lymphocytes obtained from mouse spleens and incubated with PHA (T cell mitogen, 6.25 μg/ml, 3 h) and garlic extract (0-800 μg/ml, 43 h). ↑ lymphoproliferation (peak at 150-800 μg/ml)	[7]
	Splenocytes isolated from C57BL/6 mice; allicin (0.5-1 μg/ml) stimulated uptake of 3H Thymidine by isolated splenocytes. Mechanism of lymphocyte stimulation via $p21^{ras}$ and involved ↑ ERK	[6]
	Rat thymocytes and splenocytes stimulated with Con A (0.62 or 2.5 μg/ml) and treated with garlic extract (aqueous or ethanol 1:250 – 1:1000) for 24h; higher concentrations (>1:250 of aqueous and 1:250 or 1:100 of ethanol) showed enhancement of T cell proliferation and an associated increase in IL-2 secretion. No inhibition of proliferation was seen although there was a bell-shaped curve for both extracts. Aqueous extract likely to contain allicin	[25]
	Migration/adhesion of human peripheral T cells was studied using three systems in the presence of allicin (0-100 μM): 1. Chemotactic chamber in which migration was stimulated using SDF-1α (100 ng/ml for 3 h), 2. T cells preincubated with allicin for 1 h, then exposed to SDF-1α (100 ng/ml) and allowed to adhere to fibronectin, and 3. Attachment to activated HUVEC (stimulated with 2 ng/ml of TNFα). Allicin significantly ($p < 0.05$) ↓ SDF-1α-induced migration of T cells associated with a ↓ in T cell actin polymerization. A ↓ in adherence to fibronectin was also observed and found to be mediated by a downregulation in adhesion molecules VLA-4 and VLA-5. VLA-4 also mediates adhesion to HUVEC and all doses of allicin were found to ↓ adherence of T cells to these cells using this mechanism. Lack of attachment was also associated with ↓ trans-endothelial migration.	[10]
	Human healthy PBMC incubated for 1 h with methylprednisolone (10^{-7}M) or a combination with garlic extract (10 μg/ml). T lymphocyte stimulation evaluated using PHA (25 ng/ml) and ionamycin (1 μg/ml) after 24 h; significant ($p < 0.05$) ↓ in TNFα, IL-2 and IFNγ	[19]

Table 2. (Continued)

T lymphocytes	Experimental design	Reference
In vitro	Human healthy PBMC incubated with PHA (5 μg/ml), with or without garlic extract (1 or 2 μg/ml) for 96 h; no effect was seen on lymphocyte proliferation or IL-4 secretion but a shift to ↓ Th17 cells (evidenced by drop in IL-17 secretion) occurred in the PHA-stimulated cells when incubated with garlic extract.	[26]
In vivo	Rats given garlic oil (100 or 200 mg/kg, gavage) or corn oil every other day for 14 days and cervical lymph nodes excised and stimulated with Con A (dosage); 50 mg/kg dose ↑ IFNγ relative to IL-4 100 mg/kg dose Th1 cytokines (IL-2 and IFNγ) and Th2 cytokines (IL-4 and IL-10) all expressed equally. 200 mg/kg dose significantly ↑ IL-4 and IL-10 and ↓ IFNγ	[14]
	BALB/c mice (n = 24, 6 per group) received either a normal diet, high fat diet, high fat with simvastatin (2.6 mg/kg), or high fat diet with garlic oil (12.5, 25, or 50 mg/kg) for 45 days; significant ($p < 0.05$) ↑ in $CD4^+CD25^+FOXP3$ cells (Tregs) from depletion caused by high fat diet occurred with 50 mg/kg treatment and ↑ IL-10 and TGFβ production	[15]
	C57BL/6 nude mice given a human pancreatic xenograft (n = 60, 15 per group): control, recombinant-IL-2 (20 μg i.v.), allicin alone (10 mg/kg i.v.) or allicin + recombinant-IL2 for 28 days; after 10 days significant ($p < 0.001$) ↑ T cytotoxic and T helper cells (i.e., a Th1 response). Both allicin alone or in combination with IL-2 were effective. Allicin and IL-2 appeared to be additive.	[9]
	50 BALB/c mice; allicin 10 mg/kg gastric perfusion and cyclophosphamide 60/mg/kg via injection. Assessment of tumor at 29 days; significantly ($p < 0.05$) ↑ CD3 (mature T cells) and CD4 (T helper) with respect to CD8 (T cytotoxic) cells optimally using the combination treatment	[11]
	BALB/c mice (n = 9) infected with *Plasmodium yoelii* (1×10^6 infected RBC i.p.), given allicin (3 or 9 mg/kg/day orally by gavage) for 2 days post infection and splenocytes examined; ↑ IFNγ, TNFα, IL-12p70, and NO as well as CD4 levels and $CD11c^+$ DCs, whereas it did not cause major changes in IL-4 and the level of anti-inflammatory cytokine IL-10 (i.e., it stimulated the Th1 response)	[5]
	C57BL/6J mice fed various garlic extracts including allicin (5 mg/kg/day) by gavage for 7 days; Peyers's patches removed and demonstrated to show ↑ IFNγ and IL-5 production in the presence of Con A (5 μg/ml). Also ↑ IFNγ without Con A (i.e., primarily a Th1 response.)	[12]
	Rats (n = 30, 2 groups) received either garlic solution in water (600 mg/kg/4 mL) or distilled water by gavage for 28 days; garlic-treated group demonstrated a significant ($p < 0.05$) ↓ IFNγ and ↑ IL-4 in the supernatant of PHA-stimulated (10 μg/ml) spleen lymphocytes (i.e., it stimulated a Th2 response)	[27]
	Wistar rats (n = 17, 2 groups): 8 rats received aqueous garlic extract (600 mg/kg day by gavage), and 9 rats water only for 30 days; spleens and thymuses from animals with garlic treatment demonstrated an increase in size of the argyrophilic nucleolar regions in the cells from these organs compared to controls	[28]

Abbreviations used in the table: ERK (extracellular regulated kinase), h (hour), IFNγ (interferon gamma), IL (interleukin), i.n. (intranasal), i.v. (intravenous), LPS (lipopolysaccharide), NF-κB (nuclear factor kappa beta), NO (nitric oxide), PBMC (peripheral blood mononuclear cells; typically a mixture of monocytes natural killer cells and lymphocytes), PHA (phytohemagglutinin), RBC (red blood cells), SDF-1α (stromal derived factor alpha), TGFβ (transforming growth factor beta), TNFα (tumor necrosis factor alpha).

2.2. T Lymphocytes

Fourteen studies were performed to examine the effects of allicin or garlic, either *in vitro* [6, 7,10, 19, 25, 26] or *in vivo* [5, 9, 11, 12, 14, 15, 27, 28] (see Table 2 for experimental details). The six *in vitro* studies evaluated T cells from three separate animal species; namely, mice [6, 7], rats [25], and humans [10, 19, 26]. Purified allicin was only utilized in two of these studies [6, 10], with the other four employing garlic extract [7, 19, 25, 26]. Three studies utilized isolated splenocytes or thymocytes and reported T cell proliferation when these cells were exposed to fresh garlic extract *in vitro* [6, 7, 25]. In contrast, studies that employed isolated human PBMC (a population containing T lymphocytes) reported that co-incubation with allicin [10] or garlic extract [19, 26] inhibited T cell migration [10], and/or generation of cytokines [19]. The third study of isolated human peripheral blood T cells observed no such effects, but noted a downward shift in IL-17 expression, suggestive of decreased numbers of Th17 cells [26].

At least two of the *in vitro* studies are suggestive of a mechanism by which allicin indeed interacts with T cells [6, 10]. In one study, allicin (0-100 μM) prevented the attachment and transendothelial migration of T cells across stromal-derived factor-1 alpha (SDF-1α)-activated (inflamed) HUVEC through inhibiting activation of mitogen activated kinases (MAPKs) [10]; for T cells, MAPK activation also involves phosphorylation of the protein Pyk-2, which then in turn promotes cell migration [62]. Allicin also affected the locomotor actin proteins within the T cells by preventing their polarization, as well as their expression of the β integrin proteins VLA-4 and -5 [10]. Further analysis of the effect of allicin on VLA-4 and -5 expression in this study suggested that the thiosulfinate either caused their loss or internalization in the HUVEC [10].

In the second study, allicin, at a lower dose (0.5-1 μg/ml), was able to activate the ERK pathway by activating $p21^{ras}$ [6]; of note, integrin expression is mediated by activation of c-Jun N terminal kinase (JNK) and ERK pathways [63]. In addition, mitogens binding to T cells are known to activate the proto-oncogene $p21^{ras}$, which in turn switches on ERK to stimulate these cells to remove tumors [6]. The protein $p21^{ras}$ contains a cysteine residue which allicin binds to and thereby activates the ERK pathway [6]. Activation of the $p21^{ras}$ pathway can also generate NO and may ultimately lead to death of T effector cells through p53 or caspase-induced apoptosis [64].

While these different observations in T cell responses might be ascribed to species differences, they may also be partly due to the fact that PBMC are a fairly heterogenous group of cells comprised of approximately 70-85% T lymphocytes, 5-10% B lymphocytes, and 5-20% NK cells [65]. A second aspect to consider here is the variation in dosages of allicin/garlic extract administered in these studies [6, 7, 10, 19, 25, 26]. For example, two of the rodent studies used relatively high levels of garlic extract (up to 800 μg/ml) [7, 26]. In contrast, the garlic extract doses utilized in the PBMC experiments were much lower [1-100 μg/ml) [10, 19, 26]. As previously discussed in the non-specific immunity section, allicin appears to show a bell-shaped distribution of immune cell activation, with higher doses being inhibitory [6]. Specifically, Patya and colleagues [6] observed that using concentrations of allicin below 5 μg/ml enhanced immune responses, while higher concentrations (above the 5 μg/ml) were found to be inhibitory. A similar dose-dependent effect may also be involved in the apparently disparate *in vitro* findings reported here although further dosage curves with pure allicin are necessary to elucidate this.

Analysis of the data from the eight *in vivo* rodent studies is also suggestive of several effects of allicin or garlic on the immune system [5, 9, 11, 12, 14, 15, 27, 28] (see Table 2 for further experimental details). Adminstration of allicin or garlic was via gavage in all studies but the dosages used were highly variable (3-600 mg/kg/day) as was the duration of treatment (2 - 45 days). Despite these differences, seven of the eight studies reported allicin, garlic oil, or garlic extract to induce T cell proliferation [11, 28], and increases in T cytotoxic [9] and/or T helper cells [5, 9, 11, 12, 14, 27]. In contrast, immunosuppression was observed in one study, in which garlic oil (12.5, 25, or 50 mg/kg) was given by gavage to mice on a high-fat diet for 45 days [15]. The mice in this study demonstrated a significant ($p < 0.05$) increase in anti-inflammatory cytokine-secreting $CD4^{+}CD25^{+}FOXP3+$ cells (Tregs) [15].

One possible explanation for the differing immunomodulatory effects of allicin/garlic in these *in vivo* studies has been suggested by Liu and colleagues [14]. These authors reported that different dosages of garlic oil promoted either a Th1 response (<50 mg/kg), both Th1 and Th2 equally (50-100 mg/kg), or a Th2 response (>100 mg/kg). Liu and colleagues [14] based their rationale on the levels of cytokines produced and measured; specifically, of IL-2 and IFNγ for Th1 cells, and IL-4 and IL-10 for Th2. However, like Th2 cells, Tregs also secrete the anti-inflammatory cytokine IL-10 [35] and were seen to be upregulated at the 50 mg/kg/day dosage [15]. Using the hypothesis of Liu and colleagues [14] this means that allicin/garlic at a higher concentration (50 mg/kg and above) would expand both Th1 and Th2 populations equally; an event which could need "shutting down" by the Treg population to prevent "overstimulation" of the inflammatory response.

In the context of T cell involvement in adaptive responses in an *in vivo* model of infection, allicin behaves in a typically pro-inflammatory fashion [5]. For example, the thiosulfinate is of particular utility against malaria parasites since it stimulates increases in the production of inflammatory cytokines, as well as the maturation of immature DC, and the induction of classic Th1 cells [5]. In a malaria-infected rodent model (*Plasmodium yoelli*), allicin (3 - 9 mg/kg for two days) appeared to affect the maturation of both myeloid and peripheral DC equally, allowing a widespread polarization and activation of T helper cells in these animals [5]. Increasing the level of allicin given to the animals in this model from 3 mg to a 9 mg dose resulted in the induction of immunosuppression, this time through the enhanced appearance of Treg cells [5], further providing evidence of the concentration-dependent nature of the activity of this thiosulfinate, *in vivo*. Importantly, the malaria parasite utilizes mammalian Tregs to prevent its removal, therefore the dosage of allicin is clearly influencial in balancing pro- versus anti-inflammatory effects in the context of parasitic infection [5].

Finally, extending the "bellshaped curve" observation of pro-inflammatory activity evolving into anti-inflammatory responses reported by Patya and colleagues [6], additional researchers have demonstrated similar findings *in vivo*. Specifically, when an upper level cutoff of 100 mg/kg/day is used for Th1 driven responses, the three rodent studies using allicin/garlic doses below this (namely 3, 5, 9 or 10 mg/kg/day) do indeed produce an increase in pro-inflammatory cytokine (IL-2 and IFNγ) levels [5, 9, 12] (see Table 2 for further experimental details). In contrast, the single study that used an elevated dose (600 mg/kg/day) reported a Th2 driven-response characterized by an increase in IL-4 and IL-10 secretion from splenocytes [27].

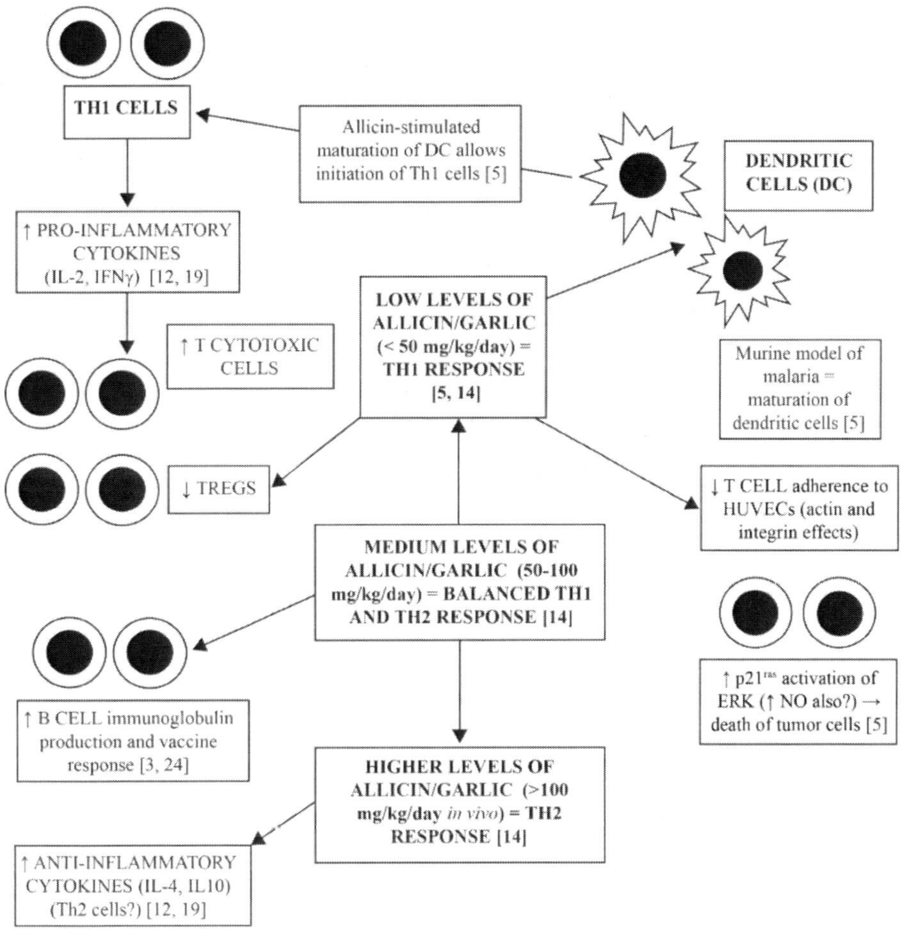

Legend: Allicin or garlic products containing allicin (extract or oil) appear to produce differential dose-dependent effects on adaptive immune system function. Lower doses are generally pro-inflammatory, especially for *in vivo* models, and improve clearance of parasites from animals by activating a Th1 response involving mature DC. Medium level doses create a balance between Th1- and Th2-driven responses, facilitate antibody production, and optimize responses to vaccines. In contrast, higher levels of allicin products create an anti-inflammatory or Th2-driven environment, which is optimal to rebalance conditions including chronic inflammatory syndromes.

Abbreviations: ERK (extracellular regulated kinase), HUVEC (human vein endothelial cells), IFNγ (interferon gamma), IL-2 (interleukin 2), IL-4 (interleukin 4), IL-10 (interleukin 10), NO (nitric oxide), Th (T helper).

References used to construct diagram: [3, 5, 6, 9-12, 14, 15, 19, 24-27].

Figure 2. Allicin/garlic's effects on adaptive immune system function.

2.3. Putting It Together: Allicin/Garlic and Adaptive Immunity

Allicin appears to have significant effects on T cells [5, 6, 9-12, 14, 15, 27] and DC [5] and modulation of cytokine production to produce either an inflammatory or immunosuppressive environment [5, 12, 14, 15, 19, 25-27]. The direct effects of allicin/garlic on B cell function are less clear, due to the paucity of investigations [3, 24]. However, since B cell function is regulated by Th2 cell activation [35], it is likely that the two *in vivo* studies in which allicin (50 mg/kg/day) or garlic extract (10 mg/kg/day) were found to stimulate immunoglobulin production are supportive of this mechanism [3, 24]. A possible schematic approach to allicin or garlic's effects on the adaptive immune system are shown in Figure 2.

If these dose-dependent effects could be replicated in humans using allicin it would indicate adaptogenic activity for the thiosulfinate. Adaptogenic activity in phytomedicines has been described since the late 1950s and are able to normalize body systems i.e., either upregulate or downregulate activity, as appropriate [66]. In a recent review of the characteristics of adaptogens, Panossian and Wagner [66] described them as "*preparations that increase attention and endurance in fatigue and stress-induced impairments and disorders related to the neuro-endocrine and immune systems.*" If allicin possesses adaptogenic qualities, this would also help to regulate immune system function rather than switching it off or on, as is the modality of current medications.

Summary and Future Directions

Allicin (or garlic products rich in allicin) has been shown in over twenty studies to exhibit direct immunomodulatory or adaptogenic effects on both innate and adaptive immune system cells (Figures 1 and 2). Analysis of these studies indicates several important effects of allicin or garlic products containing allicin, namely:

1. At low doses, these products promote the removal of a broad spectrum of bacterial, fungal, protozoal, and viral agents by being both antimicrobial [1] and increasing *in vivo* neutrophil, monocyte, and/or NK activity [3, 7-9, 17, 20-22]. Unlike classic antimicrobials, allicin reacts with cysteine residues in cell proteins, meaning that the microbes are unlikely to be able to establish resistance against the thiosulfinate [1].
2. Allicin shifts the healthy adaptive immune response towards one which decreases Tregs [5] and promotes activation of Th1 cells through stimulating DC maturation [5]. In chronic inflammation, garlic or allicin is especially effective at preventing cell attachment to inflamed endothelial cells [2, 10, 13, 16, 18], thereby preventing the perpetuation of the inflammatory response.
3. Allicin and garlic products containing allicin have the ability to promote a Th1-driven response and create a Th1:Th2 balanced environment [5, 9]. Th2-dominant responses are the hallmark of chronic inflammatory diseases that include cardiovascular, neurodegenerative, and osteodegenerative illnesses [54].
4. Allicin promotes the anti-tumor T cell-based response by activating $p21^{ras}$ and activating the cells to eliminate the tumors through classic mechanisms [6, 11].
5. Although not currently classified as an adaptogen [66], the studies in this chapter (especially those on T cells [6, 14, 15]) suggest allicin and garlic may possess adaptogenic properties.

As stated earlier, much of the issue with identifying allicin's capabilities in humans is the lack of studies done either with human cells or in healthy human subjects. Throughout this book, discussion will be made of allicin's instability and the methods currently being sought to overcome this issue. Stabilized oral [67], injectable [68], and semi-synthetic forms [69] of allicin have become available during the past decade. Several DBRPCT, being the gold standard for literature reporting of pharmaceutical efficacy [70], would need to be performed on healthy subjects to differentiate allicin's direct effects on immune system cells from its antimicrobial activities. Further studies of allicin's adaptogenic effects (if they translate to human physiology), together with an optimization of dosages for pro- versus anti-inflammatory activity, will also be needed. Adaptogens have historically been used as phytomedicines in a variety of "chronically stressed" body states, particularly including cardiovascular and neuroendocrine illnesses [66]. As will be seen in future chapters of this book, allicin is being studied for efficacy in reversing the effects of cardiovascular (chapter 10), osteodegenerative (chapter 11), and neurodegenerative (chapter 12) illnesses. It may also prove beneficial as a nutraceutical for those whose immune sytems are immunosuppressed, including those with advanced HIV-1 infection and organ transplant patients. Finally, in the elderly patient, who is likely to suffer chronic inflammatory comorbidities, allicin may have the potential to remediate the immunosenescence associated with aging. Given the global rise in immunocompromised individuals [71], especially in poorer nations, phytochemicals may provide a much needed local, economically viable, and sustainable intervention. Whether allicin will constitute one of these phytochemicals remains to be determined, but is clearly worth exploring.

REFERENCES

[1] Borlinghaus, Jan, Frank Albrecht, Martin C. H. Grulke, Ifeanyi D. Nwachukwu, and Alan J. Slusarenko. 2014. "Allicin : Chemistry and biological properties." *Molecules* 19(8) : 12591-12618.

[2] Zhang, Min, Huichao Pan, Yinjie Xu, Xueting Wang, Zhaohui Qui, and Li Jiang. 2018. "Allicin decreases lipopolysaccharide-induced oxidative stress and inflammation in human umbilical vein endothelial cells through suppression of mitochondrial dysfunction and activation of Nrf2." *Cell Physiol. Biochem.* 41 : 2255-2267.

[3] Alam, Rasha T. M., Elshaima M. Fawzi, Maha I. Alkhalf, Wafa S. Alansari, Lotfi Aleya, and Mohamed M. Abdel-Daim. 2018. "Anti-Inflammatory, Immunomodulatory, and Antioxidant Activities of Allicin, Norfloxacin, or Their Combination against Pasteurella multocida Infection in Male New Zealand Rabbits," Oxidative Medicine and Cellular Longevity, vol. 2018, Article ID 1780956, 10 pages, https://doi.org/10.1155/2018/1780956.

[4] Kang, N. S., E. Y. Moon, C. G. Cho, and S. Pyo. 2001. "Imunomodulating effect of garlic component, allicin, on murine peritoneal macrophages." *Nutrition Res* 4 : 617-626. Accessed October 16, 2018. https://eurekamag.com/pdf/003/003469471.pdf.

[5] Feng, Yonghui, Xiaotong Zhu, Quinhui Wang, Yongjun Jiang, Hong Shiang, Liwang Cui, and Yaing Cao. 2012. "Allicin enhances host pro-inflammatory responses and protects against acute murine malaria infection." *Malaria J.* 11 : 268. Accessed on September 14, 2018. doi: 10.1186/1475-2875-11-268.

[6] Patya, Miriam, Muayad A. Zahalka, Alexey Vanichkin, Aharon Rabinkov, Talia Miron, David Mirelman, Meir Wilchek, Harry M. Lander, and Abraham Novogrodsky. 2003. "Allicin stimulates lymphocytes and elicits an antitumor effect : a possible role of $p21^{ras}$." *International Immunology* 16(2) : 275-281.

[7] Haase, Hajo, Nora Hieke, Laura M. Plum, Martin C. H. Gruhlke, Alan S. Slusarenko, and Lothar Rink. 2012. "Impact of allicin on macrophage activity." *Food Chemistry* 134 : 141-148.

[8] Nya, E. J., Z. Dawood, and B. Austin. 2010. "The garlic component, allicin, prevents disease caused by *Aeromonas hydrophila* in rainbow trout, *Oncorhynchus mykiss* (Walbaum)." *Journal of Fish Diseases* 33(4): 293-300. Accessed on February 8, 2019. https://onlinelibrary.wiley.com/doi/abs/10.1111/j.1365-2761.2009.01121.x.

[9] Wang, Con-Jun, Chao Wang, Jiang Han, Yong-Kun Wang, Lin Tang, Dong-Wei Shen, Yi Zhao, Rong-Hua Xu, and Hui Xiang. 2013. "Effect of combined treatment with interleukin-2 and allicin on pancreatic cancer." *Mol. Bio. Reports* 40(12) : 6579-6585.

[10] Sela, Uri, Sharon Ganor, Iris Hecht, Alexander Brill, Talia Miron, Aharon Rabinkov, Meir Wilchek, David Mirelman, Ofer Lider, and Rami Hershkoviz. 2004. "Allicin inhibits SDF-1α-induced T cell interactions with fibrinectin and endothelial cells by down-regulating cytoskeleton arrangement, Pyk-2 phosphorylation and VLA-4 expression. " *Immunology* 111 :391-399.

[11] Gou, Yiang-Yang, Xian-Je Geng, Wen-Long Zhai, Xian-Wei Zhang, Yuan Wei, Guang-Jun Hou. 2015. "Effect of combined treatment with cyclophosphamidium and allicin on neuroblastoma-bearing mice." *Asian Pacific Journal of Tropical Medicine* 8(2) :137-141. https://doi.org/10.1016/S1995-7645(14)60304-7.

[12] Ota, Natsuko, Fumihide Takano, Shouta Muroga, Tetsuro Kawabata, Yasuhito Ishigaki, Nobuo Yahagi, Tomihisa Ohta. 2012. Garlic extract and its selected organosulphur constituents promote ileal immune responses ex vivo. *Journal of Functional Foods* 4(1): 243-252. https://doi.org/10.1016/j.jff.2011.11.003.

[13] Shih, Po-Chen, Chia-Hao Kuo, Jen-Yih Juang, Cheng-Hsien Liu, Long Hsu, and Cheng-Tzu Liu. 2010. "Effects of garlic oil on the migration of neutrophil-like cell studied by using a chemotactic gradient Labchip." *Journal of Biomedicine & Biotechnology* 2010: 319059. doi:10.1155/2010/319059.

[14] Liu, Cheng-Tzu, Hsing-Min Tsu, Chong-Kuei Lii, and Lee-Yan Sheen. 2009. Effect of supplementation of garlic oil on activity of Th1 and Th2 lymphocytes from rats. *Planta Med.* 75(3) : 205-210. doi: 10.1055/s-0028-1088396.

[15] Lestari, Sri R., and Muhaimin Rifa'i. 2018. "Regulatory T cells and anti-inflammatory cytokine profile of mice fed a high fat diet after single bulb garlic (*Allium sativum* L.) treatment." *Tropical Journal of Pharmaceutical Research* 17(11) :2157-2162. http://dx.doi.org/10.4314/tjpr.v17i11.7.

[16] Hobauer R., M. Frass, B. Gmeiner, A. D. Kaye, and E. A. Frost. 2000. "Garlic extract (*Allium sativum*) reduces migration of neutrophils through endothelial cell monolayers." *Middle East J. Anesthesiol.* 15 : 649-658.

[17] Adebolo, T. T., O. O. Adeoye, and V. O. Oyetayo. 2011. "Effect of garlic (*Allium sativum*) on *Salmonella typhi* infection, gastrointestinal flora and hematological parameters of albino rats." *African J. Biotech.* 10(35) : 6804-6808. Accessed October 11, 2018 https://academicjournals.org/journal/AJB/article-full-text-pdf/85C04D137469.

[18] Rassoul F., J. Salvetter, D. Reissig, W. Schneider, J. Thiery, and V. Reighter. 2006. "The influence of garlic (*Allium sativum*) extract on interleukin-1α expression of intracellular adhesion molecule-1and vascular cell adhesion molecule-1." *Phytomedicine* 13(4) :230-235. Accessed on October 11, 2018. https://www.sciencedirect.com/science/article/pii/S0944711305001583.

[19] Hodge, Greg, Sandy Hodge, and Ping Han. 2002. "*Allium sativum* (garlic) suppresses leukocyte inflammatory cytokine production *in vitro* : potential therapeutic use in the treatment of inflammatory bowel disease." *Cytometry* 48: 209-215. doi: 10.1002/cyto. 10133.
[20] Lau, Benjamin H. S., Takeshi Yamasaki, and Daila S. Gridley. 1991. "Garlic compounds modulate macrophage and T lymphocyte function." *Mol. Biother.* 3 :103-107.
[21] Aly, S. M., and M. F. Mohamed. 2010. "*Echinacea purpurea* and *Allium sativum* as immunostimulants in fish culture using Nile tilapia (*Oreochromis niloticus*)." *Journal of Animal Physiology and Animal Nutrition* 94: e31-e39. doi:10.1111/j.1439-0396. 2009.00971.x.
[22] Kandil, O. M., T. H. Abdullah, and A. Elkadi. 1987. "Garlic and the immune system in humans: its effect on natural killer cells." *Federation Proceedings* 46:441.
[23] Tanekhy, M., and J. Fall. 2015. "Expression of innate immunity genes in kuruma shrimp *Marsupenaeus japonicus* after *in vivo* stimulation with garlic extract (allicin)." *Veterinarni Medicina* 60(1): 39-7. https://www.agriculturejournals.cz/publicFiles/ 143005.pdf.
[24] Hanieh, Hamza, Kiyoaki Narabara, Mingzi Piao, Chaogitu Gerile, Asaki Abe, and Yasuhiro Kondo. 2010. "Modulatory effects of two levels of dietary *Alliums* on immune response and certain immunological variables, following immunization, in White Leghorn chickens." *Animal Science Journal.* 81(6):673–680. doi: 10.1111/j.1740-0929. 2010.00798.x..
[25] Čolić, M., D. Vučević, V. Kilibarda, N. Radičević, and M. Savić. 2002. "Modulatory effects of garlic extracts on proliferation of T-lymphocytes *in vitro* stimulated with concanavalin A." *Phytomedicine* 9(2): 117-124. https://doi.org/10.1078/0944-7113-00093.
[26] Moutia, Mouna, Fouad Seghrouchni, Omar Abouelazz, Annass Elouaddari, Abdellah Al Jahid, Abdelhalim Elhou, Sellama Nadafi, Jamal J. Eddine, Norddine Habti, and Abdallah Badou. 2016. "Allium sativum L. regulates *in vitro* IL-17 gene expression in human peripheral blood mononuclear cells," *BMC Complementary and Alternative Medicine* 16: 377. https://doi.org/10.1186/s12906-016-1365-9.
[27] Zamani, Alireza, Mohammad Hoseinipanah, Hasan Madadi, and Mehdi Arjipour. 2011. "Effect of garlic consumption on the argyrophilic nucleolar organiser regions (AgNORs) in splenocytes and thymocytes of rats." *Food and Agricultural Immunology* 22:4, 345-353, doi: 10.1080/09540105.2011.581271.
[28] Zamani, Alireza, Aliasghar Vahidinia, and Masoud S. Ghannad, M. S. 2009. The effect of garlic consumption on Th1/Th2 cytokines in phytohemagglutinin (PHA) activated rat spleen lymphocytes. *Phytother. Res* 23: 579-581. doi:10.1002/ptr.2700.
[29] Cundell, Diana R. 2014. Herbal phytochemicals as immunomodulators Current Immunology Reviews 2014, Volume 10 Issue 2 ISSN:1875-631X(Online), ISSN:1573-3955(Print) Accessed September 10, 2018. http://benthamscience.com/journal/index. php?journalID=cir.
[30] Winkel-Shirley, Brenda 2001. "Flavonoid biosynthesis : A colorful model for genetics, biochemistry, cells biology and biotechnology." *Plant. Phys.* 126 : 485-493. doi: https://doi.org/10.1104/pp.126.2.485.
[31] Arreola, Rodrigo, Saray Quintero-Fabián, Rocío I. López-Roa, Enrique O. Flores-Gutiérrez, Juan P. Reyes-Grajeda, Lucercia Carrera-Quintanar, and Daniel Ortuño-

Sahagún. 2015." Immunomodulation and anti-inflammatory effects of garlic compounds." *Journal of Immunology Research* 2015:401630. doi:10.1155/2015/401630

[32] Zheng, Guo-quiang, Patrick M. Kenney, and Luke K. T. Lam. 1992. "Antehofuran, carvone and limonene : potential anticancer agents from dill weed oil and caraway oil." *Planta Med* 58 :338-341.

[33] Block, Keith I, and Mark N. Mead. 2003. Immune system effects of echinacea, ginseng and astragalus: a review. *Integrative Cancer Therapies* 2(3): 247-267. doi: 10.1177/1534735403256419.

[34] Puri, Anju, R. Saxena, R. P. Saxena, K. C. Saxena, Vandita Srivastava, and J. S. Tandon. 1994. "Immunostimulant activity of *Nyctanthes arbor-tristis L.*" *Journal of Ethnopharmacology* 42(1) : 31-37. https://doi.org/10.1016/0378-8741(94)90020-5.

[35] Chaplin, David D. 2010. "Overview of the Immune Response". *The Journal of Allergy and Clinical Immunology* 125(2 Suppl 2), S3–23. Accessed September 25, 2018. http://doi.org/10.1016/j.jaci.2009.12.980.

[36] Abbas, Abul K., and Andrew H. Lichtman. Chapter 2 Innate Immunity; Cytokines of Innate immunity. In: *Basic Immunology Functions and Disorders of the Immune System*, 4th ed. Philadelphia, Saunders Elsevier Press: 2012; pp 34-35.

[37] Selders, Gretchen S., Allison E. Fetz, Marko Z. Radic, and Gary L. Bowlin. 2017. "An overview of the role of neutrophils in innate immunity, inflammation and host-biomaterial integration". *Regenerative Biomaterials* 4(1), 55–68. http://doi.org/10.1093/rb/rbw041.

[38] Vivier, Eric, David H. Raulet, Alissandro Moretta, Michael U. Caligiuri, Lawrence Zitvogel, Lewis L. Lanier, Waynde M. Yokoyama, and Sophie Ugolini. 2011. "Innate or Adaptive Immunity? The Example of Natural Killer Cells". *Science (New York, N.Y.)*, 331(6013), 44–49. http://doi.org/10.1126/science.1198687.

[39] Hirayama, Daisuke, Tomoyo Iida, and Hiroshi Nakase. 2018. "The Phagocytic Function of Macrophage-Enforcing Innate Immunity and Tissue Homeostasis."*International Journal of Molecular Sciences* 19(1): 92. http://doi.org/10.3390/ijms19010092.

[40] Amano, Keishero, Masahiro Hirayama, Eichi Azuma, Shotaro Iwamoto, Yoshitaka Keida, and Yoshihiro Komada. 2015. "Neutrophils Induced Licensing of Natural Killer Cells". *Mediators of Inflammation* 2015 747680. http://doi.org/10.1155/2015/747680.

[41] Terme, Magali, Evelyn Ullrich, Nicholas F. Delahaye, Nathalie Chaput, and Laurence Zitvogel. 2008. "Natural killer cell directed therapies : moving from unexpected results to directed therapies." *Nature Immunol.* 9 :486-494.

[42] Paul, Sourav, and Ghirdhari Lal. 2017. "The Molecular Mechanism of Natural Killer Cells Function and Its Importance in Cancer Immunotherapy." *Frontiers in Immunology* 8: 1124. http://doi.org/10.3389/fimmu.2017.01124.

[43] Dunkelberger, Jason R., and Wen-Chao Song. 2010. "The role of complement in innate and adaptive immune responses". *Cell Research* 20 : 34-50. Accessed October 10, 2018. https://www.nature.com/articles/cr2009139.

[44] Joncker, Nathalie T., Nadine C. Fernandez, Emmanuel Treiner, Eric Vivier, and David H. Raulet. 2009. "NK Cell Responsiveness is Tuned Commensurate with the Number of Inhibitory Receptors for Self MHC Class I: the Rheostat Model". *Journal of Immunology (Baltimore, Md. : 1950)*, 182(8): 4572–4580. http://doi.org/10.4049/jimmunol.0803900.

[45] Elliott, Julie M., Joseph A. Wahle, and Wayne M. Yokohama. 2010. "MHC class 1-deficient natural killer cells acquire a licensed phenotype after transferring into an MHC-class 1 sufficient environment." *J. Exp. Med.* 207 :2073. doi: 10.1084/jem.20100986.

[46] Banchereau, Jacques, Francine Briere, Christophe Caux, Jean Davoust, Serge Lebecque, Yong-Jun Liu, Bali Pulendran, and Karolina Palucka. 2000. "Immunobiology of dendritic cells". *Annu. Rev. Immunol.* 18 : 767-811.

[47] Young, James W., and Ralph M. Steinman. 1990. "Dendritic cells stimulate primary cytolytic lymphocyte responses in the absnce of CD4+ helper T cells." *J. Exp. Med.* 171 : 1315-1332.

[48] Brocker, Thomas. 1997. "Survival of mature CD4 T lymphocytes is dependent on major histocompatability complex class II-expressing dendritic cells." *J. Exp. Med.* 186 : 1223-1232.

[49] Ludewig, Burkhard, Stephan Oehnen, Federica Barchiesi, Rito A. Schwendener, Hans Hentgartner, and Rolf M. Zinkernagel. 1999. "Protective antiviral cytotoxic T cell memory is most efficiently maintained by restimulation via dendritic cells." *J. Immunol.* 163 : 1839-1844.

[50] Fayette, Jérôme, Bertrand Dubois, Stéphane Vandanabeele, Jean-Michel Bridon, Béatrice Vanbervliet, Isabelle Durand, Jacques Banchereau, Christophe Caux, and Francine Briere. 1997. "Human dendritic cells skew isotype switching of CD40-activated naive B cells towards IgA1 and IgA2." *J. Exp. Med.* 185 : 1909-1918.

[51] Piemonti, Lorenzo, Paolo Monti, Paola Allavena, Marina Sironi, Laura Soldini, Biagio E. Leone, Carlo Socci, and Valero DiCarlo. 1999. "Glucocorticoids affect human dendritic cell differentiation and maturation." *J. Immunol.* 162 : 6473-6481.

[52] Sallusto Federica, and Antonio Lanzavecchia. 2009. "Heterogeneity of $CD4^+$ memory T cells : Functional molecules for tailored immunity. *Eur. J. Immunol.* 39 : 2076-2082.

[53] Alper, Chester A., Margaret S. Kruskall, Deborah Marcus-Bagley, Donald E. Craven, Aubrey J. Katz, Stuart J. Brink, Jules L. Dienstag, Zuheir Awday, and Edmond J. Yunis. 1989. "Genetic prediction of nonresponse to hepatitis B vaccine". *N. Engl. J. Med.* 321 : 708-712.

[54] Brocker, Thomas. 1997. "Survival of mature CD4 T lymphocytes is dependent on major histocompatability complex class II-expressing dendritic cells." *J. Exp. Med.* 186 : 1223-1232.

[55] Ludewig, Burkhard, Stephan Oehnen, Federica Barchiesi, Rito A. Schwendener, Hans Hentgartner, and Rolf M. Zinkernagel. 1999. "Protective antiviral cytotoxic T cell memory is most efficiently maintained by restimulation via dendritic cells." *J. Immunol.* 163 : 1839-1844.

[56] Young, James W., and Ralph M. Steinman. 1990. "Dendritic cells stimulate primary cytolytic lymphocyte responses in the absnce of CD4+ helper T cells." *J. Exp. Med.* 171 : 1315-1332.

[57] Satyal, Prabodh, Jonathan D. Craft, Noura S. Dosoky, and William N. Setzer. 2017. "The Chemical Compositions of the Volatile Oils of Garlic (*Allium sativum*) and Wild Garlic (*Allium vineale*)." *Foods* 6(8): 63. http://doi.org/10.3390/foods6080063.

[58] Chentouh, Ryme, Catherine Fitting, and Jean-Luc Cavaillon. 2018. "Specific features of human monocytes activation by monophosphoryl lipid A". *Scientific Reports* 8: 7096. http://doi.org/10.1038/s41598-018-25367-y.

[59] Berghaus, Londa J., James N. Moore, David J. Hurley, Michel L. Vandenplas, Barbara P. Fortes, Margreet A. Wolfert, and Geert-Jan Boons. 2010. "Innate immune responses of primary murine macrophage-lineage cells and RAW 264.7 cells to ligands of Toll-like receptors 2, 3, and 4". *Comparative Immunology, Microbiology and Infectious Diseases* 33(5): 443–454. http://doi.org/10.1016/j.cimid.2009.07.001.

[60] Rosa, Rafael D., Paula T. Bandeira, and Margherita A. Barracco. 2007. "Molecular cloning of crustins from the hemocytes of Brazilian penaeid shrimps." *FEMS Microbiology Letters* 274(2):287–290. https://doi.org/10.1111/j.1574-6968.2007.00866.x.

[61] Lau, Yuk-Ting, Lauren Sussman, Emmanuelle P. Espinosa, Selma Katalay, and Bassem Allam. 2017. "Characterization of hemocytes from different body fluids of the eastern oyster *Crassostrea virginica.*" *Fish and Shellfish Immunology* 71 : 372-379. Accessed on June 26, 2019 https://cpb-us-e1.wpmucdn.com/you.stonybrook.edu/dist/c/1963/files/2017/02/Lau-et-al-2017-1-virw1r.pdf.

[62] Cheresh, David A., Jie Leng, and Richard L. Klemke. 1999. "Regulation of cell contraction and membrane ruffling by distinct signals in migratory cells." *J. Cell. Biol.* 146: 1107-1116.

[63] Boisvert, Marc, Steve Gendron, Nizar Chetoui, and Fazwi Aoudjit. 2007."Alpha2beta1 integrin signaling augments T cell receptor-dependent production of interferon-gamma in human T cells." *Molecular Immunology* 44(15) : 3732-3740.

[64] Ibiza S., and J. M. Serrador. 2008. "The role of nitric oxide in the regulation of adaptive immune responses". *Immunología* 27(3) : 103-117.

[65] Kleiveland, Charlotte R. 2015. "Peripheral blood mononuclear cells." In *The impact of food additives on health*, p 161-167. Springer, Cham. Accessed on October 10, 2019. https://link.springer.com/chapter/10.1007/978-3-319-16104-4_15.

[66] Panossian, Alexander, and Hildebert Wagner. 2011. "Adaptogens : A review of their history, biological activity and clinical benefits." *HerbalGram* 90 : 52-63. Accessed on July 2, 2019 http://cms.herbalgram.org/herbalgram/issue90/Feat_Adaptogens.html.

[67] Suddek, Ghada M. 2014. "Allicin enhances chemotherapeutic response and ameliorates tamoxifen-induced liver injury." *Pharmaceutical Biology* 52(8) : 1009-1014. Accessed November 22, 2018. https://www.tandfonline.com/doi/full/10.3109/13880209.2013.876053.

[68] Feng, Fang, Li Hong, Cui Wen, and Yongsui Dong. 1999. "Treatment of hepatitis caused by cytomegalovirus with allitridin injection – An experimental study." *Journal of Tongji Medical University* 19(4) : 271-274. https://doi.org/10.1007/BF02886960.

[69] Leontiev, Roman, Nils Hohaus, Jacob Claus, Martin C. H. Gruhlke, and Alan J. Slusarenko .2018." Comparison of the Antibacterial and Antifungal Activities of Thiosulfinate Analogues of Allicin." *Scientific Reports* 6763 :8(1). Accessed on February 22, 2019 https://www.nature.com/articles/s41598-018-25154-9.

[70] Kaptchuk, Ted. J. 2001. "The double-blind, randomized, placebo-controlled trial." *Journal of Clinical Epidemiology* 54(6): 541 – 549.

[71] Kahn, Laura H. 2006. "The Growing Number of Immunocompromised." *Bulletin of the Atomic Scientists* January 6, 2008. Accessed on July 7, 2019. https://thebulletin.org/2008/01/the-growing-number-of-immunocompromised/.

In: Allicin
Editor: Diana R. Cundell

ISBN: 978-1-53617-339-0

Chapter 5

A CONTEMPORARY OVERVIEW OF ALLICIN, AN ANCIENT ANTIBIOTIC

Mary Ann Wagner-Graham**, *PhD
College of Life Sciences, Department of Biological and Chemical Sciences,
Thomas Jefferson University, Philadelphia, PA, US

ABSTRACT

The antibacterial efficacy of allicin and garlic extract is well established. Allicin is bacteriostatic and bacteriocidal to a broad range of clinically important human pathogens, including multidrug-resistant organisms. In contrast to the targeted actions of commonly used synthetic antibiotics on bacterial cells, allicin is freely permeable through the bacterial cell wall and promiscuously attacks sulfhydryl groups, resulting in global disruption of bacterial metabolism, alteration of cellular redox potential, and inactivation of toxins. Allicin is disruptive to biofilm formation, and biocidal to cells in biofilm, reducing ability of cells to colonize host tissues. Initial studies on use of allicin and garlic extract to treat gastric ulcers, prosthetic joint infections, tuberculosis, cystic fibrosis-associated lung infections, and other infections, are promising, but clinical trials are few. Recently developed applications of allicin and allicin-inspired synthetic antibiotic drugs are presented, along with a brief overview of the use of allicin and garlic extract in livestock and aquaculture.

Keywords: allicin, antimicrobial, antibacterial, antibiotic, garlic

INTRODUCTION

Throughout history, healers have found nature's pharmacoepia to be a rich trove of remedies for the inescapable afflicions of the human condition. The literature is replete with records of naturopathic therapies applied to every maladay known to humans and the

* Corresponding Author's Email: Mary.Ann.Wagner-Graham@Jefferson.edu.

domestic animals upon which they rely. Many of today's most effective and lucerative pharmaceutical products are synthetic replicas or variants of the active compounds in crude concoctions of natural products, with their chemical structures having been elucidated through application of modern analytical chemistry and separation science techniques to ancient, complex mixtures.

Consider the ancient complex mixture of a poultice made from mouldy bread. This rememdy for infected wounds most surely would have contained penicillin as an active ingredient. Penicllin, the first naturally-occuring antibiotic approved by the US Food and Drug Administration for use in patients, was first formally named when Alexander Flemming investigated the inhibition of staphylococci growing on nian agar plate by a fungal contaminant [1]. Ernst Chain and Howard Florey initially purified and characterized the structure of penicillin, while chemists in Peoria, Illinois developed a purification schema for its large-scale production, using a fungus growing on a mouldy cataloupe as the initial prodcution strain [2]. With the initial clinical deployment of penicillin, previously penicillin-sensitive bacteria experienced increased selective pressure to acquire resistance to this miraculous drug which acylates penicillin binding proteins (D-alanyl-D-alanine carboxypeptidases/transpeptidases) to prevent formation of peptidoglycan in the bacterial cell wall [3]. The Review on Antimicrobial Resistance by the Government of the United Kingdom estimates that 10,000,000 people may succumb annually to bacterial infections by the year 2050 [4], as the antibacterial drugs in our modern arsenal are deftly rendered useless by the older and wiser prokaryotic coinhabitants of our world. As the population of novel antibiotic resistant bacterial pathogens increases, the medical and scientific communities acknowledge a grave urgency to expand the repertoire of chemotherapeutic antibiotic drugs. To this end, antibacterial properties of ages-old folk remedies are scrutinized using the lens of modern chemical and biological sciences.

This review focuses upon allicin, the primary antibacterial compound in the humble, soil-bound bulb of *Allium sativum*, garlic [5]. Unlike most synthetic antibiotic drugs, which arrest bacterial growth by attacking with great specificity a handful of enzymatic targets, allicin exerts its bactericidal power through a broad, multi-target approach, attacking multiple enzymes having catalytically or structurally important sulfhydryl groups [6, 7], and altering the redox potential of the cytoplasm [8, 9, 10]. This global, broad-scope killing strategy of allicin may discourage development of bacterial resistance and prolong its clinical effectiveness, since bacteria less often become resistant to broad-acting biocidal agents [11]. The compendium of studies presented herein address two broad topics: 1) a description of the molecular basis for the antibacterial action of allicin, which support the suitability of allicin as an effective broad-spectrum antibacterial compound with potential applications to control a diversity of infections in humans, 2) an overview of novel applications of allicin and garlic extract to improve the human condition, including improvement of food supply through increased production of meat and fish.

1. Historical Perspective

For centuries, garlic, aqueous garlic extract, and garlic oil have been used as folk remedies for infectious bacterial diseases. Efforts to identify the primary antibacterial compound in garlic did not begin in earnest until the early twentieth century, as technologies for separation and chemical analysis were developed. The active component was isolated after fractional distillation of a large-scale (5 L) ethanolic extraction of 4 kg of garlic cloves and named "allicin" (*Allium* + penicillin) [5]. Confirmation that allicin was the antibacterial factor was gained as even a 1:125,000 dilution of purified allicin into meat extract broth suppressed growth of a range of disease-causing Gram-positive and Gram-negative bacteria, including *Staphylococcus aureus*, *Streptococcus hemolyticus*, *Bacillus typhosus*, *Bacillus dysenteriae*, *Bacillus typhi-murium*, and *Vibrio cholerae* [5]. Note the historical names of organisms associated with strep throat, rheumatic fever, skin infections, typhus, dysentery, and salmonellosis. A plausible structure of allicin was proposed shortly thereafter, along with the idea that allicin exerts its bacteriostatic effects by attack of sulfhydryl groups [5]. The instability, reactvitiy, and antibiotic character of allicin was attributed to its unique thiosulfinate group [12], the existence of which was definitvely confirmed in 1948 [13].

The antibacterial nature of allicin is well established. The literature is saturated with reports regarding the antimicrobial powers of garlic extracts or allicin, with PubMed returning just over 1250 results for "garlic antimicrobial," and just under 500 results for "allicin antimicrobial" for the years 1946-2018, inclusive. Studies focused on garlic powder or aqueous garlic extract greatly outnumber those which utilize either purified allicin or garlic extract in which allicin has been quantitated. Allicin content in garlic extracts varies widely, based on plant genotype/strain, growth conditions, harvest time, extract preparation method, etc., as previewed below and more fully illustrated later, so comparison and reproducibility of scientific studies is hampered.

In China, 212 different strains of garlic from broad geographic locations were sorted into groups based on allicin content; the most populated group (93 plants) contained 0.49-1.49% allicin, and the second-most populated group (82 plants) contained 1.61-2.07% allicin [14]. Even if plant strain, growth condition, and harvest time are controlled, different processing of garlic bulbs from the same source yields different results in antibacterial assays, even when using the same solvent for extraction. Ethanolic extracts of Turkish garlic were made from bulbs processed three ways: chopping without freezing, chopping while frozen, or slicing without freezing [15]. Extract made from chopped non-frozen garlic bulbs yielded more activity against *B. subtilis* DSMZ 1971 grown on Muller-Hinton Agar than extracts made using the other two methods [15].

Solvent choice influences the concentration of allicin in garlic extracts. Allicin concentration varied from 4 to 12 mM in different solvents (water, n-hexane, or ethanol at 20, 50, 70, or 100%), and there was a correlation between allicin concentration and zone of inhibition observed with *E. coli* C600 and *S. aureus* Rosenback 1884 in disk-diffusion assay on nutrient agar [16]. Further, extracts prepared in n-hexane demonstrated greater effectiveness, while those utilizing vegetable oil were less effective [16]. Keep in mind that although allicin is regarded as the most antibacteiral compound in garlic preparartions, a host of other compounds with antibacterial power are present in complex aqueous or ethanolic extracts of garlic [17, 18]. When preparing a complex mixture from the garlic clove, different solvents draw out different concentrations of not only allicin, but also other antibacterial compounds.

The notorious instability of allicin and other bio-active compounds in complex garlic extracts further complicates comparison of different antibacterial studies, as stability and therefore antibacteiral efficacy of allicin depends upon a number of factors, including type of solvent, storage temperature, and even concentration of thiosulfinates. A review of the chemical stability of allicin is presented in Chapter 2.

A medical scientist would argue that only antibacterial studies using purified, standardized preparations of allicin have value. A medical humanitarian recognizes that heterogeneous preparations of garlic extract are more accessible to large numbers of people, especially those in underdeveloped or medically underserved areas. Restricting exploration of the antibacterial activity of garlic to studies employing only purified allicin limits discovery and development of medically effective, economically attractive treatments using heterogeneous preparations, and may limit potential to improve the human condition. Consider also that gram-for-gram, garlic oil preparations show greater killing power against some Gram-negative and Gram-positive intestinal flora and pathogens, as compared to garlic powder or aqueous garlic extract, even though aqueous preparations contain a higher percentage of strongly antibacterial allicin [19]. Application of allicin or complex aqueous or oil-based garlic extracts for prophylaxis and/or treatment of infectious disease is becoming more important as the number of multidrug-resistant strains of bacteria increase. A recent review [20] presents an elegant argument focused on application of garlic extract and allicin for treatment of multidrug-resistant tuberculosis, underscoring the urgency of such application in areas where HIV and TB infections overlap – areas where natural medicines like garlic are more readily available than synthetic pharmaceuticals. Currently, there is a dearth of controlled clinical trials regarding use of either pure or well-characterized heterogenous formulations of allicin to treat bacterial disease.

2. Molecular Bases of Antibacterial Action

2.1. General Considerations

Allicin globally impedes the infectious process, directly assualting both the bacterial cell and secreted factors necessry to host invasion and virulence (Figure 1). Allicin is freely permeable through cell wall and cell membrane [21], and modifies the structure and function of proteins and enzymes by covalently modifying free thiol groups to S-allyl-mercaptocysteine residues [6, 7, 10]. Bacterial cells can be killed by allicin, or effectively recover from sub-leathal doses of allicin, as seen with *Salmonella typhimurium* [22] and *E. coli* [10]. Allicin is effective against a broad range of Gram-positive and Gram-negative organisms, as well as acid-fast mycobacteria, and reports of bacteria not affected by it are few. *Pseudomonas fluorescens* 01 [23] and *Leuconostoc mesenteroides* NCIB 8710 (Elsom et al. 2000) are rare examples of bacterial strains poorly affected by allicin or aqueous garlic extract. Some multidrug-resistant strains of *S. beta-hemolyticus*, *P. aeruginosa*, and *E. faecium* are not sensistive to allicin (LD_{50} > 100 ug/mL) [24]. *Stenotrophomonas maltophilia*, *Flavimonas oryzihabitans*, *Erwinia* sp., and *Comamonas acidovorans* isolated from skin ulcers of mice infected with *Leishmania major* were unaffected by allicin [25].

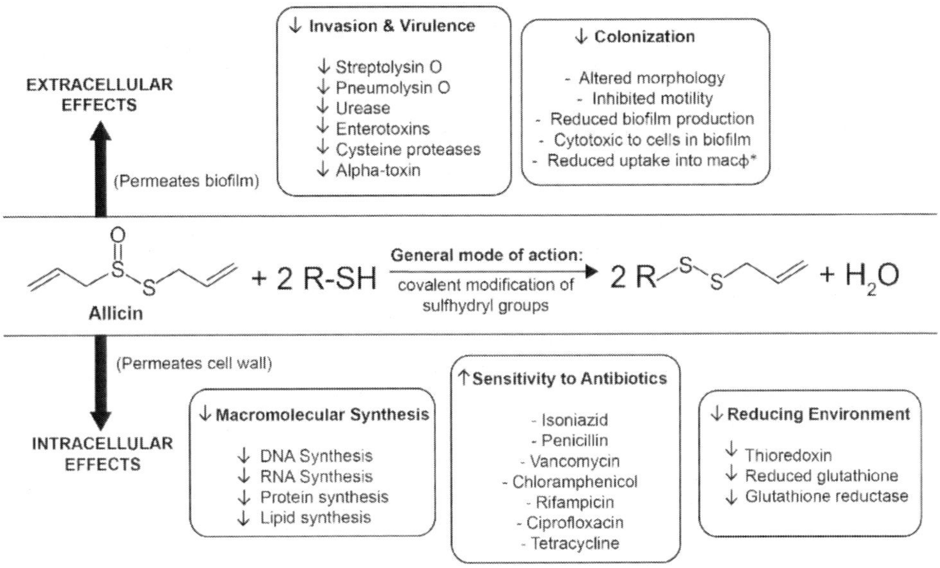

Legend: Graphical overview of the effects of antibacterial actions of allicin, based upon general themes of papers referenced in this review. See text for details. Reaction mechanism is a modification of that presented in [28]. *- Impaired uptake into macrophage likely mediated by effects on host cells [29].

Figure 1. Antibacterial actions of allicin.

The mode of action of allicin appears to be independent of whether or not bacteria are multidrug-resistant. Although details of the experimental method are not provided, both antibiotic-sensistive and multidrug-resistant *E. coli* were equally sensitive to allicin (LD_{50} = 15 ug/mL), as were methicillin-sensitive and methicillin-resistant *S. aureus* (LD_{50} = 12 ug/mL) [24]. Also, allicin in aqueous garlic extract (64% ($^{w}/_{v}$) garlic; 260 μg/mL allicin) was equally effective against both susceptible and multidrug-resistant isolates (n=28 per group) of *S. mutans* from extracted teeth, as similar distribution of zones of inhibition was observed for both groups in disk-diffusion assay on Mitis-Salivarious-Bacitracin Agar, and similar MIC values were measured in Mueller-Hinton broth (16-128 μg/mL by allicin concentration, with modal MIC = 64 μg/mL allicin) [26]. Inhibition of *Staphylococcus epidermidis* by allicin in tryptic soy broth cultures was similar regardless of sensitivity of the strains to methicillin, with an MIC 90 value of 8 μg/mL for each group (19 methicillin-sensitive or 19 methicillin-resistant strains per group) [27].

2.2. Intracellular Effects

2.2.1. Decreased Macromolecular Synthesis

Allicin at 0.3 mM in Luria broth notably but temporarily inhibited DNA, RNA, and protein synthesis in *Salmonella typhimurium* [22]. Within 15 min of addition, allicin inhibited DNA synthesis 68% relative to control, based on incorporation of tritiated thymidine, with complete recovery of DNA synthesis after 35 min [22]. Effects on RNA synthesis were more pronounced. Within 1 min of exposure to allicin, RNA synthesis was inhibited nearly 100%, measured by lack of incorporation of tritiated uridine, with recovery to only 88% of initial level after 140 min [22]. Maximal (65%) inhibition of protein synthesis was achieved after 20 min incubation with allicin, and 50 min after allicin exposure incorporation of tritiated leucine returned to a level greater than that measured in the untreated control [22]. Additionally, proteomic studies showed cysteines of the RNA polymerase alpha subunit, adenylosuccinate synthase for purine synthesis, and leucine-tRNA ligase were modified by allicin in *E. coli* cells cultured with allicin [10].

Lipid synthesis is also affected. *In vitro* assay of bacterial acetate kinase/ phosphotransacetylase revealed just over 50% inhibition of formation of acetyl-CoA from acetate by 75-100 μM allicin [30], although the bacterial source of the enzyme is not specified.

2.2.2. Increased Sensitivity to Antibiotics

Pairing a failing antibiotic with a synergistic agent may help overcome resistance and extend clinical usefulness of the antibiotic. Synergism of allicin and garlic extract with antibiotics additional to those mentioned here is presented in the section "Use Against Human Pathogens." Allicin may boost effectiveness of vancomycin against vancomycin resistant enterococci (VRE). Nine clinical isolates of *E. faecium* and one isolate of *E. durans* had MIC values of 128 - 256 μg/mL for vancomycin alone, and 64 μg/mL for allicin alone, but when incubated with vancomycin and 1-2 g/mL garlic extract or 8 - 16 μg/mL allicin, the MIC values for vancomycin decreased remarkably to 0.5 - 16 μg/mL [31]. All strains had fractional inhibitory concentration (FIC) values < 0.5 when exposed to vancomycin plus garlic or allicin, indicating a synergistic effect [31]. Two vancomycin-sensitive strains, one *E. faecalis* and the other *E. facium*, had MIC values of 32 μg/mL for pure allicin - not much lower than the MIC for the vancomycin-resistant strains - and FIC values of 0.53 for combination of allicin with vancomycin, suggesting the antibacterial effect of allicin is independent of vancomycin sensitivity, and indicating lack of synergism between allicin and vancomycin [31]. The antibiotic nature of vancomycin and garlic extract could be negated by cysteine (0.01 to 0.1%) or β-mercaptoethanol (0.001 to 0.01%) [31]. The mobile genetic element Tn1546 conveys vancomycin resistance [32]. Vancomycin-resistant *S. aureus* (VRSA) is an increasing threat in the healthcare setting, and since MRSA strains evolve to VRSA through obtainment of the Tn1546 element from VRE [33], it would be interesting to investigate efficacy of allicin against VRSA.

One of the Tn1546 gene products, D-lactate dehydrogenase (VanH), has several important cysteine residues, and its activity is dependent upon a reducing environment [34]. Allicin could attack VanH in two ways, as the cysteine residues of VanH are attractive targets for modification, and allicin depletes the reducing environment of the cell [8, 9, 10]. VanX is a possible but unlikely target of allicin, as there is only one conserved cysteine for VanX from *E. faecium* and *E. faecalis* [35]. The MIC for allicin against VRE was 64 μg/mL, and 32 μg/mL for vancomycin-sensitive strains [31], so allicin may attack a protein target not conferred by Tn1546. Another possible allicin target is UDP-N-acetylglucosamine enolpyruvyl transferase (MurA). MurA is required for biofilm formation and contains a catalytically important cysteine, Cys115, which is modified by fosfomycin [36]. It would be interesting to examine whether fosfomycin-resistant VRE are still susceptible to allicin, since fosfomycin-resistant VRE have aspartate instead of cysteine in this position in MurA [37].

Aqueous garlic extract can increase effectiveness of antibiotics even against multidrug resistant bacteria. Aqueous garlic extract (2 g freshly prepared garlic powder / 1 mL water, and diluted 1:10 just prior to use) enhanced the antibiotic activity of ciprofloxacin, but not ampicillin, against 12 multi-antibiotic resistant clinical isolates of *E. coli*, *S. aureus*, and *P. aeruginosa*, as measured in the Kirby-Bauer disc-diffusion method [38]. Even though the three *P. aeruginosa* isolates in this study were unaffected by garlic extract alone, garlic extract still enhanced the antibacterial efficacy of ciprofloxacin against these strains [38], indicating that potentiation of antibiotics by allicin is possible even if allicin alone is not antibacterial. Similarly, effectiveness of ceftoxamine against ten clinical isolates of MDR *Acinetobacter* spp. from skin and soft tissue infections was enhanced by aqueous garlic extract *in vitro* [39].

Enhanced sensitivity to antibiotics is not limited to planktonic cells, but also extends biofilm-associated cells. This is an important point, since biofilm-embedded bacteria are often more resistant to antibiotics than planktonic cells, and bacterial biofilms are implicated in multiple infections [40]. Garlic extract (1%) supplied continuously to three-day cultures of *P. aeruginosa* potentitated killing of biofilm-embedded bacteria by tobramycin (340 μg/mL, for 24 hours) [41].

Enhanced potency of antibiotics is also seen against a potential biological warfare agent. Aqueous garlic extract enhanced activity of penicillin, rifampicin, and tetracycline against *B. anthracis* Sterne 34F2 ($pXO1^+$, $pXO2^-$) in a 96-well plate growth assay in MHB [42].

Even though allicin might not act synergistically with standard antibiotic drugs, it may increase efficacy of drugs used concurrently for treatment of some infections. Although fresh aqueous garlic extract (12.3 mg/mL allicin) did not enhance activity of amoxicillin, clarithromycin, or metronidazole against *H. pylori* in agar dilution testing in blood agar medium, garlic extract increased activity of omeperazole against *H. pylori* in brain heart infusion broth cultures [43].

In addition to acting synergistically with antibiotics *in vitro*, allicin and garlic extract increase killing power of antibiotics *in vivo*, and may protect host tissues allowing tolerance of higher doses. When combined with isoniazid treatment of C57BL/6 mice infected with *M. tuberculosis* H37Rv *via* aerosol exposure, garlic extract (5 mg/kg/d i.p.) cleared the infection 15 days faster than isoniazid alone [29]. Allicin (50 mg/kg p.o.) protects against gentamicin-induced kidney damage in Wistar albino rats [44].

Allicin (50 mg/kg/d p.o., for five days) combined with norfloxacin (100 mg/kg, p.o., single dose) was found to be more effective than norfloxacin alone or allicin alone in treating New Zealand White rabbits (10 per treatment group) infected intranasally with *Pasturella multocida* Type b (2×10^5 CFU in 1 mL), with mortality rates 5 days p.i. for the three groups at 10%, 30%, or 40%, respectively [45]. As an added benefit, rabbits receiving allicin alone or in combination with norfloxacin experienced a modest amount of hepatoprotection based on standard chemistry values for liver function [45].

Finally, garlic extract and allicin are synergistic not only with antibiotics, but also with other traditional herbal antibacterials. Aqueous garlic extract (34.5 g juice from 55 g bulb tissue, diluted in water to 6.25, 12.5, 25, and 50% concentrations) combined with honey promoted greater zones of inihibition than 30 μg of chloramphenicol, when tested using well-diffiusion assays of most tested organisms (*S. typhi, L. monocytogenes, S.aureus, S. flexneri, P. vulgaris, S. dysenteriae, Salmonella*, and *S. pneumonia*), except for *E. coli* [46].

Table 1. Studies showing synergism with antibiotics *in vitro*, unless otherwise specified

Organism(s)	Allicin or extract?	Antibiotic(s)	Reference
VRE (*E. faecium, E. durans*)	Allicin	vancomycin	[31]
P. aeruginosa	Extract	tobramycin	[41]
B. anthracis	Extract	penicillin, rifampicin, tetracycline	[42]
MDR *E. coli, S. aureus, P. aeruginosa*	Extract	ciprofloxacin	[38]
Acinetobacter spp.	Extract	ceftoxamine	[39]
M. tuberculosis	Extract	isoniazid	[29]*
Pasturella mutocida	Allicin	norfloxacin	[45]*

*- animal models.

2.2.3. Decreased Reducing Environment

Allicin is freely permeable through biological membranes, as determined using red blood cells and synthetic DMPC/cholesterol 3:1 or PC/cholesterol 5:1 vesicles, and allicin does not appear to disrupt integrity of the biological membranes [21]. Uptake of garlic-derived organosulfur compounds into *Campylobacter jejuni* was confirmed with a novel combination of Raman and FT-IR spectroscopy [47]. Allicin oxidizes glutathione (GSH) to S-allylmercaptoglutathione (GSSA) [21]. Since GSH is converted to GSSA, and not glutathione disulfide (GSSG), glutathione reductase (GR) cannot recharge the cytoplasm with GSH [10]. Paradoxically, the ratio of GSH:GSSG increases five-fold when *E. coli* cells are grown in MOPS minimal media with 0.79 mM allicin, as allicin more profoundly reduces the population of GSSG as compared to that of GSH, and the reduction potential of the cytoplasm increases slightly, from – 257 mV to – 270 mV [10]. In the same study, glutaredoxin 3 and 3-phosphoglycerate dehydrogenase were found to be modified by allicin in proteomic analysis [10]. 3-Phosphoglycerate dehydrogenase is required for manufacture of serine from 3-phosphoglycerate [48], and serine is required for manufacture of glutathione.

Interestingly, GR from *Saccharomyces cerevisiae* appears to use GSSA (K_m = 0.50 mM) as a substrate *in vitro*, although not nearly as well as GSSG (K_m = 0.07 mM) [49]. Caution is advised in comparing these Michaelis constants, since the K_m for GSSG was determined by following rate of accumulation of 2-nitro-5-thiobenzoate, and the K_m for GSSA was measured by following rate of depletion of NADPH; further, the greatest decrease in $A_{340\ nm}$ was just under 0.09 over a 50 min reaction with 1.25 mM GSSA as substrate [49]. A γ-glutamylcysteine synthetase deficient yeast strain incapable of making GSH from γ-glutamylcysteine and glycine can be resuced by addition of GSSA, suggesting GR makes GSSH from GSSA *in vivo* [49]. Regardless, glutaredoxin and thioredoxin, key proteins for maintaining the level of GSH in cells, both rely upon a catalytically important cysteine and can therefore be poisoned by allicin [50].

2.2.4. Other Intraceullular Effects

Since allicin is a thiol-modifying agent, it reacts with a broad range of thiol-dependent enzymes in the cell. Some important thiol-dependent enzymes are critical for central metabolic pathways and fermentation. The reduction of enzyme activity by allicin has been demonstrated against triose phosphate dehydrogenase, lactate dehydrogenase, and succinate dehydrogenase [6]. Several thiol-dependent proteins key for central metabolism were modified by allicin in *E. coli* cells growing in broth culture, as determined by proteomic studies: glyceraldehyde-3-

phosphate dehydrogenase, phosphoglycerate kinase, and isocitrate lyase [10]. Impairment of these pathways would weaken the health of the cells.

2.3. Extracellular Effects

2.3.1. Decreased Invasion and Virulence

Allicin attacks not only bacterial cells directly, but also toxins responsible for invasion of the host and production of disease symptoms. In addition to direct inactivation of the toxins, allicin can reduce toxin production. Note, though, that a correlation between growth inhibition and reduction of virulence characteristics such as biofilm production is not assured. *Streptococcus mutans* was most highly inhibited in disc-diffusion testing on brain heart infusion agar wtih full-strength garlic juice, compared to *E. faecalis*, *S. gordonii*, *S. sanguinis*, and *S. sobrinus*, while in broth dilution assay, the MIC values were 32 mg/mL for *S. mutans*, 64 mg/mL for *S. sobrinus*, and 128 mg/mL for the other strains [51]. Despite this growth inhibition, the amount of biofilm growing on stainless steel orthodontic wire in broth culture with 16 mg/mL garlic extract was increased, as measured by ATP quantitation, live cell counts, and biofilm visualization with SEM, along with increased transcription of glucosyltransferase genes [51].

2.3.2. Inhibition of Streptolysin O and Pneumolysin O; Cholesterol-Dependent Cytolysins

The cholesterol-dependent cytolysin (CDC) family of pore-forming toxins is important in pathogenic invasion of the mammalian host; the primary sequence of the CDC's is highly conserved, and contains a single cysteine residue within an essential 11 residue sequence (ECTGLAWEWWR) in the immunuoglobulin-like domain (domain 4) near the C-terminus in most CDC toxins of Gram-positive bacteria [52]. Human pathogens containing these toxins include *Listeria monocytogenes* (Listeriolysin O, LLO), *Streptococcus pyogenes* (Streptolysin O, SLO), *Streptococcus penumoniae* (Pneumolysin, PLY), *Bacillus anthracis* (Anthrolysin O, ALO), *Bacillus cereus* (Cereolysin O, CLO), and various species of Clostridia (*C. tetani*, Tetanolysin, TLY; *C. botulinum*, Botulinolysin: BLY; *C. perfringens*, Perfringolysin O, PFO) [52]. Notably, many of these bacteria are foodborne pathogens. Recently, CDCs have been described in *Desulfolobus propionicus* and *Enterobacter lignolyticus* (a plant pathogen), both Gram-negative bacteria not associated with disease in animals [53]. The proteins from *E. lignolyticus* and *D. propionicus* have a conserved cysteine residue as mentioned above [53], and therefore may be sensistive to inactivation by allicin.

The cysteine residue in the undecapeptide is present in most, but not all, CDC toxins, and those without a conserved cysteine are likely to be unaffected by allicin. Pyolysin from *Arcanobacterium pyogenes* lacks this cysteine [54], as does intermedilysin of *Streptococcus intermedius* [55]. Intermedilysin activity was not destroyed by sulfhydryl-specific reagents N-ethylmaleimide or 5,5'-dithio-bis(2-nitrobenzoic acid) [55], lending support to the likelihood of its imperviousness to allicin.

Streptolysin O (SLO) contains a single cysteine residue at position 530 [56] required for SLO function, as replacement of this residue by glycine nearly abolished hemolysis of sheep RBCs, and greatly reduced binding to A549 human lung epithelial cells [57]. Allicin may modify Cys530. SLO from Group A Streptococci was completely inhibited in Todd-Hewitt

Broth culture supernatant by 35 μg of pure allicin, and by aged aqueous garlic extract (49 days at 4°C; total 25 μg allicin applied), measured by absorbance of released hemoglobin at 541 nm [58]. The increased activity of garlic extract (25 μg allicin) compared to pure allicin (35 μg) againt SLO may be accounted for by presence of sterols in heterogenous mixture of garlic extract [18], as SLO and other similar lytic toxins are inhibited by sterols [56].

The activity of pneumolysin O in lysate of a clinical isolate of *S. pneumoniae* (standardized at 2 hemolytic units/mL) against human RBCs was 50% reduced after 25 min incubation with 0.28 μM/mL allicin, and completely inhibited by 0.61 μM/mL [59]. Pneumolysin activity was 50% reduced upon 1 h incubation of intact cells wtih 0.31 μM/mL allicin, and completely inhibited at 1.84 μM/mL allicin [59].

2.3.3. Inhibition of Urease

Urease generates two molecules of ammonia and one molecule of carbonic acid from each molecule of urea substrate, and is involved in many processes which further infectious disease in humans and animals, such as elevation of pH in local environment to foster host colonization in stomach lumen, promotion of crystallized biofilm formation in the bladder lumen, or inhibition of host enyzmes and impairment of immune responses [60]. Allicin (7 μg in 15 μL bacterial lysate at 1.7 mg protein/mL) destroys activity of urease from *P. mirabilis*, with activity restored by 5 mM dithiothreitol (DTT) [61], a common reducing agent which can repair thiols oxidized by allicin. Comparatively, full obliteration of urease activity in intact cells required a 30 min incubation of *P. mirabilis* with 50 μg pure allicin prior to lysis by sonication [61]. The cysteine (Cys319) proposed to be modified by allicin [62] is conserved in sequences of alpha-subunits of urease from other bacterial pathogens: *H. pylori* (Cys 221), *U. urealyticum* (Cys225), *P. vulgaris* (Cys315), and *K. aerogenes* (Cys315) [63]. Urease is ubiquitous in the microbial world, present in Gram-positive and Gram-negative pathogens, including plant and animal pathogens as well as environmentally important organisms [60], providing ample opportunities to explore novel applications for allicin.

2.3.4. Inhibition of Enterotoxins

In *Staphylococcus aureus*, garlic powder (1.5% ($^{w}/_{v}$) in BHI broth) suppressed production of staphylococcal enterotoxin A (SEA) from strain ATCC 13565, SEB from strain ATCC 14458, and SEC_1 from strain FRI 137, as all were undetectable by sandwhich ELISA up to 72 hours of growth, but SED expression from strain ATCC 23235 was not suppressed [64]. In the same study, 2% ($^{w}/_{v}$) garlic powder in BHI media inhibited thermonuclease activity from all but the SEA producing strain.

2.3.5. Inhibition of Cysteine Proteases

During infection with *Porphyromonas gingivalis*, a great deal of damage to host tissue is caused by the cysteine proteases lysine gingipain and arginine gingipain [65], which can be inhibited by allicin [66]. Streptococcal pyrogenic exotoxin B (SpeB), produced by Group A streptococci, is responible for advancement of infection by degradation of host connective tissue matrix proteins and even destruction of cardiac tissue [67]. Allicin (48 μg/mL) inhibited conversion of immature SpeB to its active form, and caused 82.4% reduced activity of mature SpeB [67]. *S. pyogenes* avoids opsonization by host IgG through action of IdeS, a cysteine protease whose ability to cleave human IgG *in vitro* was blocked by small molecules commonly used to inhibit cysteine proteases [68]. Perhaps allicin can inhibit IdeS, or a related cysteine protease in *Staphylococcus epidermidis*, EcpA, which attacks IgA and IgM [69].

2.3.6. Inhibition of Alpha-Toxin

Allicin inhibits pore-forming toxins that don't share homology with SLO or PLY. Greater alpha-toxin activity is associated with increased morbidity in Staph infections, and allicin reduces alpha-toxin production by *S. aureus*, including an oxacillin/methicillin resistant clinical isolates [70]. All 4 alpha-toxin producing strains had MIC values of 64 μg/mL for allicin in broth culture, and at only 16 μg/mL allicin a substantial inhibition (78 - 100%, relative to control) of hemolysis of rabbit RBC's was observed in culture supernatants, as well as significant reduction in *hla* and *agrA* gene transcripts, as determined by RT-PCR; *agrA* is part of the regulatory system thought to govern *hla* production [70]. Note that alpha-toxin protein is devoid of cysteine [71], and unlikely to be a direct chemical target of allicin. The C-terminal portion of *P. mirabilis* hemolyisn has 35% sequence similarity to *S. aureus* alpha-toxin by local alignment with Water at EMBL-EBI [72]. Allicin (5-20 μg/mL) added to lysate of *P. mirabilis* only slightly (about 10%) reduced the hemolysis of human RBCs, and the effect was neither dose-dependent nor statistically significant compared to hemolytic activity of lysate without allicin [61]. It would be of interest to determine if *P. mirabilis* grown in presence of allicin exhibits a reduction in hemolysin activity similar to that observed with *S. aureus*.

2.3.7. Effects of Allicin or Garlic Extract on Other Bacterial Toxins

Table 2. Studies examining suppression of toxin activity or production

Organism(s)	Toxin	Summary	Reference
Group A Streptococci	Streptolysin O	Allicin in garlic extract more potent at inhibiting SLO in GAS lysate than pure allicin.	[58]
S. pneumoniae	Pneumolysin O	Allicin inhibits PLY in lysate and intact cells.	[59]
P. mirabilis	Urease	Allicin inhibits urease in lysate and intact cells.	[61]
S. aureus	SEA, SEB, SEC_1, SED, thermonuclease	Garlic powder reduces toxin production in BHI.	[64]
Porphyromonas gingivalis	Lysine gingipain, arginine gingipain	Allicin inhibits action of cysteine proteases.	[66]
Porphyromonas gingivalis	Trypsin-like protease	Allicin in garlic extract strongly inhibits activity in culture lysate.	[77]
Group A Streptococci	SpeB	Allicin inhibits conversion of toxin to active form.	[67]
S. aureus	Alpha-toxin	Allicin reduces production of alpha-toxin.	[70]

While allicin broadly inhibits an array of pathogenic bacteria and their toxins, some words of caution are in order. Garlic powder at 2.3 or 4.7 mg/mL did not suppress toxin production in *Clostridium difficile* strains NCTC 13366, R11446, or ATCC 43598, although toxicity of these strains toward Vero cells in culture was reduced [73]. Alarmingly, commercially packaged chopped garlic supplied in soybean oil and stored at room temperature supported the growth of *C. botulinum* Type A and B, with concommitant production of dangerous amounts of botulinum toxin in challenge experiements at a loading of only 5 spores per gram of product, while remaining acceptable in odor and appearance [74]. Interestingly, garlic extract contains a Kunitz-family-like 15 kDa protein that acts as a trypsin inhibitor [75]. Staphylococcal exfoliative toxins A and B are trypsin-like serine proteases responsible for the severe morbity of staphylococcal scalded skin syndrome [76], and pose possible targets for inhibition by this 15 kDa protease inhibitor. Allicin (55 µg/mL, in garlic extract) reducted trypsin-like protease activity in *P. gingivalis* culture lysate by 93% [77].

2.4. Decreased Colonization of the Host

2.4.1. Killing of Cells in Biofilm

Allicin destroys bacterial cells within established biofilms, but required minimum effective concentrations are greater than those biocidal to planktonic cells. The minimal allicin concentration to inhibit *P. mirabilis* ATCC 12453 growing in biofilm was 256 µg/mL (64 µg/mL in Muller Hinton Broth), and the minimal concentration to kill *P. mirabilis* in biofilm was 512 µg/mL (128 µg/mL in MHB) [61].

Garlic extract (2%) added to cultures of *P. aeruginosa* PAO1 did not negatively affect growth *in vitro*, but did effect changes that permitted polymorphonuclear cells applied to the biofilm to execute a respiratory burst; although this effect was most likely mediated by supression of quarum sensing in *P. aeruginosa*, further studies are required to determine whether any effects were due to actions of the extract on the phagocytic cells directly [78].

2.4.2. Impaired Biofilm Formation

In *Pseudomonas aeruginosa*, garlic extract alters production of genes required for virulence and invasion and promotes changes in biofilm structure similar to those observed in quarum-sensing deficient *P. aeruginosa* [41]. The inhibition of biofilm formation in *P. aeruginosa* by suppression of quarum sensing is attributed to S-phenyl-L-cysteine sulfoxide [79].

The mode of action of allicin in inhibition of biofilm production by *Staphylococcus epidermidis* (~95% suppression at half the MIC concentration of allicin) is likely through attack of sulfhydryl groups, as similar biofilm suppression was observed wtih iodoacetic acid [27]. *S. epidermidis* ATCC 35984 biofilm production in tryptic soy broth was substantially lessened by inclusion of 4 µg/mL allicin, and possible targets may include cysteine-containing proteins IcaA and/or IcaD, both required for biofilm formation [80]. The minimal inhibitory concentration and minimal biofilm inhibitory concentrations were identical for *S. epidermidis* ATCC 12228 and ATCC 35984, with MIC and MBIC of 12.5 µg/mL for pure allicin, and much lower MIC and MBIC values for aqueous garlic extract (1.56 µg allicin/mL) and ethanolic garlic extract (0.78 µg allicin/mL), where allicin content was standardized by HPLC [81]. This result strongly suggests that a biofilm-inhibitory compound more potent than allicin, or synergistic to allicin, is present in homogenous garlic preparations. A notable decrease in *icaA* expression, intercellular adhesion gene A, was also observed [81].

Allicin reduced biofilm formation in a dose-dependent manner, and a 26 - 35% reduction in biofilm production was observed when *P. mirabilis* clinical isolates were grown with 32 µg/mL allicin [61]. Dose-dependent inhibition of biofilm was also promoted by methanolic or ethanolic extractions of garlic powder added to broth cultures of clinical isolates of *B. cereus*, *S. aureus*, *S. pneumoniae*, *P. aeruginosa*, *E. coli*, and *K. pneumoniae* [82].

Table 3. Summary of selected studies examining effects of allicin on biofilm

Organism(s)	Allicin or extract?	Summary	Reference
P. mirabilis ATCC 12453 and *P. mirabilis* clinical isolates	Allicin	Allicin biocidal to cells in biofilm, and biofilm reduction by allicin is dose-dependent.	[61]
P. aeruginosa PAO1	Extract	Garlic extract associated with respiratory burst in PMN's applied to biofilm.	[78]
P. aeruginosa PAO1	Extract	Garlic extract appears to suppress biofilm production via disruption of quorum sensing.	[41]
Staphylococcus epidermidis ATCC 35984	Allicin	Biofilm inhibition by allicin may involve modification of –SH groups.	[27]
Staphylococcus epidermidis ATCC 35984	Allicin	Allicin may modify IcaA and/or IcaD to reduce PIA formation.	[80]
S. epidermidis ATCC 12228 and ATCC 35984	Allicin and extract	Garlic extract almost 10 times more effective at suppressing biofilm than allicin.	[81]

2.4.3. Altered Morphology and Motility

Garlic oil (129 μg/mL) impeded the swimming behavior of *H. pylori* 107018, and shifted the cells toward a spherical morphology, rather than a spiral rod [83]. Aqueous garlic extract (1.9%) impaired ability of *B. anthracis* vegetative cells to form chains in Muller Hinton broth culture [42]. Although not allicin, diallyl sulfide (5 μM) promoted alteration in cell wall and loss of membrane integrity in *Campylobacter jejuni*, as observed with SEM [47].

2.4.4. Decreased Entry into Host Macrophages

Allicin strongly limited uptake of *M. tuberculosis* H37Rv into murine peritoneal macrophages in culture, with these effects likely mediated by action of allicin on the host cells, which were not harmed even at 40 μg/mL allicin [29].

3. Difficulties in Comparing Results of Different Studies

Some bacterial species appear differently sensitive in different studies, due to variation in garlic source, extraction method, test method, and/or differences in bacterial strains. In disk-diffusion assay on nutrient agar, ethanolic extract of garlic (200 μg/mL in 95% ethanol) from Tamil Nadu, India, produced the largest zone of inhibition against multidrug-resistant clinical isolates of *P. aeruginosa*, followed by *E. coli*, *Bacillus* sp., *S. aureus*, *Enterobacter* sp. and *Proteus* sp. (tied), and finally *Klebsiella* sp. [84]. In a different study, 100% garlic juice (4 mL juice from 10 g garlic) from Gujarat, India, was applied to 25 samples each of multidrug-resistant clinical isolates of *E. coli*, *K. pneumoniae*, *P. mirabilis*, *P. aeruginosa*, and *S. aureus* [85]. In well-diffusion assay on Muller Hinton Agar, 100% garlic juice was most effective against *P. mirabilis* (zone of inhibition (ZoI = 28 mm), followed by *E. coli* and *S. aureus* (ZoI = 26 mm), *K. pneumoniae* (ZoI = 21 mm), and least effective against *P. aeruginosa* (ZoI = 12.5 mm) [85].

Even the same laboratory, using the same testing method and bacterial strains, may conclude different relative efficacies of allicin, dependent upon delivery method. In Muller Hinton broth dilution assay, the same six bacterial strains were screened for sensitivitiy to pure allicin, solubilized garlic powder, or a novel throat lozenge (15% garlic powder with menthol)

[86]. Pure allicin (1 mg/mL in 1:1 DMSO:water) was most effective (MIC = 6.25 ug/mL) against *P. aeruginosa*, *B. subtilis*, *S. aureus*, and *M. flavus*, but garlic powder (15 mg/mL in 1:1 DMSO:water) was most effective (MIC = 2.5 mg/mL) against *S. aureus*, *M. flavus*, and *E. coli*, and least effective (MIC = 5.0 mg/mL) against *P. aeruginosa*, *B. subtilis*, and *E. faecalis* [86]. A novel lozenge (1 mg allicin total; amount of menthol not disclosed) dissolved at 15 mg/mL in water showed the best activity against *E. faecalis* and *B. subtilis* (MIC = 1.87 mg/mL), while the lozenge was remarkably least effective (MIC = 15 mg/mL) against *P. aeruginosa* [86].

Differing results can be observed when the same preparations of garlic extract are used in different test methods. Neither ethanolic nor methanolic extract of garlic powder (10 g powder extracted into 100 mL solvent, dried, and resuspended at 100 mg/mL in 1% DMSO) showed any antibacterial effect against clinical isolates of *S. aureus*, *S. pneumoniae*, *P. aeruginosa*, *E. coli* or *K. pneumoniae* in the disk-diffusion assay on Muller Hinton Agar, but reasonable MIC and MBC values for both methanolic (MIC = 0.156 - 1.25 mg/mL; MBC = 0.625 - 5 mg/mL) and ethanolic (MIC = 0.078 - 2.5 mg/mL; MBC = 0.312 - 5 mg/mL) preparations were obtained in nutrient broth for all strains, including *B. cereus* [82]. *B. cereus* was the only tested strain inhibited in the Muller Hinton Agar disk-diffusion assay [82]. Of course this difference could be attributed to different media formulations used for the agar plates or broth cultures.

Further complicating determination of effectiveness of garlic extracts or allicin against bacteria is the use of different growth media. A recent review [87] meticulously shows that measured MIC values for allicin are strongly influenced by media type. Allicin and other disulfide-containing active components of garlic are inactivated by sulfhydryl groups, so media containing any appreciable quantity of sulfhydryl compounds would decrease the available amount of allicin and its antibacterial allies, thus increasing the measured MIC or MBC values. Cysteine, coenzyme A, and glutathione destroy antibacterial activity of allicin [88], as does β-mercaptoethanol [31]. Redox potentials of sterile microbiological media are different, depending on media type, and change at variable rates and magnitudes throughout the course of bacterial growth, dependent upon characteristics of the organism [89]. Consider also that anaerobic bacteria often require addition of reducing agents like thioglycollate, β-mercaptoethanol, or dithiothreitol to the culture media, and these thiols scavenege and deplete allicin. Aqueous garlic extract (1% $^{w}/_{v}$), bactericidal against *B. anthracis* in normal saline, only slowed bacterial growth in MHB [42]. Greater MIC values were measured by well-diffusion assay on BHI agar, as compared to dilution in BHI broth, against numerous Gram-positive and Gram-negative organisms, and notedly less antibacterial power was seen on media containing horse blood [77]. When tryptone powder (up to 15 g/L) or cysteine (10 mM, 25 mM) was added into minimal salt broth with 2.75 mg/mL garlic oil, the survival of *Enterobacter aerogenes* was increased [19].

At 35°C, *Campylobacter jejuni* in saline was completely eradicated in only 5 hours with 25 μg/mL garlic juice, but complete killing by 25 μg/mL garlic juice in nonselective campylobacter broth required 24 hours [47]. Temperature of incubation is equally important in assessment of antibacterial efficacy. In both saline and complex media, lower incubation temperatures protected *C. jejuni* against the effects of the garlic extract [47].

Even bacterial load affects measurements of allicin's antibacterial properties, as the antibacterial effect of allicin was greater when less *S. typhimurium* cells were present in culture [22]. This is not terribly surprising, as a common theme in bacterial control is that greater biological loads require higher biocide concentration, longer contact time, and longer heat sterilization times for full reduction. Consider also that bacterial growth changes redox potential of the media [89] - as nutrients are depleted and metabolic wastes accumulate, the killing power of allicin could be weakened.

4. USE AGAINST HUMAN PATHOGENS

Overwhelming evidence shows allicin and garlic extracts are wildly effective against a broad swath of pathogenic bacteria *in vitro*. Infections on the skin, in the oral cavity, the lungs, and the gastrointestinal tract are natural first choices for development of allicin as a clinical antibacterial therapy, due to ease of delivery of allicin to the affected site. The literature contains very few reports of studies deploying allicin as a primary or supplemental antibiotic therapy in animal and/or human trials.

4.1. Infections in the Oral Cavity

In vitro experiments show garlic extract holds great promise in killing five different clinical isolates of Aggregatibacter actinomycetemcomitans, the causative agent of localized aggressive periodontitis, which is developing antibiotic resistance [90]. Even the low concentration of 0.01 μg/mL allicin applied for 2 hours statistically reduces living *A. actinomycetemcomitans*, and when used at 0.1, 1.0 and 10 μg/mL, the killing is total [90]. Allicin may be further active against not just the bacterium itself, but also the toxins which promote and extend invasion into host cell tissue [90]. Gram-negative oral pathogens seemed to be more affected by allicin (MIC = 4.1 μg/mL in garlic extract), while Gram-positive oral pathogens seem to be less affected (MIC = 22.7 μg/mL), and in time-kill assays, *Porphyromonas gingivalis* was more rapidly killed compared to *S. mutans* [77].

4.2. Infections of the Gastrointestinal Tract

Complete killing of a clinical isolate of *E. coli* O157 from a pediatric patient in Japan was achieved after 6 h with a 1% aqueous solution ($^{w}/_{v}$) of fresh garlic powder, and after 24 h incubation with the same solution of a powder prepared from a one-year old bulb of garlic [91]. Garlic powder (2% ($^{w}/_{v}$) in nutrient agar) completely inhibited growth of a clinical isolate of *E. coli* O157, and growth of lab strains (not specified) of *E. coli* and *Salmonella enteritidis* [91]. Allicin, quantified and delivered in aqueous garlic extract, suppressed the growth of six different *Salmonella* species isolated from foods and environmental sources in Tunisia, with MIC values of 8.1 - 10.1 μg/mL and MBC values 10.5 - 12.1 μg/mL [92].

Not only did fresh aqueous garlic extract (12.3 mg/mL allicin) potentiate the anti-*H. pylori* effects of omeperazole in brain heart infusion broth [43], but the gastric H^+/K^+ ATPase has important cysteines which are targeted by omeperazole [93] and can likely also be targeted by allicin. It has been estimated 1 g of garlic powder diluted to 1 L within the gastric milieu may be sufficient to initiate killing of *H. pylori* in the stomach [83]. However, twenty gastric ulcer patients randomly assigned to receive either garlic oil capsules alone (three capsules per day,

800 μg allicin each), or garlic oil capsules at the same dose, plus 20 mg omeperazone capsules twice daily for two weeks, showed no statistically significant changes in clinical assessment, symptoms, or *H. pylori* load between the two groups [94]. Another study found more encouraging results. A large study in Turkey enrolled 210 patients, 30 patients in each of 7 treatment groups, and examined effects of ascorbic acid, allicin, and standard antibiotic treatment on *H. pylori* infection [95]. As determined by histological examination of biopsy tissue taken from 6 locations within the stomach within 4 weeks after a two week treatment regime, 66.7% of patients in the group receiving standard antibiotic therapy (all drugs b.i.d: lansoprazol, 30 mg; clarithromycin, 500 mg; amoxicillin, 1 g) had undetectible *H. pylori*, while 90% of patients receiving antibiotic therapy plus 1200 μg/mL per day of allicin had no detectible *H. pylori* [95]. In the group receiving allicin alone, only 24.4% of patients had undetectable *H. pylori* [95].

4.2.1. Effects on the Gut Flora

If allicin and garlic extracts are effective against gastrointestinal pathogens, are they disruptive to our healthly gut flora? One study in mice suggests that garlic powder reduces total numbers of gut bacteria. The total numbers of gut bacteria in BALB/c mice (n = 5) was reduced from $5.4 \pm 2.3 \times 10^6$ CFU/feces to $2.3 \pm 1.9 \times 10^5$ CFU/feces upon consumption of 1 mL of 1% garlic powder in water per day for 3 days [96].

In a comprehensive *in vitro* screen of the activity of garlic powder against human intestinal flora and human intestinal pathogens, no difference was seen in the MIC values (3.13 – 12.5 mg/mL after 24 h incubation) between the two groups of bacteria in the well-diffusion assay [19]. In the same study, the MIC values for garlic oil applied to intestinal flora were between 0.02 and 0.68 mg/mL after 24 h incubation, while MIC values for most pathogenic species were 0.32 – 5.5 mg/mL, suggesting that the "good" bacteria were more susceptible to garlic oil *in vitro* than the "bad" bacteria [19]. Still, some enteric pathogens had MIC values below those of most normal flora, including *Bacillus cereus*, *Vibro* spp. (*metschnikovii*, *parahaemolyticus*), *Yersinia enterocolitica*, *Listeria monocytogenes*, and *Campylobacter jejuni*, *E. coli*, and *C. lari*. [19]. *E. coli* and *Lactobacillus acidophilus* were the two most garlic oil tolerant members of the normal flora [19].

Ethanolic extract of *A. sativum* powder, evaporated and resuspended in DMSO at 100 mg/mL, was ineffective in well-diffusion assay on Muller Hinton Agar against clinical isolates of beta-lactamase positive multidrug-resistant *E. coli* (2 isolates), *Shigella dysenteriae* (1 isolate), and also reference strain *E. coli* K-12, but did show weak inhibitory effect against an ampicillin-sensitive clinical isolate of *Shigella sonnei* [97]. Both methanolic and aqueous extracts of garlic were effective against 68 clinical isolates of *Shigella flexneri*, 27 of *S. sonnei*, and 5 of *S. boydii*, including some drug-resistant strains, but methanolic extracts were more effective, and heating reduced antibacterial efficacy in both extract types [98].

4.3. Infections Common in Cystic Fibrosis

Allicin is more effective than many antibiotics against multidrug-resistant clinical isolates from cystic fibrosis patients: allicin was inhibitory at 0.03-0.06 mg/mL and biocidal at 1 mg/mL for *Achromobacter ruhlandii* 155B and *P. aeruginosa* 48B, and biocidal at 0.03-0.06 mg/mL against *B. cenocepacia* 122, measured in Mueller-Hinton broth [99]. In disk-diffusion assay on

Muller-Hinton Agar, allicin at 20 μg/disc provided the greatest zone of inhibition (ZoI) against *A. ruhlandii* 155B (30 mm), *B. cenocepacia* 122 (25 mm), and the smallest ZoI for *P. aeruginosa* 48 B (10 mm); notably the antibacterial action of allicin was strongly dependent upon bacterial load [99].

Pseudomonas aeruginosa colonization in the lungs of cystic fibrosis patients is notoriously resistant to clearance, due to biofilm formation and decreased sensitivity to antibiotics [100]. Ten BALB/c mice were injected subcutaneously with garlic extract (0.3 g total) each day for two days prior to dosing intratracheally with 1 x 10^7 CFU *P. aeruginosa* PAO1 per lung, and daily dosing with garlic extract was continued until the animals were sacrificed on day 5 post infection [78]. Remarkably, the lungs of all but one animal that received garlic extract were free of *P. aeruginosa*, while the average bacterial load in the control animals was 1 x 10^5 CFU/lung [78]. When the same dosing of garlic extract was applied, but the load of *P. aeruginosa* was increased to 2 x 10^7 CFU per lung, 21 mice in the treatment group survived, compared to only 9 in the control group [78]. In this study, garlic extract was prepared by homogenizing 150 g garlic and extracting into 300 mL toluene overnight, before filtering and then extracting aqueous compounds into 150 mL water [41]. The authors stress that a parallel dose of garlic extract translates to 50 cloves of garlic per day for an average-sized 176-pound human, providing impetus for isolation of the active component(s) for pharmaceutical development [78].

A clinical trial evaluating ability of garlic oil to inhibit quorum sensing molecule production by *P. aeruginosa* in cystic fibrosis patients (median age 18) in the UK found minor but statistically nonsignificant improvements in clinical aspect of patients who took a single capsule of garlic oil (656 mg garlic oil with 10 mg cardamom oil) compared to those who took a daily placebo capsule (656 mg olive oil with 10 mg cardamom oil), but a difference in blood or sputum levels of quorum sensing molecules N-(3-oxododecanoyl) homoserine lactone (blood and sputum) and N-butanoylhomoserine lactone (sputum only) could not be detected [101]. Favorable clinical outcomes in the treatment group included more stable weight, increased forced expiratory volume, and lower Jensen scores, but seven patients in this group received a course of intravenous antibiotics during the study, as compared to five patients in the control group [101].

A review of infections in cystic fibrosis patients highlights *Burkholderia cepacia* complex bacteria as common causes of chronic, severe, life-threatening lung infections [102]. Interestingly, *Burkholderia cepacia* spp. were first isolated on onion, *Allium cepa* [103], and *Allium*-derived factors like allicin may be useful in their treatment. *Burkholderia* spp. are increasingly resistant to multiple antibiotic drugs, via a range of antibiotic resistant mechanisms [104, 105]. Aqueous garlic extract (1 g/mL water; ~16.9 mg/mL allicin) at final concentrations of 8 - 62 μg/mL culture, inhibited growth of several *Burkolderia cepacia* complex members, while 31-62 μg/mL was bactericidal [106].

4.4. Tuberculosis

Garlic extract is antibacterial toward at least 17 different species of *Mycobacterium*, with MIC values on Middlebrook 7H10 Agar plates of 1.34-3.35 mg/mL reported [107]. Fifteen multidrug-resistant, and five sensitive, clinical isolates of *M. tuberculosis* were fully inhibited at 3 mg/mL ethanolic garlic extract in 7H9 Middlebrook medium [108]. In an *in vitro* broth dilution assay in Middlebrook 7H9-S broth, allicin-rich extract of garlic was more effective at killing *M. tuberculosis* H37 Rv (MIC = 0.97-1.95 μg/mL) than either isoniazid (MIC = 15.62 - 31.25 μg/mL) or ethambutol (31.25 - 62.5 μg/mL), and similarly effective to rifampicin (≤ 0.1 μg/mL) [109].

M. tuberculosis 85B protein is a mycolyl transferase associated with building of bacterial cell-wall and is also antigenic, inducing TNF-α production by the host; 500 ng/mL allicin arrested production of 85B mRNA and accumulation of 85B protein within cultured *M. tuberculosis*-infected human monocytes, although this effect may be mediated by effects of allicin on the host cell [110]. Garlic extract (5 mg/kg/d i.p.), administered at the time of infection with extremely-multi-drug resistant *M. tuberculosis*, protected against ulceration of the skin and permitted survival of the mice for as long as 90 days, whereas control animals perished on day 15 post infection and suffered severe skin ulceration [29].

The sulfur compounds of garlic are volatile and have a characteristic odor. Allicin and other thiosulfinate compounds (dimethyl-, diethyl-, and dipropyl-thiosulfinate) were all active in gas phase against *E. coli*, *P. syringe*, and *M. luteus* when 20 μL of 80 mM preparations were added to the lids of inverted Petri dishes of lawn cultures [23]. Similarly, vapor from allicin in a 20 μL drop inhibited growth of a host of pathogens grown as surface lawns or as suspensions in agar: 357 μg/20 μL was active against *P. aeruginosa* PAO1 and PAO25, *S. pyogenes*, *S. agalactiae*, and *S. dysgalactiae*; 130 μg/20 μL was inhibitory toward *S. pneumoniae* strains, including MDR strains Spain^{23F}-1 and Poland^{23F}-16; 185 μg/20 μL was effective against *S. aureus* [111]. Thus, use of allicin as a vaporized inhalant may be efficacious against lung infections.

4.5. Other Infections

4.5.1. MRSA

Stabilized allicin in aqueous garlic extract (128 μg/mL, manufactured by Allicin International Limited) was biocidal toward 88% of 30 clinical isolates of MRSA, and effective against all isolates at 256 μg/mL [112]. A recent compendium of literature reviews the emerging issue of mupirocin resistance in MRSA, which may be as high as 81% [113]. At low levels (62.5 – 125 μg/mL), allicin was more effective at killing mupirocin-resistant MRSA, as compared to MRSA strains intermediate or sensitive to mupirocin [112]. This suggests that the same mutation which confers resistance to mupirocin confers sensitivity to allicin. A single oral dose (200 uL) of aqueous garlic extract (50% or 100%), diallyl sulfide (DAS; 5% or 10% in mineral oil), or diallyl disulfide (DADS; 0.5% or 1% in mineral oil) at 16 h post intravenous infection of BALBc/A mice with MRSA (10^7 CFU total) out-performed 1% vancomycin in reducing bacterial load recovered from kidney, liver, and blood from mice sacrificed 24 h post-infection; reduction of bacterial load recovered from spleen was also seen, but not as dramatic [114]. In addition to reduction of bacterial load, levels of fibronectin, necessary for bacterial attachment and colonization, and interleukin-6, a driver of inflammation, were also reduced [114]. Effects of allicin on inflammation pathways are comprehensively described in Chapter 3.

4.5.2. Prosthetic Joint Infections

Joint replacements are at risk for colonization with *Staphylococcus epidermidis* and *Staphylococcus aureus*, organisms which build biofilms useful for adherence to materials of the prostheses and also reduction of antibiotic effectiveness [115]. *Staphylococcus epidermidis* RP62A (1 mL of 1 x 10^4 CFU/mL) was seeded into the knee joint of thirty-two New Zealand White rabbits after implantation of a stainless-steel surgical screw and polyethylene washer into the lateral femoral condyle [116]. Two weeks post-surgery, the rabbits were divided equally into four groups and began treatment with continuous intracapsular lavage (1-1.5 mL/min) of saline, 20 μg/mL vancomycin, 4 μg/mL allicin, or vancomycin and allicin combined; animals were sacrificed after three days and implants were removed [116]. Bacteria adherent to surgical screws were released by sonication in sterile saline, and the treatment group receiving allicin alone had a lower bacterial load recovered than the group treated with vancomycin alone, but the rabbits receiving the combination of vancomycin and allicin had the greatest reduction in bacterial load [116]. Biofilm on the polyethylene washer was assessed by SEM, and almost no biofilm was observed on washers recovered from the vancomycin plus allicin treatment animals [116].

4.5.3. Tubercular Lymphadenitis

In the treatment of tubercular lymphadenitis, the serum of patients receiving garlic extract in combination with standard antitubercular therapy (ATT) (n=25), had significantly increased antitubercular activity relative to the serum of healthy persons (n=3), as compared to serum of patients receiving only standard ATT (n=26) [117]. All patients received standard ATT for 45 days during the experimental period, and those in the treatment group were given garlic extract supplied in capsules (3-6 per day divided, as tolerated, 250 mg garlic each) on days 31-45, while patients in the control group did not receive garlic capsules; serum used for *M. tuberculosis* H37Rv challenge testing in Youmans and Karlson's liquid medium was drawn on day 45 [117].

4.5.4. Skin Ulcers of Leishmaniasis

Skin ulcers caused by the protozoan parasite *Leishmania* spp. are prone to secondary infection with a diverse collection of bacteria, and over 48 different types of bacteria were isolated from ulcers of mice infected with *L. major* [25]. In a study of BALB/c mice with *L. major* infection, allicin (0.30 μM) and ciprofloxacin (10 mg/mL) administered over four weeks promoted healing of skin ulcers, and allicin was effective *in vitro* against a large number (over 40) of diverse bacteria isolated from the ulcers [25].

Table 4. Studies showing efficacy of allicin or garlic extract against human pathogens

Pathogen(s)	Infectious disease(s)	Comment	Reference
Aggregatibacter actinomycetem-comitans	Aggressive periodontitis	Allicin is bactericidal at low concentrations.	[90]
Multiple oral pathogens	Periodontitis, gingivitis, dental caries	Garlic extract of known allicin content is more effective against Gram-negative oral pathogens *in vitro*.	[77]
E. coli O157, *Salmonella enteritidis*	Hemolytic uremic syndrome	Garlic extract suppresses growth in vitro.	[91]

Table 4. (Continued)

Pathogen(s)	Infectious disease(s)	Comment	Reference
Salmonella spp.	Salmonellosis	Garlic extract of known allicin content suppresses growth in vitro.	[92]
H. pylori	Gastric ulcers	Garlic extract of known allicin content synergistic with omeperazole *in vitro*.	[43]
H. pylori	Gastric ulcers	Allicin combined with antibiotic treatment more effective than antibiotic treatment alone *in vivo*.	[95]
B. cereus, Vibrio spp. Y. enterocolitica, L. monocytogenes, C. jejuni, E. coli, C. lari	Various food-borne illnesses; diarrheal illnesses	Garlic oil more antibacterial to some intestinal pathogens than members of normal flora *in vitro*.	[19]
Shigella sonnei	Shigellosis	Ethanolic garlic extract weakly effective *in vitro*.	[97]
Shigella flexneri, S. sonnei, S. boydii	Shigellosis	Aqueous and methanolic garlic extracts effective *in vitro*.	[98]
Achromobacter rhulandii, P. aeruginosa, B. cenocepacia	Cystic fibrosis-associated pathogens	Allicin effective *in vitro*.	[99]
P. aeruginosa	Cystic fibrosis-associated pathogen	Garlic extract sub-Q improves outcome with *P. aeruginosa* infection in rabbits.	[78]
P. aeruginosa	Cystic fibrosis-associated pathogen	Garlic oil improved clinical markers in cystic fibrosis patients, but outcomes were not statistically significant. No difference in quorum-sensing molecules observed.	[101]
Burkholderia cepacia complex	Cystic fibrosis-associated pathogens	Known amount of allicin in garlic extract inhibited growth *in vitro*.	[106]
M. tuberculosis	Tuberculosis	Garlic extract inhibitory toward multiple strains *in vitro*.	[107]
M. tuberculosis	Tuberculosis	Ethanolic garlic extract inhibitory even toward MDR strains *in vitro*.	[108]
M. tuberculosis	Tuberculosis	Allicin-rich extract more effective *in vitro* than common antibiotics.	[109]
M. tuberculosis	Tuberculosis	Allicin suppresses 85B protein accumulation and entry of *M. tuberculosis* into macrophages.	[110]
M. tuberculosis	Tuberculosis	Garlic extract delivered i.p. improved survival of mice and protected against skin ulcers.	[29]
M. tuberculosis	Tubercular lymphadenitis	Garlic extract plus standard antibiotic therapy promotes anti-tubercular activity in patient serum.	[117]
MRSA, multiple clinical isolates	Skin infections, cellulitis, joint infections	Allicin is biocidal *in vitro*, even against mupirocin-resistant strains.	[112]
MRSA	Skin infections, cellulitis, joint infections	Garlic extract p.o. 16 h p.i. more effective than vancomycin against i.v. challenge with MRSA in mice.	[114]
S. epidermidis	Skin infections, cellulitis, joint infections	Intracapsular lavage with allicin and vancomycin reduced bacterial load in rabbit prosthesis infection model.	[116]

5. Differentia of Allicin as an Antibiotic

5.1. Effects against Eukaryotic Host Cells

Ideal antibiotic drugs are toxic to pathogens and not host cells. A number of literature reports suggest that allicin and garlic extract at low concentrations do not harm mammalian cells. Baby hamster kidney (BHK) cells experienced only 10% destruction of the cellular monolayer at 50 μM allicin [118]. Allicin (1.2 mg/mL) had no deleterious effects on Vero cells in culture [73]. At 0.16 mM, allicin did not affect viability of human lung A549 cells in culture [23]. Allicin was toxic to cultured human cell lines Beas-2B (EC50 = 800 μM), A549 (EC50 = 250 μM), and Caco-2 cells (EC50 = 120 μM), but cytopathic effects could be avoided and these concentrations of allicin could be at least doubled by inclusion of 1 mM GSH [111]. *In vivo*, aqueous garlic extract, even at 100 g/100 mL, had no negative effect on survival of healthy BALBc/A mice [114].

5.2. Comparison of Allicin and Garlic Extracts with Commonly Used Antibiotics

Allicin potentiates several synthetic antibiotic drugs, but how does allicin fare when used on its own, without standard antibiotics? Pure allicin was effective against multiple clinical isolates *in vitro*, with LD_{50} values of 3-15 μg/mL against *E. coli*, *S. aureus*, P. *mirabilis*, *A. baumanii*, *K. pneumoniae*, but rather ineffective against and *S. β hemolyticus*, *E. faecium*, and *P. aeruginosa* (LD_{50} >100 ug/mL) [24]. Three MDR strains of *S. pneumoniae* (CSR^{14}-10, S.Africa^{18A}-13, Poland^{23F}-16) had MIC values of 64 μg/mL for allicin, while MIC values of all 3 strains were ≥ 256 μg/mL for erythromycin and clindamycin in broth dilution assay [111].

Aqueous garlic extract was effective against 41 multidrug-resistant clinical isolates of *Acinetobacter* spp. from skin and soft tissue infections, with MIC of 2.5 - 10 mg/mL in Muller Hinton Agar dilution assay, where the aqueus garlic extract contained 0.20 percentage by weight allicin [39]. Commercially available *A. sativum* essential oil at 0.05% was highly effective at killing *Borrelia burgdorferi* B31 5A19 in BSK-H medium [119]. Allicin killed intracellular multidrug resistant *M. tuberculosis* in murine macrophage culture [29].

In a disc-diffusion assay, aqueous garlic extract showed antibacterial activity equal to or greater than four common antibiotics (ceftazidime, ciprofloxacin, norfloxacin, or cephotaxime) against *V. cholerae*, *V. parahaemolyticus*, and a dozen environmental isolates of multidrug-resistant non-O1 (non-cholera toxin-producing) *V. cholera* [120].

Aqueous garlic extract (1.9%) caused a 6-log reduction in viable vegetative cells in both MHB and saline growth media, and aqueous garlic extract (100 uL, 40% ($^{w}/_{v}$)) inhibited growth of *B. anthracis* Sterne 34F2 better than rifampicin (20 uL, 90 ug/ml) and cefixime (20 uL, 20 000 U/mL) in well-diffusion assay on Muller Hinton Agar [42]. Garlic powder alone is also effective; garlic powder (1% in water) alone killed 10^7 CFU/mL vegetative cells of *B. anthracis*, and also prevented growth in nutrient agar [96]. Garlic extract containing allicin at 128 μg/mL cleared other important weaponizable pathogens, *Brucella melitensis* Rev 1 and *Brucella abortus* S19, from mouse peritoneal macrophages in RPMI with 10% fetal calf serum [121].

In Muller Hinton Agar disk-diffusion assay, clinical isolates of MRSA resistant to effects of cefoxitin, oxacillin, or piperacillin could be inhibited by aqueous garlic extract alone or when mixed with the aforementioned antibiotics [122]. In the same study, aqueous garlic extract was effective against clinical *P. aeruginosa* isolates resistant to cefotaxime, levofloxacin, ceftriaxone, cefazolin, and ampicillin, either alone or in combination with the antibiotics [122].

Garlic oil was more effective than several antibiotics against 60 clinical isolates of MRSA in Muller-Hinton Broth, with a measured mean MIC of 32 mg/mL for garlic oil, and MIC values greater than 64 mg/mL for methicillin, penicillin, ceftoxime, and tetracycline; the level of allicin in the garlic oil was not determined and pure allicin was not used in the study [123]. Note garlic oil was not more effective than methicillin, penicillin, ceftoxime, or tetracycline in the killing of non-methicillin-resistant *S. aureus* [123].

Ethanolic garlic extract (500 mg/mL in 96% ethanol) inhibited growth of several different multidrug-resistant strains of bacteria, both Gram-positive (*S. aureus, S. epidermidis, S. sciuri, E. faecalis*) and Gram-negative (*E. coli, K. pneumoniae, S. enteritidis, P. aeruginosa, A. baumannii*), in Muller Hinton Agar well-diffusion assay, and also enhanced the killing potential of multiple antibiotics against each of these strains [124]. Ethanolic garlic extract (50 mg/mL in 95% ethanol) added to nutrient broth culture was effective against multi-drug resistant clinical isolates of *E. coli*, *Enterobacter* sp., *P. aeruginosa*, *Proteus* sp., *Klebsiella* sp. *S. aureus*, and *Bacillus* sp., with the greatest effectiveness against *P. aeruginosa* (MIC = 58.5 μg/mL in broth culture) and least effectiveness against *Klebsiella* sp., MIC = 160.2 μg/mL) [84].

Some clinical isolates are less sensitive to allicin and garlic extract, compared to lab strains. *Proteus mirabilis* isolated from UTI patients at Imam Hospital in Iran had a much higher MIC 90 (64-128 μg/mL) and MBC 90 (128-512 μg/mL) values, as compared to *P. mirabilis* ATCC 12453, for which the values were MIC 90 = 64 μg/mL and MBC = 128 μg/mL [61].

Some reports show standard antibiotics are still more effective than allicin and/or garlic extract. Metronidazole remained more effective than aqueous extract of freshly prepared garlic powder at killing isolates of nosocomially acquired bacteria, when aqueous garlic extract (100 mg/mL) was applied to killing *S. aureus* (MBC = 75 mg/mL), *S. pneumoniae* (MBC = 100 mg/mL), *E. coli* (MBC = 125 mg/mL) and *P. aeruginosa* (MBC = 150 mg/mL) [125]. In disk-diffusion assay on nutrient agar, similar amounts of pure allicin and aqueous garlic extract (adjusted according to allicin content) were less effective than streptomycin and vancomycin against *S. aureus* NBRC 12732, and not nearly as effective compared to streptomycin and colistin on *E. coli* C600; no synergistic effect was seen when allicin was combined with any of these antibiotics [88].

5.3. Comparison of Allicin with Other Antibacterial Compounds in Garlic

Aqueous garlic extract outperformed pure allicin in inhibition of methicillin-sensitive *S. aureus* NBRC 12732, but there was no appreciable difference in relative activity against *E. coli* C600 in the disk-diffusion assay on nutrient agar [88].

The relative antibacterial power of allicin (MIC and MBC) was compared with that of other dithiosulfinates present naturally in garlic (dimethyl-, diethyl-, and dipropyl-thiosulfinate), and allicin was equal in effectiveness to dipropylthiosulfinate against *E. coli* K-12 (MIC and MBC = 32 μg/mL), equal in effectiveness to dimethylthiosulfinate against *P. syringae* 4612 (MIC and MBC = 16 μg/mL), but relatively ineffective against *P. fluorescens* 01 (MIC = 128 μg/mL;

MBC = 256 μg/mL) [23]. All thiosulfinates showed dose-dependent antibacterial activity in agar well diffusion testing; of the strains tested, *M. luteus* was most susceptible and *P. fluorescenes* 01 was most resistant [23].

The mean MIC values for pure diallyl mono-, di-, tri-, and tetra-sulphide against clinical isolates of MRSA in Muller-Hinton broth were seen to decrease with increasing number of sulfur atoms: 32, 12, 8, and 2 mg/L, respectively [123]. A similar trend of decreasing MIC values with increasing number of sulfur atoms was seen in experiments using *Helicobacter pylori* NCTC 11637; the MIC for diallyl monosulphide was 2074 μg/mL, and that for diallyl tetrasulphide was 3-6 μg/mL [83]. The effectiveness of allicin and diallyl tetrasulphide are comparable, as similar MIC and MBC values (6-12 μg/mL vs 3-6 μg/mL, respectively) were obtained for both allicin and diallyl tetrasulfide when used against multiple strains of *H. pylori* [83]. Pure allicin solubilized in 20% DMSO yielded an MIC of 2.3 - 4.7 mg/mL against four strains of *Clostridium difficile* (NCTC 13366, R11446, ATCC 43598, ATCC 700057), with MBCs greater than 75 mg/mL; aqueous bulb extract was effective with MIC of 0.8% ($^{v}/_{v}$) and MBC of 50% ($^{v}/_{v}$) for all four strains [73].

6. Use as an Antibiotic against Animal Pathogens

The use of garlic to treat maladies of domesticated animals is an ancient practice. Garlic extracts are currently applied to modern animal husbandry and aquaculture (see below). Just as studies examining use of allicin and garlic extracts to treat human pathogens suffer from a lack of standardized, quantitated preparations of allicin and garlic extract, so do the studies with animals. However, there are more *in vivo* studies on use of garlic extract in livestock than in humans. Below is a non-exhaustive summary of current reports.

6.1. In Domestic Livestock

Ground garlic bulbs mixed with butter and provided orally are a long-standing folk-remedy for treatment of mastitis in cows and buffaloes in Pakistan [126]. Holstein calves divided into two groups at birth were provided with a natural product called Enteroguard (allicin, fructo-oligo-saccharides, and probiotics) or standard antibiotics (oxytetracycline and neomycin) for the first five weeks of life [127]. There were no statistically significant differences in weight or overall health performance of the two groups (23 in allicin group; 22 in antibiotic group) after 5 weeks of supplementation, suggesting that the natural allicin-containing product may be an attractive alternative to traditional antibiotics [127]. As an added benefit, garlic alters composition of gut bacteria in ruminants and may help lessen production of methane [128].

Supplementation of broiler chicken feed with 1% dried garlic (from a local market in Gujarat, India) by weight was shown to be an attractive alternative to inclusion of antibiotics, as judged by return on feed cost, weight gain, and promoting healthy morphology of the small intestine [129]. An *in vivo* study involved Ross broiler chickens separated into two groups upon hatching: 33 birds were supplied with 25 mg/kg allicin in their drinking water, while 36 birds were in the control group [130]. All birds were inoculated by mouth with *Campylobacter jejni* MB 4185 when they were 14 days old, and sacrificed two days later [130]. There was no statistical difference in the total cecal load of *C. jejuni* between the two groups, but total level of *C. jejuni* in the treatment group was lower [130].

6.2. In Aquaculture

Antibiotic resistance of fish pathogens is increasing, and a recent review lists multiple plants, including *A. sativum*, which may be sources of novel antibiotic substances in aquaculture [131]. Aqueous garlic extract (0.5, 1.0, or 2% in food) supplied to *Oncorhynchus mykiss* resulted in greater survival compared to untreated controls upon challenge with *Aeromonas salmonicida*, but food supplementation with garlic extract above 2.5% promoted macrophage migration into kidney tissue and was associated with increased inflammation [132]. Supplementation of *O. mykiss* diet with 1, 1.5, and 2% garlic extract changes relative populations of members of the gut flora, and improves health of the fish [133]. A 20% methanolic extract of garlic clove was most effective against *Aeromonas hydrophila*, and less effective against *Vibrio anguillarum*, *V. alginolyticus*, and *V. harveyi*, in disc-diffusion agar on tryptic soy agar [134]. Garlic extract (1%) was fed to shrimp at 0.5% of diet for 5 days before exposure to multidrug-resistant *V. harveyi*; after 15 days the control group experienced 91% mortality, but the treatment group had 60% less mortality than the control group [135]. Silver nanoparticles incorporating garlic extract were effective in disc-diffusion assay against *P. aeruginosa* PB112 and *Bacillus licheniformis* $PKBMS_{16}$, both fish pathogens. Remarkably, aqueous garlic extract alone had no activity against *P. aeruginosa*, but when combined with silver nanoparticles, anti-*Pseudomonas* activity was prounouced [136]. European sea bass provided with Garlen® (a commercial product containing 25% allicin) in their diet experienced an increase in total gut flora but a decrease in total *Vibrio* spp. counts, and these effects even more pronounced when Garlen® was combined with Bactozyme® alone or Bactozyme® with Diamond V XPC® [137]. Garlic extract provided to diet of brown trout was protective against *Yersinina ruckeri* [138]. Methanolic extract of garlic was more effective than levofloxacin against *E. faecalis* infection in *O. niloticus*, with regard to survival rate [139].

7. Future Directions and Summary

7.1. Suggestions to Improve Future Studies

The antibacterial prowess of allicin and garlic extract is firmly established by existing studies. Reproducibility and comparison of studies is hampered by several factors, as outlined earlier. Towards improving translation of findings across research groups, and standardization of efforts to design clinical therapies, it is suggested that all studies quantitate the amount of allicin in their preparations. Given that low-tech methods are available for quantitation of allicin by simple UV-VIS spectroscopy, determination of allicin in homogenous garlic preparations should be standard protocol. Allicin bleaches the absorbance of 4-mercaptopyridine at 324 nm [140], and 2-nitro-5-thio-benzoic acid at 412 nm [141]. Great variability in composition of commercial garlic powder supplements on the European market was documented by HPLC, and argues for standarization of garlic supplements [142]. Ultimately, metabolomic and proteomic technologies can be applied to fully characterize complex mixtures of garlic extract, to determine identity and relative concentrations of components. This is most important, since some formulations of garlic extract contain compounds which are more effective or additive to the antibacterial effects of allicin.

A greater number of *in vivo* studies is needed. Just because a novel formulation containing allicin performs well in *in vitro* testing, does not mean efficacy translates fully to use *in vivo*. In agar well diffusion testing, allicin (900 μg/mL) plus chlorhexidine (0.05%) showed stronger inhibition of methicillin-sensitive *S. aureus* ATCC 25923 than chlorhexidine alone [143, 144]. Additionally, allicin and chlorhexidine soaked polypropylene mesh applied to a bacterial lawn of *S. aureus* ATCC 25923 produced the greatest zone of inhibition and also prevented adherence of *S. aureus* to the material *in vitro* [143], so allicin and chlorhexidine soaked polypropylene mesh was tested for its ability to suppress growth of *S. aureus* upon implantation into New Zealand White rabbits (n = 7 in each of 3 treatment groups) in mock abdominal hernia surgury [144]. The 2 x 5 cm polypropylene meshes were soaked in either 0.05% chlorhexidine alone or 900 μg/mL allicin and 0.05% chlorhexidine combined, while the Dual Mesh Plus material was not pre-soaked, and implants were seeded with *S. aureus* (10^6 CFU/mL, 0.5 mL) before closing [144]. Shockingly, the allicin and chlorhexidine soaked polypropylene implants were covered with large amounts of purulent material and permitted the most *S. aureus* growth compared to the other two types of implants, and a lesser amount of macrophages (although not statistically significant) was observed [144].

7.2. Allicin-Inspired Antibiotics and Antibacterial Products

Caution is in order when using commercially available supplements to suppress bacterial growth. Of ten commercially available garlic pills, crushed and solubilized in water, 50% showed no measurable inhibition of *E. cloacae* or *K. oxytoca*, but one commercial brand afforded similar zones of inhibition to meropenem antibiotic in agar-well diffusion assay on Muller-Hinton Agar [145]. The commercial product out-performed fresh aquous garlic extract (1 g/mL) [145].

Only 7 commercial preparations, standardized according to garlic content and extracted into water for 15 min, showed activity (MIC ≤ 100 mg/mL) in broth culture against *Neisseria gonorrheae* WHO V, and only 3 of these products showed any activity against *S. aureus* ATCC 29213 or *E. faecalis* ATCC 29212 [146]. One study reports that exposure of *S. aureus* and *E. coli* to commercial garlic supplements increased the MIC values of these organisms to ampicillin and norfloxicin [147].

Allicin (0.5 mg/mL) in an aqueous cream suitable for topical application was effective against 30 clinical isolates of MRSA in Muller Hinton Agar well-diffusion assay, even through many isolates were resistant to mupirocin, commonly found at 2 mg/mL in topical gels [112].

The thiosulfinate (-SS=O-) functional group of allicin was inspiration for a novel class of synthetic compounds that combines a variation of the thiosulfinate group with the familiar molecular skeleton of the sulfonamide antibiotics, and these compounds exhibit broad antimicrobial activity in disc-diffusion agar plate or serial dilution broth cultures of *A. faecalis*, *B. subtilis*, *B. mesentericus*, *E. coli*, *M. luteum*, *P. aeruginosa*, *S. aureus*, and *P. vulgaris* [148]. The *in vitro* minimial inhibitiory concentrations against *Burkholderia cepacia* are 0.41, 3.86, or 3.69 μM, for R= $-CH_3$, $-C_2H_5$, or $–C_3H_5$, respectively [148]. Another novel antibacterial compound, S-(octylthio)-2-pyridine, lacks a sulfinate or sulfonate group, but has many of the same properties as allcin: modification of coenzyme A, synergistism with vancomycin, and efficacy against MRSA, as well as VISA and VRSA [149].

Both woven and non-woven fabrics finished with nanoparticles made by combination of cerium oxide with allicin showed antibacterial effects against *E. coli* and *S. aureus*, and these novel materials may be useful in making antibacterial bandages [150]. A 2.5% agar gel containing 10% aqueous garlic extract was effective against four representative skin pathogens, listed here in order of greatest to least sensitivity as measured in an agar diffusion assay: *S. aureus*, *S. epidermidis*, *S. pyogenes*, and *P. aeruginosa* [151].

An innovative use of garlic extract (3% juice from blended cloves resuspended in water) for controlling *S. mutans* on toothbrushes looks promising, as there was a 100% reduction from baseline loads of *S. mutans* recovered from toothbrushes (n = 30) used by dental students twice a day for two weeks after soaking the brushes for 12 h in 3% garlic extract [152]. This result was far better than that seen with other disinfectants (water, 0.2% tea tree oil, 0.2% chlorhexidine, 0.05% cetylpyridinium chloride, and even a commercially available UV toothbrush sanitizer) in the same double-blind, randomly assigned paralell group study [152].

Mouthwash containing 2.5% ($^{w}/_{v}$) aqueous garlic extract selectively reduced *S. mutans* after 1 week of use (10 mL, once per day), and the bacterial load of *S. mutans* remained low for two weeks after treatment [153]. At conclusion of the treatment week, the bacterial load of *S. mutans* declined from from 1.4 x 10^5 CFU/mL to 4.3 x 10^4 CFU/mL, while total mircoorganisms declined to 2.2 x 10^5 CFU/mL from 4.8 x 10^5 CFU/mL; interestingly, total organisms fell to 7.2 x 10^4 CFU/mL one week post reduction of *S. mutans* was observed [153]; perhaps loss of *S. mutans* resulted in less biofilm for adherence of other organisms.

Powdered nanostructured porous silicon material obtained from nodal joints of bamboo shoots mixed in a 6:1 ratio by weight with oil from crushed garlic cloves afforded greater antibacterial activity against *S. aureus* compared to the same amount of garlic oil alone, both in disk-diffusion assay on LB agar plates and in LB broth turbidity assay [154]. Furthermore, combination with nanostructured porous silicon stabilized the anti-*S. aureus* activity of the garlic oil stored in the dark for up to 4 weeks at 4 °C or at room temperature, in addition to preserving antibacterial activity of the garlic oil upon UV irradiation [154]. The combination of garlic oil with porous nanostructured silicon from bamboo is a sustainable, stable, and powerful novel antibiotic.

A novel gel preparation of AEAllicin (500 mg/L) was effective against 76 vaginal isolates of Group B streptococci, with average zone of inhibition 23 ± 6 mm, which was slightly greater compared to same concentration of AEAllicin in water, 21 ± 6 mm [155]. AEAllicin is a stabilized aqueus preprartion of allicin produced by Allicin International. The slightly greater inhibition observed in the gel preparation may be due to presence of aloe extract and geraniol in the gel matrix, which are antibacterial toward streptoccoci [156].

7.3. Everything Old Is New Again

Bald's eyesalve is a medieval remedy for infections, and can be prepared with garlic, onion, leek, wine, cow bile, combined and aged in a brass vessel 9 days before use [157]. The antibacterial potency of the eyesalve is dependent upon aging, and was assessed by measuring ability to kill *S. aureus* Mu-infected wound tissue excised 4 days post-infection from Swiss-

Webster mice; in this system, a four hour submersion of infected tissue in Bald's eyesalve was a significantly more effective treatment than vancomycin [157].

Bald's eyesalve formulation "ES-GBBr" was made with garlic, pino grigio, and bovine bile salts, and aged for 9 days at 4 C in a glass bottle with 15 cm^2 sheets of brass [158]. The preparation was fractionated based on chemical properties, and fractions antibacterial to *S. aureus* and *P. aeruginosa* were analyzed by 1D ^1H NMR to determine the active component was allicin [158]. In formulation ES-GBBr, allicin was present at a concentration of 1476.6 μg/mL, but addition of onion to the eyesalve preparation reduced the allicin concentration to only 836.2 μg/mL, although the absolute amount of allicin produced in all six eyesalve formulations tested was 50.0-74.4 mg, as long as garlic was included in the formulation [158]. Furthermore, addition of cysteine to the eyesalve preparation was able to negate the antibacterial property of the eyesalve [158]. Study authors suggest that metal of the brass could leach copper and zinc into the solution, activating alliinase enzyme in the garlic, but Cu^{++} ion at 2.5 mM inhibits purified garlic alliinase [159].

Adjusted for allicin content, Bald's eyesalve was more potent against the antibiotic resistant wound isolate *P. aeruginosa* PA215 (MIC = 48.7 μg/mL) than pure allicin (MIC = 97.4 μg/mL), but eyesalve was less effective against methicillin-resistant *S. aureus* LAC (MIC = 24.3 μg/mL) than pure allicin (MIC = 12.2 μg/mL), so there are likely factors other than allicin in the eyesalve which are synertistic toward killing of *P. aeruginosa* but inhibitory toward killing of *S. aureus* [158].

Allicin, a highly-active component of garlic extract, has been used to treat bacterial diseases for hundreds of years, and bacteria are still sensitive to its effects, suggesting that bacteria truly are at a disadvantage to developing effective resistance mechanisms. With further study and development, there is a strong chance that allicin, and other compounds isolated from the humble garlic clove, can provide treatments to avoid or delay the rapidly approaching post-antibiotic era.

REFERENCES

[1] Fleming A. 1929. "On the antibacterial action of cultures of a penicillium with special reference to their use in the isolation of *B. influenzae*." *British Journal of Experimental Pathology* 10: 226–236.

[2] Kardos, Nelson and Arnold L. Demain. 2011. "Penicillin: the medicine with the greatest impact on therapeutic outcomes." *Applied Microbiology and Biotechnology* 92 (4): 677-687. doi: 10.1007/s00253-011-3587-6.

[3] Yocum, R. R., J. R. Rasmussen, and J. L. Strominger. 1980. "The mechanism of action of penicillin. penicillin acylates the active site of *Bacillus stearothermophilus* D-alanine carboxypeptidase." *Journal of Biological Chemistry* 255 (9): 3977.

[4] O'Neill, Jim. 2016. *Tackling Drug-Resistant Infections Globally: Final Report and Recommendations*: Government of the United Kingdom.

[5] Cavallito, Chester J. and John Hays Bailey. 1944. "Allicin, the antibacterial principle of *Allium sativum*. I. Isolation, physical properties and antibacterial action." *Journal of the American Chemical Society* 66 (11): 1950-1951.

[6] Wills, E. D. 1956. "Enzyme inhibition by allicin, the active principle of garlic." *The Biochemical Journal* 63 (3): 514-520.

[7] Rabinkov, Aharon, Talia Miron, Leonid Konstantinovski, Meir Wilchek, David Mirelman, and Lev Weiner. 1998. "The mode of action of allicin: trapping of radicals and interaction with thiol containing proteins." *BBA - General Subjects* 1379 (2): 233-244.

[8] Gruhlke, Martin C. H., Daniela Portz, Michael Stitz, Awais Anwar, Thomas Schneider, Claus Jacob, Nikolaus L. Schlaich, and Alan J. Slusarenko. 2010. "Allicin disrupts the cell's electrochemical potential and induces apoptosis in yeast." *Free Radical Biology and Medicine* 49 (12): 1916-1924.

[9] Borlinghaus, Jan, Frank Albrecht, Martin C. H. Gruhlke, Ifeanyi D. Nwachukwu, and Alan J. Slusarenko. 2014. Allicin: Chemistry and biological properties. *Molecules (Basel, Switzerland)* 19 (8): 12591-618.

[10] Müller, Alexandra, Jakob Eller, Frank Albrecht, Pascal Prochnow, Katja Kuhlmann, Julia Elisabeth Bandow, Alan John Slusarenko, and Lars Ingo Ole Leichert. 2016. "Allicin induces thiol stress in bacteria through S-allylmercapto modification of protein cysteines" *Joural of Biological Chemistry* 291(22): 11477-11490. doi: 10.1074/jbc.M115.702308.

[11] Williamson, Deborah A., Glen P. Carter, and Benjamin P. Howden. 2017. "Current and emerging topical antibacterials and antiseptics: agents, action, and resistance patterns." *Clinical Microbiology Reviews* 30 (3): 827-860. doi: 10.1128/CMR.00112-16.

[12] Small, LaVerne D., John Hays Bailey, and Chester J. Cavallito. 1947. "Alkyl thiosulfonates." *Jorunal of the American Chemical Society* 69(7), pp 1710–1713. doi: 10.1021/ja01199a040.

[13] Stoll, A. and E. Seebeck. 1951. "Chemical investigations on alliin, the specific principle of garlic." *Advances in Enzymology and Related Subjects of Biochemistry* 11: 377-400.

[14] Wang, Haiping, Xixiang Li, Di Shen, Yang Oiu, Jiangping Song. 2014. "Diversity evaluation of morphological traits and allicin content in garlic (*Allium sativum* L.) from China." Euphytica. 198:243-254. doi: 10.1007/s10681-014-1097-1.

[15] Yetgin, Ali, Kerem Canlı, and Ergin Murat Altuner. 2018. "Comparison of antimicrobial activity of *Allium sativum* cloves from China and Taşköprü, Turkey." *Advances in Pharmacological Sciences* 2018: 9302840-5. doi: 10.1155/2018/9302840.

[16] Fujisawa, Hiroyuki, Kaoru Suma, Kana Origuchi, Hitomi Kumagai, Taiichiro Seki, and Toyohiko Ariga. 2008. "Biological and chemical stability of garlic-derived allicin." *Journal of Agricultural and Food Chemistry* 56 (11): 4229-4235.

[17] Hughes, Bronwyn G. and Larry D. Lawson. 1991. "Antimicrobial effects of *Allium sativum* L. (Garlic), *Allium ampeloprasum* L. (Elephant Garlic), and *Allium cepa* L. (Onion), garlic compounds and commercial garlic supplement products." *Phytotherapy Research* 5 (4): 154-158.

[18] Lanzotti, Virginia, Giuliano Bonanomi, and Felice Scala. 2013. "What makes *Allium* species effective against pathogenic microbes?" *Phytochemistry Reviews* 12 (4): 751-772.

[19] Ross, Z. M., E. A. O'Gara, D. J. Hill, H. V. Sleightholme, and D. J. Maslin. 2001. "Antimicrobial properties of garlic oil against human enteric bacteria: evaluation of methodologies and comparisons with garlic oil sulfides and garlic powder." *Applied and Environmental Microbiology* 67 (1): 475-480. doi: 10.1128/AEM.67.1.475-480.2001.

[20] Dini, Catia, Alessia Fabbri, and Andrea Geraci. 2011. "The potential role of garlic (*Allium sativum*) against the multi-drug resistant tuberculosis pandemic: a review." *Annali Dell'Istituto Superiore Di Sanita* 47 (4): 465-473.

[21] T. Miron, Rabinkov A, Mirelman D, Wilchek M, Weiner L. 2000. "The mode of action of allicin: its ready permeability through phospholipid membranes may contribute to its biological activity." *Biochimica et Biophysica Acta* 1463(1):20-30. doi: 10.1016/S0005-2736(99)00174-1.

[22] Feldberg, R. S., S. C. Chang, A. N. Kotik, M. Nadler, Z. Neuwirth, D. C. Sundstrom, and N. H. Thompson. 1988. "*In vitro* mechanism of inhibition of bacterial cell growth by allicin." *Antimicrobial Agents and Chemotherapy* 32 (12): 1763-1768.

[23] Leontiev, Roman, Nils Hohaus, Claus Jacob, Martin C. H. Gruhlke, and Alan J. Slusarenko. 2018. "A comparison of the antibacterial and antifungal activities of thiosulfinate analogues of allicin." *Scientific Reports* 8 (1): 1-19.

[24] Serge Ankri and David Mirelman. 1999. "Antimicrobial properties of allicin from garlic." *Microbes and Infection* 2:125-129.

[25] Yehia, Hany M., Ebtesam M. Al-Olayan, Manal F. El-Khadragy, and Dina M. Metwally. 2017. "In vitro and in vivo control of secondary bacterial infection caused by Leishmania major." *International Journal of Environmental Research and Public Health* 14 (7): 777.

[26] Fani, M. M., J. Kohanteb, and M. Dayaghi. 2007. "Inhibitory activity of garlic (*Allium sativum*) extract on multidrug-resistant *Streptococcus mutans*." *Journal of the Indian Society of Pedodontics and Preventive Dentistry* 25 (4): 164-168.

[27] Pérez-Giraldo, C., G. Cruz-Villalón, R. Sánchez-Silos, R. Martínez-Rubio, M. T. Blanco, and A. C. Gómez-García. 2003. "*In vitro* activity of allicin against *Staphylococcus epidermidis* and influence of subinhibitory concentrations on biofilm formation." *Journal of Applied Microbiology* 95 (4): 709-711.

[28] Miron, Talia, Irving Listowsky, and Meir Wilchek. 2010. "Reaction mechanisms of allicin and allyl-mixed disulfides with proteins and small thiol molecules." *European Journal of Medicinal Chemistry* 45 (5): 1912-1918.

[29] Dwivedi, Ved Prakash, Debapriya Bhattacharya, Mona Singh, Ashima Bhaskar, Santosh Kumar, Parveen Sobia, Luc Van Kaer, and Gobardhan Das. 2018. "Allicin enhances antimicrobial activity of macrophages during *Mycobacterium tuberculosis* infection." *Journal of Ethnopharmacology*. doi: 10.1016/j.jep.2018.12.008.

[30] Focke, Manfred, Andrea Feld, and Hartmut K. Lichtenthaler. 1990. "Allicin, a naturally occurring antibiotic from garlic, specifically inhibits acetyl-CoA synthetase." *FEBS Letters* 261 (1): 106-108. doi: 10.1016/0014-5793(90)80647-2.

[31] Jonkers, D., J. Sluimer, and E. Stobberingh. 1999. "Effect of garlic on vancomycin-resistant *Enterococci*." *Antimicrobial Agents and Chemotherapy* 43 (12): 3045-3045.

[32] Arthur, M., C. Molinas, F. Depardieu, and P. Courvalin. 1993. "Characterization of Tn1546, a Tn3-related transposon conferring glycopeptide resistance by synthesis of depsipeptide peptidoglycan precursors in *Enterococcus faecium* BM4147." *Journal of Bacteriology* 175 (1): 117-127.

[33] Périchon, Bruno and Patrice Courvalin. 2009. "VanA-type vancomycin-resistant *Staphylococcus aureus*." *Antimicrobial Agents and Chemotherapy* 53 (11): 4580-4587.

[34] Stoll, V. S., A. V. Manohar, W. Gillon, E. L. MacFarlane, R. C. Hynes, and E. F. Pai. 1998. "A thioredoxin fusion protein of VanH, a D-lactate dehydrogenase from

Enterococcus faecium: cloning, expression, purification, kinetic analysis, and crystallization." *Protein Science: A Publication of the Protein Society* 7 (5): 1147.

[35] Bussiere, Dirksen E., Steven D. Pratt, Leonard Katz, Jean M. Severin, Thomas Holzman, and Chang H. Park. 1998. "The structure of VanX reveals a novel amino-dipeptidase involved in mediating transposon-based vancomycin resistance." *Molecular Cell* 2 (1): 75-84.

[36] Eschenburg, Susanne, Melanie Priestman, and Ernst Schönbrunn. 2005. "Evidence that the fosfomycin target Cys115 in UDP-N-acetylglucosamine enolpyruvyl transferase (MurA) is essential for product release." *Journal of Biological Chemistry* 280 (5): 3757-3763.

[37] Guo, Yan, Adam D. Tomich, Christi L. McElheny, Vaughn S. Cooper, Amelia Tait-Kamradt, Minggui Wang, Fupin Hu, Louis B. Rice, Nicolas Sluis-Cremer, and Yohei Doi. 2017. "High-level fosfomycin resistance in vancomycin-resistant *Enterococcus faecium*." *Emerging Infectious Diseases* 23 (11): 1902-1904.

[38] Salah Salman Zain Al-abdeen, Iman Tajer Abdullah and Sohaib Sabah Al-Salihi. 2013. "The synergism effect of aqueous garlic extract and ciprofloxacin against some multi-resistant bacteria." *J. Microbiol. Biotech. Res.* 3(3):136-142.

[39] Shah, Pratibha Jinesh, Manita T. Williamson, Sejal J. Rathod. 2016. "Antibacterial activity of aqueous garlic extract on beta-lactamase producing *Acinetobacter* isolates from skin and soft tissue infections." *Asian Journal of Pharmaceutical and Clinical Research* 9 (6): 152-156.

[40] Wolfmeier, Heidi, Daniel Pletzer, Sarah C. Mansour, and Robert E. W. Hancock. 2018. "New perspectives in biofilm eradication." *ACS Infectious Diseases* 4 (2): 93-106.

[41] Rasmussen, Thomas Bovbjerg, Thomas Bjarnsholt, Mette Elena Skindersoe, Morten Hentzer, Peter Kristoffersen, Manuela Köte, John Nielsen, Leo Eberl, and Michael Givskov. 2005. "Screening for quorum-sensing inhibitors (QSI) by use of a novel genetic system, the QSI selector." *Journal of Bacteriology* 187 (5): 1799-1814.

[42] Kaur, Rajinder, Atul, Tiwari, Manish Manish, Indresh K. Maurya, Rakesh Bhatnagar, Samer Singh. 2017. "Common garlic (*Allium sativum* L.) has potent anti-*Bacillus anthracis* activity." *BioRxiv. The preprint server for biology*. Cold Spring Harbor Laboratory. doi: 10.1101/162214.

[43] Jonkers, D. M. A. E., E. van den Broek, I. M. A. van Dooren, C. T. M. Thijs, E. Dorant, G. J. Hageman, and E. E. Stobberingh. 1999. "Antibacterial effect of garlic and omeprazole on *Helicobacter pylori*." *Journal of Antimicrobial Chemotherapy* 43 (6): 837-839. doi:10.1093/jac/43.6.837.

[44] El-Kashef, Dalia H., Asmaa E. El-Kenawi, Ghada M. Suddek, and Hatem A. Salem. 2015. "Protective effect of allicin against gentamicin-induced nephrotoxicity in rats." *International Immunopharmacology* 29 (2): 679-686.

[45] Alam, Rasha T. M., Elshaima M. Fawzi, Maha I. Alkhalf, Wafa S. Alansari, Lotfi Aleya, and Mohamed M. Abdel-Daim. 2018. "Anti-inflammatory, immunomodulatory, and antioxidant activities of allicin, norfloxacin, or their combination against *Pasteurella multocida* infection in male New Zealand Rabbits." *Oxidative Medicine and Cellular Longevity* 2018: 1780956-10.

[46] Berhanu Andualem. 2013. Combined antibacterial activity of stingless bee (*Apis mellipodae*) honey and garlic (*Allium sativum*) extracts against standard and clinical

pathogenic bacteria. *Asian Pacific Journal of Tropical Biomedicine*. 3(9): 725-731. doi: 10.1016/S2221-1691(13)60146-X.

[47] Lu, Xiaonan, Barbara A. Rasco, Jamie M. F. Jabal, D. Eric Aston, Mengshi Lin, and Michael E. Konkel. 2011. "Investigating antibacterial effects of garlic (*Allium sativum*) concentrate and garlic-derived organosulfur compounds on *Campylobacter jejuni* by using fourier transform infrared spectroscopy, raman spectroscopy, and electron microscopy." *Applied and Environmental Microbiology* 77 (15): 5257-5269.

[48] Zhang, Jing, Cong Quan, Cheng Wang, Hui Wu, Zhimin Li, and Qin Ye. 2016. "Systematic manipulation of glutathione metabolism in *Escherichia coli* for improved glutathione production." *Microbial Cell Factories* 15 (38): 38-38.

[49] Horn, Tobias, Wolfgang Bettray, Alan J. Slusarenko, and Martin C. H. Gruhlke. 2018. "S-Allylmercaptoglutathione is a substrate for glutathione reductase (E.C. 1.8.1.7) from yeast (*Saccharomyces Cerevisiae*)." *Antioxidants (Basel, Switzerland)* 7 (7): 86. doi:10.3390/antiox7070086.

[50] Nagahara, Noriyuki. 2011. "Catalytic site cysteines of thiol enzyme: sulfurtransferases." *Journal of Amino Acids* 2011: 709404-7.

[51] Lee, Heon-Jin, Hyo-Sang Park, Kyo-Han Kim, Tae-Yub Kwon, and Su-Hyung Hong. 2011. "Effect of garlic on bacterial biofilm formation on orthodontic wire." *The Angle Orthodontist* 81 (5): 895-900.

[52] Alouf, Joseph E., Stephen J. Billington, B. Helen Jost. 2006. "Repertoir and general features of the family of cholesterol-dependent cytolysins." (Ch 36) in: *The Comprehensive Sourcebook of Bacterial Protein Toxins*. Edited by Alouf and Popoff. Elsevier Ltd. pp. 643-648.

[53] Hotze, Eileen, M., Huynh . Le, Jessica R. Sieber, Christina Bruxvoort, Michael J. McInerney, Rodney K. Tweten. 2013. "Identification and characterization of the first cholesterol-dependent cytolysins from Gram-negative bacteria." *Infection and Immunity*. 81(1): 216-225.

[54] Billington, S. J., B. H. Jost, W. A. Cuevas, K. R. Bright, and J. G. Songer. 1997. "The *Arcanobacterium (Actinomyces) pyogenes* hemolysin, pyolysin, is a novel member of the thiol-activated cytolysin family." *Journal of Bacteriology* 179 (19): 6100-6106.

[55] Nagamune, Hideaki, Robert A. Whiley, Takatsugu Goto, Yasuko Inai, Takuya Maeda, Jeremy M. Hardie, and Hiroki Kourai. 2000. "Distribution of the intermedilysin gene among the anginosus group streptococci and correlation between intermedilysin production and deep-seated infection with *Streptococcus intermedius*." *Journal of Clinical Microbiology* 38 (1): 220-226.

[56] Kehoe, M. A., L. Miller, J. A. Walker, and G. J. Boulnois. 1987. "Nucleotide sequence of the streptolysin O (SLO) gene: structural homologies between SLO and other membrane-damaging, thiol-activated toxins." *Infection and Immunity* 55 (12): 3228-3232.

[57] Chiarot, Emiliano, Cristina Faralla, Nico Chiappini, Giovanna Tuscano, Fabiana Falugi, Gabriella Gambellini, Annarita Taddei, Sabrina Capo, Elena Cartocci, Daniele Veggi, Alessia Corrado, Simona Mangiavacchi, Simona Tavarini,a Maria Scarselli, Robert Janulczyk, Guido Grandi, Immaculada Margarit, Giuliano Bensia. 2013. "Targeted amino acid substitutions impair streptolysin O toxicity and Group A *Streptococcus* virulence." mBio 4(1):e00387-12. doi:10.1128/mBio.00387-12.

[58] Arzanlou, Mohsen and Shahab Bohlooli. 2010. "Inhibition of streptolysin O by allicin - an active component of garlic." *Journal of Medical Microbiology* 59 (Pt 9): 1044-1049. doi: 10.1099/jmm.0.019539-0.

[59] Arzanlou, M., S. Bohlooli, E. Jannati, and H. Mirzanejad-Asl. 2011. "Allicin from garlic neutralizes the hemolytic activity of intra- and extra-cellular pneumolysin O *in vitro*." *Toxicon* 57 (4): 540-545. doi: 10.1016/j.toxicon.2010.12.009.

[60] Mobley, H. L. and R. P. Hausinger. 1989. "Microbial ureases: significance, regulation, and molecular characterization." *Microbiological Reviews* 53 (1): 85-108.

[61] Ranjbar-Omid, Mahsa, Mohsen Arzanlou, Mojtaba Amani, Seyyedeh Khadijeh Shokri Al-Hashem, Nour Amir Mozafar, Hadi Peeri Doghaheh. 2015. "Allicin from garlic inhibits the biofilm formation and urease activity of *Proteus mirabilis in vitro*." *FEMS Microbiology Letters*. 362(9): doi: 10/1093/femsle/fnv049.

[62] Sriwanthana, B. and H. L. Mobley. 1993. "*Proteus mirabilis* urease: histidine 320 of UreC is essential for urea hydrolysis and nickel ion binding within the native enzyme." *Infection and Immunity* 61 (6): 2570-2577.

[63] Todd, M. J. and R. P. Hausinger. 1991. "Identification of the essential cysteine residue in *Klebsiella aerogenes* urease." *Journal of Biological Chemistry* 266 (36): 24327-24331.

[64] González-Fandos, E., M. L. García-López, M. L. Sierra, and A. Otero. 1994. "Staphylococcal growth and enterotoxins (A—D) and thermonuclease synthesis in the presence of dehydrated garlic." *Journal of Applied Bacteriology* 77 (5): 549-552. doi:10.1111/j.1365-2672.1994.tb04400.x.

[65] Hočevar, Katarina, Jan Potempa, and Boris Turk. 2018. "Host cell-surface proteins as substrates of gingipains, the main proteases of *Porphyromonas gingivalis*." *Biological Chemistry* 399 (12): 1353-1361.

[66] Bachrach, Gilad, Areen Jamil, Ronit Naor, Golan Tal, Zvi Ludmer, and Doron Steinberg. 2011. "Garlic allicin as a potential agent for controlling oral pathogens." *Journal of Medicinal Food* 14 (11): 1338-1343.

[67] Arzanlou, Mohsen. 2016. "Inhibition of streptococcal pyrogenic exotoxin B using allicin from garlic." *Microbial Pathogenesis* 93: 166-171.

[68] Berggren, Kristina, Björn Johansson, Tomas Fex, Jan Kihlberg, Lars Björck, Kristina Luthman. 2009. "Synthesis and biological evaluation of reversible inhibitors of IdeS, a bacterial cysteine protease and virulence determinant." *Bioorganic Medicinal Chemistry* 17 (9): 3463-3470.

[69] Martínez-García, Sergio, Sandra Rodríguez-Martínez, Mario E. Cancino-Diaz, and Juan C. Cancino-Diaz. 2018. "Extracellular proteases of *Staphylococcus epidermidis*: roles as virulence factors and their participation in biofilm." *Apmis* 126 (3): 177-185.

[70] Leng, Bing-Feng, Jia-Zhang Qiu, Xiao-Han Dai, Jing Dong, Jian-Feng Wang, Ming-Jing Luo, Hong-En Li, et al. 2011. "Allicin reduces the production of α-toxin by *Staphylococcus aureus*." *Molecules (Basel, Switzerland)* 16 (9): 7958-7968.

[71] Xiao, Meng, Rui Zhao, Qi Zhang, Xin Fan, Matthew V. N. O'Sullivan, Dong-Fang Li, Xin-Ying Wang, Hong-Long Wu, Fanrong Kong, and Ying-Chun Xu. 2016. "Genotypic diversity of *Staphylococcus aureus* α-hemolysin gene (Hla) and its association with clonal background: implications for vaccine development." *PloS One* 11 (2): e0149112-e0149112.

[72] Madeira, Fábio, Young Mi Park, Joon Lee, Nicola Buso, Tamer Gur, Nandana Madhusoodanan, Prasad Basutkar, et al. 2019. "The EMBL-EBI search and sequence analysis tools APIs in 2019." *Nucleic Acids Research.*

[73] Roshan, Niloufar, Thomas V. Riley, Daniel R. Knight, and Katherine A. Hammer. 2018. "Effect of natural products on the production and activity of *Clostridium difficile* toxins *in vitro.*" *Scientific Reports* 8 (1): 15735-9.

[74] Solomon, Haim M. and Donald A. Kautter. 1988. "Outgrowth and toxin production by *Clostridium botulinum* in bottled chopped garlic." *Journal of Food Protection* 51 (11): 862-865.

[75] Shamsi, Tooba Naz, Romana Parveen, Mohd Amir, Mohd Affan Baig, M. Irfan Qureshi, Sher Ali, and Sadaf Fatima. 2016. "*Allium sativum* protease inhibitor: A novel kunitz trypsin inhibitor from garlic is a new comrade of the serpin family." *PloS One* 11 (11): e0165572. doi:10.1371/journal.pone.0165572.

[76] Plano, L. R., D. M. Gutman, M. Woischnik, and C. M. Collins. 2000. "Recombinant *Staphylococcus aureus* exfoliative toxins are not bacterial superantigens." *Infection and Immunity* 68 (5): 3048-3052.

[77] Bakri, I. M. and C. W. I. Douglas. 2005. "Inhibitory effect of garlic extract on oral bacteria." *Archives of Oral Biology* 50 (7): 645-651. doi: 10.1016/j.archoralbio.2004. 12.002.

[78] Bjarnsholt, Thomas, Peter Ostrup Jensen, Thomas B. Rasmussen, Lars Christophersen, Henrik Calum, Morten Hentzer, Hans-Petter Hougen, et al. 2005. "Garlic blocks quorum sensing and promotes rapid clearing of pulmonary *Pseudomonas aeruginosa* infections." *Microbiology* 151 (12): 3873-3880.

[79] Cady, Nathaniel C., Kurt A. McKean, Jason Behnke, Roman Kubec, Aaron P. Mosier, Stephen H. Kasper, David S. Burz, and Rabi A. Musah. 2012. "Inhibition of biofilm formation, quorum sensing and infection in *Pseudomonas aeruginosa* by natural products-inspired organosulfur compounds." *PloS One* 7 (6): e38492.

[80] Cruz-Villalón, G. and C. Pérez-Giraldo. 2011. "Effect of allicin on the production of polysaccharide intercellular adhesin in *Staphylococcus epidermidis*: effect of allicin on the PIA production." *Journal of Applied Microbiology* 110 (3): 723-728.

[81] Wu, Xueqing, Regiane R. Santos, and Johanna Fink-Gremmels. 2015. "Analyzing the antibacterial effects of food ingredients: model experiments with allicin and garlic extracts on biofilm formation and viability of *Staphylococcus epidermidis.*" *Food Science Nutrition* 3 (2): 158-168.

[82] Mohsenipour, Zeinab and Mehdi Hassanshahian. 2015. "The effects of *Allium sativum* extracts on biofilm formation and activities of six pathogenic bacteria." *Jundishapur Journal of Microbiology* 8 (8): e18971.

[83] O'Gara, E. A., D. J. Hill, and D. J. Maslin. 2000. "Activities of garlic oil, garlic powder, and their diallyl constituents against *Helicobacter pylori.*" *Applied and Environmental Microbiology* 66 (5): 2269-2273.

[84] Ponmurugan Karuppiah Shyamkumar Rajaram. 2012. "Antibacterial effect of *Allium sativum* cloves and *Zingiber officinale* rhizomes against multiple-drug resistant clinical pathogens." *Asian Pacific Journal of Tropical Biomedicine* 2 (8): 597-601.

[85] Yadav, Seema, Niyati A. Trivedi, and Jagat D. Bhatt. 2015. "Antimicrobial activity of fresh garlic juice: an *in vitro* study." *Ayu* 36 (2): 203-207.

[86] Kundaković, Tatjana D., Ana D. Ćirić, Marina D. Soković, Marina T. Milenković, Vesna D. Nikolić, Goran S. Nikolić. 2011." Antimicrobial activity of lozenge with garlic bulb powder." *Hemijska Industrija* 65 (5): 607-610. doi: 10.2298/HEMIND 110414048K.

[87] Rad, Imani, Hamed, Mohsen Arzanlou, Mahsa Ranjbar Omid, Saber Ravaji, and Hadi Peeri Doghaheh. 2017. "Effect of culture media on chemical stability and antibacterial activity of allicin." *Journal of Functional Foods* 28: 321-325.

[88] Fujisawa, Hiroyuki, Kazuhiro Watanabe, Kaoru Suma, Kana Origughi, Hiroshi Matsufuji, Taiichiro Seki, and Toyohiko Ariga. 2009. "Antibacterial potential of garlic-derived allicin and its cancellation by sulfhydryl compounds." *Bioscience, Biotechnology, and Biochemistry* 73 (9): 1948-1955.

[89] Oblinger, J. L. and A. A. Kraft. 1973. "Oxidation-reduction potential and growth of *Salmonella* and *Pseudomonas fluorescens*." *Journal of Food Science* 38 (7): 1108-1112.

[90] Kabilan Velliyagounder, Krishnaraj Ganeshnarayan, Senthil Kumar Velusamy, and Daniel H. Fine. 2012. "*In vitro* efficacy of diallyl sulfides against the periodontopathogen *Aggregatibacter actinomycetemcomitans*." *Antimicrobial Agents and Chemotherapy*. P. 2397-2407. doi: 10.1128/AAC00020-12.

[91] Sasaki, Jin-ichi, Takeshi Kita, Kunio Ishita, Hidemitsu Uchisawa, Hajime Matsue. 1999. "Antibacterial activity of garlic powder against Escherichia coli O-157." *Journal of Nutritional Science and Vitaminology*, 45(6), 785–790. doi:10.3177/jnsv.45.785.

[92] Belguith, H., F. Kthiri, A. Chati, A. Abu Sofah, J. Ben Hamida, and A. Landoulsi. 2010. "Study of the effect of aqueous garlic extract (*Allium sativum*) on some *Salmonella* serovars isolates." *Emirates Journal of Food and Agriculture* 22 (3): 189.

[93] Sachs, G., J. M. Shin, C. Briving, B. Wallmark, and S. Hersey. 1995. "The pharmacology of the gastric acid pump: The H^+,K^+ ATPase." *Annual Review of Pharmacology and Toxicology* 35 (1): 277-305.

[94] Aydin, Ahmet, Galip Ersöz, Oktay Tekesin, Eren Akçiçek, and Müge Tuncyürek. 2000. "Garlic oil and *Helicobacter pylori* infection." *The American Journal of Gastroenterology* 95 (2): 563.

[95] Koçkar, C., M. Oztürk, and N. Bavbek. 2001. "*Helicobacter pylori* eradication with beta carotene, ascorbic acid and allicin." *Acta Medica (Hradec Kralove)* 44 (3): 97-100.

[96] Sasaki, Jin-ichi and Jyun-ichi Kita. 2003. "Bacteriocidal activity of garlic powder against *Bacillus anthracis*." *Journal of Nutritional Science and Vitaminology* 49 (4): 297-299.

[97] Ahmad, Iqbal and Farrukh Aqil. 2007. "*In Vitro* efficacy of bioactive extracts of 15 medicinal plants against ES βL-producing multidrug-resistant enteric bacteria." *Microbiological Research* 162 (3): 264-275.

[98] Sadeghian, A., and K. Ghazvini. 2002. "Antimicrobial activity of garlic extract against *Shigella*." *Iranian Journal of Medical Sciences* 27(3): 142-144.

[99] Kulikova, V. V., M. Yu Chernukha, E. A. Morozova, S. V. Revtovich, A. N. Rodionov, V. S. Koval, L. R. Avetisyan, et al. 2018. "Antibacterial effect of thiosulfinates on multiresistant strains of bacteria isolated from patients with cystic fibrosis." *Acta Naturae* 10 (3): 77-80.

[100] Malhotra, Sankalp, Jr Hayes Don, and Daniel J. Wozniak. 2019. "Cystic fibrosis and *Pseudomonas aeruginosa*: The host-microbe interface." *Clinical Microbiology Reviews* 32 (3). pii: e00138-18. doi: 10.1128/CMR.00138-18.

[101] Smyth, Alan R., Paramita M. Cifelli, Catharine A. Ortori, Karima Righetti, Sarah Lewis, Penny Erskine, Elaine D. Holland, et al. 2010. "Garlic as an inhibitor of *Pseudomonas aeruginosa* quorum sensing in cystic fibrosis - a pilot randomized controlled trial." *Pediatric Pulmonology* 45 (4): 356.

[102] LiPuma, John J. 2010. "The changing microbial epidemiology in cystic fibrosis." *Clinical Microbiology Reviews* 23 (2): 299-323. doi: 10.1128/CMR.00068-09.

[103] Burkholder, W. 1950. "Sour skin, a bacterial rot of onion bulbs." *Phytopathology* 40: 115–117.

[104] Rhodes, Katherine A. and Herbert P. Schweizer. 2016. "Antibiotic resistance in *Burkholderia* species." *Drug Resistance Updates* 28: 82-90. doi: 10.1016/j.drup.2016.07.003.

[105] Scoffone, Viola C., Laurent R. Chiarelli, Gabriele Trespidi, Massimo Mentasti, Giovanna Riccardi, and Silvia Buroni. 2017. "*Burkholderia cenocepacia* infections in cystic fibrosis patients: drug resistance and therapeutic approaches." *Frontiers in Microbiology* 8: 1592.

[106] Wallock-Richards, Daynea, Catherine J. Doherty, Lynsey Doherty, David J. Clarke, Marc Place, John R. W. Govan, and Dominic J. Campopiano. 2014. "Garlic revisited: antimicrobial activity of allicin-containing garlic extracts against Burkholderia Cepacia Complex." *PloS One* 9 (12): e112726-e112726. doi:10.1371/journal.pone.0112726.

[107] Delaha, E. C. and V. F. Garagusi. 1985. "Inhibition of *Mycobacteria* by garlic extract (*Allium sativum*)." *Antimicrobial Agents and Chemotherapy* 27 (4): 485-486.

[108] Hannan, Abdul, Muhammad Ikram Ullah, Muhammad Usman, Shahid Hussain, Muhammad Absar, and Khursheed Javed. 2011. "Anti-mycobacterial activity of garlic (*Allium sativum*) against multi-drug resistant and non-multi-drug resistant *Mycobacterium tuberculosis*." *Pakistan Journal of Pharmaceutical Sciences* 24 (1): 81.

[109] Viswanathan, V., A. G. Phadatare, and Alka Mukne. 2014. "Antimycobacterial and antibacterial activity of *Allium sativum* bulbs." *Indian Journal of Pharmaceutical Sciences* 76 (3): 256-261.

[110] Hasan, Nazarul, Mashiat Ullah Siddiqui, Zahra Toossi, Saba Khan, Jawed Iqbal, and Najmul Islam. 2007. "Allicin-induced suppression of *Mycobacterium tuberculosis* 85B mRNA in human monocytes." *Biochemical and Biophysical Research Communications* 355 (2): 471-476.

[111] Reiter, Jana, Natalja Levina, Mark van der Linden, Martin Gruhlke, Christian Martin, and Alan J. Slusarenko. 2017. "Diallylthiosulfinate (allicin), a volatile antimicrobial from garlic (*Allium sativum*), kills human lung pathogenic bacteria, including MDR strains, as a vapor." *Molecules (Basel, Switzerland)* 22 (10): 1711.

[112] Cutler, R. R. and P. Wilson. 2004. "Antibacterial activity of a new, stable, aqueous extract of allicin against methicillin-resistant *Staphylococcus aureus*." *British Journal of Biomedical Science* 61 (2): 71-74.

[113] Poovelikunnel, T., G. Gethin, and H. Humphreys. 2015. "Mupirocin resistance: Clinical implications and potential alternatives for the eradication of MRSA." *The Journal of Antimicrobial Chemotherapy* 70 (10): 2681-2692. doi: 10.1093/jac/dkv169.

[114] Tsao, Shyh-ming, Cheng-chin Hsu, and Mei-chin Yin. 2003. "Garlic extract and two diallyl sulphides inhibit methicillin-resistant *Staphylococcus aureus* infection in BALB/cA Mice." *The Journal of Antimicrobial Chemotherapy* 52 (6): 974-980.

[115] Widmer, Andreas F. 2001. "New developments in diagnosis and treatment of infection in orthopedic implants." *Clinical Infectious Diseases* 33 (5): S94.

[116] Zhai, Haohan, Jianchao Pan, En Pang, and Bo Bai. 2014. "Lavage with allicin in combination with vancomycin inhibits biofilm formation by *Staphylococcus epidermidis* in a rabbit model of prosthetic joint infection." *PloS One* 9 (7): e102760.

[117] Gupta, R. L., Sundeep Jain, V. Talwar, H. C. Gupta, and P. S. Murthy. 1999. "Antitubercular activity of garlic (*Allium sativum*) extract on combination with conventional antitubercular drugs in tubercular lymphadenitis." *Indian Journal of Clinical Biochemistry* 14 (1): 12-18.

[118] Ankri, S., T. Miron, A. Rabinkov, M. Wilchek, and D. Mirelman. 1997. "Allicin from garlic strongly inhibits cysteine proteinases and cytopathic effects of *Entamoeba histolytica*." *Antimicrobial Agents and Chemotherapy* 41 (10): 2286-2288.

[119] Feng, Jie, Wanliang Shi, Judith Miklossy, Genevieve M. Tauxe, Conor J. McMeniman, and Ying Zhang. 2018. "Identification of essential oils with strong activity against stationary phase *Borrelia burgdorferi*." *Antibiotics (Basel, Switzerland)* 7 (4): 89.

[120] Sharma, Anjana, and Virendra Kumar Patel. 2009. "*In vitro* screening of the antibacterial activity and identification of bioactive compounds from plants against selected *Vibrio* spp. pathogens." *Turkish Journal of Biology* 33 (2): 137-144.

[121] Shapoury, Reza, Morteza Sattari, and Zuhair M. Hassan. 2006. "Studies on the antimicrobial effect of allicin on the intra macrophages *Brucella*." *Pakistan Journal of Biological Sciences* 9 (10): 1935-1939.

[122] Li, Guoliang, Xudong Ma, Lisha Deng, Xixi Zhao, Yuejiao Wei, Zhongyang Gao, Jing Jia, Jiru Xu, and Chaofeng Sun. 2015. "Fresh garlic extract enhances the antimicrobial activities of antibiotics on resistant strains *in vitro*." *Jundishapur Journal of Microbiology* 8 (5): e14814.

[123] Tsao Shyh-ming and Mei-chin Yin. 2001. "*In-vitro* antimicrobial activity of four diallyl sulphides occurring naturally in garlic and Chinese leek oils." *Journal of Medical Microbiology* 50 (7): 646-649.

[124] Ćirković, Ivana, M. Jovalekić, and B. Jegorović. 2012. "*In vitro* antibacterial activity of garlic and synergism between garlic and antibacterial drugs." *Arch. Biol. Sci., Belgrade*, 64(4): 1369-1375.

[125] Abubakar, El-Mahmood Muhammad. 2009. "Efficacy of crude extracts of garlic (*Allium sativum* Linn.) against nosocomial *Escherichia coli*, *Staphylococcus aureus*, *Streptococcus pneumoniae* and *Pseudomonas aeruginosa*." *Journal of Medicinal Plants Research* 3(4): 179-185.

[126] Mussarat, Sakina, Rahila Amber, Akash Tariq, Muhammad Adnan, Naser M. AbdElsalam, Riaz Ullah, and Roqaia Bibi. 2014. "Ethnopharmacological assessment of medicinal plants used against livestock infections by the people living around Indus River." *BioMed Research International* 2014: 616858-14.

[127] Donovan, D. C., S. T. Franklin, and C. C. L. Chase. 2002. "Growth and health of Holstein calves fed milk replacers supplemented with antibiotics or Enteroguard." *Journal of Dairy Science* 85 (4): 947-950.

[128] Kamra, D. N., N. Agarwal, P. C. Sakthivel, and L. C. Chaudhary. 2012. "Garlic as a rumen modifier for eco-friendly and economic livestock production." *Journal of Applied Animal Research* 40 (2): 90-96.

[129] Karangiya, V.K., H.H. Savsani, Shrikant Soma Patil, D.D. Garg, K.S. Murthy, N.K. Ribadiya, S.J. Vekariya. 2016. "Effect of dietary supplementation of garlic, ginger and their combination on feed intake, growth performance and economics in commercial broilers." *Veterinary World* 9(3):245-250. doi: 10.14202/vetworld.2016.245-250.

[130] Robyn, J., G. Rasschaert, D. Hermans, F. Pasmans, and M. Heyndrickx. 2013. "Is allicin able to reduce *Campylobacter jejuni* colonization in broilers when added to drinking water?" *Poultry Science* 92 (5): 1408-1418.

[131] Stratev, Deyan, Georgi Zhelyazkov, Xavier Siwe Noundou, and Rui W. M. Krause. 2018. "Beneficial effects of medicinal plants in fish diseases." *Aquaculture International* 26 (1): 289-308.

[132] Breyer, Kate E., Rodman G. Getchell, Emily R. Cornwell, Gregory A. Wooster, H. George Ketola, and Paul R. Bowser. 2015. "Efficacy of an extract from garlic, *Allium sativum*, against infection with the *Furunculosis bacterium*, *Aeromonas salmonicida*, in rainbow trout, *Oncorhynchus mykiss*." *Journal of the World Aquaculture Society* 46 (3): 273-282.

[133] Etyemez Büyükdeveci, Miray, José L. Balcázar, İbrahim Demirkale, and Suat Dikel. 2018. "Effects of garlic-supplemented diet on growth performance and intestinal microbiota of rainbow trout (*Oncorhynchus mykiss*)." *Aquaculture* 486: 170-174.

[134] Natasya-Ain, R., N. Eirna-Liza, M. Jasmin, Murni Karim. 2018. "Antibacterial activity of garlic extracts on fish pathogenic bacteria." *Journal of Environmental Biology* 39 (5(SI)): 808-812.

[135] Vaseeharan, B., G. Sai Prasad, P. Ramasamy, and G. Brennan. 2011. "Antibacterial activity of *Allium sativum* against multidrug-resistant *Vibrio harveyi* isolated from black gill–diseased *Fenneropenaeus indicus*." *Aquaculture International* 19 (3): 531-539.

[136] Saha, Mandira and Probir Kumar Bandyopadhyay. 2019. "Green biosynthesis of silver nanoparticle using garlic, *Allium sativum* with reference to its antimicrobial activity against the pathogenic strain of *Bacillus* sp. and *Pseudomonas* sp. infecting goldfish, *Carassius auratus*." *Proceedings of the Zoological Society* 72 (2): 180-186.

[137] Goda, A. M., E. A. Omar, T. M. Srour, A. M. Kotiet, E. El-Haroun, and Simon J. Davies. 2018. "Effect of diets supplemented with feed additives on growth, feed utilization, survival, body composition and intestinal bacterial load of early weaning european seabass, *Dicentrarchus labrax* post-larvae." *Aquaculture International* 26 (1): 169-183.

[138] Zaefarian, Azadeh, Sakineh Yeganeh, and Batoul Adhami. 2017. "Dietary effects of garlic powder (*Allium sativum*) on growth, blood indices, carcass composition, and lysozyme activity in brown trout (*Salmo caspius*) and resistance against *Yersinia ruckeri* infection." *Aquaculture International* 25 (6): 1987-1996.

[139] Rahman, Muntasir, Md Mahbubur Rahman, Suzan Chandra Deb, Md Shahanoor Alam, Md Jahangir Alam, and Md Tofazzal Islam. 2017. "Molecular identification of multiple antibiotic resistant fish pathogenic *Enterococcus faecalis* and their control by medicinal herbs." *Scientific Reports* 7 (1): 3747-11.

[140] Miron, Talia, Irina Shin, Guy Feigenblat, Lev Weiner, David Mirelman, Meir Wilchek, and Aharon Rabinkov. 2002. "A spectrophotometric Assay for allicin, alliin, and alliinase (alliin lyase) with a chromogenic thiol: reaction of 4-mercaptopyridine with thiosulfinates." *Analytical Biochemistry* 307 (1): 76-83.

[141] Miron, Talia, Aharon Rabinkov, David Mirelman, Lev Weiner, and Meir Wilchek. 1998. "A spectrophotometric assay for allicin and alliinase (alliin lyase) activity: Reaction of 2-nitro-5-thiobenzoate with thiosulfinates." *Analytical Biochemistry* 265 (2): 317-325.

[142] Arnault, I., T. Haffner, M. H. Siess, A. Vollmar, R. Kahane, and J. Auger. 2005. "Analytical method for appreciation of garlic therapeutic potential and for validation of a new formulation." *Journal of Pharmaceutical and Biomedical Analysis* 37 (5): 963-970.

[143] Pérez-Köhler, Bárbara, Francisca García-Moreno, Yves Bayon, Gemma Pascual, and Juan Manuel Bellón. 2015. "Inhibition of *Staphylococcus aureus* adhesion to the surface of a reticular heavyweight polypropylene mesh soaked in a combination of chlorhexidine and allicin: An *in vitro* study." *PloS One* 10 (5): e0126711.

[144] Pérez-Köhler, Bárbara, Francisca García-Moreno, Thierry Brune, Gemma Pascual, and Juan Manuel Bellón. 2015. "Preclinical bioassay of a polypropylene mesh for hernia repair pretreated with antibacterial solutions of chlorhexidine and allicin: an *in vivo* study." *PloS One* 10 (11): e0142768-e0142768.

[145] Choules, Lucinda, Dennis A. Gravatt, Stephen M. Kosovich, Wei Yuan, Wang Ping, and Ron Havner. 2016. "Inhibition of *Enterobacter cloacae* and *Klebsiella oxytoca* by garlic (*Allium sativum* L.) and garlic pills" *Pharmaceuticl Crops* 6:1-12. doi: 10.2174/2210290601606010001.

[146] Ruddock, Patrick S., Mingmin Liao, Brian C. Foster, Larry Lawson, John T. Arnason, and Jo-Anne R. Dillon. 2005. "Garlic natural health products exhibit variable constituent levels and antimicrobial activity against *Neisseria gonorrhoeae*, *Staphylococcus aureus* and *Enterococcus faecalis*." *Phytotherapy Research* 19 (4): 327-334.

[147] P.M.L, Ward, Fasitsas S, and Katz S.E. 2002. "Inhibition, resistance development, and increased antibiotic and antimicrobial resistance caused by nutraceuticals." *Journal of Food Protection* 65 (3): 528-533.

[148] Lubenets, Vira, Sofiya Vasylyuk, Nataliya Monka, Khrystyna Bolibrukh, Olena Komarovska-Porokhnyavets, Diana Baranovych, Rostyslav Musyanovych, et al. 2017. "Synthesis and antimicrobial properties of 4-acylaminobenzenethiosulfoacid S-esters." *Saudi Pharmaceutical Journal* 25 (2): 266-274. doi: 10.1016/j.jsps.2016.06.007.

[149] Sheppard, Jordan G., Jeremy P. McAleer, Pushkar Saralkar, Werner J. Geldenhuys, and Timothy E. Long. 2018. "Allicin-inspired pyridyl disulfides as antimicrobial agents for multidrug-resistant *Staphylococcus aureus*." *European Journal of Medicinal Chemistry* 143: 1185-1195.

[150] Rajan, S. Thanka, M. Karthika, U. Balaji, A Muthappan, B. Subramanian. 2017. "Functional finishing of medical fabrics using CeO2allicin nanocomposite for wound dressings." *Jounal of Alloys and Compounds*. 695:747-752. doi: 10.1016/j.jallcom.2016.06.241.

[151] Abdulrahman, Dadile, Abdullahi Daskum, Kura Abdulrahim, Abubakar Dadile, and Hajja Amma. 2017. "Antibacterial potency of garlic extract against certain skin pathogenic bacteria." *Novel Research in Microbiology Journal* 1 (1): 3-13.

[152] Chandrdas, Dithi, H. L. Jayakumar, Mahesh Chandra, Lavleen Katodia, and Athira Sreedevi. 2014. "Evaluation of antimicrobial efficacy of garlic, tea tree oil, cetylpyridinium chloride, chlorhexidine, and ultraviolet sanitizing device in the decontamination of toothbrush." *Indian Journal of Dentistry* 5 (4): 183-189.

[153] Groppo, F. C., J. C. Ramacciato, R. P. Simões, F. M. Flório, and A. Sartoratto. 2002. "Antimicrobial activity of garlic, tea tree oil, and chlorhexidine against oral microorganisms." *International Dental Journal* 52 (6): 433-437.

[154] Le, Nguyen T., Jhansi R. Kalluri, Armando Loni, Leigh T. Canham, and Jeffery L. Coffer. 2017. "Biogenic nanostructured porous silicon as a carrier for stabilization and delivery of natural therapeutic species." *Molecular Pharmaceutics* 14 (12): 4509-4514.

[155] Cutler, Ronald R., Michel Odent, Hussein Hajj-Ahmad, Sunil Maharjan, Norman J. Bennett, Peter D. Josling, Vanessa Ball, Paulette Hatton, and Martino Dall'Antonia. 2009. "*In Vitro* activity of an aqueous allicin extract and a novel allicin topical gel formulation against Lancefield Group B Streptococci." *Journal of Antimicrobial Chemotherapy* 63 (1): 151-154.

[156] Inouye, S., H. Yamaguchi, and T. Takizawa. 2001. "Screening of the antibacterial effects of a variety of essential oils on respiratory tract pathogens, using a modified dilution assay method." *Journal of Infection and Chemotherapy* 7 (4): 251-254.

[157] Harrison, Freya, Aled E. L. Roberts, Rebecca Gabrilska, Kendra P. Rumbaugh, Christina Lee, and Stephen P. Diggle. 2015. "A 1,000-year-old antimicrobial remedy with antistaphylococcal activity." *Mbio* 6 (4): e01129-e01129.

[158] Fuchs, Amanda L., Jr Weaver Alan J, Brian P. Tripet, Mary Cloud B. Ammons, Martin Teintze, and Valérie Copié. 2018. "Characterization of the antibacterial activity of Bald's eyesalve against drug resistant *Staphylococcus aureus* and *Pseudomonas aeruginosa*." *PloS One* 13 (11): e0208108-e0208108.

[159] Mazelis, M. and L. Crews. 1968. "Purification of the alliin lyase of garlic, *Allium sativum* L." *The Biochemical Journal* 108 (5): 725-730.

In: Allicin
Editor: Diana R. Cundell
ISBN: 978-1-53617-339-0

Chapter 6

ANTIFUNGAL ACTIVITY OF ALLICIN

Beth M. French-Arthur*[*]*, PhD
Notre Dame of Maryland University, Baltimore, MD, US

ABSTRACT

Allicin was first isolated in the 1940s as an antibacterial agent, and ten years later it was discovered to possess antifungal activity. In 12 separate studies, researchers have found at least six different fungi, infecting human/animals or plants, for which allicin can inhibit all *in vitro* and two *in vivo*. There is a pressing need for new human antifungal agents as resistance is rising against the current treatments. Available antifungal treatments also have many side effects due to the similarities between these eukaryotes and other cells. In addition, mortality rates associated with fungal disease are high as these microbes frequently target immunosuppressed patients. Fungal infections of plants are no less of an issue as they destroy much of the world's food crops. Allicin has been shown to be effective in either treatment alone or together with antifungal drugs (Amphotericin B or flucytosine) to treat human diseases. Allicin is also effective treatment alone against fungal infections of plants. Therefore, it may provide a more effective and cheaper treatment, especially in developing nations. Future effects of allicin treatment will be considered in this chapter as well as possible delivery systems.

Keywords: antifungal, plant pathogens

INTRODUCTION

Garlic has long been documented as an antimicrobial, anticancer, antidiabetic, antiviral agent [1]. Use of crushed garlic bulbs has also been reported to have effects on the growth of receiver plants and to help those plants overcome cropping obstacles in eggplants, cucumbers and pepper [1]. In 1944 the active antibacterial principle was found to be allicin which, although

* Corresponding Author's Email: beth.m.french@gmail.com.

relatively unstable, exhibited a wide spectrum of potency. As allicin is the main biologically active component of garlic clove extracts, it has been found to have anti-oxidant properties which may be the cause of anti-bacterial activity [2, 3].

The first discovered antifungal activity of allicin was against plant-associated microbes, in the 1950s [4]. When juice from crushed garlic was applied to the soil near the roots of plants it led to a drastic decrease in the number of microorganisms [4]. This suggested that perhaps there was something specific in crushed garlic that could possibly be anti-microbial [4]. Appleton and Tansey added to the evidence and found inhibition of growth within several fungi, specifically communicable fungi, by an extract from garlic [5]. These early studies marked the beginning of an exploration into the antifungal nature of allicin that would eventually expand from plants into human disease [4-5].

Fungal infections have provided a challenge to treatment in humans, animals and plants since these microbes were discovered. Although this large kingdom is primarily involved in recycling available complex organic molecules, there are a few important species that can result in morbidity and mortality of multicellular organisms. Common and widespread human fungal diseases include aspergillosis, candidiasis, and cryptococcosis [6,7]. Plant diseases include rice blast fungi *Magnaporthe oryzae* and tree pathogens such as *Ophiostoma ulmi* which causes Dutch Elm Disease [8, 9].

Treatment strategies for human fungal diseases have included polyene antifungals that include amphotericin B and Nystatin which bind with sterols in the fungal cell membrane, specifically ergosterol [10]. When these antifungal agents bind they change the temperature of the cell membrane, which causes ions and small organic molecules to be able to leak out [10]. Animal cells contain cholesterol instead of ergosterol making them less susceptible to this drug. However, amphotericin B may bind to cholesterol causing the drug to become human toxic with many harmful side effects [10]. A second major class of antifungals are azoles such as imidazole and fluconazole. These are effective by inhibiting the enzymes needed by fungi to convert lanosterol to ergosterol and if there is not enough ergosterol the structure of the membrane is disrupted [10]. Much like the polyene antifungals there are serious side effects associated with these drugs such as anaphylaxis [10]. Fungal cells are similar in structure to their human hosts so most available antifungal agents have significant side effects [11]. Limited varieties of fungal treatments have also resulted in the evolution of a large amount of resistance against these agents [12]. For example, antifungal resistance is a problem with *Candida* infections [12]. The CDC reports that the proportion of *Candida* strains resistance to fluconazole has remained constant over the past 20 years but resistance to echinocandin has recently emerged [12]. Mortality rates of plant fungal infections also remains high despite the availability of new antifungal agents [11]. For example, T4 *Fusarium* infections are killing the multi-billion-dollar industry's Cavendish banana crop and there are no current interventions for this strain of fungus or banana variant [13]. The Cavendish banana is the most significant commercially grown banana and has no reasonable replacement. Therefore, there is a large need for better treatments for fungal infections, with less side effects or capacity to generate resistance both in humans as well as plants.

Natural products, such as apple cider vinegar, baking soda and chamomile tea, are now being used to treat fungal infections on plants, especially in developing nations or by organic gardeners [14]. Many of these natural products have been made into sprays that can be used as pre-treatment/treatment for plants [15]. Recently, interest in natural product-based screening for human fungal treatments has also been on the rise [15]. Researchers have found valuable features of natural products due to improvements in structure-identification, separation and target identification [15]. Two of the three major classes of antifungals (polyenes and echinocandins) are already derived from natural products and researchers are looking for more [15].

Given the need for new agents to intervene with both human and animal fungal infections, the next question is why allicin? Although only a small body of research has been done on garlic/allicin as a treatment it has hopes of being effective. Several observations about allicin's effects, which will be discussed in detail later, point towards its potential uses. First, researchers believe that allicin targets thiol enzymes much like antifungal drugs [16]. It has been found that allicin, due to its chemical reaction with thiol groups of various enzymes, like alcohol dehydrogenase or thioredoxin, can negatively affect fungal metabolism [16]. Allicin could also potentiate the entry of existing medications into fungal cells [7]. Studies by Akira Ogita [17] have shown that allicin could help antifungal drug amphotericin B (AmB) kill fungi through altering the fungi's plasma membrane permeability. Finally, allicin or allicin-enriched garlic extracts possess broad spectrum antifungal activity i.e., the nature of the infective agent would need to be identified. Allicin or allicin-enriched garlic extracts have been shown to have *in vitro* efficacy against 11 fungi and *in vivo/in planta* against 4 fungi [16, 18-23, 38-41]. This chapter will discuss these studies, the importance of these fungi and the potential mechanism through which allicin impairs them. Possible delivery or combination therapies for allicin will also be suggested.

ALLICIN OR GARLIC AND HUMAN FUNGAL PATHOGENS

Allicin/garlic extracts have been shown to be effective against five human pathogens using *in vitro* or *in vivo* models [16, 18-23]. The results of these studies are summarized in Tables 1 and 2 below.

Allicin was more effective against *Candida albicans* than the standard antifungal treatments (Itraconazole and Fluconazole) and this efficiency increased when allicin was combined with these agents [18]. Allicin was also combined with flucytosine and amphotericin B [19]. Allicin alone and when combined resulted in a >40% survival [19]. *In vivo* alcoholic extracts of garlic were given to diabetic rats that were infected with *Candida albicans* and this reduced the infection [23]. They found that if rats were given alcoholic extracts of garlic, the *C. albicans* concentrations were significantly reduced in the infected control and diabetic rats [23]. *Trichophyton rubrum* was treated with allicin and garlic extract and pure allicin caused the inhibition of hyphal cells [20]. The minimum inhibitory concentration (MIC) of allicin extract against 1×10^5 organisms of *Cryptococcus neoformans* ranged from 6 to 12 μg/mL [16]. When the extract was used synergistically with amphotericin B it demonstrated fungistatic activity against all isolates of *C. neoformans* [16]. The MIC and minimum fungicidal concentration (MFC) of pure allicin against 31 clinical isolates of *Aspergillus* were between 8 and 32 mg/L [21]. An *in vivo* study showed that *Aspergillus fumigatus* infected mice that were given allicin increased the mean survival from 7.7 days to 21.3 days (iv treatment) and 13.9 days (oral treatment) [21]. Using the agar dilution method to test antifungal efficacy, the MIC of allicin after 5 days was 6.25 μg/ml for *Candida*, 3.13 μg/ml for *Cryptococcus*, 1.57 μg/ml for *Trichophyton*, 0.78 μg/ml for *Epidermophyton* and 1.57 μg/ml for *Microsporum* [22]. In the broth dilution method, the MIC after 5 days was 6.25 μg/ml for *Candida*, 3.13 μg/ml for *Cryptococcus,* 6.25 μg/ml for *Trichophyton*, 3.13 μg/ml for *Epidermophyton* and 6.25 μg/ml for *Microsporum* [22]. The MICs of allicin against *Candida* and *Cryptococcus* remained constant after more than 3 days of incubation [22]. Allicin seems to be very efficient at killing *C. albicans* not only in several *in vitro* experiments but also *in vivo*. Allicin also seems to be most efficient at killing *Aspergillus* as it increases survival of infected rats from mean survival 7.7 days to 21.3 days (intravenous treatment) and 13.9 days (oral treatment) [21]. Although the other fungi do seem to be affected by allicin/garlic more studies (especially *in vivo*) would need to be done to prove the efficiency.

Table 1. Allicin/garlic extracts *in vitro* studies against human fungal pathogens

Fungi	Results	Reference
Candida albicans	Disk Diffusion: Zones of inhibition for Fresh garlic extract: 25 mm Itraconazole: 12.5 mm Fluconazole: 15 mm Fresh garlic with fluconazole: 30 mm Fresh garlic with itraconazole: 28 mm.	[18]
	Tested combination of flucytosine and amphotericin B (AmB) (0.1 μg/ml and 1 μg/ml) with allicin in vitro. After 24 hours of treatment: allicin alone or in combination with one of the other drugs resulted in a >40% survival in *C. albicans*. Allicin appeared to inhibit both the germination of spores and the growth of the hyphae of the *C. albicans*.	[19]
Trichophyton rubrum	Treated with allicin and garlic extract. Allicin treated group: Hypha were rough and granular on the surface and irregularly shaped. The hyphal cytoplasm disintegrated, and the cell wall and membrane broke down. Garlic extract treated group: Hypha was irregularly shaped, exhibiting a rough and fluffy surface. The cytoplasm was also found to be degraded and the cell wall and membrane were similarly broken down. Pure allicin was more effective in inhibiting the growth of hyphal cells compared to the garlic extract.	[20]
Cryptococcus neoformans	Allicin extract had a potent fungistatic and fungicidal activity against three different isolate of *C. neoformans*. The MIC of the extract against 1×10^5 organisms ranged from 6 to 12 μg/mL. When the extract was used synergistically with amphotericin B it demonstrated fungistatic activity against all isolates of *C. neoformans*.	[16]
Aspergillosis	Pure allicin against 31 clinical isolates of *Aspergillus*. MIC and MFC were between 8 and 32 mg/L. Time kill studies showed that allicin exerts its fungicidal activity within 2 to 12 hours of administration.	[21]
Candida, Cryptococcus, Trichophyton, Epidermophyton, and *Microsporum*.	Allicin treatment was tested using the agar dilution and broth dilution methods. Using the agar dilution method to test antifungal efficacy, the MIC of allicin after 5 days was 6.25 μg/ml for *Candida*, 3.13 μg/ml for *Cryptococcus*, 1.57 μg/ml for *Trichophyton*, 0.78 μg/ml for *Epidermophyton* and 1.57 μg/ml for *Microsporum*. In the broth dilution method, the MIC after 5 days was 6.25 μg/ml for *Candida*, 3.13 μg/ml for *Cryptococcus*, 6.25 μg/ml for *Trichophyton*, 3.13 μg/ml for *Epidermophyton* and 6.25 μg/ml for *Microsporum*. The MICs of allicin against *Candida and Cryptococcus* remained constant after more than 3 days of incubation. As the inoculum size decreased, the susceptibility to allicin treatment increased for all fungi. The antifungal activity against allicin was particularly potent on agar at pH 5.6 compared to media with a pH of 6.0 or higher.	[22]

Abbreviations used in the table: MIC: Minimum Inhibitory Concentration; MFC: Minimal Fungicidal Concentration

Table 2. Allicin/garlic extracts *in vivo* studies against human fungal pathogens

Fungi	Results	Reference
Candida albicans	Streptozotocin-induced diabetic rats. Six different groups: Control rats (3 groups) Diabetic rats (3 groups). Some infected with *C. albicans* (4 groups) others were not (2 groups). Some were treated with garlic extract (2 groups) others were not (4 groups). If rats were given alcoholic extracts of garlic, the *C. albicans* concentrations were significantly reduced in the infected control and diabetic rats.	[23]
Aspergillosis	Immunocompetent mice infected with *Aspergillus fumigatus*. Allicin was administered through IV once daily for 5 days post-infection, or orally for 5 days pre-infection and 10 days post-infection. Allicin treatment prolonged survival of infected mice from mean survival 7.7 days to 21.3 days (IV treatment) and 13.9 days (oral treatment).	[21]

Abbreviations used in the table: IV (intravenous).

Allicin/Garlic Extract and Candida Albicans

Three *in vitro* studies were performed on *C. albicans* [18, 19, 22]. The study by Guoliang Li and colleagues [18] study, they used the disk diffusion method to see the effect of fresh garlic extract and the combination of antibiotics and fresh garlic extract against *C. albicans* [18]. Clinical isolates of *C. albicans* were used, and the samples/discs were given one of the following: deionized water, fresh garlic extract, antibiotics, or antibiotics with fresh garlic extract [18]. The antifungal activity was measured by determining the diameter of inhibition zones [18]. Fresh garlic extract displayed inhibition properties and the potential to improve the effect of antifungal agents on resistant pathogens [18]. It was found that the zones of inhibition were larger for fresh garlic extract (25 mm) than itraconazole (12.5 mm) or fluconazole (15 mm) [18]. The synergism of fluconazole and itraconazole with fresh garlic extract yielded larger sized inhibition zones compared to those without fresh garlic extract [18]. Fresh garlic with fluconazole had zones of inhibition at 30 mm and fresh garlic with itraconazole had zones of inhibition at 28 mm [18]. This suggests that fresh garlic extract can improve the antibiotic sensitivity of *C. albicans* to some antibiotics and may be a candidate for the treatment of infection by multi-drug resistant strains [18].

A second *in vitro* study tested the effect of allicin on *C. albicans* as well as its synergistic effect with the antifungal drugs flucytosine and amphotericin B (AmB) [19]. Young-Sun Kim et al. [19] treated *C. albicans* with allicin both alone and together with an antifungal drug for 24 hours [19]. They then observed the fungus with a scanning electron microscope and an atomic force microscope to measure cell death [29]. After 24 hours of treatment, allicin alone, or in combination with one of the other drugs (either AmB or flucytosine), resulted in a >40% survival in *C. albicans* [19]. However, when *C. albicans* was treated with combinations of more than two of these drugs, the survival decreased to less than 32% [19]. Upon further observation, allicin appeared to inhibit both the germination of spores (blastoconidia) and the growth of the hyphae of the *C. albicans* [19]. Allicin was also found to increase oxidative stress and reduce glutathione levels [19]. Both traits are part of the pathway that antifungal drugs take against fungal infections. Allicin was also found to inhibit biofilm formation in *C. albicans* [19]. This shows that allicin is just as effective in its inhibition of C. albicans as typical antifungal drugs. Additionally, researchers found that the outer membranes of cells treated with allicin and AmB were destroyed [19]. These results demonstrate that allicin can enhance the activity of the antifungal drugs by increasing the permeability of the fungal cell membrane [19]. The ability of allicin to increase the efficacy of AmB and flucytosine is promising and can potentially be used to decrease the dosages of the antifungal drugs used to treat *C. albicans* infections.

The third *in vitro* study tested the effect of allicin treatment on *Candida,* using agar and broth dilution methods [22]. Using the agar dilution technique, the MIC of allicin after 5 days was 6.25 μg/ml [22]. In the broth dilution method, the MIC after 5 days was 6.25 μg/ml for *Candida* [22]. The MICs of allicin against *Candida,* remained constant after more than 3 days of incubation [22]. As the inoculum size decreased, the susceptibility to allicin treatment increased for all fungi [22]. The antifungal activity against allicin was particularly potent on agar at pH 5.6 compared to media with a pH of 6.0 or higher [22]. The decreased susceptibility of allicin in pH of more than 5.6 may be a consequence of degradation of allicin at a pH value higher than 5.6 [22].

One *in vivo* study investigated the effect of garlic extract on *Candida* infections in streptozotocin-induced diabetic rats [23]. The rats were divided into 6 different groups with control rats (3 groups) and diabetic rats (3 groups) [23]. Some groups were infected with *C. albicans* (4 groups) and others were not (2 groups) [23]. Finally, some rats were treated with garlic extract (2 groups) and others were not (4 groups) [23]. Livers and kidneys were homogenized to measure the *C. albicans* levels following infection and treatment [23]. They found that if rats were given alcoholic extracts of garlic, the *C. albicans* concentrations were significantly reduced in the infected control and diabetic rats [23]. These results demonstrate that garlic extract can be used to decrease Candida infections, even in diabetic patients.

C. *albicans* is a normal component of the human flora/microbiome and different factors can allow the fungus to grow out of control causing infections [24]. The patients that have the most issues with C. *albicans* becoming pathogenic are immunocompromised adults such as HIV-infected patients [25]. A mortality rate of 40% has been reported for patients with systemic candidiasis from *C. albicans* [25]. Along with immunocompromised patients, *C. albicans* is also commonly isolated from biofilms in implanted medical devices or on human tissue [26].

Patients who are immunocompromised or undergoing cancer chemotherapy (which can be highly immunosuppressive) are likely to develop invasive fungal infections. The mortality rates from candidemia (~24%) is higher in patients with cancer [27]. AmB is typically used for the control of serious fungal infections [27]. However, the use of AmB is limited by the toxic side effects as well as the fact that many drug-resistant strains of fungus to AmB have recently emerged [27]. AmB kills fungi by altering the plasma membrane ion permeability due to its binding to ergosterol on the plasma membrane [27]. As mentioned in the beginning of this chapter, egosterol is found only on the membrane of fungi and protozoa [27]. AmB binds physically to ergosterol within the membrane, thus creating a polar pore in fungal membranes [27]. This causes ions and other molecules to leak out, which will kill the cell [27]. Additionally, researchers have recently found that AmB could also have a vacuole disruptive action when used in combination with allicin in treating *Saccharomyces cerevisiae* and *C. albicans* infections [27]. The normal cellular response to prevent disintegration of the vacuole membrane is to traffic ergosterol from the plasma membrane to the vacuole membrane [27]. AmB and allicin together inhibit ergosterol-trafficking, resulting in the breakdown of the vacuole membrane [27]. The fungal vacuole is very important because it helps the fungi with cellular homeostasis, degradation of intracellular components, and storage of ions and molecules therefore, if the vacuole is broken down this will greatly hinder the fungi [27]. The synergistic activity of AmB and allicin highlights the potential of developing vacuole-targeting treatments against fungal infections.

Allicin/Garlic Extract and Trychophyton Rubrum

Allicin treatment was tested using the agar dilution and broth dilution methods against *Trychophyton rubrum* [22]. Using the agar dilution method to test antifungal efficacy, the MIC of allicin after 5 days was 1.57 μg/ml [22]. In the broth dilution method, the MIC after 5 days was 6.25 μg/ml [22]. In another *in vitro* study researchers treated *T. rubrum* with allicin and garlic extract (allicin: 12.5; garlic extracts: 4.0), then used a scanning electron microscope and transmission electron microscopy to assess morphological changes between the two treatments [20]. In the allicin treated group, they found that the *T. rubrum* hypha were rough and granular on the surface and irregularly shaped [20]. It was also observed that the cytoplasm of the hypha had disintegrated, and the cell wall and membrane were broken down [20]. Much like the treatment with allicin, the hypha treated with the garlic extract was irregularly shaped, exhibiting a rough and fluffy surface [20]. The cytoplasm was also found to be degraded and the cell wall and membrane were similarly broken down [20]. Overall it was found that pure allicin was more effective in inhibiting the growth of hyphal cells compared to the garlic extract [20]. This demonstrates that garlic extract or allicin could be alternative methods of treatment that are cheaper and less likely to cause resistance for diseases caused by *T. rubrum.*

T. rubrum is one of the most common causes of fungal infections worldwide [28]. It colonizes the upper layers of dead skin, known as epidermis, in humans [28]. However, deeper infections are possible. Approximately 80-93% of chronic fungal infections in the developed world are caused by *T. rubrum* [28]. Diseases caused by infections of *T. rubrum* include athlete's foot, infection of the nail, jock itch and ringworm [28]. Infections of *T. rubrum* can manifest as both chronic and acute forms [28]. There are various treatment options depending on the number of affected nails and severity of the infection, but most treatments involve terbinafine for 2 or 3 months [29]. Athlete's foot can be treated with over the counter topical medications including clotrimazole, econazole or ketoconazole [30]. In severe cases a doctor may prescribe a more powerful oral antifungal medication such as terbinafine or itraconazole [30]. To treat ringworm on the scalp a patient will take oral medication for 1 to 3 months of either terbinafine, itraconazole or fluconazole [31]. Some patient groups, such pregnant women, children and elderly, require modified treatments due to the likelihood of adverse effects [29]. One issue with these treatments is that patients often do not complete the long course [29-31]. This means that the condition never clears up completely and has also led to the development of fungal resistance to many standard therapies [29-31].

Allicin/Garlic Extract and Cryptococcus Neoformans

An *in vitro* study investigated concentrated allicin extract that had 34% allicin, 44% total thiosulfinates and 20% vinyldithiins [16]. The extract had a potent fungistatic (inhibit fungal growth) and fungicidal (killing) activity against three different isolates of *C. neoformans* [16]. The minimum inhibitory concentration (MIC) of the extract against 1×10^5 organisms ranged from 6 to 12 μg/ml [16]. Further, when the extract was used synergistically with amphotericin

B (the normal treatment for *C. neoformans* infections) it demonstrated in-vitro fungistatic activity against all isolates of *C. neoformans* [16]. This lends support for the use of concentrated garlic extracts to treat crypotococcal infections [16]. A second study with *C. neoformans* [22], tested allicin treatment with agar and broth dilution methods. Using the agar dilution method to test antifungal efficacy, the MIC of allicin after 5 days was 3.13 μg/ml for *Cryptococcus* [22]. In the broth dilution method, the MIC after 5 days was 3.13 μg/ml for *Cryptococcus* [22]. The MIC of allicin remained constant after more than 3 days of incubation [22].

C. neoformans is an obligate aerobe that can live in both plants and animals, although only producing animal-based disease [32]. Most infections with C. neoformans occur in the lungs [32]. However, fungal meningitis and encephalitis, especially as a secondary infection for AIDS patients, are often caused by *C. neoformans* [32]. Patients with cryptococcal meningitis tend to have recurrences of infection [33]. Researchers have found strong evidence that clinical recurrences of cryptococcal meningitis result from persistence of the original infecting strain [33]. An estimated 220,000 cases of cryptococcal meningitis occur among people with HIV/AIDS worldwide each year, resulting in nearly 181,000 deaths [34]. Cryptococcal meningitis is one of the leading causes of death in HIV/AIDS patients in sub-Saharan Africa, where it may kill more people each year than tuberculosis [34]. Reduced availability of fungicidal drugs continues to compromise outcomes in high-burden countries. Therefore, a cheaper treatment like allicin/garlic could be very useful, especially since it seems to be as effective as the normal treatments.

Allicin and Aspergillus Species

A single study tested the efficacy of pure allicin against 31 clinical isolates of *Aspergillus* [21]. The MIC and MFC for allicin were between 8 and 32 mg/L [21]. This shows that it may be an effective fungicide *in vitro* against *Aspergillus* [21]. Time kill studies showed that allicin exerts its fungicidal activity within 2 to 12 hours of administration *in vitro* [24]. The same researchers also assessed the *in vivo* efficacy of allicin in immunocompetent mice infected with *Aspergillus fumigatus* [21]. Allicin was administered through IV once daily for 5 days post-infection, or orally for 5 days pre-infection and 10 days post-infection [21]. Allicin treatment prolonged survival of infected mice from mean survival 7.7 days to 21.3 days (iv treatment) and 13.9 days (oral treatment) [21]. Allicin IV treatment led to a 10-fold hyphal reduction of the fungus. This shows that allicin could be used as a treatment for *Aspergillosis* [21].

Aspergillus consists of a few hundred fungi species found in various climates worldwide [35]. Some *Aspergillus* species cause serious disease in humans and animals/plants [35]. *A. funmigatus* and *A. flavus* (which produces alflatoxin - a toxin and a carcinogen) can contaminate foods such as nuts [35]. *Aspergillus* species also cause disease on many grain crops, especially maize [35]. Aspergillosis of the air passages is frequently reported in birds, and certain species have been known to infect insects [35]. *A. fumigatus* infections can cause primary pulmonary infections (such as paranasal sinus infections and allergic bronchopulmonary aspergillosis) and can potentially become necrotizing pneumonia or spread widely through the body [35]. Usually only patients that are immunocompromised or who suffer other lung conditions are susceptible [35]. Treatment strategies for this fungus are available for patients in the form of prescription antifungal medication, usually voriconazole. Other antifungal medications used to treat aspergillosis include lipid amphotericin formulations, posaconazole, isavuconazole, itraconazole, caspofungin, and micafungin. Whenever possible, immunosuppressive medications should be discontinued or decreased. People who have severe cases of aspergillosis may need surgery [36]. Aspergillus can be spread to humans through infections of plants [37]. Some chemical fungicides like Metalaxyl, reduces the growth of this fungus on plant materials [37].

Allicin or Garlic and Plant Fungal Pathogens

Allicin/garlic extracts have been shown to be effective against six plant pathogens using *in vitro* or *in planta* models [38-41]. The results of these studies are summarized in Tables 3 and 4 below.

Table 3. Allicin/garlic extracts *in vitro* studies against plant fungal pathogens

Fungi	Results	Reference
Fusarium oxysporum	Aqueous extracts of garlic inhibited germination of microconidia (spores) and hyphal extension. The inhibitory effects were reversible unless high concentrations of garlic (500 mg/ml) were used and then it was fungicidal. Extract has MIC of 160 μl/ml compared to fluconazole which had a MIC of 100 μl/ml.	[38, 39]
Alternaria brassisicola, Botrytis cinerea, Plectosphaerella cucumerina and *Magnaporthe grisea*	Using 280 μg of allicin zones of inhibition were reported for all fungi tested. It was also shown that spore germination by *Alternaria* was also inhibited.	[40]

Abbreviations used in the table: MIC (minimum inhibitory concentration).

Table 4. Allicin/garlic extracts *in planta* studies against plant fungal pathogens

Fungi	Results	Reference
Magnaporthe grisea	Disease reduction *in planta* was shown for *Magnaporthe grisea*-infected rice. Rice leaves were sprayed with approximately 0.7 mg/ml of allicin 24 hours before inoculation with spore of *Magnaporthe grisea*. There was a five-fold reduction in the severity of the disease.	[40]
Alternaria brassisicola	Carrot seeds infected with *Alternaria* were disinfected by treatment with garlic juice that was comparable to a commercial seed-disinfection product. Germination and seedling development of pathogen infested wheat seeds were enhanced by treatment with garlic juice as well.	[41]

Garlic extracts were shown to have a MIC of 160 μl/ml on *Fusarium oxysporum* compared to fluconazole (an antifungal treatment) which had a MIC of 100 μl/ml [38,39]. 280 μg of allicin was shown to inhibit *in vitro* growth of *Alternaria brassisicola, Botrytis cinerea, Plectosphaerella cucumerina* and *Magnaporthe grisea* [40]. Using 0.7 mg/ml of allicin spray pretreatment on rice there was a reduction in the severity of the disease caused by *Magnaporthe grisea* [40]. *Alternaria brassisicola* infected carrot seeds were disinfected by treatment with garlic juice which was comparable to the commercial seed-disinfection [41]. This data shows that allicin/garlic could be used for pretreatment of plants to prevent them from being infected with fungal infection. However, only one study has been performed using each of the fungal infections so more studies would need to be done to confirm these findings.

Allicin and Plant Infections

Researchers tested *in vitro* the effect of aqueous extracts of garlic on *Fusarium oxysporum* (*F. oxysporum*) [38]. V.N. Tariq and colleagues [38] reported that extracts (500 mg/ml) inhibited germination of microconidia (spores) and hyphal extension of the *Fusarium.* [38]. The inhibitory effects were reversible unless high concentrations of garlic (500 mg/ml) were used and then it was fungicidal [38]. Other researchers found that allicin had MIC of 160 μl/ml against *F. oxysporum* compared to fluconazole (which is the normal treatment for this infection) which had a MIC of 100 μl/ml [39]. *Fusarium* are fungi found in soil and associated with plants [42]. Some species produce mycotoxins in crops that can affect human and animal health [42]. For example, *F. graminearum* infects barley which can have a large economic impact on the malting and brewing industries [42]. As described earlier, *F. oxytocum* can cause Panama disease of bananas (also called wilt) and is one of the most destructive plant diseases of modern times [43].

The effectiveness of garlic extract against multiple plant pathogenic organisms was tested in a single study *in vitro* and *in planta* [40]. Anti-fungal activity was shown *in vitro* against *Alternaria brassisicola, Botrytis cinerea, Plectosphaerella cucumerina and Magnaporthe grisea* [40]. Using 280 μg of allicin zones of inhibition were shown for all the fungi studied [40]. Hannah Curtis and colleagues [40] also reported that spore germination by *Alternaria* was inhibited [40]. Disease reduction *in planta* was shown for *Magnaporthe grisea*-infected rice [40]. Rice leaves were sprayed with approximately 0.7 mg/ml of allicin 24 hours before inoculation with spore of *Magnaporthe grisea.* [40]. There was a five-fold reduction in the severity of the disease and loss of plants [40].

Other studies showed that allicin can also help with seed-disinfection [41]. Carrot seeds infected with *Alternaria* were disinfected by treatment with garlic juice that was comparable to a commercial seed-disinfection product [41]. Germination and seedling development of pathogen infested wheat seeds were enhanced by treatment with garlic juice as well [41].

Conclusion and Further Directions

Allicin has potential use against at least 5 fungal infections of both humans and plants. For *Candida albicans* allicin has been shown to be able to inhibit alone or synergistically with flucytosine or AmB [18, 19]. This natural thiosulfinate can either act alone or synergistically with AmB to inhibit Crytococcus neoformans [16]. Allicin alone has been found to be able to inhibit *Trichophyton rubrum* and *Aspergillus fumigatus* as well as plant fungi *Fusarium oxysporum, Magnaporthe grisea and Alternaria brassisicola* [20, 38-41]. Although the number of studies on allicin/ garlic are relatively few, these fungi do need new interventions as resistant strains have evolved to nearly all the current strategies (Table 5).

Table 5. Current treatments/interventions for fungal infections

Fungus	Treatment	Reference
Candida albicans	Fluconazole/Flucytosine in combination with amphotericin B (AmB)	[44, 45]
Trichophyton rubrum	Oral terbinafine	[46]
Cryptococcus neoformans	Amphotericin B	[16]
Fungus	Treatment	Reference
Aspergillus fumigatus	Azoles	[36]
Fusarium oxysporum	Breeding for resistance	[14]
Magnaporthe grisea	None	[40]
Alternaria brassisicola	Fungicides with active ingredients Iprodione and Strobilurins	[47]

Although *C. albicans* is a normal component of the human microbiome individuals with compromised immune systems commonly develop candidemia or candidiasis [48]. Candidiasis is encouraged by the ability of the yeast to colonize sites like indwelling catheters and produce antifungal-resistant biofilms [48]. Allicin has been shown to prevent biofilm formation in bacteria [49] and potentiate the effects of antifungal agents [18], suggesting it may also destroy fungal biofilms.

Currently one in three of the 46,000 U.S. patients with invasive candidiasis currently dies from these biofilm-forming strains despite conventional medications [48]. A combination therapy with allicin might at least improve the efficacy of the existing medications at penetrating these biofilms as well as attack the biofilm itself.

T. rubrum is another common fungus and causes 80-93% of the fungal infections in the developed world such as athlete's foot and ringworm [28]. Much like *C. albicans* infections the available antifungal treatments for *T. rubrum* can cause side effects and are expensive [28]. Allicin and garlic extract have been found to degrade *T. rubrum* [20, 22] and could be used as an alternative, natural method for treatment. *C. neoformans*, which infects both plants and animals, can cause serious diseases in both immunocompetent and immunocompromised patients [16]. One study reported that allicin extract had a potent fungistatic/fungicidal activity at a low concentration against *C. neoformans,* which increased further when used in combination with AmB [16]. A fourth human fungal agent that allicin/garlic was able to inhibit was Aspergillus. Pure allicin inhibited over 31 isolates of Aspergillus within 2-12 hours of administration [21]. The same study also reported that allicin had in-vivo effects as well against *A. fumigatus* [21]. Aspergillus can grow on and in many places producing diseases of humans, plants, and is known to play a major role in sick building syndrome [21].

Allicin also was found to have antifungal activity against several plant pathogenic fungi [38-41]. Each year *Magnaporthe grisea* is estimated to destroy enough rice to feed more than 60 million people and is known to occur in 85 countries worldwide [50] and allicin was found to inhibit this fungal infection on rice [40]. *Fusarium* produces mycotoxins which can infect plants like barley which then can make humans sick [42]. This has had a serious economic impact on the malting and brewing industries [42]. *Fusarium* can also cause Panama disease (wilt) in bananas which is a hugely destructive disease of our time [43]. Allicin was found to inhibit *Fusarium* in an *in vitro* infection [38, 39]. *Alternaria brassicicola* causes black spot disease on plants such as broccoli, cabbage, canola and mustard. In addition, infection with Alternaria results in 20-25% yield reductions in crop [51]. Carrot and wheat seeds were disinfected from Alternaria by treatment with garlic juice [41]. These results suggest the possibility of developing treatment procedures with garlic extracts in horticultural or agricultural situation where other treatments are prohibited (such as in organic farming) [40]. However, the potential drawbacks, such as tainting the material with unwanted odor or taste, have yet to be investigated [40]. Allicin could have potential for seed-disinfection programs both in ecological agriculture of in developing countries who need a more low-tech technique. Since garlic/allicin is easy to obtain, a plant protection plan can be put in place where developing countries are shown how to make their own pesticides. Garlic treatment could help us with the large amounts of crops that are lost to disease worldwide and help to resolve hunger issues.

Allicin's antibacterial activity has been thoroughly researched in multiple studies. The study of allicin's antifungal activity has not been quite as elucidated but the need for this research has been discovered. The positive effects of using allicin/garlic for treatment against fungal infections both in humans as well as plants are immense. Garlic is already in use in Ayurvedic and Traditional Chinese Medicine systems and well accepted in many developing countries [52]. Adding allicin to alone or synergistically with existing medications could dampen or eliminate side effects as well as making the treatment regimen less expensive.

Allicin could also be used to treat a variety of common plant fungal infections and would have the added advantage of providing a broad-spectrum fungicide against at least 5 common fungi [37-41]. Organic farmers already use garlic spray to keep insects off plants [53] and this would add a second layer to the treatment. Developing nation farmers have no access to commercial anti-fungal treatments [53] for crops so some type of garlic product could be a cheaper treatment to help them keep their much-needed crops. This could have potential for seed-disinfection programs and to help preserve crops in developing countries. Garlic is easy to obtain, growing in most climates around the world and could provide locally sourced, inexpensive material.

Interest in allicin and garlic has already been spurred by the reports in the literature discussed in this chapter. There have already been at least two patents involving the use of allicin or garlic extract to treat fungal infections [54, 55]. One patent involves a device that can be used for the topical administration of allicin to an infection site [54]. The premise is to use separate carriers of dry alliin and alliinase, which are activated by a wetting agent at their point of contact [54]. This process generates allicin *in situ* and avoids issues with stability [54]. A second patent has been established using allicin as a combination insect repellent and insecticide for commercial crops [55]. This invention described both the use of allicin to prevent crop attack as well as spraying harvested fruits and vegetables after harvesting [55]. This latter component to the patent would be expected to prevent fungal growth in addition to its insecticidal value based on the studies discussed in this chapter.

There are products that are also readily available which use stable allicin/garlic extracts as treatments or supplements [49, 56, 57]. Allimax is an encapsulated form of allicin that has been already studied for efficacy against tumor cells and can be safely ingested [56]. Recent studies have also created nanoparticulate formulations which could be incorporated easily into topical creams [57]. Since most strains of *C. albicans* and *T. rubrum* require topical treatments [27, 28], this strategy could also prove effective. Synthetic or semi-synthetic forms of allicin might also produce a stable and consistent approach to studying its anti-fungal activity. Two recently published studies are already examining allicin's potential in this respect [58, 59]. Leontiev and colleagues [58] synthesized a series of four analogs of allicin (diethyl-, dimethyl-, dipropany- and dibenzyl-thiosulfinates) and compared them with the parent molecule for *in vitro* antibacterial and antifungal activity. Apart from allicin, dimethyl-thiosulfinates (DMTS) was the most effective against gram negative bacteria and all analogs were effective against bakers yeast (*Saccharomyces cerevisiae).* Allicin was most toxic to the plant pathogenic fungus *Alternaria* but impaired the growth of seedlings [58]. DMTS was the least toxic to the plants and most toxic to the pathogen [58]. A second group was also able to generate twenty four esterified aminobenzene sulfur acids and demonstrated a hierachy of *in vitro* anti-bacterial and anti-fungal activities [59]. Lubenets and colleagues [59] observed the most efficacy with cycloalky and arly esters of 4-acylaminobenzenethiofulfoacids at very low (nanomolar) concentrations.

All the research that has been shown is very promising however, more trials are needed. Although there are *in vivo* trials there are no human clinical trials yet and the cost of developing new medicines remains are high [60]. Using allicin/garlic to treat plant fungal diseases may be feasible but, to date, only a few studies have been published and it is unclear as to whether experimenter bias was involved. For both human and plant treatment multiple, large scale trials that are both double blind and placebo controlled would prevent such investigator bias and give more credibility towards using garlic/allicin as an antifungal treatment.

Phytomedicines are regularly used in treating fungal infections in many developing nations with around eighty percent of the world's population fulfilling its general medicinal needs from locally sourced plants [61]. In a recent review of potential antifungal phytomedicines, Murtaza and colleagues described nearly thirty species of plants with reported *in vitro* or *in vivo* animal model efficacy [61]. Many of these plants have efficacy against *C. albicans, Aspergillus* and *Fusarium* species [61], which are common causes of human illness. But what of developed nations: would consumers there be receptive? Interestingly, current surveys suggest that in the U.S. only around fifteen percent of patients rely entirely on prescription advice from medical practitioners [62]. Many individuals are increasingly drawn to herbal medicines, including garlic, saw palmetto and ginkgo for relief of inflammation, or to improve general well-being [63]. At least 40% of the U.S. population now reporting they use one or more herbal agents as they consider these safe nutraceuticals with few to no side effects [63]. This latter statement shows that the world is ready for herbal antifungal agents and supports the idea that further research into using garlic/allicin should be performed.

REFERENCES

[1] Hayat, Sikandar, Zhihui Cheng, Husain Ahmad, Muhammad Ali, Xuejin Chen, and Mengyi Wang. 2016. "Garlic, from Remedy to Stimulant: Evaluation of Antifungal Potential Reveals Diversity in Phytoalexin Allicin Content among Garlic Cultivars; Allicin Containing Aqueous Garlic Extracts Trigger Antioxidants in Cucumber." *Frontiers in Plant Science* 7: 1235. doi: 10.3389/fpls.2016.01235.

[2] Reiter, Jana, Natalja Levina, Mark Van Der Linden, Martin Gruhlke, Christian Martin, and Alan Slusarenko. 2017. "Diallylthiosulfinate (Allicin), a Volatile Antimicrobial from Garlic (Allium Sativum), Kills Human Lung Pathogenic Bacteria, Including MDR Strains, as a Vapor." *Molecules* 22(10): 1711.

[3] Rabinkov, Aharon, Talia Miron, Leonid Konstantinovski, Meir Wilchek, David Mirelman, and Lev Weiner. 1998. "The Mode of Action of Allicin: Trapping of Radicals

and Interaction with Thiol Containing Proteins." *Biochimica Et Biophysica Acta (BBA) - General Subjects* 1379(2): 233-44.

[4] Timonin, M. I., and R. H. Thexton. 1951. "The Rhizosphere Effect of Onion and Garlic on Soil Microflora1." *Soil Science Society of America Journal 15(C)*: 186.

[5] Appleton, Judith A., and Michael R. Tansey. 1975. "Inhibition of Growth of Zoopathogenic Fungi by Garlic Extract." *Mycologia* 67(4): 882-885.

[6] Nielsen, Kirsten, and Joseph Heitman. 2007. "Sex and Virulence of Human Pathogenic Fungi." *Fungal Genomics Advances in Genetics* 57: 143-73.

[7] Brakhage, Axel. 2005. "Systemic Fungal Infections Caused by Aspergillus Species: Epidemiology, Infection Process and Virulence Determinants." *Current Drug Targets* 6(8): 875-86.

[8] Talbot, Nicholas J. 2003. "On the Trail of a Cereal Killer: Exploring the Biology of Magnaporthe Grisea." *Annual Review of Microbiology* 57(1) :177-202.

[9] Paoletti, Mathieu, Kenneth W. Buck, and Clive M. Brasier. 2005. "Selective Acquisition of Novel Mating Type and Vegetative Incompatibility Genes via Interspecies Gene Transfer in the Globally Invading Eukaryote Ophiostoma Novo-ulmi." *Molecular Ecology* 15(1): 249-62.

[10] Ghannoum, Mahmoud A., and Louis B. Rice. 1999. "Antifungal Agents: Mode of Action, Mechanisms of Resistance, and Correlation of These Mechanisms with Bacterial Resistance." *Clinical Microbiology Reviews* 12(4): 501-17.

[11] Spellberg, Brad. 2011. "Vaccines for Invasive Fungal Infections." F1000 *Medicine Reports* 3:13 doi: 10.3410/M3-13.

[12] "*Antifungal Resistance | Fungal Diseases | CDC*." Centers for Disease Control and Prevention. https://www.cdc.gov/fungal/antifungal-resistance.html. Accessed July 10, 2019.

[13] "Fusarium Wilt: Symptoms, Treatment and Control." *Planet Natural.* https://www.planetnatural.com/pest-problem-solver/plant-disease/fusarium-wilt/. Accessed July 10, 2019.

[14] Esther. "Treating Plant Diseases Naturally." *Off The Grid News.* May 16, 2013. Accessed April 25, 2019. https://www.offthegridnews.com/food/treating-plant-diseases-naturally/.

[15] Roemer, T., and D. J. Krysan. 2014. "Antifungal Drug Development: Challenges, Unmet Clinical Needs, and New Approaches." *Cold Spring Harbor Perspectives in Medicine* 4(5): a019703. doi: 10.1101/cshperspect.a019703.

[16] Ankri, Serge, and David Mirelman. 1999. "Antimicrobial Properties of Allicin from Garlic." *Microbes and Infection* 1(2): 125-29.

[17] Ogita, Akira, Ken-Ichi Fujita, and Toshio Tanaka. 2012. "Enhancing Effects on Vacuole-Targeting Fungicidal Activity of Amphotericin B." *Frontiers in Microbiology* 3:100. doi: 10.3389/fmicb.2012.00100.

[18] Li, Guoliang, Xudong Ma, Lisha Deng, Xixi Zhao, Yuejiao Wei, Zhongyang Gao, Jing Jia, Jiru Xu, and Chaofeng Sun. 2015. "Fresh Garlic Extract Enhances the Antimicrobial Activities of Antibiotics on Resistant Strains in Vitro." *Jundishapur Journal of Microbiology* 8(3):e14814. doi: 10.5812/jjm.14814.

[19] Kim, Young-Sun, Kyung Sook Kim, Ihn Han, Mi-Hyun Kim, Min Hyung Jung, and Hun-Kuk Park. 2012. "Quantitative and Qualitative Analysis of the Antifungal Activity of Allicin Alone and in Combination with Antifungal Drugs." *PLoS ONE* 7(6): e38242. doi: 10.1371/journal.pone.0038242.

[20] Aala, F., UK Yusuf, R. Nulit, and S. Rezaie. 2014. "Inhibitory Effect of Allicin and Garlic Extracts on Growth of Cultured Hyphae." *Iran J Basic Med Sci* 17(3): 150-54.

[21] Shadkchan, Y. 2004. "Efficacy of Allicin, the Reactive Molecule of Garlic, in Inhibiting Aspergillus Spp. in Vitro, and in a Murine Model of Disseminated Aspergillosis." *Journal of Antimicrobial Chemotherapy* 53(5): 832-36.

[22] Yamada, Y., and K. Azuma. 1977. "Evaluation of the In Vitro Antifungal Activity of Allicin." *Antimicrobial Agents and Chemotherapy* 11 (4): 743-49.

[23] Bokaeian, M., A. Nakhaee, Bita Moodi, A. Farhangi, and Azim Akbarzadeh. 2010. "Effects of Garlic Extract Treatment in Normal and Streptozotocin Diabetic Rats Infected with Candida Albicans." *Indian Journal of Clinical Biochemistry* 25(2): 182-87.

[24] Erdogan, Askin, and Satish S. C. Rao. 2015. "Small Intestinal Fungal Overgrowth." *Current Gastroenterology Reports* 17(4):16. doi: 10.1007/s11894-015-0436-2.

[25] Arendrup, Maiken C. 2010. "Epidemiology of Invasive Candidiasis." *Current Opinion in Critical Care* 16(5): 445-52.

[26] Seneviratne, Chaminda Jayampath. "Candida Biofilms." *Microbial Biofilms*, 103-28. 1st ed. CRC Press, 2017.

[27] Gow, Neil A. R., and Bhawna Yadav. 2017. "Microbe Profile: Candida Albicans: A Shape-changing, Opportunistic Pathogenic Fungus of Humans." *Microbiology* 163(8): 1145-147.

[28] Woodfolk, J. A. 2005. "Allergy and Dermatophytes." *Clinical Microbiology Reviews* 18(1): 30-43.

[29] Tosti, Antonella. 2017. "Diseases of Hair and Nails." *Goldmans Cecil Medicine*: 2551-556. doi:10.1016/b978-1-4377-1604-7.00450-4.

[30] Nordqvist, Christian. "Athlete's Foot: Symptoms, Causes, and Treatments." *Medical News Today*. February 27, 2017. https://www.medicalnewstoday.com/articles/261244.php. Accessed July 10, 2019.

[31] "Treatment & Outcomes of Dermatophytes | Ringworm | Types of Diseases | Fungal Diseases | CDC." Centers for Disease Control and Prevention. https://www.cdc.gov/fungal/diseases/ringworm/treatment.html. Accessed July 10, 2019.

[32] Tripathi, Kaushlendra, Visesato Mor, Narendra K. Bairwa, Maurizio Del Poeta, and Bidyut K. Mohanty. 2012. "Hydroxyurea Treatment Inhibits Proliferation of Cryptococcus Neoformans in Mice." *Frontiers in Microbiology* 3: Article 187. https://doi.org/10.3389/fmicb.2012.00187.

[33] Spitzer, E.d., S.g. Spitzer, L.f. Freundlich, and A. Casadevall. 1993. "Persistence of Initial Infection in Recurrent Cryptococcus Neoformans Meningitis." *The Lancet* 341(8845): 595-96.

[34] "C. Neoformans Infection Statistics | Fungal Diseases | CDC." *Centers for Disease Control and Prevention*. https://www.cdc.gov/fungal/diseases/cryptococcosis-neoformans/statistics.html. Accessed July 10, 2019.

[35] Garcia-Giraldo, Ana María, Barbara Lucia Mora, Jorge Mario Loaiza-Castaño, Jorge Andrés Cedano, and Fernando Rosso. 2019. "Invasive Fungal Infection by Aspergillus Flavus in Immunocompetent Hosts: A Case Series and Literature Review." *Medical Mycology Case Reports* 23: 12-15.

[36] "Treatment | Aspergillosis | Types of Fungal Diseases | Fungal Diseases | CDC." *Centers for Disease Control and Prevention*. https://www.cdc.gov/fungal/diseases/aspergillosis/treatment.html. Accessed July 10, 2019.

[37] Sharma, R. 2012. "Pathogenecity of Aspergillus Niger in Plants." *Cibtech Journal of Microbiology* 1(1): 47-51.

[38] Tariq, V.-N., and A.c. Magee. 1990. "Effect of Volatiles from Garlic Bulb Extract on Fusarium Oxysporum F. Sp. Lycopersici." *Mycological Research* 94(5): 617-20.

[39] Parvu, M., L. Barbu-Tudoran, O. Rosca-Casian, and L. Vlase. 2010. "Ultrastructural Changes in Fusarium Oxysporum F. Sp. Tulipae Hyphae Treated In Vitro with Allium Fistulosum Plant Extract." *Annals of the Romanian Society for Cell Biology* 15 (2): 65-72.

[40] Curtis, Hannah, Ulrike Noll, Judith Störmann, and Alan J. Slusarenko. 2004. "Broad-spectrum Activity of the Volatile Phytoanticipin Allicin in Extracts of Garlic (Allium Sativum L.) against Plant Pathogenic Bacteria, Fungi and Oomycetes." *Physiological and Molecular Plant Pathology* 65(2): 79-89.

[41] Borlinghaus, Jan, Frank Albrecht, Martin Gruhlke, Ifeanyi Nwachukwu, and Alan Slusarenko. 2014. "Allicin: Chemistry and Biological Properties." *Molecules* 19(8): 12591-2618.

[42] Mastanjević, Kristina, Vinko Krstanović, Krešimir Mastanjević, and Bojan Šarkanj. 2018. "Malting and Brewing Industries Encounter Fusarium Spp. Related Problems." *Fermentation* 4(1): 3.

[43] Nelson, P. E., M. C. Dignani, and E. J. Anaissie. 1994. "Taxonomy, Biology, and Clinical Aspects of Fusarium Species." *Clin Microbiol* 7(4): 479-504.

[44] Vermes, A. 2000. "Flucytosine: A Review of Its Pharmacology, Clinical Indications, Pharmacokinetics, Toxicity and Drug Interactions." *Journal of Antimicrobial Chemotherapy* 46(2): 171-79.

[45] Gallis, Harry A., Richard H. Drew, and William W. Pickard. 1990. "Amphotericin B: 30 Years of Clinical Experience." *Clinical Infectious Diseases* 12(2): 308-29.

[46] "Fungal Nail Infections | Fungal Diseases | CDC." *Centers for Disease Control and Prevention*. https://www.cdc.gov/fungal/nail-infections.html. Accessed on July 10, 2019.

[47] Nowicki, Marcin, Marzena Nowakowska, Anna Niezgoda, and Elżbieta Kozik. 2012. "Alternaria Black Spot of Crucifers: Symptoms, Importance of Disease, and Perspectives of Resistance Breeding." *Vegetable Crops Research Bulletin* 76(1): 5-19.

[48] "Statistics | Invasive Candidiasis | Candidiasis | Types of Diseases | Fungal Diseases | CDC." *Centers for Disease Control and Prevention*. https://www.cdc.gov/fungal/diseases/candidiasis/invasive/statistics.html. Accessed on July 10, 2019.

[49] Marchese, Anna, Ramona Barbieri, Ana Sanches-Silva, Maria Daglia, Seyed Fazel Nabavi, Nematollah Jonaidi Jafari, Morteza Izadi, Marjan Ajami, and Seyed Mohammad Nabavi. 2016. "Antifungal and Antibacterial Activities of Allicin: A Review." *Trends in Food Science & Technology* 52: 49-56.

[50] Choi, Jung-Sup, Daniel A. Sumner, Robert K. Webster, and Christopher A. Greer. "Economic Consequences of a New Exotic Pest: The Introduction of Rice Blast Disease in California." *Exotic Pests and Diseases*, Chapter 14: 215-24. doi:10.1002/9780470290125.

[51] *Home - Alternaria Brassicicola*. https://genome.jgi.doe.gov/Altbr1/Altbr1.home.html.

[52] "*Garlic: The Pungent Panacea*." 1998. Dr. Christopher Hobbs. https://www.christopherhobbs.com/library/articles-on-herbs-and-health/garlic-the-pungent-panacea/. Accessed on July 10, 2019.

[53] "Garlic Barrier: Natural Garlic Extract Used to Repel Insects." *Garlic Barrier: Natural Garlic Extract Used to Repel Insects*. https://www.garlicbarrier.com/. Accessed on July 10, 2019.

[54] US20110027341A1- Device for in situ production and topical administration of allicin. *Google Patents*. https://patents.google.com/patent/US20110027341 Accessed July 10, 2019.

[55] WO2003090537A2- Use of allicin as insect repellent and insecticide in agricultural crops. *Google Patents*. https://patents.google.com/patent/WO2003090537A2 Accessed July 10, 2019.

[56] Suddek, Ghada M. 2014. "Allicin enhances chemotherapeutic response and ameliorates tamoxifen-induced liver injury." *Pharmaceutical Biology* 52(8) : 1009-1014. Accessed November 22, 2018. https://www.tandfonline.com/doi/full/10.3109/13880209.2013.876053.

[57] Soumya, R. S., S. Sherin, K. G. Raghu, and Annie Abraham. 2018." Allicin functionalized locust bean gum nanoparticles for improved therapeutic efficacy: An *in silico*, *in vitro* and *in vivo* approach." *International Journal of Biological Macromolecules* 109(1):740-747. https://doi.org/10.1016/j.ijbiomac.2017.11.065.

[58] Leontiev, Roman, Nils Hohaus, Jacob Claus, Martin C.H. Gruhlke, and Alan J. Slusarenko. 2018."Comparison of the Antibacterial and Antifungal Activities of Thiosulfinate Analogues of Allicin." *Scientific Reports* 6763:8(1). Accessed on February 22, 2019 https://www.nature.com/articles/s41598-018-25154-9.

[59] Lubenets, Vira, Sofiya Vasylyuk, Nataliya Monka, Khrystina Bolibrukh, Olena Komarovska-Porokhnyavets, Diana Baranovych, Rostyslav Musyanovych, Ewa Zaczynska, Anna Czarny, Urszula Nawrot, and Volodymyr Novikov. 2016. "Synthesis and antimicrobial properties of 4-acylaminobenzenethiosulfoacid S-esters." *Saudi Pharmaceutical Journal: SPJ: The Official publication of the Saudi Pharmaceutical Society*25(2), 266-274. doi: 10.1016/j.jsps.2016.06.007.

[60] "A Tough Road. Cost To Develop One New Drug Is $2.6 Billion; Approval Rate for Drugs Entering Clinical Development Is Less Than 12%." *Policy & Medicine*. https://www.policymed.com/2014/12/a-tough-road-cost-to-develop-one-new-drug-is-26-billion approval-rate-for-drugs-entering-clinical-de.html. Accessed July 10, 2019.

[61] Murtaza, Ghulam, Muhammed Mukhtar, and Aysha Sarfraz. 2015. "A review : antifungal potentials of medicinal plants. *Journal of Bioresource Management* 2(2) : 23-31. https://pdfs.semanticscholar.org/6c57/b4c4513ae952b1c24f9c4b7e6f266e125ab6.pdf Accessed July 10, 2019.

[62] Eisenberg, David M., Roger B. Davis, Susan L. Ettner, Scott Eppel, Snja Wilkey, Maria Van Rompey, and Ronald C. Kessler. 1998. "Trends in alternative medicine use in the United States, 1990-1997: results of a followup survey." *JAMA* 280(18):1569-75.

[63] Quato, Dima M., G. Caleb Alexander, Rena M. Conti, Michael Johnson, Phil Schumm, and Stacy T. Lindau. 2008. "Use of prescription and over-the-counter medications and dietary supplements among older adults in the United States." *JAMA* 300:2867-78. doi: 10.1001/jama.2008.892.

In: Allicin
Editor: Diana R. Cundell

ISBN: 978-1-53617-339-0

Chapter 7

ANTIPROTOZOAN AND ANTI-HELMINTHIC ACTIVITY OF ALLICIN

Beth M. French-Arthur*[*]*, PhD
Notre Dame of Maryland University, Baltimore, MD, US

ABSTRACT

Garlic has been used to treat infectious diseases including what would later be identified as worm infestations for thousands of years. Allicin, as the major antimicrobial principle of garlic, was discovered in 1944 and first determined to be antiprotozoal and antihelminthic fifty years later. Since this time 14 studies have been performed focusing on 6 common protozoal infections and helminths, including *Schistosoma mansoni* and *Trematodes*. Diagnosis and mortality rates associated with parasitic diseases remain high despite anti- parasitic treatments as the treatments are expensive or of poor duration and developing countries cannot afford to either give or maintain treatment. These infections are associated with significant morbidity and mortality and exert a tremendous economic burden in countries where they remain endemic. New strategies are urgently needed and for some researchers this has led the way to phytomedicines. Garlic/allicin has been shown to be effective in several animal models as a treatment to treat parasitic infections. Therefore, it may provide a more effective and economical treatment compared to the treatments given now. Potential mechanisms for using allicin together with already patented products will be discussed in this chapter.

Keywords: antiprotozoan, antihelminthic, allicin

INTRODUCTION

The first written records of parasitic infections were in Egypt between 3000 to 400 BC [1]. Due to the large size of helminths (such as roundworms and tapeworms) it is believed that our earliest ancestors were aware of these worms and sought methods of treatment [1]. Paulis

* Corresponding Author's Email: beth.m.french@gmail.com.

Aegineta (AD 625- 690) was the first to clearly describe these worms and gave good clinical descriptions of the infections they caused [1]. Between 1674 and 1716 Anton van Leeuwenhoek was the first person to see protozoa using microscopes [2]. He described free-living protozoa, parasitic species from animals and *Giardia lamblia* from his own stools [2].

Plant products have been sources for treatment of parasitic infections, as they are naturally sourced and therefore readily available to populations that need them [3]. For example, the first drugs to treat malaria came from the bark of the *Cinchona officinalis* tree [3]. *Cinchona* bark was found by chemists to contain the alkaloid quinine and served as a lead structure for the synthesis of several antimalarial drugs [3]. Interestingly, the *C. officinalis* tree is native to tropical and subtropical areas where malaria is endemic and was discovered because the plant was used by traditional healers [4].

Within many ancient cultures, it was well-known that crushed garlic had anti-parasitic effects [5]. Albert Schweizer, a famous physician, used crushed garlic to treat people suffering from dysentery or intestinal worms [5]. Traditional Chinese medicine for intestinal disease is an alcoholic extract of crushed garlic cloves [5]. Chapter 1 previously discussed that in Mesopotamia garlic was used to treat parasites that were common in that area [6, 7]. In early times medical practitioners in both India and Egypt also utilized garlic for similar purposes to remove parasite infections [8, 9, 10]. At the same time in ancient Greece garlic was used to treat parasites such as helminths [10, 11]. Even today developing nations still rely on plant-based healing such as India and Nigeria who use garlic to treat malaria. Anti-parasitic effects of allicin have been previously confirmed against multiple parasites including *Entamoeba, Cryptosporidium, Giardia, Plasmodium, Leishmania, Trypanosoma, Trichomonas, Schistosoma* [5, 12-24]. Interestingly, allicin or allicin-enriched garlic extracts have been shown to have *in vitro* efficacy against 4 such parasites [5, 12-16] and *in vivo* against 7 separate parasitic infections [12, 14-15, 17-20, 21, 22].

We now know that a parasite lives on or in a host organism and gets its food very often at the expense of its host. Protozoa are one-celled organisms that can be free-living or parasitic [23]. Parasitic protozoa are unicellular organisms specialized for transmission from one host to another either directly or via insect vectors [23]. Some parasitic protozoa are found in the intestines of humans. The spread of these protozoa to another human occurs through a fecal-oral route [23]. This occurs through contaminated food or water or person-to-person contact [23]. In 2010, there was an estimated 357 million causes of illness with one of three of these 3 enteric protozoa, *Entamoeba, Cryptosporidium and Giardia* [24]. These cases caused 33,900 deaths [24]. These infections can be asymptomatic or cause diarrhea, abdominal pain and/or weight loss [16]. There are also protozoa that live in the blood or tissue of humans that are transmitted to other humans by an arthropod vector (such as a mosquito or a sand fly) [23]. *Leishmania* can be transmitted by sand flies and *Plasmodium* (which causes malaria) is transmitted by mosquitos. These types of protozoa cause the most widespread protozoal disease; malaria.

Helminths are multicellular organisms that are also either free-living or parasitic. In adult form, helminths cannot multiply in humans [23]. The three main groups of helminths are flatworms (flukes and tapeworms), thorny-headed worms, and roundworms (nematodes) [23]. In this chapter we will mainly talk about flatworms (flukes/trematodes). Humans can get this disease from eating infected animals or when drinking, bathing or swimming in contaminated water [23]. Flatworms live in the intestines, blood or tissues and there are several species [23].

One important flatworm disease is Schistosomiasis, which infects people worldwide and is second only to malaria in its global impact [23].

Anyone can get a parasitic infection, however, there are some who are at greater risk [25]. Most patients have either a compromised immune system, live in a tropical/subtropical area, lack a clean supply of drinking water, swim in lakes, rivers or ponds where parasites such as Giardia are common, work in childcare, work with soil, or are in contact with feces [25]. In developed nations, parasitic infections can usually be effectively treated with pharmaceutical agents, but these are expensive and out of reach for many patients [26]. Ironically, parasitic infections are more common in developing countries where considerations of cost and access mean many individuals are chronically colonized [27]. For example, albendazole and mebendazole have been given to whole populations to control worms [27]. Researchers looked at data from four communities from the Ivory Coast between March 1997 and September 2010 [27]. They stimulated different treatment scenarios and found that community-wide treatment programs were worth the investment [27]. However, this is not only very costly, but both children and adults become re-infected within a few months [28]. In addition, repeated courses of these medications have already led to drug resistance [28]. These issues raise the idea that another less costly, possibly locally treatment option is necessary. For some researchers a return to plant-based medicines would seem optimal as they have proven effective in the past and, in turn, may represent a less expensive option for the future [29]. As discussed in chapter 1, garlic and other *Allium* species that contain allicin, can grow in a variety of climates and these plants may represent a good local source of potential anti-parasitic medications as a result [30].

This chapter will discuss the published anti-protozoal and anti-helminthic studies on allicin and garlic with a view to determining which show the most potential. The global importance of these parasites, current strategies used to treat them and the potential mechanism through which allicin impairs them will also be discussed. Possible delivery or combination therapies for allicin will also be suggested.

1. Allicin/Garlic and Protozoan Pathogens

Allicin/garlic extracts have been shown to be effective against five protozoa using *in vitro* or *in vivo* models [5, 12-20]. The results of these studies are summarized in Table 1 below.

1.1. Allicin/Garlic Extracts and Leishmaniasis

Most of the studies on allicin/garlic against protozoa have been performed on either *L. major* [12-14] or *L. tropica* [12]. Leishmaniasis is caused by an intracellular protozoan in the Leishmania genus. It is spread by the bite of sandflies. The diseases can either be cutaneous, mucocutaneous or visceral [29]. Cutaneous presents itself as skin ulcers [29]. Mucocutaneous presents itself as ulcers on the skin, mouth and nose [29]. The visceral form starts with skin ulcers and then with fever, low red blood cells and enlarged spleen and liver [29]. Interestingly the two forms of the disease involve different species of the *Leishmania* genus; *L. major* producing skin ulcers and nodules on the skin and *L. tropica* producing skin sores. Allicin/garlic extracts affect both species.

Table 1. Allicin/garlic extracts and antiprotozoal activity

In vitro studies	Results	Reference
Entamoeba histolytica	*Entamoeba histolytica* trophozoites can destroy monolayers of baby hamster kidney cells. This is inhibited by allicin. 30 µg/ml of allicin inhibited the growth of amoeba cultures. Even more recently it was found that that at 5 ug/ml, allicin inhibited virulence of trophozoites by 90%.	[5, 16]
Leishmania major	Aqueous garlic extract has been found to have a dose-dependent cytotoxic effect against *L. major* promastigotes. 48 hours after being treated with the garlic extract, the parasites showed cell shrinkage, immobilization, cytoplasmic condensation, and blebbing.	[12]
	The effect of aqueous garlic extract on IL-12 and IL-10 secretion levels in *L. major* infected macrophages were measured. Results showed that garlic extract treatment led to increased levels of IL-12 from infected macrophages, but the results did not show changes in the level of IL-10.	[13]
	PS externalization was measured after aqueous garlic extract was used to treat *Leishmania major*. The percentage of annexin-positive *L. major* promastigotes 36-48 hours after treatment was 65.55%and 86.11% compared to the 3.9% of the control group. DNA fragmentation was assessed in agarose gel and there was increased fragmentation with treatment of garlic extract.	[14]
Leishmania tropica	Aqueous allicin extracts on *L. tropica* showed IC50 values of 19.2 ± 2.51 µg/mL against promastigotes.	[12]
Plasmodium	At 10,25 and 50 µM allicin was not toxic to either sporozoites or mammalian cells. Allicin inhibited circumsporozoite protein processing and prevented sporozoite invasion of host cells *in vitro*.	[15]
Cryptosporidium	Cryptosporidial cysts were isolated from human stools and used to infect immunosuppressed mice. Experimental groups: received garlic two days orally before the infection, or one day following infection, and continued daily until the end of the study. Two weeks after garlic: Garlic eradicated the cysts from their stool and intestines.	[20]
Giardia	Human patients who had giardia were given garlic extracts of 1 mg/mL twice a day or .6 mg/mL of commercially prepared garlic capsules. Within 24 hours: symptoms had disappeared, and giardiasis infection was completely gone from the stool within 72 hours.	[18]

In vitro studies	Results	Reference
Leishmania major	BALB/C mice that had been infected with L major. These mice secreted Th2-related cytokines, IL-4, IL-5 and IL-10 during leishmaniasis infection and the immune response was weak. Garlic extracts stimulated a Th1- type response and enhanced the engulfment activity of macrophages in L major infected mice.	[12]
	Topical gel was prepared with active compounds of garlic and given to mice with Leishmaniasis infections to their ulcers. After six weeks: ulcers healed perfectly. Glucantime: impedance on ulcer expansion but did not suppress lesion growth. Glucantime and garlic extract combined: more effectiveness against lesions compared to when they were used alone.	[14]
	Injected mice with *Leishmania major*. Ulcers formed 2-6 weeks after the injection, and bacteria were isolated from the skin ulcer tissues. Liquid allicin, ciprofloxacin, and many other antibiotics, were able to control the L. major infection. Pure allicin: 71.43% effective against all gram positive and negative bacteria found. Allicin and ciprofloxacin: most effective against *L. major* and 92.30% of isolated bacteria	[17]
Plasmodium	Mice injected with allicin had decreased *Plasmodium* infections. If sporozoites were treated with allicin before injection into mice, the malaria infection was completely prevented. If mice were given allicin (orally or IV, 4 days) parasitemia decreased and the survival of the mice increased by 10 days.	[15]
Plasmodium voelii	Mice were treated with allicin after infection with *P. voelii*. Allicin treatment reduced the numbers of parasites. The number of pro-inflammatory mediators were increased and the numbers of CD4+ T cells, dendritic cells and macrophages were also higher	[19]

Abbreviations used in the table: IC50: half maximal inhibitory concentration; IV intravenous*; L. major: Leishmania major; L. tropica: Leishmania tropica; P. voelii: Plasmodium voelii.*

Studies have been performed to review the effectiveness and mechanisms of different garlic extracts and organosulfur compounds from garlic against *Leishmania*. Natural compounds of garlic such as allicin and ajoene result in growth inhibition of several species of *Leishmania in vitro* [12]. Aqueous garlic extract has been found to be effective against *L. mexicana* and has shown to have a dose-dependent cytotoxic (toxic to living cells) effect against *L. major* promastigotes [12]. In *Leishmania*, the life cycle stage in the vertebrate is the amastigote and, in the insect, the promastigote [12]. Forty-eight hours after being treated with the garlic extract, the parasites showed cell shrinkage, immobilization, cytoplasmic condensation, and blebbing [12]. Cytoplasmic condensation is the breakdown of intercellular interactions as the cell undergoes apoptosis (cell death). Blebbing is an emerging of a bulge on the plasma membrane of a cell. Aqueous allicin extracts on *L. tropica* showed IC50 (concentration of an inhibitor where the response of the parasite is reduced by half) values of 19.2 ± 2.51 μg/mL against promastigotes [12].

Programmed cell death (apoptosis) can be seen by several features: chromatin condensation, cell shrinkage, blebbing of plasma membrane, and phospholipid phosphatidylserine (PS) externalization [13]. In a recent study, PS externalization was measured (through annexin-V staining) after aqueous garlic extract was used to treat Leishmania major [13]. In normal viable cells, PS is located on the inside surface of the cell membrane. However, in the intermediate stages of apoptosis, PS is translocated from the inner to the outer of the membrane, exposing PS to the external cellular environment where it can be detected [13]. The percentage of annexin-positive *L. major* promastigotes 36-48 hours after treatment was 65.55% and 86.11% compared to the 3.9% of the control group [13]. DNA fragmentation was also measured in agarose gel and there was increased fragmentation with treatment of garlic extract [13].

In another study, the effect of aqueous garlic extracts on IL-12 and IL-10 secretion levels in *L. major* infected macrophages were measured [14]. IL-10 and IL-12 play very important immunoregulatory roles in host defense and immune homeostasis [14]. Being anti- and pro-inflammatory in nature, respectively, their functions are antagonistic to one another. Results showed that garlic extract treatment led to increased levels of IL-12 from infected macrophages, but the results did not show changes in the level of IL-10 [14]. This shows that the garlic extract shifted the macrophages to a more pro-inflammatory T-helper 1 (Th1) response rather than an anti-inflammatory Th2 response. Garlic/allicin's effects on cytokine production has also been shown *in-vivo* in BALB/C mice that had been infected with *L. major* [14]. These mice secreted Th2-related cytokines, IL-4, IL-5 and IL-10 during leishmaniasis infection and the immune response was weak. Garlic extracts stimulated a Th1- type response and enhanced the engulfment activity of macrophages in *L. major* infected mice. This helps cure the disease [14].

To study garlic/allicin's effect on infections in a living organism, a topical gel was prepared with active compounds of garlic (0.1 mg/mL) and was then given to mice with ulcerative leishmaniasis infections [12]. After six weeks, their ulcers healed perfectly. It was then given to human patients and 57 out of 70 patients responded to the treatment [12]. Glucantime, which is a normal treatment for *Leishmania* infections, was given to *L. major* infected mice and though there was an impedance on ulcer expansion, it did not suppress lesion growth [12]. When glucantime and garlic extract were combined into one treatment, there was more effectiveness against lesions compared to when they were used alone [12].

Leishmania infection causes skin ulcers. Those ulcers can become susceptible to bacterial infections which will cause a secondary infection which can cause a longer recovery time or higher morality [17]. Therefore, researchers have done an *in-vivo* study to look at the effect of garlic on leishmaniasis and secondary bacterial infections [17]. The researchers injected mice with *Leishmania major* by giving intramuscular injections [17]. Ulcers formed 2-6 weeks after the injection, and bacteria were isolated from the skin ulcer tissues [17]. Liquid allicin, ciprofloxacin, and many other antibiotics, were able to control the Leishmania major infection [17]. From the ulcers, 200 bacterial colonies were isolated [17]. Pure allicin exhibited antibacterial activity against a wide range of the bacteria and was 71.43% effective against all the gram positive and negative bacterial species isolated [17]. Out of 15 different antibiotics, allicin and ciprofloxacin were the most effective against *L. major* and 92.30% of isolated bacteria [17].

In a study by Jesus Corral-Caridad et al. [31] these authors hypothesized that the mechanism of action of allicin/garlic was associated with an interaction with thiol groups of some enzymes in the parasites [31]. Allicin's interference with thiol-redox proteins, like glutathione and trypanothione/trypanothione reductase was reportedly what led to damaging the *Leishmania* parasites [31]. *Leishmania* are endowed with powerful and host-independent mechanisms, which create new or regenerate reduced glutathione (GSH) as well as protect the parasites from oxidative damage [31]. Trypanothione reductase (TR) is an essential enzyme of the unique trypanothione-based thiol metabolism [31]. Antioxidant systems of glutathione and trypanothione reductase participate in the protection of *Leishmania* against the toxic effect of nitrogen-derived reactive species from macrophages [31]. Interference of allicin with these proteins could lead to amastigote destruction [31]. It is also believed that microtubule disruption is another target for allicin [12]. Shortening these microtubules converts parasites to a distinctive round shape [12]. Round parasites are incapable of invading new host cells and die [12]. A study by Prager-Khoutorsky et al. reported that the effects of allicin on cell polarization and migration are similar to the effects of micro-tubule-depolymerizing drugs such as nocodazole [32]. Treatment of fibroblasts with micromolar doses of allicin results in microtubular depolymerization in cells within minutes [32]. Some researchers have also suggested that allicin disrupts the activity of cysteine protease enzyme [12]. Cysteine proteases are essential in the degradation of host hemoglobin, the principal source of amino acids for many bloodborne parasites [12] and this may extend the efficacy of allicin to many protozoa.

1.2. Allicin/Garlic Extracts and Giardiasis

Inhibitory activity of garlic extract on *giardia* has been seen at 25 pg/mL and lethal dosage has been seen at 50 pg/mL [18]. A clinical trial was held where human patients who had *giardia* were given garlic extracts of 1 mg/mL twice a day or .6 mg/mL of commercially prepared garlic capsule [18]. Within 24 hours the patient's symptoms were gone and giardiasis was completely gone from the stool within 72 hours [18]. This research shows that garlic is efficient, safe and shortens the duration of the treatment [18].

Giardia infection is an intestinal infection marked by abdominal cramps, bloating, nausea and bouts of watery diarrhea [25]. When patients are infected with giardia but don't have symptoms they usually don't need treatment unless they are likely to spread the parasites [25]. When signs and symptoms are severe, or the infection persists doctors treat with metronidazole, tinidazole or nitazoxanide [25]. *Giardia* infection is caused by a microscopic parasite that is found worldwide, especially in areas with poor sanitation and unsafe water which makes this a larger problem in developing countries [25].

1.3. Allicin/Garlic Extracts and Malaria

The effects of allicin/ garlic extract on the malaria parasite were investigated in three studies, two *in vitro* [14, 19] and one *in vivo* [19]. Researchers believe that allicin is a cysteine protease inhibitor, which can inhibit circumsporozoite protein, (CSP) the major surface protein of *Plasmodium* sporozoites [14]. CSP is proteolytically processed by a parasite-derived cysteine protease and this is associated with sporozoite invasion of host cells [14]. Sporozoites are a motile spore like stage in the life cycle that is typically the infective agent introduced into a host. It has been shown that cysteine protease inhibitors affect sporozoite infectivity *in vitro* and *in vivo* [14]. At low concentrations allicin was not toxic to either sporozoites or mammalian cells [14]. However, at these concentrations, allicin inhibited CSP processing and prevented sporozoite invasion of host cells *in vitro* [14]. *In vivo*, mice that were injected with allicin had decreased *Plasmodium* infections [14]. If sporozoites were treated with allicin before injection into mice, the malaria infection was completely prevented. If mice were given allicin (orally or intravenously) on a 4-day regimen, the parasitemias decreased and the survival of the mice increased by 10 days [14].

During a malaria infection with *Plasmodium*, pro-inflammatory mediators including IFN-γ, TNF and nitric oxide (NO) are produced to protect against the parasites [19]. Researchers have tested *in vivo* to see if allicin can be used to treat a *Plasmodium voelii* infection [19]. Mice were treated with allicin after infection with *P. voelii*. The mortality was checked every day and the levels of parasites were checked every other day. Pro-inflammatory mediators were measured and the populations of dendritic cells, macrophages, CD4+ T and regulatory T cells were assessed [19]. CD4 T cells play a central role in immune protection by helping B cells to make antibodies, inducing macrophages, recruiting neutrophils, eosinophils and basophils to the sites of infection. They also produce cytokines and chemokines [33]. The levels of these mediators and cells help the body to fight off an infection. Allicin treatment reduced the numbers of parasites and prolonged survival of the host in a dose-dependent manner [19]. The number of pro-inflammatory mediators were increased and the numbers of CD4+ T cells, dendritic cells and macrophages were also higher. Because of this, it is predicted that allicin could partially protect a host against *P. voelii* infection [19].

Plasmodium develop in blood-feeding insect hosts (mosquitos) and then inject the parasites into a vertebrate host during a blood meal. Parasites grown in a vertebrate body tissue (most of the time in the liver) before going into the bloodstream to infect red blood cells [34]. The red blood cells are then destroyed and cause malaria [34]. These parasites can then be picked up again by blood feeding insects which continue to spread the parasite [34]. Plasmodium has been found in birds and mammals and has a large variety of hosts allowing for an easy spread of disease [34]. Quinine was used as the main antimalarial drug until widespread resistance emerged. A broad array of medications was developed; however, parasites have grown resistant to all those drugs within a few decades of the drug being developed. Therefore, new treatments need to be discovered [35].

1.4. Allicin/Garlic Extracts and Entamoeba Histolytica

Entamoeba histolytica trophozoites can destroy monolayers of baby hamster kidney cells [16]. This is inhibited by allicin (10 μM- 50 μm) [16]. At 10 μM there was 50% inhibition and at 50 μM there was 100% inhibition [16]. Trophozoites were exposed to different concentrations of allicin and then cysteine proteinase activity was determined. Short exposure to allicin (10 min at 100 μM) revealed an 80% decrease in cysteine proteinase activity [16]. Like malaria parasites, cysteine proteases are important to amebic virulence and this study extends the use of allicin to a second protozoan endemic to tropical and sub-tropical areas [16]. A second study found that *Entamoeba histolytica* is highly sensitive to allicin with 30 μg/ml of allicin inhibiting the growth of amoeba cultures [5]. At a lower dose of 5 μg/ml, allicin inhibited virulence of *E. histolytica* trophozoites by 90% [5]. Some allicin toxicity was seen on mammalian cells at concentrations above 100 μM, but the high concentrations had no damage to mammalian cells if the incubations were done in the presence of amoebic trophozoite [5]. This suggests that the affinity of the allicin is towards parasite targets [5].

E. histolytica predominantly infects humans and other primates [36]. The active (trophozoite) stage exists in the host and in loose feces. The cysts (eggs) survive outside the host in water, soils and foods and are passed to a new host following ingestion [36]. When cysts are swallowed, trophozoites are released in the digestive tract [36]. Most patients experience abdominal symptoms although for about 1 in 10 individuals the amoeba can bore into the intestinal wall causing lesions, and may reach the bloodstream, going to vital organs like the liver, lungs, brain and spleen [36]. Treatment is metronidazole, but resistance is due to altered gene expression in the parasite and now accounts for many treatment failures [37].

1.5. Allicin/Garlic Extracts and Cryptosporidiosis

The effect of allicin-containing garlic extract was only investigated using a single study [20]. Mada Reda Gaafar investigated swiss albino mice and split them into control and experimental groups [20]. Cryptosporidial cysts were isolated from human stools and used to infect the mice [20]. The experimental groups received garlic two days orally before the infection, or one day following infection, and continued daily until the end of the study [20]. Garlic was given as a crude juice of 500g of garlic bulbs were crushed and the resulting paste was diluted to obtain a 1g/ml aqueous solution [20]. The dose given was 50 mg/kg body weight. Two weeks after garlic was given, the stools of mice were examined for cryptosporidial cysts [20]. Their small intestines were then processed and examined for lesions and to count the parasites [20]. Gaafar reported that the infected immunosuppressed groups of mice had a significant increase in the number of cysts in their stool and intestines [20]. Garlic eradicated the cysts from their stool and intestines [20]. Ingestion or inhalation of *Cryptosporidium* cysts can cause a respiratory and gastrointestinal illness in both immunocompetent and immunodeficient patients [38]. Currently, nitazoxanide is the only drug approved for treatment in immunocompetent patients and there are increasing issues with insufficient and defective treatment [38]. Additional therapies are certainly needed especially given the global range of this parasite.

2. ALLICIN OR GARLIC AND HELMINTHIC PATHOGENS

Allicin/ garlic extracts have been shown to be effective against two helminths using *in vivo* models [21, 22]. The results of these studies are summarized in Table 2 below.

Table 2. Allicin/garlic extracts and antihelminthic activity

Helminth	Results	Reference
Trematodes	Daily oral administration of doses of garlic was conducted on three groups of mice: (i) before infection, (ii) after infection and (iii) both before and after infection. A fourth group of mice, not exposed to garlic, was used as control. No differences in worm recovery, fecundity and local cytokine expression profiles were found with respect to control infections. However, considerable alterations in tegument structure including swelling, furrowing and changes in secretory bodies were detected in garlic-exposed parasites.	[21]
Schistosoma mansoni	Mice were divided into 7 groups. Group 1: healthy controls. Group 2: garlic oil given orally three days a week for six weeks. Group 3: infected with S. mansoni and left untreated for six weeks. Group 4: treated with garlic oil extract from day one to day seven after being infected with S. mansoni. Group 5: treated with garlic oil extract from week two to week three after being infected. Group 6: treated with garlic oil extract from week five to week six after infection. Group 7: given garlic oil extract from the first day of infection for all six weeks of infection. Garlic oil extract showed changes in the parasite structure and decrease in the number of worms for all treatment times. It also increased the amount of pro-inflammatory cytokines.	[22]

2.1. Allicin/Garlic Extracts and Trematodes

The effect of allicin-containing garlic extract was only investigated using a single study [21]. Alba Cortes and colleagues [21], investigated 20 mice infected with trematodes. Daily oral administration of doses of garlic was conducted on three groups of mice: (i) before infection, (ii) after infection and (iii) both before and after infection [21]. A fourth group of mice, not exposed to garlic, was used as control [21]. No differences in worm recovery, fecundity (the ability to produce an abundance of new parasites) and local cytokine expression profiles were found with respect to control infections [21]. However, considerable alterations in tegument structure (outer body covering), including swelling, furrowing and changes in secretory bodies were detected in garlic-exposed parasites using scanning and transmission electron microscopy [21]. The results presented herein provide new insights in the anthelminthic activity of garlic compounds and the mode that parasites respond to toxins [21]. Trematodes (flatworms) are internal parasites of snails and vertebrates [39]. They asexually reproduce in a snail (intermediate host) and sexually reproduce in a vertebrate (primary host) [39]. Infections are most common in Asia, Africa, Latin America and the Middle East [39]. They are can be found anywhere untreated human waste is used as fertilizer [39]. Resistance to trematode's treatments is stimulating the need for developing new drugs against trematodes [39].

2.2. Allicin/Garlic Extracts and Schistosomes

The effect of allicin-containing garlic extract was only investigated using a single study [22]. Reem Kamel and colleagues [22], investigated the effect of garlic oil extract against *Schistosoma mansoni (S. mansoni)* in mice [22]. Mice were divided into 7 groups [39]. Group 1 was comprised of healthy controls [22]. Group 2 had garlic oil (100 mg/kg body weight) given orally (through an esophageal tube) three days a week for six weeks [22]. Group 3 was infected with *S. mansoni* and left untreated for six weeks [22]. Group 4 was treated with garlic oil extract from day one to day seven after being infected with *S. mansoni* [22]. Group 5 was treated with garlic oil extract from week two to week three after being infected [22]. Group 6 was treated with garlic oil extract from week five to week six after infection [22]. Group 7 was given garlic oil extract from the first day of infection for all six weeks of infection [22]. Garlic oil extract showed changes in the parasite structure and decrease in the number of worms for all treatment times [22]. It also increased the amount of pro-inflammatory cytokines. These results confirmed that garlic oil extract effect on *S. mansoni* as well as enhancing the immune system's response [22].

Schistosoma (blood flukes) are parasitic flatworms responsible for a highly significant group of infections in humans termed schistosomiasis. It is the second-most socioeconomically devastating parasitic disease (after malaria) [40]. Adult flatworms parasitize blood capillaries of the bladder and then thousands of eggs are released which reach either the bladder or the intestine [41]. These are then excreted in urine or feces to fresh water [41]. Larvae must then pass through an intermediate snail host, before the next larval stage of the parasite emerges that can infect a new mammalian host by directly penetrating the skin [41]. Those who have been infected for a long time may experience liver damage, kidney failure, infertility, or bladder cancer [41]. In children, it may cause poor growth and learning difficulty [41]. The disease is especially common among children in developing countries, as they are more likely to play in contaminated water [41]. Other high-risk groups include farmers, fishermen, and humans using unclean water during daily living [41]. In areas where the disease is common, the medication praziquantel may be given once a year [41]. There is little evidence of parasite resistance to praziquantel which is the normal treatment [40]. Side effects of praziquantel include headache, dizziness, nausea, joint/muscle pain, vomiting and loss of appetite [42]. An average treatment is between $.20-.30 but it is now available free of charge to high-disease burden countries through a donation from Merck Serono to the World Health Organization [43].

Conclusion and Further Directions

Researchers have found that allicin and ajoene from garlic can inhibit growth of several species of *Leishmania* [12-14, 17]. First, aqueous garlic extract can be used to cause apoptosis in *Leishmania major* [12-14]. In another study the effect of garlic was tested with a topical gel with garlic given to human patients with ulcers from *Leishmania* and a large percentage of the patients responded to the treatment [17]. Garlic extract has also been seen to inhibit or kill

Giardia [18]. Human patients were given garlic extract or garlic capsules and within 24 hours the symptoms from *Giardia* were gone and the *Giardia* was gone from the stool within 72 hours [18]. Allicin at low concentrations is not toxic to the *Plasmodium* however, it inhibited circumsporozoite protein (CSP), the surface protein of *Plasmodium,* which prevented sporozoite invasion of host cells *in vitro* [15]. *In vivo*, mice that were injected with allicin had decreased *Plasmodium* infections and if the sporozoites were treated with allicin before injection this prevented infection completely [15]. Immunosuppressed mice infected with *Cryptosporidium* were given garlic orally [20]. There was a significant increase in the number of cysts however, garlic eradicated the cysts from their stool and intestines [20]. Mice who were infected with *Schistosoma mansoni* were given garlic oil at different intervals. The garlic oil changed the parasite structure and decreased the number of worms [22].

These parasitic infections cause a tremendous burden of disease in both the tropics and subtropics climates [44]. The neglected tropical diseases (many of which are caused by parasites) suffer from a lack of attention by the public health community [44]. They affect over 1 billion people largely in rural and low- income countries [44]. These diseases cause a large toll on populations including losing the ability to attend school/work, retardation of growth in children, impairment of intellectual skills and serious economic burden [44]. Malaria (*Plasmodium*) in 2016 caused an estimated 216 million new cases with 445,000 death with 90% of those deaths in the African region [44]. Cutaneous leishmaniasis ranges from 700,000 to 1.2 million near cases per year [44]. Visceral leishmaniasis have approximately 100,000 new cases a year [44]. Giardiasis infects nearly 2% of adults and 6 to 8% of children in developed countries worldwide and nearly 33% of people in developing countries have giardiasis [44]. *Entamoeba histolytica* infects about 50 million people worldwide and kills around 55,000 people each year [44]. Cryptosporidiosis occurs worldwide and in the United States causes an estimated 748,000 new cases each year [44].

Most of these parasites are spread by fecal-oral route, contaminated food or water or insect vector [23]. Those with compromised immune systems or who live in tropical areas that lacks a clean supply of drinking water are more likely to develop a parasitic infection [25]. Individuals in a developing country are therefore more likely to contract a parasitic infection, and ironically least likely to afford or have access to it [42]. Unlike the plethora of antibacterial agents available antiprotozoal and antihelminthic drugs are very few [21]. One approach has been to repurpose existing antimicrobial and anti-cancer drugs, as these do not require additional clinical trials [47]. Unfortunately, conventional therapies of these kind remain cost prohibitive and access remains limited [47]. Additionally, currently available anti-parasitic medications have severe side effects including nausea, parageusia, rashes, secondary infections, peripheral neuropathy and leukopenia [48]. Several also require several treatments before effectiveness is seen [48]. These unwanted effects occur because since protozoa and helminths are eukaryotes the medications also kill/damage human cells [49].

Plants provide a wealth of metabolites which can be used as anti-parasitic [48] or anti-protozoal treatments [29]. It has been found that these plants interfere with important targets in parasites, such as DNA, membrane integrity, microtubules and others [29]. Between 1981 and 2006 1,184 drugs were registered and 28% were natural products and another 24% had functional groups derived from natural products [29]. Researchers are looking into antiparasitic natural products from traditional medicinal plants [29, 48]. One of those plants is garlic/allicin.

To develop allicin further first we require an understanding of the mechanisms behind its efficacy against parasites. Allicin is believed to interfere with thiol-redox proteins in

Leishmania parasites. These proteins participate in the protection of Leishmania against toxic effects of oxidative damage from macrophages [12]. Another target that researchers believe to target is microtubule disruption. Treatment with allicin results in microtubular depolymerization [32]. A third target for allicin is as a cysteine protease inhibitor which can inhibit circumsporozoite protein (CSP) which is a major surface protein of Plasmodium sporozoites that is associated with invasion of the parasites into host cells [16]. CSP forms a coat on the parasite surface and mediates the initial interactions between the sporozoite (parasite) and its two hosts [49]. Researchers have shown that processing of CSP by a parasite cysteine protease occurs during invasion of hepatocytes [49]. CSP-based vaccines have been a focus of the malaria vaccine effort [49]. Proteolytic processing of CSP is critical for sporozoite infectivity in the mammal host and suggests that treatments that specifically target this function, such as garlic, could be a foundation for a more effective treatment [49].

Treatment for *E. histolytica*, *Trichomonas vaginalis* and *Giardia lamblia* is metronidazole. Resistance is due to altered gene expression in the parasite and now accounts for many treatment failures [37]. Interestingly metronidazole resistance results from upregulation of iron sulfur flavoproteins. These organisms also depend on a thioredoxin system to prevent their being killed by oxidative stress [50]. Allicin could interact directly with thioredoxin and so impair growth of the protozoa this way [50].

A second issue to developing effective medical preparations has been allicin's stability [51]. Researchers have found that garlic is unstable in various aqueous and ethanolic solutions [51]. Crushed fresh garlic cloves generated antibacterial activity and detectable allicin but both declined in aqueous and ethanolic solutions at room temperature with half-lives of between 6 and 11 days [51]. At room temperature allicin in aqueous extract was most stable at pH 5-6 and degraded quickly at lower or higher pH [51, 52]. Allicin degraded quickly when the temperature was higher than 40 °C and especially higher than 70 °C [52]. However, people have been able to stabilize allicin for products to be used [53, 54]. Allitridin can be injected [53] and another stabilized version, Allimax, can be ingested [54].

Since it has become known that garlic can be used to treat parasitic infections, a few patents have been filed and products have been sold [55-57]. One patent that has been filed is for an oil that has macerated garlic [55]. This oil is applied to animals to be treated against internal and external parasites [55]. The oil will carry through the skin and internally treat the animal. This is suitable for worms in cows, sheep and horses [55]. One of the products that is on the market is ParaGuard, which has a blend of herbs including garlic bulb, which can enhance digestive flora and is a powerful cleanser for parasitic infections [56]. AniMed, a natural garlic powder horse supplement, is made of 100% concentrated garlic powder [57]. It helps maintain the intestinal tracts of horses and help with parasites and microbes, and even acts as an antihistamine [57].

Once the mechanism for allicin has been elucidated human double-blind randomized placebo-controlled trials (DBRPCT) can be performed. So far only two small animal trials have been done, one on *Giardia* and *Cryptospordium*, but both were positive [18, 20]. It is also important to note that allicin's effects on the protozoa appear to be selective and not harm host cells. The effect of allicin on helminths has only been studied in 2 studies. Both studies showed positive effects *in vivo* but more studies would need to be done to confirm allicin's effect. Many of the protozoa and helminths discussed in this chapter are an everyday occurrence for the residents of developing nations. Indigenous peoples are both familiar with traditional medicines and would be likely to be receptive to their usage. When this is coupled with a lack of financial resources to develop new medications, phytomedicines could clearly be an effective way forward. Garlic can grow in a variety of climates and could potentially generate inexpensive, locally sourced topical and systemic medicines for these currently hard to treat diseases.

REFERENCES

[1] Cox, F. E. G. 2002. "History of Human Parasitology." *Clinical Microbiology Reviews* 15(4): 595-612.

[2] Ford, Brian J. 2005. "The discovery of giardia." *Microscope* 53(4) : 147-153. http://www.brianjford.com/Giardia-14-06.pdf Accessed on July 12, 2019.

[3] Gachelin, G., P. Garner, E. Ferroni, U. Tröhler, and I. Chalmers. 2017. "Evaluating Cinchona bark and quinine for treating and preventing malaria." *Journal of the Royal Society of Medicine*, *110*(1), 31–40. https://doi.org/10.1177/0141076816681421.

[4] Achan, Jane, Ambrose O. Talisuna, Annette Erhart, Adoke Yeka, James K. Tibenderana, Frederick N. Baliraine, Philip J. Rosenthal, and Umberto Dalessandro. 2011. "Quinine, an Old Anti-malarial Drug in a Modern World: Role in the Treatment of Malaria." *Malaria Journal* 10(1):144. https://doi.org/10.1186/1475-2875-10-144.

[5] Ankri, Serge, and David Mirelman. 1999. "Antimicrobial Properties of Allicin from Garlic." *Microbes and Infection* 1 (2): 125-29.

[6] Dannesteter, J. 2003. "AVESTA: VENDIDAD: Fargard 20: The origins of medicine." Translated from *Sacred Books of the East, American Edition*. New York: The Christian Literature Company. www.avesta.org. Accessed on July 12, 2019.

[7] Heinerman, John. 1993. *"The healing benefits of garlic: from pharoahs to pharmacists."* New Caanan, CT: Keats Publishers.

[8] Bergner, Paul. 1996. "*The healing power of garlic*." Pp 3-26. Rocklin, CA: Prima Publishing.

[9] Lawson, Larry D. 1998. "Garlic: a review of its medicinal effects and indicated active compounds". In: *Phytomedicines of Europe. Chemistry and Biological ACS Symposium Series 691* (Lawson L. D. & Bauer R eds.), pp 176-209. American Chemical Society, Washington D.C.

[10] Moyers, Susan. 1996. *"Garlic in health, history and world cuisine."* pp 1-36. St. Petersberg, FL: Suncoast Press.

[11] Petrovska, Biljana B., and Svetlana Cekovska 2010. "Extracts from the history and medical properties of garlic." *Pharmacogn. Rev.*, 4(7): 106-110.

[12] Foroutan-Rad, M., K. H. Tappeh, and S. Khademvatan. 2017. "Antileishmanial and Immunomodulatory Activity of Allium Sativum (Garlic): A Review." *J Evid Based Completementary Altern Med* 22 (1): 141-55.

[13] Khademvatan, S., J. Sakil, M. Gharavi, and F. Rahim. 2011. "Allium Sativum Extract Induces Apoptosis in Leishmania Major (MRHO/IR/75/ER) Promastigotes." *Journal of Medicinal Plants Research* 5(16): 3725-732.

[14] Gharavi, M. J., M. Nobakht, S. Khademvatan, F. Fani, M. Bakhshayesh, and M. Roozbehani. 2011. "The Effect of Aqueous Garlic Extract on Interleukin-12 and 10 Levels in Leishmania Major (MRHO/IR/75/ER) Infected Macrophages." *Iran J Public Health* 40(4): 105-11.

[15] Coppi, A., M. Cabinian, D. Mirelman, and P. Sinnis. 2006. "Antimalarial Activity of Allicin, a Biologically Active Compound from Garlic Cloves." *Antimicrobial Agents and Chemotherapy* 50(5): 1731-737.

[16] Ankri, S., T. Miron, A. Rabinkov, M. Wilchek, and D. Mirelman. 1997. "Allicin from Garlic Strongly Inhibits Cysteine Proteinases and Cytopathic Effects of Entamoeba Histolytica." *Antimicrobial Agents and Chemotherapy* 41(10): 2286-288.

[17] Yehia, Hany, Ebtesam Al-Olayan, Manal El-Khadragy, and Dina Metwally. 2017. "*In Vitro* and *In Vivo* Control of Secondary Bacterial Infection Caused by Leishmania Major." *International Journal of Environmental Research and Public Health* 14(7): 777. https://doi.org/10.3390/ijerph14070777.

[18] Bayan, L., P. H. Koulivand, and A. Gorji. 2014. "Garlic: A Review of Potential Therapeutic Effects." *Avicenna J Phytomed* 4(1): 1-14.

[19] Feng, Yonghui, Xiaotong Zhu, Qinghui Wang, Yongjun Jiang, Hong Shang, Liwang Cui, and Yaming Cao. 2012. "Allicin Enhances Host Pro-inflammatory Immune Responses and Protects against Acute Murine Malaria Infection." *Malaria Journal* 11(1): 268. https://doi.org/10.1186/1475-2875-11-268.

[20] Gaafar, Maha R. 2012. "Efficacy of Allium Sativum (garlic) against Experimental Cryptosporidiosis." *Alexandria Journal of Medicine* 48(1): 59-66.

[21] Cortés, Alba, Miguel García-Ferrús, Javier Sotillo, J. Guillermo Esteban, Rafael Toledo, and Carla Muñoz-Antolí. 2017. "Effects of Dietary Intake of Garlic on Intestinal Trematodes." *Parasitology Research* 116(8): 2119-129.

[22] Kamel, Reem O. A., and Nashwa A. El-Shinnawy. 2015. "Immunomodulatory Effect of Garlic Oil Extract on Schistosoma Mansoni Infected Mice." *Asian Pacific Journal of Tropical Medicine* 8(12): 999-1005.

[23] Gonçalves, Marcelo Luiz Carvalho, Adauto Araújo, and Luiz Fernando Ferreira. 2003. "Human Intestinal Parasites in the Past: New Findings and a Review." *Memórias Do Instituto Oswaldo Cruz* 98 (1): 103-18.

[24] Burgess, Stacey L., Carol A. Gilchrist, Tucker C. Lynn, and William A. Petri. 2017. "Parasitic Protozoa and Interactions with the Host Intestinal Microbiota." *Infection and Immunity* 85:(8). doi: 10.1128/IAI.00101-17.

[25] Flanagan, P. A. 1992. "Giardia diagnosis, clinical course and epidemiology. A review." *Epidemiology and Infection* 109(1), 1–22.

[26] Monzote, Lianet., and Afshaq Siddiq. 2011. "Drug development to protozoan diseases." *The Open Medicinal Chemistry Journal* 5:1–3. doi:10.2174/1874104501105010001.

[27] News Center. "*Large-scale Treatment of Parasitic-worm Disease Cost-effective, Stanford-led Study Shows*." https://med.stanford.edu/news/all-news/2015/09/large-scale-treatment-of-parasitic-worm-disease-cost-effective.html. Accessed on July 12, 2019.

[28] Koning, Harry P. De. 2017. "Drug Resistance in Protozoan Parasites." *Emerging Topics in Life Sciences* 1(6): 627-32.

[29] Wink, Michael. 2012. "Medicinal Plants: A Source of Anti-Parasitic Secondary Metabolites." *Molecules* 17(11): 12771-2791. doi:10.3390/molecules171112771.

[30] Calvey, Elizabeth M., Kevin D. White, Jean E. Matusik, Deyou Sha, and Eric Block 1998. "Allium chemistry: identification of organosulfur compounds in ramp (Alliu tricoccum) homogenates". *Phytochemistry* 49(2): 359-364.

[31] Corral-Caridad, Ma. Jesús, Inmaculada Moreno, Alfredo Toraño, Mercedes Domínguez, and José Ma. Alunda. 2012. "Effect of Allicin on Promastigotes and Intracellular

Amastigotes of Leishmania Donovani and L. Infantum." *Experimental Parasitology* 132(4): 475-82.
[32] Prager-Khoutorsky, Masha, Igor Goncharov, Aharon Rabinkov, David Mirelman, Benjamin Geiger, and Alexander D. Bershadsky. 2007. "Allicin Inhibits Cell Polarization, Migration and Division via Its Direct Effect on Microtubules." *Cell Motility and the Cytoskeleton* 64(5): 321-37.
[33] Zhu, J., and W. E. Paul. 2008. "CD4 T Cells: Fates, Functions, and Faults." *Blood* 112(5): 1557-569.
[34] Siciliano, Giulia, and Pietro Alano. 2015. "Enlightening the malaria parasite life cycle: bioluminescent Plasmodium in fundamental and applied research." *Frontiers in Microbiology* 6: 391. doi:10.3389/fmicb.2015.00391.
[35] Blasco, Benjamin, Didier Leroy, and David A. Fidock. 2017. "Antimalarial Drug Resistance: Linking Plasmodium Falciparum Parasite Biology to the Clinic." *Nature Medicine* 23(8): 917-28.
[36] Shirley, Debbie-Ann T., Laura Farr, Koji Watanabe, and Shannon Moonah. 2018. "A Review of the Global Burden, New Diagnostics, and Current Therapeutics for Amebiasis." *Open Forum Infectious Diseases* 5(7): https://doi.org/10.1093/ofid/ofy161.
[37] Penuliar, Gil M., Kumiko Nakada-Tsukui, and Tomoyoshi Nozaki. 2015. "Phenotypic and Transcriptional Profiling in Entamoeba Histolytica Reveal Costs to Fitness and Adaptive Responses Associated with Metronidazole Resistance." *Frontiers in Microbiology* 6:354 doi: 10.3389/fmicb.2015.00354.
[38] Sponseller, J. K., J. K. Griffiths, and S. Tzipori. 2014. "The Evolution of Respiratory Cryptosporidiosis: Evidence for Transmission by Inhalation." *Clinical Microbiology Reviews* 27(3): 575-86.
[39] Doughty, Barbara. 1996. Chapter 88 Schistosomes and other trematodes. *Medical Microbiology*. 4th Edition. S.l.: University of Texas Medical Branch at Galveston.
[40] "CDC - Schistosomiasis - Treatment." *Centers for Disease Control and Prevention*. https://www.cdc.gov/parasites/schistosomiasis/treatment.html. Accessed July 12, 2019.
[41] Agbata, Eric, Rachael Morton, Zeno Bisoffi, Emmanuel Bottieau, Christina Greenaway, Beverley-A. Biggs, Nadia Montero, Anh Tran, Nick Rowbotham, Ingrid Arevalo-Rodriguez, Daniel Myran, Teymur Noori, Pablo Alonso-Coello, Kevin Pottie, and Ana Requena-Méndez. 2018. "Effectiveness of Screening and Treatment Approaches for Schistosomiasis and Strongyloidiasis in Newly-Arrived Migrants from Endemic Countries in the EU/EEA: A Systematic Review." *International Journal of Environmental Research and Public Health* 16(1): 11 https://doi.org/10.3390/ijerph16010011.
[42] "Praziquantel Oral: Uses, Side Effects, Interactions, Pictures, Warnings & Dosing." *WebMD*. https://www.webmd.com/drugs/2/drug-8873/praziquantel-oral/details. Accessed on July 12, 2019.
[43] "Strategy." *World Health Organization*. September 23, 2016. https://www.who.int/schistosomiasis/strategy/en/. Accessed on July 12, 2019.
[44] "CDC - Parasites." *Centers for Disease Control and Prevention*. https://www.cdc.gov/parasites/index.html. Accessed on July 12, 2019.
[45] Andrews, Katherine T., Gillian Fisher, and Tina S. Skinner-Adams. 2014. "Drug Repurposing and Human Parasitic Protozoan Diseases." *International Journal for Parasitology: Drugs and Drug Resistance* 4(2): 95-111.

[46] Thome, Joel, and Mary Wen. 2012. "Drug Therapy for Common Parasitic Infections within the United States." *US Pharmacist* 37(8): 2-6.

[47] Keown, Alex. "Tapeworm Drug Could Be an Effective Treatment for Certain Cancers." *BioSpace*. February 19, 2019. https://www.biospace.com/article/tapeworm-drug-could-be-an-effective-treatment-for-certain-cancers/. Accessed on July 12, 2019.

[48] Tandon, V., A. K. Yadav, B. Roy, and B. Das. 2011. "Phytochemicals as Cure of Worm Infections in Traditional Medicine Systems." *Emerging Trends in Zoology*: 351-78.

[49] Coppi, Alida, Ramya Natarajan, Gabriele Pradel, Brandy L. Bennett, Eric R. James, Mario A. Roggero, Giampietro Corradin, Cathrine Persson, Rita Tewari, and Photini Sinnis. 2011. "The Malaria Circumsporozoite Protein Has Two Functional Domains, Each with Distinct Roles as Sporozoites Journey from Mosquito to Mammalian Host." *The Journal of Experimental Medicine* 208(2): 341-56.

[50] Jeelani, Ghulam, and Tomoyoshi Nozaki. "Entamoeba Thiol-based Redox Metabolism: A Potential Target for Drug Development." 2016. *Molecular and Biochemical Parasitology* 206(1-2): 39-45.

[51] Fujisawa, Hiroyuki, Kaoru Suma, Kana Origuchi, Hitomi Kumagai, Taiichiro Seki, and Toyohiko Ariga. 2008. "Biological and Chemical Stability of Garlic-Derived Allicin." *Journal of Agricultural and Food Chemistry* 56(11): 4229-235.

[52] Wang, Haiping, Xixiang Li, Xinyan Liu, Di Shen, Yang Qiu, Xiaohui Zhang, and Jiangping Song. "Influence of PH, Concentration and Light on Stability of Allicin in Garlic (Allium Sativum) Aqueous Extract as Measured by UPLC." 2014. *Journal of the Science of Food and Agriculture* 95(9): 1838-844.

[53] Feng, Fang, Li Hong, Cui Wen, and Yongsui Dong. 1999. "Treatment of hepatitis caused by cytomegalovirus with allitridin injection – An experimental study." *Journal of Tongji Medical University* 19(4) : 271-274. https://doi.org/10.1007/BF02886960.

[54] Suddek, Ghada M. 2014. "Allicin enhances chemotherapeutic response and ameliorates tamoxifen-induced liver injury." *Pharmaceutical Biology* 52(8):1009-1014. https://www.tandfonline.com/doi/full/10.3109/13880209.2013.876053.

[55] WO1999066798A1 - Garlic Pour-on Cattle and Sheep Anthelmintic. *Google Patents*. https://patents.google.com/patent/WO1999066798A1/en?q=parasites&oq=garlic and parasites. Accessed July 12, 2019.

[56] "All Products." *Zahlers ParaGuard Liquid Comments*. https://zahlers.com/product/paraguard-liquid-4-fl-oz/15/. Accessed July 12, 2019.

[57] "Garlic Powder Pure for Horses" *Animed - Multi-Purpose | Supplements | Equine*. https://www.valleyvet.com/ct_detail.html?pgguid=148e1735-aa3e-461e-87db-73eb664cf6d5. Accessed July 12, 2019.

In: Allicin
Editor: Diana R. Cundell
ISBN: 978-1-53617-339-0

Chapter 8

VIRUCIDAL ACTIVITY OF ALLICIN

Diana R. Cundell*, PhD
College of Life Sciences, Jefferson University, Philadelphia, PA, US

ABSTRACT

The bioactive thiosulfinate allicin was isolated from garlic in the 1940s and its antiviral activity first described forty years later. Since then literature studies have reported at least ten viruses, seven affecting humans and three animal only, that can be inhibited by allicin, at least *in vitro*. More importantly six of these viruses have no effective vaccine or pharmaceutical intervention. Viruses provide a difficult target for elimination by either the immune system or targeted therapeutic agents given their need to multiply in a human host cell. Despite innovative antiviral development over the past 50 years, many still are poorly responsive to treatment or have no effective management strategies. An evaluation of the viruses allicin is able to eliminate will be combined with the known mechanisms this thiosulfinate uses, including those shared with extant antivirals. Given the benign and multi-faceted effects of allicin it may well provide a directed or complementary medicine in the treatment of some viral disease.s Issues with fully comprehending this potential, based on literature review of the available studies will also be discussed. Finally, future strategies for allicin, including effective delivery, will also be considered.

Keywords: HCMV, herpes, HPV, IBDV, NDV, REV, VSV

INTRODUCTION

Garlic and its related *Allium* species have been utilized for centuries to treat the symptoms of colds, and influenza by native peoples of Europe, Asia and the Americas [1-4]. We now know that the causes of these infections are viruses [5, 6]. Studies have shown that most episodes of the "common cold" result from one of four viruses; the human rhinovirus (HRV), coronavirus, parainfluenza and mild strains of influenza [5, 6]. With the discovery in 1944

* Corresponding Author's Email: Diana.Cundell@jefferson.edu.

that allicin was the major garlic component with antimicrobial activity [7] the scene was set to test its antiviral activity once the technology became available. In 1985, the first literature report appeared that suggested garlic and/or allicin could impair the growth of influenza, cocksackie and herpes viruses (HPV 1 and 2) *in vitro* [8]. A second study also confirmed the effects of allicin on the inflenza virus [9]. Extensive survey of the available scientific literature has also revealed a several studies exploring the effects of garlic extracts or allicin on the *in vitro* growth of other viruses including human cytomegalovirus (HCMV) [10, 11], herpes simplex (HSV-1 and HSV-2) [12], parainfluenza [12], rhinovirus [12], vaccinia [12] and vesicular stomatitis virus (VSV) [12, 13]. Foreign language literature has also reported that the thiosulfinate has efficacy against the human immunodeficiency virus (HIV) [14]. One animal model of HCMV demonstrated allicin had *in vivo* efficacy [10]. Infection with the "common cold" was also decreased in three pre-clinical studies of human volunteers taking allicin [15, 16]. A single human study reported a decrease in skin warts produced by the human papilloma virus [HPV] [17]. Finally, three individual and longer term investigations have reported positive effects of allicin aganst the poultry viruses causing infectious bursal disease (IBD) [18], Newcastle (NDV) [19] and reticuloendotheliosis virus (REV) [20].

So what does all this mean? For many researchers the combination of predominantly individual investigations and paucity of studies overall equates with a lack of antiviral efficacy for allicin. We may want to look further, however, before making that decision. There are several reasons why and they all relate to gaps in available treatment and prevention [21-31]. Viruses, have always proven notoriously difficult to culture reproducibly in the laboratory, given that they target only specific host cells [21]. This also impacts the ability to rapidly, inexpensively and easily diagnose viral illnesses as they are highly cell and host specific [22]. Additionally, there is a lack of available antiviral medications for many diseases [23]. Antiviral agents have to be considerably more targeted than other antimicrobials in order to prevent major adverse events and the range of available antivirals remains small compared with other antimicrobials as a result [23]. Reviewed in reference [23], the ninety antiviral pharmaceuticals that have been launched during the past half century focus on treating only nine human viral diseases. Medications are available for five DNA-containing viruses, namely HCMV, herpes, hepatitis B, HPV and varicella zoster (VCV) [23]. The remaining four viruses are the RNA-containing hepatitis C, HIV, influenza and respiratory syncytical virus (RSV) [23]. Several approaches have been taken but at least fifteen medications act as protease inhibitors that prevent the generation of viral capsid protein precursors [23]. Antiviral agents often have significant side effects [23]. For example the antiretroviral drugs that are an HIV mainstay medication are associated with body fat accumulation, hyperlipdemia and insulin resistance [24]. Like other antimicrobials resistance is emerging for many antivirals, necessitating new therapies [23]. Many ssRNA-containing pervasive or emerging viruses including Epstein-Barr virus (EBV) and Zika have no specific antiviral medication or vaccines and patients rely on palliative interventions [23, 25]. These medications are costly and therefore not widely available to patients who need them [23].

A third issue is that viruses that have been made vaccine-preventable are not typically selected as candidates for medication development, although there is some overlap [23, 26-28]. Vaccines are in current use against twelve viral diseases, three of which are DNA containing and nine RNA containing [23, 25-27]. Although their common use has lessened the incidence of infectious disease [23, 25-27] some may require modification as they are less than effective

[26-28]. For example, despite being multivalent, only about fifty percent of patients receiving the influenza vaccine are protected from getting the infection [28]. This means that influenza medications are still needed and continue to be developed [23].

Increasing numbers of people, who cite religious or other objections, also point to vaccine and pharmaceutical use as "unnatural" [29-31]. This growing problem has led to a decrease in vaccine frequencies in many developed countries resulting in outbreaks of measles in the United States [29] and influenza in Europe [28]. These and other individuals are now also increasingly looking to improve their immune defenses through optimizing nutrition and the use of plant-based medicines [32, 33]. At least one in three people in the United States use some type of plant supplement, with complementary medicine training increasing in Canada and Europe [32]. A large scale literature study suggests that, in developed countries, these individuals are typically more educated consumers who investigate the herbal products they are taking thoroughly [33]. At least five of the ten plants in common use and the individual phytochemicals they contain have proven efficacy at least *in vitro* and on animal models [32, 34]. Apart from garlic and soy, taken primarily for cholesterol issues, these include *Ginko biloba* (dementia and claudication), St. John's Wort (depression) and kava kava (anxiety) [34]. The diverse properties of allicin, as the major individual active moiety in garlic, are just beginning to be undertood, especially with respect to its antiviral effects [8-20]. At least ten viruses, seven affecting humans and three animal only, can be inhibited by allicin *in vitro* [8-20]. Six of these viruses have no effective vaccine or pharmaceutical intervention [8, 13, 18-20]. An in depth look at the studies on the antiviral activities of purified or stabilized allicin and its potential insertion into current treatments will be discussed in subsequent sections of this chapter.

1. ANTIVIRAL ACTIVITIES OF ALLICIN: *IN VITRO* STUDIES

Six literature studies have examined the effects of either allicin or a stabilized form (Alltridin or Alltridium) against seven viruses [8-13]. A brief description of the experimental detail and findings is provided in Table 1.

The main issue with any *in* vitro cell study is that, unless specifically stated, the investigators will have knowledge of what treatments are being used. Studies of this kind are always the first approach and should be able to demonstrate significant efficacy and reproducibility. A closer look at the studies listed indicates that data on five viruses (HSV, parainfluenza, rhinovirus, vaccinia and VSV) come from a single literature report [12]. Weber and colleagues [12] did use naturally sourced allicin but their dosage had a wide range (25-1000 µg/ml), with plaque assay effcacy only being seen at the upper doses of 500 or 1,000 µg/ml. It is also important to note that for three viruses (parainfluenza, rhinovirus and vaccinia) these reman the only literature reports on allicin's effects. This reduces the number of potential viruses to be examined further to four; HCMV, HSV, influenza and VSV.

Table 1. *In vitro* antiviral efficacy of allicin co- incubation

Virus	Cell line	Allicin and assay used	Results	Reference
HCMV	Human lung fibroblasts	*Allitridin (7.5 μg/ml) every three days, plaque assay	60% ↓growth after 14 days	[10]
		*Allitridin (25 μg/ml), MTT assay	↓viral gene expression beginning at 6 h and plateauing by 12 h. ↓ in HCMV growth ($p < 0.001$)	[11]
HPIV	HeLa	Allicin (25-500 μg/ml), plaque assay	1 log decrease in growth (500 μg/ml allicin) after 6 h	[12]
HRV	HeLa	Allicin (25-1,000 μg/ml), plaque assay	2 log ↓ in growth (1,000 μg/ml allicin) after 6 h	[12]
HSV	HeLa	Purified from *Allitridium (0.015-1.5 mg/ml), plaque assay	Significant ($p < 0.001$), dose-dependent (>2 logs) in HSV-1 growth at both 6 and 24	[8]
	Vero	Allicin (25-500 μg/ml), plaque assay	2 log ↓ in HSV-1 and HSV-2 growth (500 μg/ml allicin) after 6 h	[12]
Influenza	Chick embryos	Purified from *Allitridium (0.015-1.5 mg/ml), plaque assay	Significant ($p < 0.001$), dose-dependent ↓ (>2 logs) in influenza B growth at both 6 and 24 h	[8]
	MDCK	"Filtered fresh garlic extract" (10-100 μg/ml), MTT assay	Significant ↓ in influenza A load ($p < 0.001$) reflected as a two-fold increase in cell viability beginning as early as 1 h	[9]
Vaccinia	HeLa, Vero	Allicin (25-1,000 μg/ml), plaque assay	1 log ↓ in growth (1,000 μg/ml of allicin) after 6 h	[12]
VSV	HeLa, Vero	Allicin (25-500 μg/ml), plaque assay	1 log ↓ in growth using 1000 μg/ml, after 6 h	[12]
	Human cell lines; THP-1, MT-2 and WISH	Allicin (10-50 μg/ml), MTT assay	Significant ↓ in viral load ($p < 0.001$) and apoptosis of these cell lines after 72 h	[13]

Abbreviations used: h (hours), HCMV (human cytomegalovirus), HPIV (human parainfluenzavirus), HRV (human rhinovirus), HSV (herpes simplex virus), HPV (human papillomavirus), VSV (vesicular stomatitis virus).

*= stabilized proprietary forms of allicin/ajoene metabolite.

Further analysis, reveals that at least three variables are not consistent namely the allicin source, cell line and assessment of viral demise. Comparing the three studies in which allicin itself or extract containing allicin were employed [9, 12, 13], two achieved efficacy with lower doses of allicin (10-100 μg/ml) [9, 13], whereas the third required levels five to ten fold higher (500 or 1,000 μg/ml) [12]. Comparisons are only available for one virus, VSV, which was reduced by a ten fold lower allicin dosage (10-50 μg/ml) after 72 hours when normal human cell lines [13] versus tumor cells were employed [12]. Either the cell line used or more likely the instability of the allicin source in the Weber study [12] may be of issue here.

Stabilized allicin (Allitridium or Alltridin) was used in the remaining three studies of three viruses (HCMV, HSV and influenza) [8, 10, 11]. Alltridium is a Chinese formulation containing not allicin but is standardized to contain its major metabolite ajoene [35]. Ajoene has been suggested to be more potent as an antiviral [12]. For the *in vitro* studies it appears ten fold stronger than allicin against the herpesvirus HSV-1 [8, 12]. In contrast, against the influenza virus the two sulfur compounds appear equivalent [8, 9]. This is even more interesting given that two different types of influenza were used; influenza A and B [8, 9].-These are the most common causes of influenza and are current components of the quadrivalent and trivalent influenza vaccines [23]. Allitridin is a commercially available injectable form of allicin [11] and was effective in two separate studies, at relatively low doses (7.5 and 25 μg/ml) against HCMV [10, 11]. The first study delivered Allitridin (7.5 μg/ml) every three days for a total of fourteen days [10]. This, more long term study, showed a sixty percent drop in the viral load of the human fibroblasts at this time [10]. The herpesvirus group, which includes both HSV and HCMV as well as common illnesses such as Epstein-Barr virus (EBV), is considered highly conserved genetically [36, 37]. Variation in efficacy of allicin may be in the delieverable format i.e., stable versus unstable rather than the virus strain itself.

Another issue is the cell lines being used. Three studies employed normal, healthy cells, namely the chick embryo study of influenza B [8] and the human fibroblasts for HCMV [10, 11]. All three sudies demonstrated efficacy at low levels with the stabilized allicin metabolite ajoene. The remaining four studies used various combinations of tumor cell lines, including Vero (African Monkey Kidney) [12], human epithelial cervical carcinoma (HeLa) cells [8, 12], Madin-Darbey Canine Kidney (MDCK) cells [9] and three human tumors of monocytes (THP-1), T lymphocytic leukemia (MT-2) and amniotic cells (WISH) [13] Although it is important to be able to culture viruses the efficacy of allicin against them is blurred in these four latter studies as the thiosulfinate is also tumoricidal [14, 38] (see Chapter 13 for more details). It is particularly effective against leukemia [39], as well as kidney [40] and cervical [41] tumors. Is allicin therefore inactivating the tumor cell and thereby stopping the virus propogating? This question was also raised by the studies of Shou and colleagues [13], who observed that exposure to the thiosulfinate resulted in cytotoxicity of the three cell lines and had to reduce the dosages used for testing as a result. The observation that the lower dose of allicin they used still reduced cell apoptosis and significantly decreased viral load suggests direct antiviral effects [13]. It still means data must be interpreted with caution.

The plaque assay is usually definitive for viral-induced cell death and decrease in the number observed, expressed as logarithmic data, is the method used [42]. Since their original development plaque assays have been criticized as the data can vary by as much as ten per cent depending on the viral strain being used [42]. Three of the studies on allicin used only plaque assays [8, 10, 12]. Three of the viruses only demonstrated a one log or less decrease in growth with this technique (HCMV, parainfluenza and vaccinia), making these data questionable [8,

10, 12]. Tumor cell lines especially may grow unevenly and so the neutral red. 3-(4,5-dimethylthiazol-2-yl)-2,5-diphenyl tetrazolium bromide MTT assay [42, 43], which determines viability is now preferred [43]. MTT can detect the difference between live and dead plaques and is very sensitive for cellular apoptosis [43].

MTT assessment was performed in the remaining three studies [9, 11, 13] and was able to be used to identify mechanistic targets of allicin for HCMV [11], influenza [9] and VSV [13]. Two HCMV mutants namely a clinical strain (AD169) and a mutant that did not express an essential viral cycle protein (IE72) [11]. Growth rate of the AD169 strain over a twenty four hour period was significantly slowed by allitridin ($p < 0.001$) and less so in the mutant IE72 strain [11]. Further gene expression analysis demonstrated that allitridin targeted the synthesis of early antigen E proteins [11]. These include the DNA polymerase as ell as other proteins [11]. If allitridin does target these proteins it could be a valuable and unusual weapon against the virus, preventing it multiplying at a very early stage [11].

Influenza A growth over a twenty four hour period was significantly impaired ($p < 0.001$) on MDCK cells by "filtered fresh garlic extract"(FDE) [9]. Further analysis showed that influenza A failed to penetrate the MDCK cells when the FDE was used [9]. Hemagglutinin, which acts as an adhesin for the virus, possesses subunits linked by disulfide bonds [9]. Allicin typically targets thiol-based groups [38] and this was suggested by the authors to mediate the anti-influenza mechanism of action of the thiosulfinate [9]. Finally, VSV exerts its effects through inducing cellular apoptosis, producing lesions and scarring [44, 45]. Studies of allicin's effects on VSV colonization of three human cell lines found the thiosulfinate failed to prevent viral adherence or entry but reduced the expression of nuclear factor kappa beta (NF-κB) and caspases three, six, seven and nine [13].

Several studies examined in this chapter do seem to have merit, with HCMV, influenza and VSV providing promising data. More observer investigations using Allitridin, the MTT assay and normal human cell isolates will be needed to determine whether these will be worth pursuing further.

2. Antiviral Activities of Allicin: Animal Studies

Only four animal studies emerged from a literature search for animal models of allicin [10, 18, 19, 20]. Each has clearly not been replicated yet, as they investigate separate viruses. They were also performed unblinded but when taken as a whole do extend the *in vitro* evidence for HCMV [10] and provide novel evidence for three important, highly lethal poultry viruses [18, 19, 20]. The design and results from these studies are summarized in Table 2.

It is important to note that all these studies have used an achievable physiological concentration of allicin, as the thiosulfinate is estimated at 37 mg/g in freshly chopped garlic cloves [46]. The smallest of the studies investigated twelve immunocompromised BALB/ c mice infected with HCMV, six of whom received daily infections of stabilized allicin (Allitridin at 0.6 mg/20g) for two weeks [10]. The BALB/c mice that received Allitridin injections demonstrated a significant reduction ($p < 001$) in hepatic pathology and improved liver enzyme function [10]. Since this is an *in vivo* study, the effects of the thiosulfinate on immune cells also play into its antiviral role. BALB/c mice show defective responses to viral infections, as well as increased numbers of T helper cell-2 and macrophage-2 (Th2 and M2) subsets [47]. These cells are involved in supporting tumor development as well as preventing viral elimination [47]. Allicin has been shown to promote the shift of T helper cells and macrophages to a pro-inflammatory profile (Th1 and 1) thereby eliminating tumors and viruses [48-50]. In this mouse model it may, therefore, have a two-fold effect.

Three much larger trials examined the effects of allicin alone [18, 20] or in fresh garlic paste [19] on poultry viruses. The earliest of these studies investigated the effect of steam-distilled allicin (1.5 mg/ml) on IBDV infection in white leghorn chicks [18]. One hundred and twenty, fourteen day old chicks were divided into four experimental groups, two of which received allicin [18]. The sixty chicks receiving allicin (0.2 mg/kg or 5mg/kg) in their water demonstrated a significant decrease ($p < 0.01$) in bursal shrinkage after seven days of treatment [18]. This was accompanied by a significant increase in both IgA and IgM secreting lymphocytes ($p < 0.01$) as well as the secretion of interferon gamma (IFN-γ) [18]. Whether this would have led to the treated birds' survival is unknown as they were sacrificed to assess the bursal changes. Clearly these data are encouraging, especially given the lack of effective intervention strategies.

Table 2. Animal studies of allicin

Virus	Animal used	Allicin	Results	Reference
HCMV	[1]6 BALB/c mice	*Allitridin (0.6 g/20g)	Animals receiving the allicin daily for 14 days demonstrated ↓ liver pathology and normal liver enzymes	[10]
IBDV	120, 14-day old white leghorn chicks	Allicin (0.2 or 5 mg/kg)	Chicks receiving the allicin daily for 7 days had significant ($p < 0.001$) ↓ in bursal shrinkage and ↑IgA and IgM antibodies (indicative of animal recovery)	[18]
NDV	153, 3-day old Cobb 500 broiler chicks	"Fresh garlic paste" (0.2, 0.6 or 0.8%)	Chicks on the 0.8% allicin demonstrated improved weight gain over the other groups after 42 days Allicin treatment ↓ mortality by 20-35% at 42 days Birds vaccinated using normal regimen at days 7, 12, 21 and 28 of the study.	[19]
REV	240, day old white leghorn chicks	Allicin (300 or 600 mg/kg)	Chicks on both doses of allicin without REV infection demonstrated weight gain The two groups infected with REV demonstrated ↓ bursal shrinkage and weight loss by 14 days of treatment In REV infected chicks allicin ↓ damage by abrogating inflammatory cytokines and downregulating biochemical pathways	[20]

Abbreviations used: HCMV (human cytomegalovirus), IBDV (infectious bursal disease virus), Newcastle disease virus, REV (reticuloendotheliosis virus).
*= stabilized proprietary form of allicin;
[1]Immunosuppressed animals

A six week, randomized, controlled study of one hundred and fifty three day old chicks examined the effect of fresh garlic paste (FGP) (containing allicin) administration on survival from a second lethal virus; NDV [19]. Chicks in the treatment groups were given either 0.2, 0.6 or 0.8% FGP in their drinking water between days seven and 42 [19]. All chicks in the study were vaccinated using the live, attenuated NDV (Gumboro) vaccine at days seven, twelve, twenty one and twenty eight [19]. Chicks receiving 0.8% FGP demonstrated an increased weight gain compared with the other poultry [19]. Most importantly, FGP reduced mortality of the birds by between twenty and thirty percent over and above vaccine-based protection [19]. The study did not standardize the content of the FGP and it is also not apparent from the report whether experimenter bias could have occurred. The study, however, remains of importance as it represents the first attempts at using allicin-containing garlic as an adjunct to vaccination in this disease.

The most recent of these studies to appear in the literature investigated the effect of allicin (150 and 300 mg/kg) on inhibiting the REV-induced immunosuppression of white leghorn chicks [20]. Two hundred and forty day old chicks were divided into six groups, four of which received allicin (300 or 600 mg/kg) either with or without infection with REV [20]. The chicks were observed for five weeks and analysis of internal organs made at weekly intervals [20]. Allicin at both concentrations used, prevented the weight loss produced by REV and significantly reduced the atrophy of immune system organs, beginning by week two of administration ($p < 0.05$) [20]. Both 300 mg/kg and 600 mg/kg also decreased the pro-inflammatory cytokines that induce damage in REV-infected birds [20]. This was also reflected by a decreased in the expression of innate inflammatory pattern recognition receptors (PRR) in the spleen and thymus of the REV-infected chicks [20].

Allicin (300 or 600 mg/kg) supplementation suppressed the biochemical extrinsic receptor kinase (ERK) and NF-κB expression in the spleen but not thymus of the chicks [20]. The biochemical changes elicited by REV are similar to those seen in tumor cells and probably relate to the oncogenic nature of REV [20]. Allicin's activity against ERK and NF-κB has been documented in a variety of cellular systems [38]. For the REV infection it may prevent inflammation from reaching dangerously high levels and thereby prevent permanent host damage and tumor formation [20]. It was not apparent how the treatment affected long term survival as the birds were sacrificed to examine their internal organs [20].

Although HCMV infections are typically benign they are associated with serious mortality rates when acquired *in utero* or following bone marrow transplantation [23]. Viral resistance to current medications is rising and there is no vaccine [23]. Additionally the three poultry viruses produce mortality rates anywhere from twenty percent (REV) [51] to one hundred percent (Newcastle and IBDV virus) mortality [19, 52] and spread rapidly through bird flocks [19, 51, 52]. Further DBRPCT studies are needed to evaluate the efficacy of allicin in mediating both survival and recovery from all four of these viral infections as treatment interventions are urgently needed.

3. Antiviral Activities of Allicin: Human Trials

Only three human trials emerged from a literature search on the antiviral effects of either allicin itself [15] or stabilized garlic preparations likely to contain fully active allicin [16, 17].

Two studies are particularly of note as they are DBPCRT with the viruses being investigated are listed as "colds/ upper respiratory infections" [15, 16]. The third is more recent and examined the effect of allicin on human papillomavirus (HPV) warts [17]. Although the latter study has not been replicated, and is unblinded, it is included here as it is deemed worthy of discussion as the investigators utilized a garlic preparation likely to contain fully active allicin [17]. The design and results from these three studies are summarized in Table 3.

Table 3. Human antiviral allicin studies

Virus	Design	Allicin	Results	Reference
Cold	DBRCT; 146 adult volunteers	180 mg versus placebo	3x as many colds in placebo versus treatment group after 12 weeks	[15]
	DBRCT; 83 children (10-12 years old)	*Allicor (300 mg) versus placebo, 5 months	1.5 times as many respiratory infections in placebo versus treatment group	[16]
HPV	Unblinded trial; 32 male patients with penile warts (20-54 years of age)	10% freeze dried garlic extract compared with cryotherapy	Patients acted as their own control No significant difference in clearance of warts by garlic (68%) versus cryotherapy (79%).	[17]

Abbreviations used: HPV (human papillomavirus).
*= stabilized proprietary form of allicin.

Two large DBRPCT studies have been performed on patients with upper respiratory infections described as "colds" [15, 16]. The first was by Josling and colleagues [15] and assigned one hundred and forty six volunteers to receive either a daily allicin supplement (180 mg) or placebo for twelve weeks [15]. The authors reported nearly three times as many incidences of the common cold in the placebo compared with the treatment group ($p < 0.001$; sixty five versus twenty four) [15].

A second DBRPCT study of possible note on upper respiratory infections was performed by Andrianova and colleagues [16]. The study involved eighty three children who received either a 300 mg coated allicin-containing garlic tablet (Allicor) or placebo for five months [16]. Andrianova and colleagues [16] stated that the study found that children receiving the Allicor were 1.5 times less likely to get infections than those receiving placebo [16]. Allicor contains stabilized garlic powder and is likely thereore to possess allicin activity, although allicin levels have not been described for this preparation [16]. A major issue with both studies is trying to identify which virus or viruses the investigator was trying to prevent. A landmark Finnish study performed in the late 1990s found that of the determinable cold etiologies, the three viruses most commonly isolated were rhinovirus, coronavirus, influenza and parainfluenza virus [4]. Of these four, rhinoviruses were the most frequent isolates (90%) in the Finnish study [4]. It is likely the efficacy being studied in both investigations was primarily rhinovirus [15, 16], although it is believed influenza patients may have been included in the Russian trial [16]. Examination of literature published since 2012 has identified no DBRPCT have been performed subsequent to these studies, which are now more than a decade old.

A single unblinded Turkish study by Mousavi and colleagues [17], compared the effects of fresh dried garlic extract (10%) to cryotherapy in shrinking the sizes of penile HPV warts in thirty three male patients. After two weeks, the size of the warts was decreased equally using both treatments [17]. This study does have merit in that the researchers investigated patients with multiple similar sized warts and could therefore compare shrinkage using both techniques on the same epidermal area. Patients with genital warts face a range of painful removal techniques that include surgery and cryotherapy that result in scarring [17]. By comparison, no patients reported adverse events from the garlic extract application [17]. As this study only appeared in 2018 it is hoped that it will now be followed by additional trials that are DBRPCT in nature.

Conclusion and Future Directions for Allicin as an Antiviral

Allicin appears to have some antiviral efficacy *in vitro*, and using animal or human studies of seven viruses, namely HCMV [10, 11], influenza [8, 9], HPV [17], VSV [13], IBDV [18], NDV [19] and REV [20]. Most exciting is that two of these viruses are DNA-containing (HCMV and HPV) and the other five RNA-containing. If this is correct it might result in a unique broad-spectrum antiviral therapeutic; an entity that doesn't currently exist among pharmaceuticals [23]. Combining the information from the studies [9, 13, 20] that suggested underlying mechanisms may provide several clues to its efficacy and future developments. A possible scheme for three possible antiviral mechanisms is illustrated in Figure 1.

Thiosulfinates, including allicin, attach to and inactivate thiol groups [38]. These are present on proteins containing glutathione or cysteine residues and include many cellular enzyme systems [38]. Most interesting in this respect was the observation by Mehrbod and colleagues [9] that allicin was preventing access of influenza virus by attacking the thiol groups of the hemagglutinin receptor. If this is indeed accurate then it could provide a true effective target for a stable allicin moiety since thiol-based glycoproteins are important in the entry of many viruses to their target cells [53]. These include HCMV [53], hepatitis C [54], and NDV [55] as well as being highly conserved among other members of the paramyxovirus group [56]. Thiazolide medications, including nitazoxanide and tizoxanide, that target thiol groups are already in common use to effectively treat influenza, hepatitis C and rotavirus infections [55]. Interestingly these medications are also broad spectrum antibacterial agents [57, 58] and have antiprotozoal and anti-inflammatory [58] activities. They also appear well tolerated with only minimal side effects [57, 58].

Cysteine residues are involved in generating the structural (capsid) proteins of HIV and are present in the oncogenic proteins produced by HPV [59]. Serine proteases such as the 3C enzyme in human rhinoviruses (HRV) also contain an active site cysteine-sulfhydryl group [60], which would make this a target of any thiollation Protease inhibitors selectively attacking these structures have been suggested as a new class of broad spectrum antivirals and anticancer agents as a result [59]. Currently, however, none have completed more than pre-clinical trials [61]. Cysteine proteases are also essential to the propagation of many pathogens including protozoa such as malaria and *Schistosomula* worms [61].

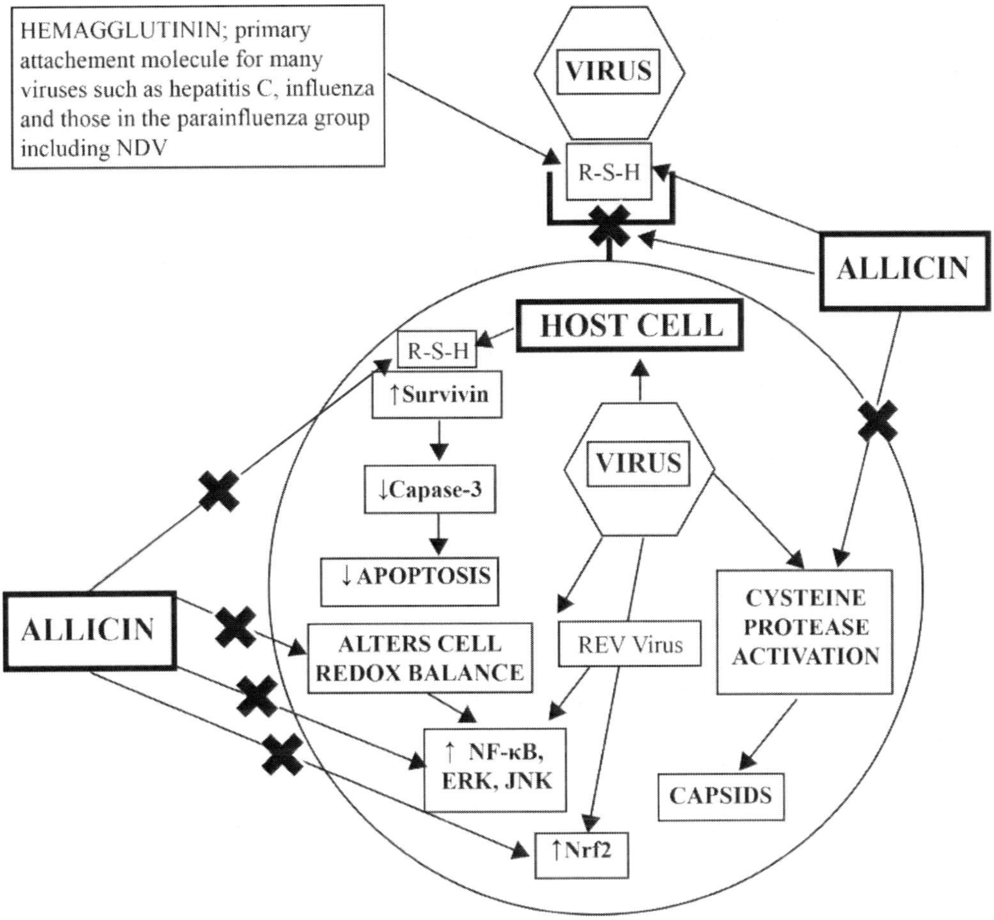

✖ = biochemical pathway points blocked by allicin.

Legend: Allicin may prevent viral entry by blocking the hemagglutinin receptor. Central biochemical pathways needed by the virus are inhibited by NF-κB impaired activation through allicin's alteration of redox balance together with Nrf2, which activates "mopping up" of ROS. Allicin also prevents cysteine protease activation to generate viral capsid proteins. Finally, the thiol group on survivin may also represent an allicin target allowing cell death to occur and viral demise.

Abbreviations used: - ERK (extracellular-initiated kinase), JNK (Jun amino-terminal kinase), NDV (Newcastle disease virus), NF-κB (nuclear factor kappa beta), Nrf2 (NF-E2, p45-related factor 2), REV (reticuloendotheliosis virus), R-S-H (thiol group).

References used to construct diagram [9, 13, 20, 53-56, 59-67].

Figure 1. Possible mechanisms of antiviral activity of allicin.

Another group of proteins containing an oxidation-susceptible, cysteinyl residue at the active site are the caspases [62]. Caspases regulate cellular apoptosis, but these were found to be *activated* by allicin, which would not occur if the thiosulfinate bound directly to these enzymes. Most virus infections need to selectively prevent apoptosis until the particles are assembled and ready to leave the host cell [63]. They achieve this by stimulating the secretion of the caspase-3 inhibitor protein survivin by the host cell [63]. By preventing caspase-3 from dimerization, survivin in turn prevents activation of the apoptosis cascade [63]. Like caspase-3, survivin contains cysteine residues but this time they are arranged in what is termed a "zinc finger" [64] which is known to be susceptible to the activity of allicin [65]. Several viruses can amplify survivin levels including hepatitis B [63] and HPV [66] and this ability may be linked to their ultimate capacity to induce tumors [63, 66]. Removal of the activity of survivin, by eliminating its block on caspase 3 activity would allow cellular apoptosis and in turn decrease the numbers of surviving particles. Given that allicin was found able to both prevent VSV proliferation [13] and eliminate cervical cancer cells [41], it may have thiol-containing survivin as a target rather than caspases.

Another third potential, albeit indirect mechanism for allicin, may be to affect the overall "redox level" of the cell, which directly relates to levels of reactive oxygen species (ROS) [62, 67]. Thiols bind to the cysteine residues in the enzyme glutathione synthetase (GSH) and this in turn results in the decrease of cellular reactive oxygen species (ROS) production. A second protein, thioredoxin, also provides a buffer system, via NADPH, to control cellular ROS levels and can directly modulate NF-κB as well as the apoptosis protein p53 [67]. Several biochemical pathways including ERK and Jun amino-terminal kinases (JNK) are also "redox" sensitive, typically via their initiating proteins [62, 67]. Finally, the NF-E2, p45-related factor 2 (Nrf2) signaling pathway contains cysteine residues that are essential to monitor cellular oxidative i.e., ROS levels [68]. Nrf2 activation switches off NF-κB and it is believed that many chronic diseases and infections are associated with a malfunction of this enzyme [68]. Allicin demonstrated efficacy against the REV virus which upregulates the Nrf2 signaling pathway and maintains an inflammatory environment via chronic NF-κB activation [20]. REV is also associated with chronic activation of all three mitogen activated protein kinase (MAPK) pathways, namely p38, ERK and JNK [20]. Could these three mechanisms be at the heart of allicin's efficacy? If so it would explain a good part of the efficacy of this thiosulfinate as well as its metabolite ajoene.

A major barrier to making allicin effective is its instability [38]. Some attempts have been made to bypass this including stabilized forms of allicin like Allitridin that can be injected [10] and Allimax that can be ingested [69]. Another approach could be to generate allicin *in vivo* at a particular target site [66]. One group was able to attach allinase and allicin separately to an ErB2 monoclonal antibody (McAb) targeting human gastrocarcinoma (N87) cells [70]. Using an N87 xenografted athymic nude mouse model, researchers observed that the modified ErB2 McAb both attached to and killed only cells of the xenograft [70]. Allicin was successfully generated *in vivo* and selectively damaged and significantly ($p < 0.001$) reduced the size of the tumors in the nude mice after three weeks of application [70]. Earlier this year researchers were also able to create a nanoparticle formulation for allicin that involved its functionalization into locust bean gum [71]. Nanoparticles created by this method were non-toxic and retained efficacy against reactive oxygen species generation *in vitro* by RAW 264.7 macrophages and *in vivo* by Sprague Dawley rats [71]. Finally, it may be that some type of derivatization of allicin may preserve its thiol and cysteine binding activities whilst increasing stability. Semi-synthetic and synthetic forms of natural products are common, especially for antimicrobial drugs, and have proven to provide the added bonus of increasing bioavailability [72].

Computational chemistry can now also examine and optimize structures for drug development and may also play a role in developing future new "allicin-like" molecules [73]. At least two groups are already examining allicin's potential in this respect [74, 75]. Leontiev and colleagues [74] synthesized a series of four analogs of allicin (diethyl-, dimethyl-, dipropany- and dibenzyl-thiosulfinates) and compared them with the parent molecule for *in vitro* antibacterial and antifungal activity. Apart from allicin, dimethyl-thiosulfinates (DMTS) was the most effective against gram negative and all analogs were effective against bakers yeast (*Saccharomyces cerevisiae).* Allicin was most toxic to the plant pathogenic fungus *Alternaria* but impaired the growth of seedlings [74]. DMTS was the least toxic to the plants and most toxic to the pathogen [74]. This group also looked at adenocarcinoma cells and found a similar trend for allicin and DMTS [74]. A second group was also able to generate twenty four esterified aminobenzene sulfur acids and demonstrated a hierachy of *in vitro* anti-bacterial and anti-fungal activities [75]. Lubenets and colleagues [75] observed the most efficacy with cycloalkyl and aryl esters of 4-acylaminobenzenethiofulfoacids at very low (nanomolar) concentrations. No viral studies have yet been attempted by either group.

If any or all these techniques are successful, the next question is which viral candidates are likely to provide the most useful candidates for treatment development? Looking first at the seven viruses that emerged from an analysis of the allicin literature it is important to see which have no existing interventions. The viruses associated with significant morbidity and mortality would also be viable candidates in this respect. All seven viruses fit into one or both of these categories and a summary of their effects is shown in Table 4.

Viral culture is expensive and complex, requiring special techniques and laboratory equipment that is therefore not readily available to all parts of the world [83]. In developed countries, sophisticated research methodologies have centered around the development of pharmaceuticals and vaccines to treat and prevent illness [23]. It is to be hoped that recent cost-effective breakthroughs in viral culture [83] may allow the search for less expensive, natural antiviral agents to broaden, potentially to include allicin.

Looking a little more closely at the viruses discussed in this Chapter reveals that some belong to two closely conserved families; herpesviruses [36, 37] and retroviruses [20, 77, 84]. Allicin appears effective against at least two herpesviruses (HCMV and HSV) [8, 10-12] and might be antiviral against others with no current interventional strategies. For example, EBV shares at least one protein with HCMV [85] and cross reactive IgM antibodies recognize both viruses [36]. EBV has no efffective vaccine and produces a pervasive illness that affects a large percentage of the population, sometimes chronically [86]. At this point a low cost alternative medication would be an important addition to an EBV treatment strategy. The retrovirus REV has often been studied as a model for the HIV [20]. At least two reports suggests that the metabolite of allicin, ajoene, can impair the entry of HIV into cells by preventing its attachment to integrins and in turn decrease viral replication [14, 87]. Retroviruses are also frequently oncogenic [25, 88] and the tumoricidal capacity of allicin has also been well established against a number of human viruses (see Chapter 13 for more details) [23]. The link between viruses and tumors is a well established one [88] and identification of an agent that inhibits oncogenic viruses would be a prime candidate for incorporation into prevention strategies.

Another issue with some viruses is their virulence in specific target populations [5, 89, 90]. Infections with the common cold, initiated by HRV and parainfluenza (HPIV) viruses, are typically self-limiting [5, 89, 90]. HRV can precipitate bronchial infections in infants, including croup, and sometimes are the cause of fatal pneumonias in elderly patients [5, 89]. Both HRV and HPIV infections have been linked to the development of asthma [5, 89, 90] and also produce exacerbations of disease in chronic obstructive pulmonary disease (COPD) and cystic fibrosis patients [5, 89, 90]. Neither has a current vaccine or medication strategy. Allicin's ability to reduce upper respiratory tract infections, including children as young as ten suggest it as a potential adjunct therapy for at-risk indviduals.

Table 4. Epidemiology and current interventions for potential viral targets for allicin

Virus	Hosts	Disease outcomes	Intervention strategies	References
HCMV	Human	Congenital infections – fatal 25% of the time, 50% of survivors have permanent impairment Often fatal to bone marrow transplant patients	No vaccine, three medications (foscamir, ganciclovir and cidofovir)	[23, 76]
HPV	Human	~5% of human tumors of cervical, anal and penile cancers and 90% of genital warts	Bivalent and tetravalent vaccines, no medications.	[23]
Influenza A	Human, pig, bird	Human (HN1, H1N2, H3N2)– highly lethal pneumonia especially to elderly; as many as ½ million deaths annually	Human – Trivalent and tetravalent inactivated, 9 medications	[23]
	Human, pig and bird	Pig – (H1N1, H3N2) pneumonia with high mortality rates in avian flu colonizing strains e.g., H1N1	Pig – vaccination of pregnant sows, no medications	[77, 78]
		Bird (H2N2, H5N1) high mortality	Bird – No vaccine, infected poultry euthanized	[79]
VSV	Human and animal	Human – zoonotic or accidental (animal handlers) "flu like" syndrome	No vaccine and only palliative treatment Infected animals euthanized	[44, 45]
Influenza A	Human, pig and bird	Pig – (H1N1, H3N2) pneumonia with high mortality rates in avian flu colonizing strains e.g., H1N1	Pig – vaccination of pregnant sows, no medications	[77, 78]
		Bird (H2N2, H5N1) high mortality	Bird – No vaccine, infected poultry euthanized	[79]
VSV	Human and animal	Human – zoonotic or accidental (animal handlers) "flu like" syndrome	No vaccine and only palliative treatment Infected animals euthanized	[44, 45]
		Cattle, horses and pigs – insect vectors spread skin lesions to mouth and teats → anorexia		
IBDV	Bird	Attacks birds < 2 months of age causing immune system failure. Death from opportunistic infections (100% mortality)	No vaccine or treatment. Infected poultry euthanized Wild birds are reservoirs	[51, 52]
NDV	Bird	Spread through fecal matter and rapidly kills young chicks or embryos. Birds display paralysis and tremors with 100% mortality	Live attenuated inactivated viruses but no treatment. Infected poultry euthanized	[19, 80]
REV	Bird	Attacks birds < 2 months of age and causes immune system failure. Death from opportunistic infections often within two weeks	No vaccine or treatment	[20, 81, 82]

Abbreviations used: HCMV (human cytomegalovirus), HPV (human papillomavirus), VSV (vesicular stomatitis virus), IBDV (infectious bursal disease virus), NDV (Newcastle Disease Virus), REV (reticuloendotheliosis virus).

As was discussed earlier, effective vaccine coverage in developed countries may still be poor due to non compliance [91]. For example, despite effective influenza vaccines being available for all age groups annual vaccine coverage remains below fifty percent in the United States [91]. In contrast, these interventions are either inacccessible to patients in developing countries or they are cost-prohibitive [23]. This is also an issue for several of the viruses discussed in this Chapter [17, 19, 23]. For example, the eighty countries that began adminstering bivalent and tetravalent HPV vaccines in 2007, have reported a decrease of over ninety percent in genital warts and at least fifty percent in abnormal cervical smears [92]. These countries are mostly affluent and had lower rates of cervical cancer and genital warts to begin with [17]. Cervical cancer has a very poor prognosis and genital warts are removed using painful cryotherapy [17, 23]. Any promising alternative treatment therefore offers hope to these patients. In the case of poultry, two vaccines have been established for prevention of NDV [80]. Areas of the world that vaccinate chicks as well as laying hens have seen a drastic decrease in NDV incidence in poultry flocks with only sporadic cases from unvaccinated backyard poultry [80]. The virus is still prevalent in developing countries as they simply cannot afford these vaccines [80].

As an affordable deliverable, stabilized allicin would provide particular benefits against other animal viruses which lack treatments such as VSV [44, 45], IBDV [18, 51, 52], avian influenza A [79] and REV [20, 81, 82]. These RNA-containing viruses have been particularly difficult to provide effective vaccines against as they mutate very rapidly due to the polymerase not "checking" the genome effectively for errors [24]. Together these viruses cause millions of dollars in lost income as a result of livestock and poultry morbidity and mortality [44, 45, 51, 52, 79, 81, 82]. Nowhere is this more keenly felt in poor agrarian communities that are reliant on animals and poultry for their survival, since they can be kept in backyards or small plots [93]. In these areas, farmers live in close proximity to their animals thereby allowing any zoonotic viruses to easily move over into the human population [94]. Clearing these viruses would thereby decrease the likelihood of their direct passage to human handlers as well as their potential epidemic spread into the population. Given that the next pandemics are expected to begin in this manner [94], prevention strategies are urgently needed.

Addition of herbal products to drinking water has already allowed several industrial groups to eliminate the use of antibiotics in rearing poultry [79]. Use of local plants such as pennyroyal, fennel, clove, rosemary and thyme for example were found to be as effective as traditional antibiotics and antifungal agents [79]. Allicin can clearly be effectively administered and absorbed the same way, as demonstrated by the three recent *in vivo* poultry studies [18-20]. These studies required simple, daily preparations of the thiosulfinate to be made [18-20] and could have widespread use in developing nations where garlic would be easy to grow and obtain [14].

REFERENCES

[1] Petrovska, Biljana B., and Svetlana Cekovska 2010. "Extracts from the history and medical properties of garlic." *Pharmacogn. Rev.*, 4(7): 106-110.

[2] Moyers, Susan. 1996. "*Garlic in health, history and world cuisine.*" pp 1-36. St. Petersberg, FL: Suncoast Press.

[3] Moerman Daniel E. 1998. "*Native American Ethnobotany.*" Portland OR : Timber Press.

[4] Hamel, Paul B., and Mary U. Chiltoskey. 1975. "*Cherokee Plants and their uses – A 400 year history.*" Herald Publishing Company, NC, USA.

[5] Mäkelä, Mika J., Tuomo Puhakka, Olli Ruuskanen, Maja Leinonen, Pekka Saikku, Marko Kimpimäki, Soile Blomqvist, Timo Hyypiä, and Perrti Arstila. 1998. "Viruses and bacteria in the etiology of the common cold." *Journal of Clinical Microbiology* 36(2):539-42. Accessed November 16, 2018. https://www.ncbi.nlm.nih.gov/pmc/articles/PMC104573/.

[6] Jacobs, Samantha E., Daryl M. Lamson, Kirsten St. George, and Thomas J. Walsh. 2013. "Human Rhinoviruses." *Clinical Microbiology Reviews* 26 (1): 135-162; doi: 10.1128/CMR.00077-12.

[7] Cavallito, Chester J., and John H. Bailey. 1944. "Allicin, the antibacterial principle of Allium sativum. Isolation, physical properties and antibacterial action." *J. Am. Chem. Soc.* 66(11) : 1950-1951. doi: 10.1021/ja01239a048.

[8] Tsai, Yen, Linda L. Cole, Larry E. Davis, Steven J. Lockwood, Victoria Simmons, and Gaynor C. Wild. 1985. "Antiviral properties of garlic : *In vitro* effects on influenza B, herpes simplex and cocksackie viruses." *Planta Medica* 5 :460-461. doi: 10.1055/s-2007-969553.

[9] Mehrbod, P. E. Amini, and M. Tavassoti-Kheiri. 2009. "Antiviral activity of garlic extract on influenza virus." *Iranian Journal of Virology* 3(1): 19-23. Accessed November 16, 2018. https://www.sid.ir/en/journal/ViewPaper.aspx?ID=168987.

[10] Feng, Fang, Li Hong, Cui Wen, and Yongsui Dong. 1999. "Treatment of hepatitis caused by cytomegalovirus with allitridin injection – An experimental study." *Journal of Tongji Medical University* 19(4) : 271-274. https://doi.org/10.1007/BF02886960.

[11] Zhang, Ju, Hui Wang, Zhi-Dan Xiang, Sei-Nan Shu, and Feng Fang 2013. "Allitridin inhibits human cytomegalovirus replication *in vitro*." *Molecular Medicine Reports* 7(4): 1343-1349. https://doi.org/10.3892/mmr.2013.1328.

[12] Weber, Norbert D., Douglas O. Andersen, James A. North, Byron K. Murray, Larry D. Lawson, and Bronwyn G. Hughes. 1992. "*In vitro* virucidal effects of *Allium sativum* garlic extracts and compounds." *Planta Med* 58(5) : 417-423. doi: 10.1055/s-2006-961504.

[13] Shou, Chunchui, Nanchuan Weng, Xichun Chang, Lei Feng, Hangping Yao, and Nanping Wu. 2015. "Effect of allicin on THP-1, MT-2 and WISH cell apoptosis induced by vesicular stomatitis virus (VSV) and the molecular mechanism involved." *African Journal of Biotechnology* 10(36) : 7040-7047. doi : 10.5897/AJB11.184.

[14] Bayan, Leila, Peir H. Koulivand, and Ali Gorji. 2014. "Garlic : a review of potential therapeutic effects." *Avicenna Journal of Phytomedicine* 4(1) : 1-14.

[15] Josling, Peter. 2001. "Preventing the common cold with a garlic supplement : a double-blind, placebo-controlled study."*Advances in Therapy* 18(4) :189-193. Accessed November 21, 2018. http://www.bravacorp.com/garlic%20and%20the%20common%20cold.pdf.

[16] Andrianova, I.V., I.A. Sobenin, E.V. Sereda, L.I. Bodina, and M.I. Studenkin. 2003. "Effect of long acting tablets "allicor" on the incidence of acute respiratory viral infections in children." *Ter. Arkh.* 75(3) : 53-56. PMID:12718222.

[17] Mousavi, Zahra B., Abolfath Mehrabian, Fereshteh Golfakhrabadi, and Foroogh Namjoyan. 2018. "A clinical study of efficacy of garlic extract versus cryotherapy in the

treatment of the male penile genital wart." *Dermatologica Sinica* xxx: 1-4. Accessed November 20, 2018 https://www.sciencedirect.com/science/article/pii/S1027811718300612.

[18] Zhao, Sufen, Yuanyuan Jia, Weiwei Zhang, Lili Wang, Yunfei Ma, and Kedao Teng. 2015. "Oral administration of *Allium sativum* extract protects against infectious bursal disease in chickens." *Front. Agr. Sci. Eng.* 2(4) : 318-326. doi: 10.15302/J-FASE-2015080.

[19] Gautam, Gokarna, Nabaraj Shrestha, and Shishir Bhandari. 2017. "Effect of *Allium sativum* on immune status against Newcastle Disease virus and productive performance of broiler chicken." *International Journal of Poultry Science* 16(12) : 515-521. doi:10.3923/ijps.2017.515.521.

[20] Wang, Liyuang, Hongchao Jiao, Jinpeng Zhao, Xiaojuan Wang, Shuhon Sun, and Hai Lin. 2017. "Allicin alleviates reticuloendotheliosis virus-induced immunosuppression via ERK/mitogen-activated protein kinase pathway in pathogen-free chickens" *Frontiers in Immunology*, 8:1856. Accessed November 16, 2018. doi: 10.3389/fimmu.2017.01856.

[21] Woolhouse, Mark, Fiona Scott, Zoe Hudson, Richard Howey, and Margo Chase-Topping. 2012. "Human viruses: discovery and emergence." *Philosophical Transactions of the Royal Society of London. Series B, Biological Sciences* 367(1604): 2864-71. doi: 10.1098/rstb.2011.0354.

[22] Storch, Gregory A. 2000. "Diagnostic Virology." *Clinical Infectious Diseases* 31(3): 739–751, https://doi.org/10.1086/314015.

[23] De Clerq, Eric, and Guangdi Li. 2016. "Antiviral drugs developed over the last 50 years." *Clinical Microbiology Reviews* 29(3) :695-747. Accessed November 14, 2018. https://cmr.asm.org/content/cmr/29/3/695.full.pdf.

[24] Carrasco-Hernandez, R., Rodrigo Jácome, Yolanda L. Vidal, and Samuel Ponce de León. 2017. "Are RNA viruses candidates for the next viral pandemic ? A review." *ILAR Journal* 58(3) 15: 343–358. https://doi.org/10.1093/ilar/ilx026.

[25] Roush, Sandra W., Trudy Murphy, and the Vaccine Preventable Disease Table Working Group. 2007. "Historical comparisons of morbidity and mortality for vaccine-preventable diseases in the United States." *JAMA* 298(18) :2155-2163. doi:10.1001/jama.298.18.2155.

[26] Ogholikhan, Sina, and Kathleen B. Schwarz. 2016. "Hepatitis Vaccines." *Vaccines* 4(1), 6. doi:10.3390/vaccines4010006.

[27] Basu, Partha, Dipanwita Banerjee, Priyanka Singh, Chandrani Bhattacharya, and Jaydip Biswas. 2013. "Efficacy and safety of human papillomavirus vaccine for primary prevention of cervical cancer: A review of evidence from phase III trials and national programs." *South Asian Journal of Cancer* 2(4): 187-92. doi: 10.4103/2278-330X.119877.

[28] Simonds, Anita K. 2018."Influenza news from the frontline : what's happening ?"*ERK Open Research* 4 :0020-2018. doi: 10.1183/23120541.00020-2018.

[29] Phadke, Varun K., Robert A. Bednarczyk, Daniel A. Salmon, and Saad B. Omer. 2016. "Association between Vaccine Refusal and Vaccine-Preventable Diseases in the United States: A Review of Measles and Pertussis." *JAMA* 315(11): 1149-58. doi:10.1001/jama.2016.1353..

[30] Panneraj, Pia. 2018. "U.S. vaccine outbreaks catalyzed by vaccine hesitancy." *Healio Infectious Diseases in Children.* April 2018 Accessed November 14, 2018. https://www.

healio.com/pediatrics/vaccine-preventable-diseases/news/print/infectious-diseases-in-children/%7B8073077c-43e9-407a-8766-4752884bb162%7D/us-measles-outbreaks-catalyzed-by-vaccine-hesitancy.

[31] Pullin, Daniel. 2018. “Dramatic drop in public confidence after Philippines dengue vaccine controversy.” *Taylor and Francis Group Press Release*, 11 October. Accessed November 18, 2018. https://www.eurekalert.org/pub_releases/2018-10/tfg-ddi101118.php.

[32] Cundell, Diana R. 2014. Herbal phytochemicals as immunomodulators. *Current Immunology Reviews* 2014, Volume 10 Issue 2 ISSN: 1875-631X(Online), ISSN:1573-3955(Print) Accessed September 10, 2018. http://benthamscience.com/journal/index.php?journalID=cir.

[33] Frass, Michael, Robert P. Strassl, Helmut Friehs, Michael Müllner, M., Kundi, and Alan D. Kaye. 2012. “Use and acceptance of complementary and alternative medicine among the general population and medical personnel: a systematic review.” *The Ochsner Journal* 12(1), 45-56. Accessed on February 19, 2019. https://www.ncbi.nlm.nih.gov/pmc/articles/PMC3307506/.

[34] Bent Stephen. 2008. Herbal medicine in the United States: review of efficacy, safety, and regulation: grand rounds at University of California, San Francisco Medical Center. *Journal of General Internal Medicine* 23(6), 854-9. doi: 10.1007/s11606-008-0632-y.

[35] Davis, Stephen R. 2005. “An overview of the antifungal properties of allicin and its breakdown products – the possibility of a safe and effective antifungal prophylactic.” *Mycoses* 48: 95-100. doi:10.1111/j.1439-0507.2004.01076.x.

[36] Lang, Dieter, Rolf Vornhagen, Markus Rothe, Walter Hinderer, Hans-H. Sonneborn, and Bodo Plachter. 2001.”Cross reactivity of Eptein-Barr virus-specific immunoglobulin M antibodies with cytomegalovirus antigens containing glycine homopolymers.” *Clin. Diagn. Lab Immunol.* 8 (4): 747-756; doi: 10.1128/CDLI.8.4.747-756.2001.

[37] Odumade, Oludare A, Kristin A. Hogquist, and Henry H. Balfour Jr. 2011.”Progress and problems in understanding Epstein Barr virus infections.” *Clinical Microbiology Reviews* 24 (1): 193-209. doi: 10.1128/CMR.00044-10.

[38] Borlinghaus, Jan, Frank Albrecht, Martin C. H. Grulke, Ifeanyi D. Nwachukwu, and Alan J. Slusarenko. 2014. “Allicin : Chemistry and biological properties.” *Molecules* 19(8) : 12591-12618.

[39] Patya, Miriam, Muayad A. Zahalka, Alexey Vanichkin, Aharon Rabinkov, Talia Miron, David Mirelman, Meir Wilchek, Harry M. Lander, and Abraham Novogrodsky. 2004. “Allicin stimulates lymphocytes and elicits an antitumor effect: a possible role of $p21^{ras}$.” *International Immunology* 16(2) : 275-281. https://doi.org/10.1093/intimm/dxh038.

[40] Song, Bin, Shu Ying, Cui Tianlei, and Fu Ping. 2015.”Allicin inhibits human renal clear cell carcinoma progression vi suppressing HIF pathway.” *Int. J. Clin. Exp. Med.* 8(11):20573-20580. Accessed on January 1, 2019. http://www.ijcem.com/files/ijcem0015487.pdf.

[41] Ooommen, Suby, Ruby J. Anto, Gopal Srinivas, and Devarajan Karunagaran. 2004. “Allicin (from garlic) induces caspase-mediated apoptosis in cancer cells.” *Eur. J. Pharmacol.* 485: 97-103.Accessed January 4, 2019 https://pdfs.semanticscholar.org/5193/eeeda4e2d9d812b2409edc012c13f7171a0f.pdf.

[42] Baer, Alan, and Kylene Kehn-Hall. 2014. "Viral concentration determination through plaque assays: using traditional and novel overlay systems." *Journal of Visualized Experiments JoVE* (93): e52065. doi:10.3791/52065.

[43] Garg, Sukant, Hu Huifu, Sunil C. Kaul, and Renu Wadhwa. 2018. "Integration of conventional cell viability assays for reliable and reproducible read-outs: experimental evidence." *BMC Research Notes* 11(1):403. doi:10.1186/s13104-018-3512-5.

[44] Reis, Janildo L., Danny Mead, Luis L. Rodriguez, and Corrie C. Brown. 2009. *"Transmission and pathogenesis of vesicular stomatitis viruses."* Accessed on November 18, 2018. https://bjvp.org.br/wp-content/uploads/2015/07/V.2-N.1-12-20881_2009_12_30_29_6.pdf.

[45] Knight-Jones, T. J., and J. Rushton. 2013. "The economic impacts of foot and mouth disease - what are they, how big are they and where do they occur?" *Preventive Veterinary Medicine* 112(3-4): 161-73. doi: 10.1016/j.prevetmed.2013.07.013.

[46] Rahman, Mohammad S. 2007. "Allicin and other functional active components in garlic: health benefits and bioavailability." *Int J Food Properties* 10 : 245-268.

[47] Sellers, R. S., C. B. Clifford, P. M. Treuting, and C. Brayton. 2012. "Immunological Variation Between Inbred Laboratory Mouse Strains: Points to Consider in Phenotyping Genetically Immunomodified Mice." *Veterinary Pathology* 49(1), 32–43. https://doi.org/10.1177/0300985811429314.

[48] Feng, Yonghui, Xiaotong Zhu, Quinhui Wang, Yongjun Jiang, Hong Shiang, Liwang Cui, and Yaing Cao. 2012. "Allicin enhances host pro-inflammatory responses and protects against acute murine malaria infection." *Malaria J.* 11: 268. Accessed on September 14, 2018. doi: 10.1186/1475-2875-11-268.

[49] Kang, N. S., E. Y. Moon, C. G. Cho, and S. Pyo. 2001. "Imunomodulating effect of garlic component, allicin, on murine peritoneal macrophages." *Nutrition Res* 4: 617-626. Accessed October 16, 2018. https://eurekamag.com/pdf/003/003469471.pdf.

[50] Alam, Rasha T. M., Elshaima M. Fawzi, Maha I. Alkhalf, Wafa S. Alansari, Lotfi Aleya, and Mohamed M. Abdel-Daim. 2018. "Anti-Inflammatory, Immunomodulatory, and Antioxidant Activities of Allicin, Norfloxacin, or Their Combination against Pasteurella multocida Infection in Male New Zealand Rabbits," *Oxidative Medicine and Cellular Longevity,* vol. 2018, Article ID 1780956, 10 pages, https://doi.org/10.1155/2018/1780956.

[51] Qin, Yao, and Shijun J. Zheng. 2017. "Infectious Bursal Disease Virus-Host Interactions: Multifunctional Viral Proteins that Perform Multiple and Differing Jobs." *International Journal of Molecular Sciences* 18(1): 161. doi: 10.3390/ijms18010161.

[52] Ailke, Tamiru N., and Silke Rautenschlein. 2016. "Infectious bursal disease virus in poultry : current status and future prospects." *Veterinary Medicine Research and Reports* 7 :9-18. doi: https://doi.org/10.2147/VMRR.S68905.

[53] Mirazimi, Ali, Mehrdad Mousavi-Jazz, Vivi-Anne Sundqvist, Lehnart Svensson L. 1999. "Free thiol groups are necessary for infectivity of human cytomegalovirus." *J. Gen. Virol.* 80(11):2861-2865 doi:10.1099/0022-1317-80-11-2861.

[54] McCaffrey Kathleen, Irene Boo Kevin Tewierek, Mark L. Edmunds, Pantelis Poumbourios and, Heidi E. Drummer. 2012."Role of conserved cysteine residues in hepatitis C virus glycoprotein e2 folding and function." *J Virol.* 86(7) 3961-3974. doi:10.1128/JVI.05396-11.

[55] Jain, Surbhi, Laurie W. McGinnes, and Trudy G. Morrison. 2008. "Role of thiol/disulfide exchange in newcastle disease virus entry." *Journal of Virology*, *83*(1), 241-9. doi: 10.1128/JVI.01407-08.

[56] Piacentini, Sara, Simone La Frazzia, Anna Ricchio, Jens Z. Pedersen, Alessandra Topai, Orazzio Nicolotti, Jean-Francois Rossignol, and Gabriela Santoro. 2018. "Nitazoxanide inhibits paramyxovirus replication by targeting the Fusion protein folding: role of glycoprotein-specific thiol oxidoreductase ERp57." *Scientific Reports* 8: Article number: 10425. Accessed on February 21, 2019 https://www.nature.com/articles/s41598-018-28172-9.

[57] Pankuch, Glenn A., and Peter C. Appelbaum. 2006. "Activities of tizoxanide and nitazoxanide compared to those of five other thiazolides and three other agents against anaerobic species." *Antimicrobial Agents and Chemotherapy* 50(3), 1112-7. doi: 10.1128/AAC.50.3.1112-1117.2006.

[58] Hemphill, Andrew, Joachim Mueller, and Marco Esposito. 2006. "Nitazoxanide, a broad-spectrum thiazolide anti-infective agent for the treatment of gastrointestinal infections." *Expert Opinion on Pharmacotherapy* 7:7, 953-964, doi: 10.1517/14656566.7.7.953.

[59] Casini, Angela, Andrea Scozzafava, and Claudiu Supuran. 2002. "Cysteine-modifying agents: a possible approach for effective anticancer and antiviral drugs." *Environmental Health Perspectives* 110(5):801-6. doi: 10.1289/ehp.02110s5801.

[60] Patick, A. K., and K. E. Potts. 1998. "Protease inhibitors as antiviral agents." *Clinical Microbiology Reviews* 11(4), 614-27. Accessed on February 21, 2019 https://www.ncbi.nlm.nih.gov/pmc/articles/PMC88900/.

[61] Verma, Sonia, Dixit Rajnikant and Kailash C. Pandey. 2016. Cysteine Proteases: Modes of Activation and Future Prospects as Pharmacological Targets. *Frontiers in Pharmacology* 7 : Article 107. doi: =10.3389/fphar.2016.00107.

[62] Klomsiri, Chananat, P. Andrew Karplus, and Leslie B. Poole. 2011. "Cysteine-based redox switches in enzymes." *Antioxidants & Redox Signaling* 14(6): 1065-77. doi: 10.1089/ars.2010.3376.

[63] Marusawa, Hiroyuki, Shu-Ichi Matsuzawa, Kate Welsh, Hua Zou, Robert Armstrong, Ingo Tamm, and John C. Reed. 2003. "HBXIP functions as a cofactor of survivin in apoptosis suppression." *The EMBO Journal* 22(11), 2729-40. doi: 10.1093/emboj/cdg263.

[64] Altieri, David C. 2015. "Survivin - The inconvenient IAP." *Seminars in Cell & Developmental Biology* 39: 91-6. doi: 10.1016/j.semcdb.2014.12.007.

[65] Ganjipoor, Naji, S. Eghbalnia, P. Khodabakshsh, M. Daustany, and Tahereh Naji. 2016. "The effect of allicin on ZNF703 gene expression in GCC lines." *Proceedings of 2016 International Conference on Cellular and Molecular Biology and Medical Sciences.* ISBN 978-93-84468-71-2. https://doi.org/10.17758/URUAE.AE0916405.

[66] Borbély Ágnes, Melinda Murvai, József Kónya, Zoltán Beck Z, Lajos Gergely, Fengzhi Li, and Gyorgy Veress. 2006. "Effects of human papilloma virus type 16 oncoproteins on survivin gene expression." *Gen. Virol.* 87(2):287-294. doi:10.1099/vir.0.81067-0.

[67] Cross, Janet V., and Dennis J. Templeton.2006. "Regulation of cysteine transduction through protein cysteine oxidation." *Antioxidants & Redox Signaling* http://doi.org/10.1089/ars.2006.8.1819.

[68] He, Xiaoqing, and Quiang. 2009. "NRF2 cysteine residues are critical for oxidant/electrophile-sensing, Kelch-like ECH-associated protein-1-dependent

ubiquitination-proteasomal degradation, and transcription activation." *Molecular Pharmacology* 76(6), 1265-78. doi: 10.1124/mol.109.058453.

[69] Suddek, Ghada M. 2014. "Allicin enhances chemotherapeutic response and ameliorates tamoxifen-induced liver injury." *Pharmaceutical Biology* 52(8) : 1009-1014. Accessed November 22, 2018. https://www.tandfonline.com/doi/full/10.3109/13880209.2013.876053.

[70] Miron, Talia, Marina Mironchik, David Mirelman, Meir Wilchek, and Aharon Rabinkov. 2003. "Inhibition of tumor growth by a novel approach : *in situ* allicin generation using targeted alliinase delivery." *Molecular Cancer Therapeutics* 2 (12) :1295-1301. http://mct.aacrjournals.org/content/molcanther/2/12/1295.full.pdf.

[71] Soumya, R. S., S. Sherin, K. G. Raghu, and Annie Abraham. 2018." Allicin functionalized locust bean gum nanoparticles for improved therapeutic efficacy: An *in silico*, *in vitro* and *in vivo* approach." *International Journal of Biological Macromolecules* 109(1):740-747. https://doi.org/10.1016/j.ijbiomac.2017.11.065.

[72] Wright, Peter M., Ian B. Seiple, and Andrew G. Myers. 2014. "The evolving role of chemical synthesis in antibacterial drug discovery." *Angewandte Chemie (International ed. in English) 53*(34): 8840-69. doi: 10.1002/anie.201310843.

[73] Leelananda, Sumudu P. and Steffen Lindert, S. 2016. "Computational methods in drug discovery." *Beilstein Journal of Organic Chemistry* 12:2694-2718. doi:10.3762/bjoc.12.267.

[74] Leontiev, Roman, Nils Hohaus, Jacob Claus, Martin C. H. Gruhlke, and Alan J. Slusarenko .2018."Comparison of the Antibacterial and Antifungal Activities of Thiosulfinate Analogues of Allicin." *Scientific Reports* 6763 :8(1). Accessed on February 22, 2019 https://www.nature.com/articles/s41598-018-25154-9.

[75] Lubenets, Vira, Sofiya Vasylyuk, Nataliya Monka, Khrystina Bolibrukh, Olena Komarovska-Porokhnyavets, Diana Baranovych, Rostyslav Musyanovych, Ewa Zaczynska, Anna Czarny, Urszula Nawrot, and Volodymyr Novikov. 2016. "Synthesis and antimicrobial properties of 4-acylaminobenzenethiosulfoacid S-esters." *Saudi Pharmaceutical Journal: SPJ: The Official publication of the Saudi Pharmaceutical Society* 25(2), 266-274. doi: 10.1016/j.jsps.2016.06.007.

[76] Dollard, Sheila C., Scott D. Grosse, and David S. Ross. 2007. "New estimates of the prevalence of neurological and sensory sequelae and mortality associated with congenital cytomegalovirus infection." *Rev. Med. Virol.* 17 :355-363. http://dx.doi.org/10.1002/rmv.544.

[77] Janke, H., B. 2014. "Influenza A Virus Infections in Swine: Pathogenesis and Diagnosis." *Veterinary Pathology* 51(2): 410–426. https://doi.org/10.1177/0300985813513043.

[78] Thacker, Eileen, and Bruce Jancke. 2008. "Swine influenza virus : zoonotic potential and vaccination strategies for the control of swine and avian influenzas." *J. Clin. Microbiol.* 197: S19-S24. Accessed November 22, 2018. https://academic.oup.com/jid/article/197/Supplement_1/S19/841647.

[79] Mehdi, Yousef, Marie-Pierre Létourneau-Montminy, Marie-Lou Gaucher, Younez Chorfi, Gayatri Suresh, Tarek Rouissi, Santinder K. Brar, Caroline Côté, Antonio A. Ramirez, Stéphane Godbout. 2018. "Use of antibiotics in broiler production : Global impacts and alternatives." *Animal Nutrition* 4(2) :170-178. Accessed November 22, 2018. https://www.sciencedirect.com/science/article/pii/S2405654517302512.

[80] Brown, Vienna R., and Sarah N. Bevins. 2017. "A review of virulent Newcastle disease viruses in the United States and the role of wild birds in viral persistence and spread." *Veterinary Research* 48(1):68. doi: 10.1186/s13567-017-0475-9.

[81] Bi, Yulin, Lu Xu, Yingling Qiu, Shasha Wang, Xiangping Liu, Yani Zhang, Yang Chen, Yang Zhang, Qi Xu, Guobin Chang, and Guohong Chen. 2018. "Reticuloendotheliosis virus inhibits the immune response acting from lymphocytes in peripheral blood of chicken." *Front. Physiol.* 23 January 2018. Accessed November 20, 2018. https://www.frontiersin.org/articles/10.3389/fphys.2018.00004/full.

[82] Okoye, J. O. A., W. Ezema, and J. N. Agoha. 1993. "Naturally occurring clinical reticuloendotheliosis in turkeys and chickens." *Avian Pathology* 22 :237-244. Accessed November 18, 2018. https://www.tandfonline.com/doi/pdf/10.1080/0307945 9308418917.

[83] Leland, Diane S., and Chrstine C. Ginocchiom. 2007. "Role of cell culture for virus detection in the age of technology." *Clinical Microbiology Reviews* 20(1): 49-78. doi: 10.1128/CMR.00002-06.

[84] Niewiadomska, Anna M and Robert J. Gifford. 2013. "The Extraordinary Evolutionary History of the Reticuloendotheliosis Viruses." *PLoS Biol* 11(8): e1001642. https://doi.org/10.1371/journal.pbio.1001642.

[85] Donaghy, G., and R. Jupp. 1995. "Characterization of the Epstein-Barr virus proteinase and comparison with the human cytomegalovirus proteinase." *Journal of Virology* 69(2), 1265-70.

[86] Gallagher, K. E., D. S. LaMontagne, and D. Watson Jones. 2018. "Status of HPV vaccine introduction and barriers to country uptake." *Vaccine* 36(32A): 4761-4767. https://doi.org/10.1016/j.vaccine.2018.02.003Get rights and content.

[87] Walder, R., Z. Kalvatchev, D. Garzaro, M. Barrios, and R. Apitz-Castro. 1997. "In vitro suppression of HIV replication by ajoene [(e)-(z)-4,5,9-trithiadodeca-1,6,11-triene-9 oxide]." *Biomedicine Pharmacotherapy* 51(9) : 397-403.

[88] Luo, Guangxiang G., and Jing-Hsiung J Ou. 2015. "Oncogenic viruses and cancer." *Virologica Sinica* 30(2): 83–84. http://doi.org/10.1007/s12250-015-3599-y.

[89] Henrickson, Kelly D. 2003. "Parainfluenza viruses." *Clinical Microbiology Reviews* 16(2):242-64. doi: 10.1128/CMR.16.2.242-264.2003.

[90] Jacobs, Samantha E., Daryl M. Lamson, Kirsten St. George, and Thomas J. Walsh. 2013. "Human Rhinoviruses." *Clinical Microbiology Reviews* 26 (1): 135-162; doi: 10.1128/ CMR.00077-12.

[91] Santibanez, Tammy A., and Erin D. Kennedy. 2016. "Reasons given for not receiving an influenza vaccination, 2011-12 influenza season, United States." *Vaccine* 34(24): 2671-8.doi: 10.1016/j.vaccine.2016.04.039.

[92] Basu, Partha, Dipanwita Banerjee, Priyanka Singh, Chandrani Bhattacharya, and Jaydip Biswas. 2013. "Efficacy and safety of human papillomavirus vaccine for primary prevention of cervical cancer: A review of evidence from phase III trials and national programs." *South Asian Journal of Cancer* 2(4): 187-92. doi: 10.4103/2278-330X.119877.

[93] Padhi, Mahendra K. 2016 "Importance of Indigenous Breeds of Chicken for Rural Economy and Their Improvements for Higher Production Performance," *Scientifica* 2016, Article ID 2604685.https://doi.org/10.1155/2016/2604685.

[94] Johnson, Christine K., Peta L. Hitchens, Tierra S. Evans, Tracey Goldstein, Kate Thomas, Andrew Clements, Damien O. Joly, Nathan F. Wolfe, Peter Daszak, William B. Karesh, and Jonna K. Mazet. 2015. "Spillover and pandemic properties of zoonotic viruses with high host plasticity." *Scientific Reports* 5: Article 14830. Accessed on February 26, 2019. https://www.nature.com/articles/srep14830.

In: Allicin
Editor: Diana R. Cundell

ISBN: 978-1-53617-339-0

Chapter 9

INSECTICIDAL AND ANTI-PEST ACTIVITY OF ALLICIN AND THE EVOLUTIONARY ORIGINS OF THE ALLICIN TRAIT

Jeffrey A. Klemens**, PhD
Department of Biological and Chemical Sciences, Thomas Jefferson University, Philadelphia, PA

ABSTRACT

The biological activity of Allicin and its metabolites manifests in a wide range of anti-pest activity. Garlic extracts in various forms have been shown to be effective against insects and nematodes in diverse agricultural settings and situations. Insect repellent activity of garlic is widely invoked but has little justification in the scientific literature. Studies of anti-pest activity in garlic are limited by methodological differences in extraction and application; progress in this field will require a standardization of methods. Bioinformatic investigation of the origin of the allicin trait suggests that allicin production is derived from a modification of an auxin biosynthesis pathway and not from a more ancient anti-herbivore defense.

INTRODUCTION

The biocidal properties of allicin and its principal metabolites result in a wide range of anti-pest activity, which is unsurprising given its documented anti-microbial, anti-fungal, anti-protozoal and anti-helminthic activity (see Chapters 5-7). This chapter will review several aspects of this anti-pest activity.

* Corresponding Author's Email: Jeffrey.Klemens@jefferson.edu.

1. INSECTICIDAL ACTIVITY OF ALLICIN

Allicin extracts have been shown to interact with pest insects across the life cycle, reducing larval growth, causing direct mortality of adults, and reducing rates of oviposition on target crops. Anwar et al. recently reviewed the literature on the effects of allicin on insect pests [1]. They documented anti-insect activity against a a range of insects including Orthopterans (grasshoppers, crickets, and locusts), Hemipterans (true bugs), Thysanopterans (thrips), Coleopterans (beetles), Lepidopterans (moths and butterflies), and Dipterans (flies). As shown in Figure 1, these insects do not form a unified, monophyletic group and are broadly distributed across the insect family tree [2]. This indicates that the observed activity of allicin may be quite general, but should also raise a caution about the potential for non-target effects of allicin-based agricultural interventions.

Since this review, several studies have documented additional effects of allicin on pests. In a test of an experimental allicin-based biopesticide the house fly (*Musca domestica*) was shown to be sensitive to allicin at several life stages, including increases in egg, larval, and adult mortality and decreases in oviposition rate on allicin treated substrates [3]. Importantly, this study compared the effect of the allicin treatment to an existing biopesticide, Vectobac, derived from *Bacillus thuringiensis.* By using a commercially prepared extract with known allicin concentration, this study represents a good starting point for further explorations of allicin as an agricultural pesticide.

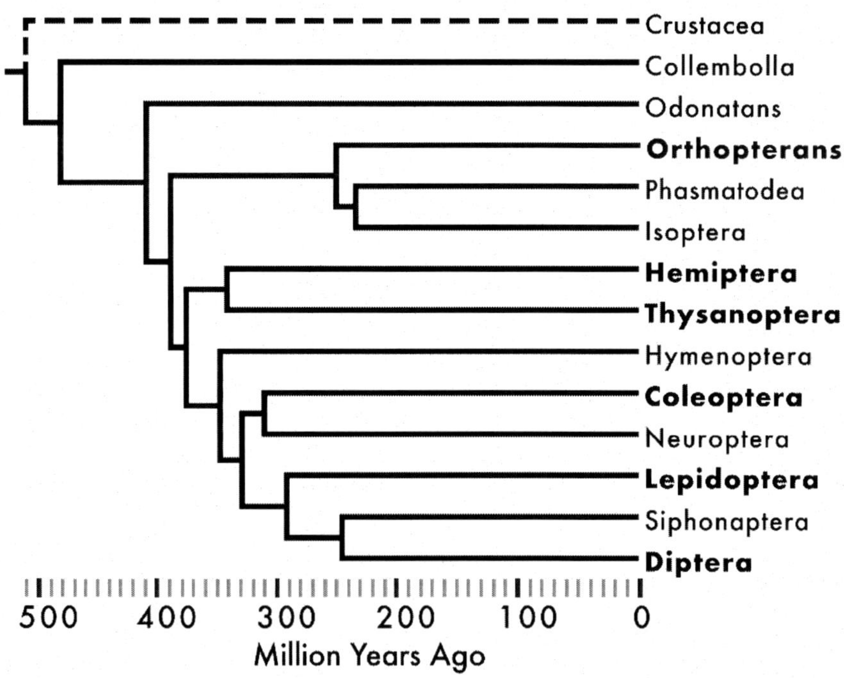

Legend: The phylogenetic relationships among major insect orders with Crutaceans included as an outgruop. Orders highlighted in **bold** text have documented sensitivity to garlic extract in some form. Tree constructed from data on group divergence times as estimated in supplementary material to [2], data on senstivity from [1].

Figure 1. Phylogenetic relationships of insect groups with documented sensitivity to allicin.

A study of the effects of garlic essential oils on the mealworm beetle (*Tenebrio molitor*) was notable for its attribution of insecticidal activity to different components of the garlic extract, specifically diallyl disulfide and diallyl sulfide, in a range of concentrations [4]. Although diallyl disulfide was more toxic than diallyl sulfide, both compounds, as well as the unseparated essential oil, "induced symptoms of intoxication in larvae and adults of *T. molitor*, such as progressive paralysis, reduced food consumption, and regurgitation. Necrosis was observed in larvae, pupae and adults on the area applied, mainly in mouthparts, pronotum, legs, abdomen segments, and anus" [*ibid.*]. Essential oils, diallyl disulfide, and diallyl sulfide were also shown to be repellent to the insects. The authors concluded that there was high potential for garlic extract to function as a a pesticide to be deployed as a fumigant against insect pests of stored grains.

In a simulated mushroom production system garlic oil extract was shown to have a repellent effect on two species of flies, reducing oviposition rates on the substrate [5]. The species differed in the degree to which emergence of larvae was affected by allicin, however, with one species showing sensitivity across a range of extract concentrations and the other showing sensitivity only at the highest concentration of garlic oil extract employed.

In a unique study, garlic extract was incorporated as the toxic element in an attractive toxic sugar bait (ATSB) study on *Anopheles* mosquitos in Israel [6]. Using a measure of biting pressure (the rate at which mosquitos attack a human 'bait') showed high efficacy of garlic oil in the ATSB system, and suggested that due to the low residence time of the compound in the environment it could serve as an effective mosquito control agent, particularly in areas where repeated applications were feasible.

Very little information exists on the effect of garlic extract on non-target species. In integrated pest management, pesticides are often combined with other factors such as the introduction of natural predators of the pest. Two studies on the effect of garlic extract on the pentatomid bug *Podisus maculiventris* found that garlic extract did slightly reduce growth and survival of this insect predator, but was "reasonably safe" to the predator [7] even at rates that were effective for the control of insect pests [8]. This is clearly an area that will need much more attention if the use of allicin begins to increase, particularly if it is to be deployed at the scale of agricultural production.

Anwar et al. concluded that allicin had high potential as an alternative pesticide [1]. They cautioned, however, that one of the challeges moving forward from our current understanding of Allicin's anti-pest activity to the development of marketable products based on Allicin chemistry would be in the interpretation of the diverse studies that have been undertaken to date:

> *one should be cautious when comparing the efficacy of garlic extracts against different pathogens given that the tests have been conducted in different labs ... as different garlic extract preparation methods from different garlic sources can significantly influence the composition of the organosulfur bioactives. Many of the previously published studies conducted with crude extract and oils of garlic do not report the composition of biologically active constituents in the test materials [1].*

This call for standardization of methods among studies is something we will see repeated below in the context of allicin's nematocidal effects.

2. Repellent Activity of Allicin

Garlic is reputed to be an effective insect repellent for humans [9]. There is very little evidence to back up this assertion, however. The single placebo-controlled study of garlic as a mosquito repellent found no effect of garlic consumption on rates of moquito bite [10]. Nevertheless, there are many products on the market today that describe themselves as natural insect and pest repellents. These yard sprays are described as being derived from a mixture of essential oils and based on customer reviews of the post-application scent seem to contain a large garlic component. If rigorous studies of these products' effectiveness exist they have yet to be make their way into the scientific literature.

3. Nematocidal Activity

Given the effects of allicin on growth and development of insects, it is unsuprising to discover that allicin also affects the other major Ecdysozoan clade, the nematodes. Nematodes are root pests of many commercial crops, including the Alliums. Numerous studies have been performed on the effect of allicin on nematodes [1]. These generally fall into two categories: the effects of allicin on phytopathogens that attack crop plants and the effects of allicin on nematodes that infect the guts of livestock.

3.1. Effect of Allicin on Phytopathogens

Root-knot nematodes (*Meloidogyne sp.*) are a major agricultural pest world-wide [11]. Several studies have investigated the effect of allicin on infection by root-knot nematodes, particularly on tomatoes. Cetintas et al. [12] found that application of garlic extracts to tomato seedlings reduced gall formation and the number of egg masses produced, and increased plant growth performance compared to other essential oil treatments. Experimental results have been mixed, however. Studies in which tomato seedlings were dipped in a garlic extract with the goal of protecting roots against *Meloidogyne* infection have generated conflicting results, with one study showing a protective effect [13] and others showing no effect [14]. Gong et al. [15] reviewed the literature and described experimental treatments in which garlic extracts were used in soil emendation with and without fertilizer and plastic sheeting. They found promising but complex effects of garlic extract on tomato production, in part due to allelopathic effects of the garlic extract on plant growth.

3.2. Effects of Allicin as Deworming Treatment

The anti-helminthic properties of garlic were intuited by traditional people, and garlic has historically been included in animal forage as a deworming agent for livestock. For example, summarizing historical reports from the Nordic countries, Waller et al. [16] included four *Allium* species on a list of plants "known" to be useful in deworming livestock.

Evidence for the effectiveness of including Alliums in forage is mixed, however. Some evidence has shown that the anti-helminthic properties of allicin persist when fed to organims *in vivo*. For example, garlic extract showed activity against *Haemonchus contortus*, the barber-pole worm, in a gerbil model system [17].

Velkers et al. found sparse evidence for anti-helminthic effects in birds in their review of the literature, and were unable to demonstrate experimentally an effect of garlic extract on *Ascaridia* infections in chickens [18]. A review of phytotherapy in organic sheep and goat farming systems reviewed several studies and found no anti-helminthic effect of *Allium* [19], however a 2010 study showed strong anti-helminthic effects against nematode parasites in sheep [20]. In evaluating *Allium* species for agricultural use it must also be kept in mind that the use of garlic in forage has long been known to influence the flavor of animal products, particularly milk [21], which may explain why the research on this topic is not more extensive.

All of these studies of nematocidal activity have reatively small sample sizes, and there were differences in how the *Allium* was administered to the target organisms. These different modes of extraction and delivery of the phytochemicals have been shown to have large effects on the efficacy of a particular extract [22]. Furthermore all *Allium* extracts are not created equal, and extracts of different Alliums may have different *in vivo* and *in vitro* effects [*ibid.*]. In order to make further progress on the potential of *Allium* in organic agriculture larger scale studies must be undertaken and standardization of application protocols among experiments will probably be necessary to generate interpretable, generalizable results.

4. Alliinase and the Evolutionary Origin of Insecticidal Activity in Allicin

An interesting question with regard to the anti-pest properties of allicin is the evolutionary origin of this trait. Specifically, is the allicin production system a modified anti-pest system or does it have its origin elsewhere?

Understanding the evolutionary origin of allinase requires an understanding of the gentically encoded components of the system. The primary focus of inquiry might therefore be the alliinase enzyme itself. The production of allicin is not found outside of the Allium group, and is thus a key shared derived characteristic of these plants. The allinase enzyme is highly conserved among the Alliums, in particular the three dimensional structure determined by the three disulfide bridges that give shape to the enzyme's active site [23].

To get a first-pass understanding of the evolutionary origins of a particular protein we can examine amino acid sequence alignments using BLAST and then use the PFAM database to determine the protein family to which it belongs. PFAM is a database that organizes proteins and protein functional domains by relatedness [24]. A protein family represents a group of related proteins as determined by a sequence alignment algorithm that is weighted towards the highly conserved sites that are more likely to be important structural and functional elements of a particular protein.

A BLAST search of the UNIPROTKB database using the amino acid sequence of the protein Alliin lyase 1 derived from *Allium sativum* (UNIPROT ID Q01594) and Alliinase (UNIPROT ID D2CXG4) revealed a number of Alliinase sequences from other species in the genus Allium. As would be expected, where good alignments were obtained, sequence identify was > 80% for these proteins. More interestingly, there were also extensive shared sequences between the Alliinase protein in *A. sativum* and a number of other proteins that occur throughout the plant kindom. Many of these proteins are characterized as tryptophan aminotransferases or tryptophan aminotransferase related proteins.

Similarly, PFAM indicates that Allinase consists of two major families of protein domains, Alliinase EGF-like domain (EGF_alliinase, PF04863) and Allinase C (Aliinase_C, PF04864). Both of these domains are widely distributed in the plant kingdom and the Alliinase C domain is a component of several proteins characterized as tryptophan aminotransferases (e.g., dicots W9S717 (*Morus notabilis*) and A0A0B2S7V1 (*Glycine soja*) as well as monocots AOA199V6R7 (*Ananas ananas*) and M7Z4Z7 (*Triticum uratu*)). Alliinase C is itself part of a super family known as the PLP dependent aminotransferases. Most of the proteins in this family or superfamily seem be part of normal anabolic metabolism and none are known to function in plant defense (although there are many proteins within the family of uncharacterized function).

In *Arabidopsis* Alliinase C is related to the TAA/TAR proteins, these proteins have been shown to function in a tryptophan-dependent auxin biosynthesis pathway [25, 26]. A recent phylogenetic analysis showed that TAA/TAR and their precursors, the YUC proteins, are widespread in plants and likely arose in the charophytes [27]. The Allinase related genes are in turn descended from these more ancient TAA/TAR proteins [28].

Given the evidence available to date, it seems most likely that the production of allicin by the Alliums is a trait which arose from non-defense-related biosynthetic pathways, specifically the auxin biosynthetic pathway, rather than a co-option or elaboration of existing plant defense mechanisms. It is likely that this trait was a key innovation in the common ancestor of the alliums and contributed to the evolutionary success of this group.

REFERENCES

[1] Anwar, Awais., Emma, Gould., Ryan, Tinson., Murree, Groom. & Chris, J. Hamilton. (2016). "Think Yellow and Keep Green – Role of Sufanes from Garlic in Agriculture". *Antioxidants*, *6*(1) https://www.mdpi.com/2076-3921/6/1/3.

[2] Misof, B., Liu, S., Meusemann, K., Peters, R. S., Donath, A., Mayer, C., Frandsen, P. B., Ware, J., Flouri, T., Beutel, R. G., Niehuis, O., Petersen, M., Izquierdo-Carrasco, F., Wappler, T., Rust, J., Aberer, A. J., Aspöck, U., Aspöck, H., Bartel, D., Blanke, A., Berger, S., Böhm, A., Buckley, T. R., Calcott, B., Chen, J., Friedrich, F., Fukui, M., Fujita, M., Greve, C., Grobe, P., Gu, S., Huang, Y., Jermiin, J. S., Kawahara, A. Y., Krogmann, L., Kubiak, M., Lanfear, R., Letsch, H., Li, Y., Li, Z., Li, J., Lu, H., Machida, R., Mashimo, Y., Kapli, P., McKenna, D. D., Meng, G., Nakagaki, Y., Navarrete-Heredia, J. L., Ott, M., Ou, Y., Pass, G., Podsiadlowski, L., Pohl, H., von Reumont, B. M., Schütte, K., Sekiya, K., Shimizu, S., Slipinski, A., Stamatakis, A., Song, W., Su, X., Szucsich, N. U., Tan, M., Tan, X., Tang, M., Tang, J., Timelthaler, G., Tomizuka, S., Trautwein, M., Tong, X., Uchifune, T., Walzl, M. G., Wiegmann, B. M., Wilbrandt, J., Wipfler, B., Wong, T. K. F., Wu, Q., Wu, G., Xie, Y., Yang, S., Yang, Q., Yeates, D. K., Yoshizawa, K., Zhang, Q., Zhang, R., Zhang, W., Zhang, Y., Zhao, J., Zhou, C., Zhou, L., Ziesmann, T., Zou, S., Li, Y., Xu, X., Zhang, Y., Yang, H., Wang, J., Wang, J., Kjer,

K. M. & Zhou, X. (2014). "Phylogenomics resolves the timing and pattern of insect evolution." *Science*, *346*(6210), 763-767. https://doi.org/ 10.1126/science.1257570.

[3] Howard, A. Bell., Andrew, G. Cuthbertson. & Neil, Audsley. (2016)."The potential use of allicin as a biopesticide for the control of the house fly, *Musca domestica* L." *International Journal of Pest Management*, *62*, 2, 111-118, doi: 10.1080/09670874. 2015.1120363.

[4] Plata-Rueda, Angelica., Luis, Carlos Martinez., Marcello, Enrique Dos Santos., Flavío, Lames Fernandez., Carlos, Frederico Wilcken., Marcus, Alverenaga Soares., José, Eduardo Serrão. & José, Cola Zenuncio. (2017). "Insecticidal activity of garlic essential oil against the mealworm beetle, *Tenebrio molitor* Linneus (Coleoptora: Tenebrionidae). *Scientific Reports*, *7*, Article number, 46406, (2017). https://www.nature.com/ articles/srep46406.

[5] Jess, S. J. M., Kirbas, A. W. Gordon. & Murchie, A. K. (2017). "Potential for use of garlic oil to control Lycoriella ingenua (Diptera: Sciaridae) and Megaselia halterata (Diptera: Phoridae) in commercial mushroom production." *Crop Protection*, *102*, 1-9. ISSN 0261-2194 https://doi.org/10.1016/j.cropro.2017.08.003.

[6] Revay, Edita E., Yosef, Schlein., Onie, Tsabari., Vasiliy, Kravchenko., Whitney, Qualls., Rui, De-Xue., John, C. Beier., Sekou, F. Traore., Seydou, Doumbia., Axel, Hausmann. & Günter, C. Müller. (2015). "Formulation of attractive toxic sugar bait (ATSB) with safe EPA-exempt substance significantly diminishes the Anopheles sergentii population in a desert oasis." *Acta Tropica*, *150*, 29-34. ISSN 0001-706X. https://doi.org/10. 1016/j.actatropica.2015.06.018.

[7] Mamduh, Ziba., Vahid, Hosseininaveh., Hossein, Allahyari. & Khalil, Talebi-Jahromi. (2017). "Side effects of garlic extract on the life history parameters of the predatory bug, Podisus maculiventris (Say) (Hemiptera: Pentatomidae)." *Crop Protection*, 100, 65-72. ISSN 0261-2194. https://doi.org/10.1016/j.cropro.2017.05.029.

[8] Mamduh, Ziba., Vahid, Hosseininaveh., Fazeli, M. Movhedi. & Jahromi, K. Tahebi. (2018). "Toxicity of garlic extract on spined soldier bug Podisus maculiventris (Hemiptera: Pentatomidae) in comparison to its two hosts." *Journal of Crop Protection*, *7*(1), 93-107.

[9] Natural mosquito repellants and bite rememdics. Old Farmer's Almanac https://www. almanac.com/content/how-deter-mosquitoes-and-treat-bug-bites.

[10] Rajan, T. V., Hein, M., Porte, P. & Wikel, S. (2005). "A double-blinded, placebo-controlled trial of garlic as a mosquito repellant: a preliminary study." *Medical and Veterinary Entomology*, *19*, 84-89. doi:10.1111/j.0269-283X.2005.00544.x.

[11] Anwar, S. A. & McKearney, M. V. (2010). " Incidence and Reproduction of Meloidogyne incognita on Vegetable Crop Genotypes." *Pakistan J. Zool.*, *42*(2), 135-141. Accessed on October 10, 2019. http://zsp.com.pk/pdf/135-141%20(5).pdf.

[12] Cetintas, Ramazan. & Mehmet, Yasum Yarba. (2010). " Nematicidal Effects of Five Plant Essential Oils on the Southern Root-Knot Nematode, Meloidogyne incognita Race 2." *Journal of Animal and Veterinary Advances*, *9*(2), 222-225. http:// www.medwelljournals.com/abstract/?doi=javaa.2010.222.225.

[13] Gupta, R. & Sharmaj, N. K. (1993). "A study of the nematicidal activity of allicin—an active principle in garlic, *Allium sativum* L., against root-knot nematode, *Meloidogyne incognita* (Kofoid and White, 1919) Chitwood, 1949," *International Journal of Pest Management*, *39*, 4, 390-392, doi: 10.1080/09670879309371828.

[14] Sardari, A. Asadi., Hojat Jalali, A. A., Bahraminejad, S. & Safaee, D. (2015). "Effect of plant extracts on the mortality of root-knot nematodes' J_2, *Meloidogyne javanica.*" *Archives of Phytopathology and Plant Protection*, *48*, 4, 365-375, doi: 10.1080/03235408.2014.889342.

[15] Gong, Biao., Sean, Bloszies., Xiu, Li., Min, Wei., Fengjuan, Yang., Qinghua, Shi. & Xiufeng, Wang. (2013). "Efficacy of garlic straw application against root-knot nematodes on tomato." *Scientia Horticulturae*, *161*, 49-57. ISSN 0304-4238. https://doi.org/10.1016/j.scienta.2013.06.027.

[16] Waller, P., Bernes, P., Thamsborg, S., Sukura, A., Richter, S. H., Ingebrigsten, K. & Höglund, J. (2001). "Plants as De-Worming Agents of Livestock in the Nordic Countries: Historical Perspective, Popular Beliefs and Prospects for the Future." *Acta Vet Scand*, *42*, 31 doi:10.1186/1751-0147-42-31.

[17] Palacios, Landin J., Gives, P., Salinas, D., López, M., Hernández, E Liébano. Velázquez, V. M. & Valladares-Cisneros, M. (2016). "*In vitro* and *in vivo* Nematocidal Activity of Allium sativum and Tagetes erecta Extracts Against Haemonchus contortus." *Turkish Journal of Parasitology*, *39*, 260–264. https://doi.org/10.5152/ tpd.2015.4523.

[18] Velkers, F. C., Dieho, K., Pecher, F. W. M., Vernooij, J. C. M., van Eck, J. H. H. & Landman, W. J. M. (2011). "Efficacy of allicin from garlic against Ascaridia galli infection in chickens." *Poultry Science*, *90*(2), 364–368. https://doi.org/10.3382/ps.2010-01090.

[19] Rahmann, G. & Seip, H. (2007). "Bioactive forage and phytotherapy to cure and control endo-parasite diseases in sheep and goat farming systems–a review of current scientific knowledge." *Landbauforschung Völkenrode*, 285–295.

[20] Masamha, B., Gadzirayi, C. & Mikutirwa, I. (2010). "Efficacy of Allium Sativum (Garlic) in Controlling Nematode Parasites in Sheep." *Intern. J. Appl. Res. Vet. Med.*, *8*, 161–169.

[21] Rossi, G., Schiavon, S., Lomolino, G., Cipolat-Gotet, C., Simonetto, A., Bittante, G. & Tagliapietra, F. (2018). "Garlic (Allium sativum L.) fed to dairy cows does not modify the cheese-making properties of milk but affects the color, texture, and flavor of ripened cheese." *Journal of Dairy Science*, *101*(3), 2005–2015. https://doi.org/10.3168/ jds.2017-13884.

[22] Klimpel, S., Abdel-Ghaffar, F., Al-Rasheid, K. A. S., Aksu, G., Fischer, K., Strassen, B. & Mehlhorn, H. (2011). "The effects of different plant extracts on nematodes." *Parasitology Research*, *108*(4), 1047–1054. https://doi.org/10.1007/s00436-010-2168-4.

[23] Weiner, L., Shin, I., Shimon, L. J. W., Miron, T., Wilchek, M., Mirelman, D., Frolow, F. & Rabinkov, A. (2009). "Thiol-disulfide organization in alliin lyase (alliinase) from garlic (Allium sativum)." *Protein Science: A Publication of the Protein Society*, *18*(1), 196–205. https://doi.org/10.1002/pro.10.

[24] Finn, R. D., Mistry, J., Tate, J., Coggill, P., Heger, A., Pollington, J. E., Gavin, O. L., Gunasekaran, P., Ceric, G., Forslund, K., Holm, L., Sonnhammer, E. L. L., Eddy, S. R. & Bateman, A. A. (2010). "The Pfam protein families database." *Nucleic Acids Research*, *38*, (Database issue), D211–D222. https://doi.org/10.1093/nar/gkp985.

[25] Tao, Y., Ferrer, J. L., Ljung, K., Pojer, F., Hong, F., Long, J. A., Li, L., Moreno, J. E., Bowman, M. E., Ivans, L. J., Cheng, Y., Lim, J., Zhao, Y., Ballaré, C. L., Sandberg, G., Noel, J. P. & Chory, J. (2008). "Rapid Synthesis of Auxin via a New Tryptophan-

Dependent Pathway Is Required for Shade Avoidance in Plants." *Cell*, *133*(1), 164–176. https://doi.org/10.1016/j.cell.2008.01.049.

[26] Mano, Yoshihiro. & Keiichiru, Nemoto. (2012). "The pathway of auxin biosynthesis in plants." *Journal of Experimental Botany*, *63*(8), 2853-2872. https://academic.oup.com/jxb/article/63/8/2853/734272.

[27] Poulet, Axel. & Verena, Kriechbaumer. (2017). "Bioinformatics Analysis of Phylogeny and Transcription of TAA/YUC Auxin Biosynthetic Genes." *International Journal of Molecular Sciences*, *18*(8), 1791. https://doi.org/10.3390/ijms18081791.

[28] Matthes, Michaela S., Norman, B. Best., Janlo, M. Robil., Simon, Malcomber., Andrea, Gallavotti. & Paua, McSteen. (2019). "Auxin EvoDevo: Conservation and Diversification of Genes Regulating Auxin Biosynthesis, Transport, and Signaling." *Molecular Plant*, *12*(3), 298–320. https://doi.org/10.1016/j.molp.2018.12.012.

In: Allicin
Editor: Diana R. Cundell

ISBN: 978-1-53617-339-0

Chapter 10

CARDIOVASCULAR DISEASE AND ALLICIN

Diana R. Cundell*, PhD and Anne H. Bower, PhD
College of Life Sciences, Jefferson University, Philadelphia, PA

ABSTRACT

Garlic has been used for at least three thousand years as a natural phytochemical for the control of heart and blood pressure issues. With atherosclerosis-induced cardiovascular disease (CVD) now reaching epidemic proportions globally new strategies of management and prevention need to be developed. This is especially true as many of the new patients will be residents of developing countries, where cost and accessibility of classic pharmaceuticals are already major issues. Several components underpin the development of CVD including hyperlipidemia, periodontal disease and blood vessel damage through atherosclerotic plaque formation These combine to produce hypertension and thrombi resulting in significant morbidity and mortality. Literature studies appearing within the past two decades suggest that allicin, as well as active, fresh garlic preparations, are able to affect cholesterol biosynthesis, improve oral health and suppress the biochemical pathways leading to atherosclerosis. Several studies have also reported effects of allicin on blood sugar levels in hyperlipidemic animals suggesting a potential role for this phytochemical in type II diabetes. This chapter will review the currently available data on allicin together with suggesting future delivery systems for this thiosulfinate in both conditions.

Keywords: atherosclerosis, cardiovascular disease, type II diabetes

INTRODUCTION

Garlic has a long history of use in various cultures for the control of cardiovascular issues [1-5]. Dating back as far as 1500 BC in the *Codex Ebers* there is evidence of Egyptian healers prescribing the ingestion of crushed garlic cloves for cardiovascular disease [1-3]. The Ayurvedic practitioners in India suggested its use in circulatory disorders in the written text of

* Corresponding Author's Email: Diana.Cundell@jefferson.edu.

the *Vedas* [1]. Hippocrates in Greece observed diurectic properties [4] while Dioscorides in Rome from 40 to 100 AD described using garlic to "*clean the arteries*" in *De Materia Medica* [2, 3, 5]. Unlike the doctors of the Ancient World we now know that CVD is a complex, progressive, chronic inflammatory disease with a series of risk factors that include hyperlipidemia, hypertension, diabetes, smoking and genetics [6]. Recent studies have also added dysregulation of the microbiota of the gut [7] and oral cavity [8] to this equation. For example, patients with severe periodontal disease are more likely to have atherosclerosis as well as experience a resulting cerebral or myocardial infarct [8].

CVD symptoms appear only following significant disruption of the endothelial cell lining (intima) of arterial blood vessels and the heart tissue that they feed [6]. Most cardiologists now agree that initiating events involve the generation of atherosclerotic plaques, which begin to form after low density cholesterol (LDL) is deposited on blood vessel walls as "fatty streaks" [6]. Disruption of intimal integrity initiates a cycle of inflammatory processes, resulting in narrowed blood vessels (seen clinically as hypertension) [6]. Chronic hyperlipidemia also triggers the dysfunction of several important biochemical pathways [9-11]. A microenvironment in which nitric oxide (NO)[9] and reactive oxygen species (ROS) [10] synthesis is increased and their inactivator NF-E2, p45-related factor 2 (Nrf2) is impaired [9, 11] is now considered to be central to the develoment and perpetuation of the atheroslerotic plaque [9-11]. Endothelial damage results in an irregular surface, promoting platelet activation and clot formation uneven nature of with formation of blood clots (thrombi), which may break off (emboli) and travel far from their point of origin or block local vessels [6]. Two major pathologies result from these effects [6]. Cardiac muscle cells cannot be replaced once injured or deprived of blood flow and eventual left ventricular failure then triggers a myocardial infarction (heart attack) as a result [6]. Traveling emboli may lodge in major vessels supplying the brain, resulting in a cerebral infarction (stroke) [6]. Myocardial or cerebral infarctions are often fatal on the first occasion so the current interventional strategies for the at-risk patient are to avoid these exacerbations of the disease [6].

Prevention methods currently focus on exercise, smoking cessation and maintenance of good nutrition; ironically most clinicians recommend the Mediterranean diet, which already contains garlic! [12]. Patients are usually identified when atherosclerotic insults begin to produce elevated blood pressure changes [6] or when annual blood work reveals hyperlipidemia or hyperglucosemia [13]. Once diagnosed, pharmacological therapies are then the typical "go to" for patient management if diet change, smoking cessation or exercise do not moderate blood pressure, lipids or glucose after three to six months [13, 14]. These interventions do not address the underlying atherosclerotic plaques that have already formed but seek to prevent new endothelial damage and resulting clot formation, hence avoiding the fatal sequelae of the disease [6, 13, 14]. In addition, no current interventions address the biochemical changes that are occurring at the molecular level in the endoethelial cells of the blood vessels and myocardium.

So, are these management strategies effective for the CVD patient? The answer, sadly, may often be no although for some patient is does work. Patients in developed countries have access to a plethora of medications but their cost and side effects may bar many patients from taking them [15]. Despite advanced management techniques, current studies report that around forty percent of people in developed countries are likely to die from CVD and its compications [16]. The situation in developing countries, where the incidence of CVD and hypertension is increasing and where cardiac issues occur as sequelae of valve infection, malaria and Chagas' disease is far worse [16]. Poor documentation, management and access to medications is especially an issue in rural areas where nearly one in three people die from CVD [16]. As with the other conditions discussed in this book, new sustainable strategies need to be identified that are less expensive to consumers and have lower side effects [15, 16]. Phytomedicines have resurfaced as realistic complementary medicine therapies for a variety of conditions [17]. Garlic and, to a lesser extent its thiosulfinate allicin, has been researched relatively extensively in CVD prevention with *in vitro*, animal and human double blind, placebo-controlled (DBRPCT) clinical trials appearing in the literature [18-20]. This chapter will evaluate the role that allicin could potentially play in managing patients with CVD as well as exploring its effects on the associated condition of type II diabetes. Evidence for allicin's molecular interventions on the hyperlipidemia, endothelial cell damage and platelet activation that lead to atherosclerosis will be evaluated. Finally, other downstream ameliorating effects of allicin and allicin-enriched garlic preparations on lipid metabolism by gut flora in CVD patients as well as periodontal plaque will be explored.

1. Basic Mechanisms Involved in Cardiovascular Disease

As previously stated, cardiovascular disease is a chronic cascade of damaging events involving hyperlipidemia, endothelial inflammation and damage and finally blood vessel narrowing and clot formation [6]. Each of these components has its own associated mechanisms and are described in the following sections.

1.1. Hyperlipidemia as an Initiating Event in Atherosclerosis

Under normal circumstances, LDL transports cholesterol in the bloodstream and this allows its widespread distribution to LDL receptors [21, 22]. Plaque formation in atherosclerosis is initiated when cholesterol is chronically elevated and LDL begins depositing it in the blood vessel walls [21, 22]. Initially seen as "fatty streaks" of immobile LDL-cholesterol, deposition of blood vessel wall fats are detected by circulating monocytes that attempt to remove them [21]. Accumulation of these lipids transforms the monocyes into "foam cells" which, if they cannot rid themselves of their burden, die thereby releasing their intracellular enzymes and initiating damage processes [21]. Monocytes rid themselves of LDL-bound cholesterol by reverse cholesterol transport in which ATP-binding cassette transporter A1 (ABCA1) deposits the cholesterol onto HDL [21]. Defects in ABCA1 genes are associated with rapid, early atherosclerosis lesions initiated by dysregulated monocyte foam cells [21].

The human body manufactures approximately 25% of its own cholesterol; an effect that cannot be moderated by diet or exercise [21]. The cholesterol pathway requires the substrate of acetyl coenzyme A (Acetyl CoA), which is manufactured from coenzyme A and acetate using acetyl CoA synthase [23]. At least three important steps are then involved [23, 24]. The initial convertion of Acetyl coenzyme A (Acetyl CoA) to mevalonic acid using the enzyme beta-hydroxy-beta-methylglutaryl coenzyme A (HMG-CoA reductase) [21-24]. Interestingly, HMG-CoA reductase is the target of the pharmaceutical statins) [21, 22, 24]. Mevalonic acid is then converted to farnosylpyruvate (FP) through, in part, the actions of mevalonate kinase

[23]. Finally FP is converted to squalene, lanosterol and cholesterol [23, 24]. The latter component of the pathway involves the enzyme squalene monooxygenase, which converts squalene to the cholesterol precursor 2,3 oxidosqualene [23, 24].

Circulating cholesterol doesn't remain free but is transferred to high density lipoprotein (HDL) where it is converted to a cholesterol ester form by lecithin cholesterol ester acyl transferase (LCAT) to allow its effective transport [25]. This is termed reverse cholesterol transport (RCT)[25]. Cholesterol esters then return to the liver by two mechansisms [25]. Primary carriage is by HDL, which transfers cholesterol esters to hepatocyte LDL receptors for final absorption and excretion in bile [25]. Cholesterol esters can also be transferred to LDL proteins by cholesterol ester transfer proteins (CETP) and follow the same route [25].

Cholesterol esters are also generated by a second enzyme, Acyl-CoA cholesterol acyltransferase (ACAT) [26]. ACAT is present in all cells and its activation prevents excess toxic cholesterol accumulation [26]. Catabolism of cholesterol esters results from the activation of a a second enzyme; cholesterol ester hydrolase (CEH) [26]. Cellular cholesterol levels determine which of these two enzymes are activated; if low CEH and if high ACAT [26]. Saturated fatty acids in the circulation can also influence cholesterol secretion, absorption and LDL manufacture [26]. Finally, in a feedback loop when free cholesterol levels fall liver biosynthesis is initiated through a sterol regulatory element binding pathway (SREBP) [26]. SREBP activates HMG-CoA synthase and upregulates LDL receptor gene transcription [27]. Putting this together, CETP and SREBP are central regulatory elements in controlling blood cholesterol levels [25, 27].

1.2. Role of Dysregulation of Gastrointestinal and Oral Flora in CVD

Dysregulation of the gut biome typically involves a decrease in beneficial (probiotic) bacteria combined with a decrease in the overall diversity of species [7]. Diets high in refined sugars and fats contribute to the gut floral dysbiosis [7] and result in overgrowth of opportunists such as *Clostridium difficile* and *C. perfringens* [7, 28]. Ingestion of complex carbohydrates results in more beneficial bacteria including *Bifidobacterium* species [25]. When the bacterial population is composed of fewer species, such as occurs in an omnivorous diet, they are more likely to secrete trimethylamine or trimethylamine *N*-oxide (TMAO) metabolites of phosphatidylcholine [7, 28]. Elevated TMAO levels are associated with an increased risk of atherosclerosis and a more "pro-inflammatory" gut biome [7, 28]. Animal studies have shown that TMAO reduces RCT and impair the sequestration of cholesterol into bile [7]. TMAO also upregulates inflammatory receptors on endothelial cells [7]. Studies have also reported that administration of TMAO inhibitors reduces the CVD symptoms of cardiac hypertrophy and fibrosis [7].

Observations that oral plaque-forming bacteria, including *Streptococci* and *Porphyromonas gingivalis* were isolated from atherosclerotic lesions provided an early link between oral health and CVD [7, 8]. Periodontal infections are now widely accepted to result in the entry of these bacteria into the bloodstream where they can attach to and damage endothelial cells [8]. Their role in the persistence of atherosclerotic plaques still remains unclear, although some researchers speculate they may either allow other infections to take place or exacerbate lipid-induced damage [8]. These strains can also directly interact with platelets and, either directly or indirectly, induce local thrombus formation [8]. Thus, oral bacteria that become residents of atherosclerotic plaques are likely to contribute to their persistance, at least at the local level [8].

1.3. Atherosclerotic Lesions Lead to Platelet Activation and Hypertension

Atherosclerotic lesions are by their very nature pro-inflammatory and associated with activation of the endothelial cell lining of the blood vessels [29].

Several inflammatory molecules are expressed as a result including ROS and NO [9, 10, 29]. ROS contribute to these lesions in several ways, First, in combination with NO, superoxide ROS can produce peroxynitrite which results in platelet aggregation via LDL [9, 10]. Human atherosclerotic lesions generate large amounts of peroxynitrite which perpetuates their maintentance [9, 10, 29]. Second, circulating monocytes in this milieu express elevated mitochondrial levels of ROS, which they are unable to compensate for, and an increased tendency to migrate into the lesions due to overexpression of macrophage chemotactic factor (MCP)[9]. Monocytes stay in this inflamed area as activated endothelial cells upregulate their expression of adhesion molecules, including vascular cell adhesion molecule-1 (VCAM) and intracellular adhesion molecule-1 (ICAM), thereby allowing attachment of passing monocytes [29]. Thirdly, animals deficient in pathways that can attenuate ROS, including Nrf2, are unable to protect smooth muscle cells from the effects of ROS and therefore develop atherosclerotic plaques [9].

By regulating ROS, Nrf2 also plays a major role in preventing cardiac myopathy [30]. Current studies of cardiac illness allocate a primary role to oxidative stress and ROS in the development of scar (fibrotic) tissue resulting from high blood pressure [30]. Further support from this concept comes from the finding that some antioxidants stimulate Nrf2 and are cardioprotective as a result [30]. When the stimulus is elevated blood glucose Nrf2 appears to be activated during early metabolic syndrome, which limits cardiac damage [31]. As the disease progresses, the extracellular initiated kinase (ERK) cardiomyocyte pathway becomes activated suppresses Nrf2 and at this point the heart muscle becomes insulin- resistant and eventually functionally impaired [31]. Here is seen the first connection between hyperglucosemia and the perpetuation of cardiac disease. Nrf2 can also directly inhibit the secretion of inflammatory-induced NO from endothelial cells [11].

Interestingly, in atherosclerosis, the macrophages that play a primary role in initating and propogating the endothelial plaques demonstrate desensitization to Nrf2 [30]. It is important to note at this point that NO plays a dual role with respect to endothelial activation [32]. When derived from constitutionally expressed endothelial nitric oxide synthase (eNOS) low levels of NO maintain intimal health [32]. Activation or inflammation of the endothelial cells results in inducible nitric oxide synthase (iNOS) and elevated NO levels [32]. Regulation of eNOS and iNOS enzymes is mediated by a phosphatidylinositol-3-OH-kinase (PI3K)-dependent mechanism involving protein kinase B (Akt) [33].

Damage to blood vessel endothelial cells by the above mechanisms, results ultimately in the creation of an uneven blood vessel wall surface capable of initiating platelet binding [34]. Platelet binding results in an initial shape change then leading to aggregation and granule release [34]. Platelet granule release and subsequent thromboxane A_2 (TXA_2) generation are both central to the final formation of a solid fibrin clot (thrombus) [34]. At this point blood vessels either narrow or become blocked entirely, contributing to the detectable feature of hypertension [6].

2. Allicin, Garlic and Hyperlipidemia

In total over a hundred studies have been performed to investigate the effects of whole garlic preparations containing allicin on models of hyperlipidemia and DBRCT of human patients [35-43, 47-63, 66-73]. Since not all garlic preparations contain allicin, data will only be analyzed from those studies in which this thiosulfinate is likely to be present namely garlic powder or garlic oil [74].

2.1. Effects of Allicin and Garlic on Hyperlipidemia; *In Vitro* Models

Nine *in vitro* studies [35-43] have sought to determine the effects of either allicin or garlic preparations containing allicin on the biochemical pathways involved in the generation of lipids as shown in Table 1.

Table 1. Effects of allicin or garlic containing allicin on *in vitro* or *ex vivo* lipid pathways

Study design	Result	Reference
Rat hepatocytes or HepG2 cells incubated with garlic extract (0-125 mg/ ml) or alliin (expected allicin of 1.66 mg/ml) for 2 h;	↓ manufacture of sterols (assessed by C^{14} acetate incorporation) above 10 mg/ml garlic or with the allicin with an IC_{50} of 90 μg/ml	[35]
Rat hepatocytes incubated with water soluble garlic extracts (0-100 mM) for 2 h	Allicin was chief effector of ↓in manufacture of sterols particularly cholesterol (assessed by C^{14} acetate uptake) and produced these effects as low as 5 μM	[36]
Rat hepatocytes incubated with various garlic extracts (0-100 mM) including allicin for 2 h;	↓ Manufacture of sterols (assessed by C^{14} acetate incorporation) and target of inhibition for allicin (IC_{50} 17 μM) identified as HMGCoA- reductase	[37]
Rat hepatocytes incubated with garlic extract (1g/L) for 30 min and squalene monoxidase assessed	↓ Squalene monooxidase enzyme	[38]
Rat hepatocytes incubated with water soluble garlic extract (1.25 g/L) for 4 h	↓ Triglyceride and cholesterol synthesis; may constitute fatty acid synthesis inhibition also	[39]
Mitochondria isolated from bovine heart and incubated with allicin (10-100 μM) for 1 h	↓ Acetyl-CoA synthase enzyme	[40]
Human HepG2 cells treated with 1,3 DCP (100 μM, 1 h) and incubated with allicin (0- 80 μM) for 23 h	↓ Triglycerides, free cholesterol in cells and downregulated SREBP-1 and 2	[41]
Ex vivo: Human subendothelial smooth muscle cells (2-3 hr deceased cadavers from MI) incubated with 0.6% allicin for 24 h	↓ Triglycerides, free cholesterol and cholesterol esters in cells from patients' plaques and normal endothelium ↓ Acyl-CoA cholesterol acyltransferase and ↑ cholesteryl ester hydrolase; this ↓ cholesteryl ester levels	[42]
Ex vivo; 5-week old broiler chickens fed polar fractions of garlic (1-8% of feed) for 3 weeks, hepatocytes from animals incubated with 6% fresh garlic for 15 min	↓50-70% hepatic HMG-CoA reductase and fatty acid synthetase	[43]

Abbreviations used: 1,3 DCP (1,3 dichloropropanol), HMG-CoA (beta-hydroxy-beta-methylglutaryl coenzyme A), h (hour), IC_{50} (concentration used to produce a 50% decrease in function), MI (myocardial infarction), SREBP (sterol regulatory element binding protein)

Most of the *in vitro* studies employed rat hepatocytes [35-39] and all reported that allicin [35, 37] or garlic extracts containing allicin [36, 38, 39] inhibited cholesterol [35-37, 39] synthesis. An *in vitro* study using the human hepatocyte tumor line HepG2 reported allicin (0-48 μM) decreased production of cholesterol and triglycerides following lipid perturbation by 1,3-dichloropropanol (1,3-DCP) treatment [41]. Decreased cholesterol manufacture was also seen two further *ex vivo* studies using human cadaver blood vessel smooth muscle cells [41] and hepatocytes from garlic fed broiler chickens [43].

Six of the studies determined that the effects of garlic containing allicin [38, 43] or pure allicin [37, 40-42] affected the functionality of enzymes in the cholesterol biosynthesis pathway. Two studies also reported garlic inhibited fatty acid synthesis [39, 43], possibly through impairment of fatty acid synthase [43]. Garlic preparations containins allicin as well as pure allicin has been reported to inhibit four separate cholesterol enzymes namely HMG-CoA reductase [37, 43] squalene monooxidase [38], Acetyl-CoA synthase [30] and Acyl-CoA cholesterol acyltransferase [42]. As previously described, the cholesterol biosynthesis pathway is initiated by two steps: acetyl CoA synthesis by Acetyl-CoA synthase and mevalonic acid synthesis by HMG-CoA reductase [30]. Squalene monooxidase is then at the terminal end of the cholesterol biosynthesis pathway [30]. The fourth enzyme suggested as a target for allicin, namely ACAT [42], is not in the cholesterol biosynthesis pathway but involved in its conversion to cholesterol esters [33]. The same study found that allicin was able to stimulate the enzyme involved in decreasing cholesterol ester levels; CEH [42].

2.1.1. Possible Mechanisms; Evidence from In Vitro Models

So how is garlic, and allicin as its major component, simultaneously affecting numerous cholesterol-generating enzymes? More likely is that there is an individual target, which is in turn impairing the formation of substrates for the enzymes that come after it e.g., squalene monooxidase. Several findings support this target being the SREBP [34, 37, 41-43]. The recent report by Lu and colleagues [41] of allicin's capacity to impair SREBP would explain the inhibition of HMG-CoA reductase seen in a further two studies [37, 43]. As the first step in the biosynthetic pathway this block would prevent any synthesis and create a decreased hepatocyte cholesterol level. As previously stated, low levels of cellular cholesterol would activate CEH to catabolize cholesterol esters and inhibit ACAT; results reported by Orekhov and colleagues [42].

Interestingly, SREBP controls both cholesterol and fatty acid synthesis, with the two pathways both being activated by a decrease in cholesterol [44]. Garlic was shown to simultaneously inhibit fatty acid and cholesterol synthesis in one *in vitro* study in which a similar hypothesis was suggested by the researchers [39]. Allicin, ajoene and alliin were found in a recent study to be share the same docking target as statins, namely the fatty acid synthase enzyme [45]. The three sulfur moieties were equipotent [35]. Finally, allicin belongs to a family of neutral cysteine proteases, [46] at least one member of which (ALLN) has been shown to inhibit SREBP [44]. Borlinghaus [46] in his review also suggested that allicin might directly attach to the thiol group on unbound CoA, thus sequestering it from acetylation to acetyl CoA and removing the substrate.

2.2. Effects of Allicin and Garlic on Hyperlipidemia; Animal Studies

Seventeen *in vivo* animal studies [47-63] investigated the effects of allicin or garlic preparations containing allicin on blood lipid profiles as shown in Table 2.

Table 2. Effects of allicin or garlic containing allicin on animal lipid profiles

Study design	Result	Reference
Wistar rats (n = 8) fed a diet containing 1% cholesterol, 46.8% glucose with or without 5 g garlic (1 week) and injected with C^{14} sucrose or acetate	↓ Liver triglycerides and FFA as well as total serum lipid but no effect on abdominal fat pads. Garlic also ↓ serum glucose, ↑ serum insulin and liver glycogen.	[47]
Sprague Dawley rats (n = 9 per group) fed 1% cholesterol diet with or without whole/ autoclaved garlic (2 or 4%, 4 weeks)	Whole garlic ↓ serum and liver cholesterol ↓ serum LDL. Liver glucose-6-phosphate activity also ↓	[48]
Sprague Dawley rats (n =10 per group) fed 1% cholesterol or 15% lard diet with or without lyophilized garlic (2 or 4%, 4 weeks)	Garlic ↓HDL and ↑ LDL ↓ Liver cholesterol and total lipids by 30% ↓ Liver glucose-6-phosphate activity	[49]
Sprague Dawley rats (n = 90; 3 groups) fed fructose-rich diet (60%) and blood taken at day 0, 3 weeks and 5 weeks, one group was given allicin for last 2 weeks (8 mg/kg/day, orally) and comparison made with control group and those given enalapril (20 mg/kg/day, orally)	Allicin ↓ serum triglycerides; effects were especially evident on weeks 3-5.	[50]
Male spontaneously hypertensive rats (n =20; 2 groups) treated with or without allicin (80 mg/kg/ day orally) for 6 weeks	Allicin ↓ serum triglycerides No effect on cholesterol, insulin or adiponectin	[51]
Hypercholesterolemic Wistar rats (n = 6 per group) fed freeze-dried garlic powder (0.5, 1.0, 2.0 and 3.0%) or commercial garlic pearls (0.15% garlic) for 9 weeks	Garlic (2 and 3%) ↑ HDL and ↓ LDL. Rats fed garlic pearls significantly decreased serum and liver cholesterol levels	[52]
Sprague Dawley rats (n =30, 3 groups) fed normal or high cholesterol (2%) diet with or without garlic (50 mg/kg containing 0.6% allicin) for 6 weeks	Levels of triglycerides fell below level of rats with control diet! ↓ total cholesterol	[53]
Rabbits (n =36; 3 groups) fed high cholesterol diet for 12 weeks, with one group receiving garlic oil (0.5 mg/kg)	Animals receiving garlic oil showed ↑ HDL and ↓ in aortic lipids as well as 50% fewer aortic lesions	[54]
Albino rabbits (n =16) fed high cholesterol (0.5 g/kg/day) for 8 weeks, with one group receiving raw, garlic (1 g/kg gavage)	Plasma cholesterol similar in garlic versus untreated group Cholesterol: phospholipid ratio was lower in garlic group Atherosclerotic lesions 50% lower in garlic group	[55]
New Zealand White rabbits (n = 19) fed cholesterol-rich (0.25%) diet for 18 weeks then allicin (3 mg/kg, orally) for 10 weeks	↓ LDL and total cholesterol ↑ HDL	[56]
New Zealand White Rabbits (n = 6 per group) fed 1% cholesterol diet for 12 weeks with or without 1% garlic	↓ LDL, triglycerides and CETP ↑ HDL	[57]
Rabbits (n = 42) fed 0.5% cholesterol diet for 16 weeks with or without garlic (0.25 g)	↓ cholesterol, triglycerides and atherosclerotic plaques	[58]
C57/BL/6 mice (n = 60) fed Paigen diet (17% fat, 1.25% cholesterol for 15 weeks) with or without allicin (9 mg/kg) for 15 weeks	50% decrease in aortic fatty streaks in allicin treated group but no effect on total blood lipids	[59]
LDL-R-/- (n= 13 per group) and apoE-/- mice (n = 12 per group) fed high (15.7%) fat diet with or without allicin (3 or 9 mg/kg) for 6 weeks	Allicin (9 mg/kg) ↓ atherosclerotic lesions by ~ 70% in the LDL receptor knockout mice and ~ 50% in the apoE knockout mice. No effect on total blood lipids	[60]

Study design	Result	Reference
ApoE*3-Leiden mice (n = 12 per group) fed high (15.7%) fat diet with or without allicin (0.28 g/L), DADS (0.27 g/kg) or Kwai garlic (42 g/kg) for 8 weeks	None of the garlic preparations investigated had any effect on total blood lipids	[61]
White Leghorn chicken pullets (n = 8 laying chickens and 6 broilers per group) fed diet containing either 3.8% garlic paste, solvent extract of the paste or garlic oil for 4 weeks	Significant ($p < 0.01$) ↓ in HMG-CoA reductase, cholesterol 7 alpha-hydroxylase, fatty acid synthetase and in representative pentose-phosphate pathway. Significant ↓ in serum lipids in response to the feeding of garlic fractions: serum total cholesterol by 20-25%, LDL by 28-41% and triglycerides by 10-26%; HDL failed to respond	[62]
Hy laying hens fed diet containing allicin (0-150 mg/kg) for 6 weeks	Dose-dependent allicin ↓ of serum triglyceride and cholesterol levels	[63]

Abbreviations used: CETP (cholesterol ester transfer protein), DADS (diallyldisulfide), FFA (free fatty acids), HDL (high density lipoprotein), HMGCoA (beta-hydroxy-beta-methylglutaryl coenzyme A), LDL (low density lipoprotein)

Of the seventeen studies, ten employed rodent models that displayed spontaneous [51, 52] or induced hypercholesterolemia [47-50, 53, 58-60]. The efficacy on reducing lipid levels appeared to vary depending on whether garlic [47-49, 52, 53] or allicin [50, 51, 58-60] was used. All five of the rodent studies that administered oral whole garlic for between four and six weeks reported either decreased circulating [48, 52, 53] or liver cholesterol [48, 49, 53] levels. Several of these rodent studies also reported changes in circulating free fatty acids [47], total lipids [49] or triglycerides [53] following whole garlic administration for between one and six weeks. Similar results were also seen following whole garlic administration in rabbit [57, 58] and chicken [62] models of hyperlipidemia.

The five rodent studies performed using allicin [50, 51, 58-60] produced differential efficacy. Two studies demonstrated beneficial effects on plasma lipids, namely falls in plasma triglycerides [50, 51] after five or six weeks of allicin administration, but with no apparent corresponding effect on cholesterol [50, 51]. Three murine studies further reported that allicin (9 mg/kg for 6 or 15 weeks) had no effects on circulating lipids [58-60]. In contrast a rabbit study of allicin (3 mg/kg for 10 weeks) reported a decrease in serum cholesterol as well as decreased LDL and increased HDL [56]. Decreases in serum cholesterol and triglycerides were also seen following allicin (0-150 mg/kg for 6 weeks) administration to laying hens [63].

Interestingly studies in which either oral garlic oil [54] or whole garlic [48, 49, 52, 56] were administered for between 4 and 12 weeks also reported a decrease in LDL and or increase in HDL levels. Finally, four studies looked at the generation of atherosclerotic plaques on the blood vessel walls of either mice [59, 60] or rabbits [54, 55, 58]. All four reported a sharp decrease in lesions after between ten and fifteen weeks of administration of either whole garlic [54, 58], garlic oil [55] or allicin [59-61] for between eight and fifteen weeks.

2.2.1. Possible Mechanisms; Evidence from In Vivo Animal Models

So, the question is why is there this difference in findings? Mice seemed unresponsive to the allicin in all three studies [59-61] but are known to be a good model for hyperlipidemia [64]. It is important also to note that rodents and rabbits are both considered to have similar cardiovascular physiology to humans, but are more difficult for the study of atherosclerotic lesions [64]. Dosages of whole garlic also varied from 50 mg/kg [53] to 5 g [47], resulting in a lack of standardization. A second issue that has arisen repeatedly in this book is the instability of allicin [46], which could also be a contributing factor. More important might be the length of time the animals received the garlic or allicin preparation. No weekly monitoring of the effects of garlic was done, excepting in one study, that reported maximal efficacy at between three and five weeks of garlic administration [50]. Additional benefits on atherosclerosis only appeared after eight weeks [54, 55, 58-61], suggesting an extension to the length of these studies. Finally, garlic contains a variety of entities which could be acting synergistically to impair lipid and cholesterol synthesis [39]. Both S-allyl-cysteine (SAC) and diallyldisulfide (DADS), the major metabolities of allicin are also known to impair cholesterol synthesis for example [39].

But if garlic and or allicin is not working directly against hyperlipidemia, what other mechanisms could be involved? One hypothesis was suggested by two groups [54, 55] namely that garlic "*mobilized cholesterol*" from the vessels, possibly through elevating HDL [54]. Circulating cholesterol levels might therefore initially rise following garlic treatment, later falling as has been suggested by these authors [54, 55]. Again, this underlines the need for longer observations even in animal-based studies. HDL levels undergo feedback regulation through CETP; inhibition of this molecule in turn decreases LDL levels and increases HDL [25]. A study of hypercholesteremic rabbits fed 1% garlic for 12 weeks demonstrated a simultaneous decrease in LDL and CETP expression together with significant ($p < 0.01$) elevations of HDL in these animals [56]. More recent studies have provided yet another pathway for allicin to affect, namely ABCA1 transporter [64]. As previously stated, ABCA1 transporters are responsible for moving cell cholesterol and phospholipids onto HDL, thereby preventing the initiation of atherosclerosis [21]. Allicin (2.5-40 g/L for 24 hours) pretreatment of human monocyte (THP-1)-induced foam cells (phorbol myristate acetate-induced) was found to decrease total lipids, free cholesterol and cholesterol ester levels in these cells [65]. Further analysis revealed the effects to be mediated by allicin's inhibition of peroxisome proliferator-activated receptor γ (PPARγ) signaling and increased expression of ABCA1 [64]. Studies by Gonen and colleagues [60] also demonstrated that allicin was able to bind to the thiol groups of LDL, preventing its uptake by monocytes and macrophages. If reflected in other cell types, this latter effect might go some way to explaining the reductions in overall lipids seen in garlic and allicin-treated animals.

2.3. Effects of Allicin and Garlic on Hyperlipidemia; Human Studies

Although there were four meta analyses of garlic's efficacy on hyperlipidemia in the 1980s and 1990s [66], three more recent studies during the past decade were selected for review in this section [19, 67, 68]. Both meta analyses only examined studies which were original (i.e., not duplicate publications), double blind randomized and placebo controlled design and extracted these using PubMed, EMBASE and Cochrane Library databases [19, 67, 68]. Studies that did not report initial and final lipid values or document changes were not evaluated [19, 67, 68].

Khoo and colleagues [67] produced the earliest of the three meta analyses and identified thirteen trials from over 1,200 papers that matched the criteria listed above. Statistical analyses did not uncover any differences between either serum cholesterol or triglyerides when garlic was administered for between twelve weeks and six months [67]. Two of the trials are notable as they involved completely healthy individuals, which might explain some of the lack of efficacy, and there was no standardization as to the "garlic" preparations used

Some four years later, Ried and colleagues [68] evaluated garlic's efficacy based on thirty seven studies, but closer examination indicates that eight of these involved aged Kyolic garlic which has S-allyl cysteine (SAC) as the major bioactive ingredient. Garlic preparations used were primarily powder or oil although Allicor was used in two studies. Ried and colleagues [68] determined that garlic was effective "*in patients with elevated cholesterol ((< 200 mg/dL) when used for at least two months or longer)*". They did not find any effect of garlic on HDL or triglyceride levels [68].

Sun and colleagues [19] produced the most recent of the meta analyses which was based on fourteen papers that were also double blinded (from an original of nearly one thousand) published between 1981 and 2016 that met the criteria. One of the included studies was, however, on aged black garlic reducing the number to thirteen studies in this review. Several variables were noted for the studies including a differing preparations (garlic powder or oil), a wide range of doses (0.3g to 20 g/day) and various study durations (one to twelve months) [19]. Despite these variations, Sun and colleagues [19] reported statistically significant ($p < 0.01$) decreases in cholesterol and LDL and increases in HDL across the studies [19]. No differences in triglycerides were seen.

Dyslipidemia is also a major issue in other conditions particularly type II diabetes [69]. Interestingly a recent meta analysis of DBRPCT trials of garlic's effects on type II diabetes patients was similarly positive [69]. Similar databases and criteria were used as for the three meta analyses discussed above, but the authors also employed MagIran and Irandoc to identify the thirty three of twenty three thousand papers that were evaluated [69]. Shabani and colleagues [69] reported that garlic (500-20,000 mg) significantly reduced cholesterol, triglycerides and LDL when utilized for between two and one hundred and eighty two days. Interestingly, there was also a corresponding significant decrease ($p < 0.01$) in fasting blood glucose and HbA_{1c} in patients taking garlic [69]. The diabetic patients in these thirty three studies had high hyperlipidemia (> 200 mg/dL) [69].

Most of the crititicisms from authors conducting these meta analyses have been a reliance on the use of garlic powder (which has a highly variable allicin content) as well as the differential constructs of the trials. In fact, a highly publicized DBRPCT study by Gardner and colleagues [70] in 2005 threatened to deter any future garlic trials when it reported no effects on any lipids in patients after six months of administration. The study of 192 patients with moderate hypercholesterolemia (130-150 mg/dL LDL) compared three preparations of garlic, namely raw, powdered-stabilized allicin (Garlicin) and aged garlic (Kyolic), which had been assessed ahead of delivery for allicin or SAC content [70].

Since then two, DBRPC trials of slow release allicin (Allicor) on patients with hypercholesterolemia have been performed yielding positive results [71, 72]. In their first trial, Sobenin and colleagues [71] investigated forty two patients with mild hypercholesterolemia who received either Allicor (600 mg) or placebo for eight to twelve weeks. The second trial [72] investigated fifty two patients with high hypercholesterolemia who received Allicor (300 mg) versus placebo for twelve months. In both studies, all patients in the Allicor group demonstrated statistically ($p < 0.05$) lower LDL levels than those in the placebo group [71, 72]. Interestingly, male patients demonstrated statistically significant ($p < 0.001$) changes in cholesterol and triglycerides, including HDL improvement, at the end of the study [71, 72].

While Sobenin's studies are both smaller it is to be noted that they were conducted for twice as long, with patients exhibiting high lipid levels and with a garlic preparation that is "slow release" [71, 72]. Support for enteric coated tablets as providing the continuous supply of allicin needed to reduce blood lipids comes from a second DBRPCT [73]. Forty six patients with high cholesterol (6.5-9.0 mmol/L) were given either an enteric garlic tablet (non-commercial equivalent to 2.6 g garlic) or placebo for twelve weeks [73]. At the end of the study the garlic treated group exhibited significant reductions ($p < 0.05$) in cholesterol and LDL compared with placebo subjects [73]. These latter three human studies on allicin-based products raise more questions than they provide answers, but do underline the need for similarly structured DBRPCT that investigate different levels of hyperlipidemia and evaluate patients more regularly during the trials rather than at the beginning and the end.

3. Allicin, Garlic and Endothelial Cell Inflammation

Twelve *in vitro* [75-82] or animal studies [83-86] have sought to determine the effects of either allicin or garlic preparations containing allicin on endothelial cell activation pathways as shown in Table 3. Since not all garlic preparations contain allicin, data will only be analyzed from those studies in which this thiosulfinate is likely to be present namely garlic powder or garlic oil [74].

Ten of the twelve studies employed allicin [75-82, 85, 86] and reported similar data as was seen using fresh garlic [83, 84]. Allicin and fresh garlic produced their anti-inflammatory effects through downregulation of ROS [75-78, 84, 86] or NO [79-81, 83, 85] generation through activation of Nrf2 [84-86] and the P13K/Akt pathways [82]. Decreases in ROS and NO seen in these studies was also associated with a decrease in general vascular activation resulting in depressed nuclear kappa beta (NF-κB) expression [76, 77, 84]. These data are in keeping with the findings for allicin as an antioxidant, anti-inflammatory and Nrf2 activator in other organ systems (see Chapter 3 for details). The ability of allicin (25-100 μM) to increase the activation of the phosphatidylinositol-3-OH-kinase/protein kinase B/mammalian target of rapamycin pathway (P13K/Akt/MTOR) *in vitro* [82] adds further support for an SREBP-mediated mechanism for the thiosulfinate. mTOR is now understood to be known to be a regulator of SREBP, although the exact mechanism remains unclear [87]. No human trials on allicin's effects on underlying CVD inflammation have yet been undertaken.

4. Allicin, Garlic, Platelet Activation and Fibrinolytic Activity

Four literature *in vitro* studies have appeared that discuss allicin directly and its effects on human platelet aggregation [88-91]. Interestingly Apitz-Castro and colleagues [92], as well as subsequent authors, have described that a second principle from garlic, ajoene was also anti-aggregatory [66, 92]. The first studies of allicin extracted it from garlic oil (1-13 mM) and reported an inhibition of aggregation but with no effect on either the precursor arachidonic acid (AA) or thromboxane A (TXA_2) formation. They hypothesized allicin affected calcium uptake preventing platelet granule mobilization [88]. Later studies by Makheja and Bailey [89] reported similar findings as those of Mayeux but made no suggestion as to a mechanism of action.

Table 3. CVD inflammatory pathways affected by allicin or garlic

In vitro studies	Experimental design	Reference
ROS	HUVECs pre-treated with allicin (30 and 100 μg/ml) and then exposed to oxidized LDL (ox-LDL 150 μg/ml) for 24 h; ↓ ROS by suppressing NADPH oxidase activity and death of cells (↓ caspase 3 induction)	[75]
NF-κB, ROS	HUVECs treated with allicin (40 μg/ml) and LPS (1 μg/ml) for 24 h: ↓ NF-κB also ROS	[76]
NF-κB, ROS	Isolated high glucose (25 mmol/L)-stimulated murine vein endothelial cells treated with allicin (10 μg/ml) for 24 h; ↓ NF-κB, ROS and oxidative stress through Nox4 and PKC inhibition	[77]
ROS, lipid peroxidation	Methyl linoleate (144 mm) oxidation in AMVN (0.5 mM) was ↓ in presence of allicin (100 μg/ml) after 12 minutes AMVN (0.5 mM) when dissolved in acetonitrile and exposed to air → peroxyl radicals; ↓ radical generation in presence of allicin (100 μg/ml) after 12 minutes	[78]
NO synthesis	H9c2 cells pre-treated with allicin (0.2, 0.5 and 1 μM 1 h) and exposed to hypoxic stress (5% CO_2, 95% N_2) for 12 h; ↑ eNOS-derived NO	[79]
NO synthesis	HUVEC incubated with TNF-α (5 ng/ml) in the presence or absence of allicin (500 μg/ml) for 20 h; ↓ NO release	[80]
NO synthesis	Myocytes from neonatal Wistar rats stimulated with LPS (10 μg/ml) in presence or absence of allicin (10, 40, 50 or 200 μM) for 24 hours; allicin ↓ iNOS at higher concentrations (200 μM) and ↑ at lower concentrations (50 μM)	[81]
P13K/Akt/ MTOR	Neonatal rat cardiomyocytes (Wistar rats) incubated with angiotensin (100 nM, 48 h) then treated with either allicin (25, 50 or 100 μM) or control for a further 48 h; ↑ phosphorylation of ERK, Akt and P13K (50 μM) Effects of 50 μM allicin were reversed by rapamycin (1 μM) indicating these effects are mediated through the P13K/Akt/MTOR pathway following allicin treatment compared with that in angiotensin-treated cardiomyocytes	[82]
***In vivo* studies**	**Experimental design**	**Reference**
NO synthesis	Congestive heart failure Wistar rats (n = 8-10 per treatment) fed with raw garlic extract (1 g orally) for 3 weeks or 1 days before treatment with monocrotaline (60 mg/kg i.p.), euthanized 3 weeks later and coronary arteries isolated and contracted by raising intraluminal pressure; raw garlic preserved the ability of the right coronary arteries to respond to acetylcholine via eNOS derived NO.	[83]
NF-κB, antioxidant enzymes, Nrf2 (Keap)	Fructose fed (65% of feed) Sprague Dawley rats (n = 7) also supplemented 250 mg/ kg/day fresh garlic homogenate for 8 weeks; ↓ NF-κB and Keap ↑ GSH, GpX of cardiac tissue	[84]
Nrf2	Sprague Dawley rats (n=9) infused with angiotensin (250 mg/kg via osmotic pump) for 14 days and fed allicin (180 mg/kg) for 8 weeks; ↑ Nrf2 in cardiac tissue compared with control animals without angiotensin	[85]
Antioxidant enzymes, Nrf2, NO	Wistar rats (n = 6 per group) CKD model created by kidney ablation and administered allicin (40 mg/kg orally) for 6 weeks; allicin ↓ angiotensin 1 receptor expression in the heart ↑ Nrf2, CAT, SOD and GpX and ↓Keap compared with CKD animals that had not received allicin	[86]

Abbreviations used: AMVN (2, 2' Azobis (2, 4 dimethylvaleronitrile), CAT (catalase), CD (chronic kidney disease), eNOS (endothelial nitric oxide synthase), ERK (extracellular initiated kinase), GpX (glutathione peroxidase), GSH (glutathione synthase), HUVEC (human vein endothelial cells), iNOS (inducible nitric oxide synthase), Keap (Kelch-like ECH-associated protein 1), LDL (low density lipoprotein), LPS (lipopolysaccharide), NADPH (nicotinamide adenine dinucleotide phosphate), NF-κB (nuclear factor kappa beta), NO (nitric oxide), Nrf2 (NF-E2, p45-related factor 2), NF-κB (nuclear factor kappa beta), P13K/Akt/MTOR (phosphatidylinositol-3-OH-kinase/ protein kinase B/ mammalian target of rapamycin), PKC (protein kinase C), ROS (reactive oxygen species), SOD (superoxide dismutase)

Briggs and colleagues [90] compared four garlic thiosulfinates for their ability to impair human platelet aggregation *in vitro*. They reported that allicin was the strongest of the thiosulfinates tested [90]. Allicin at 0.4 mM inhibited platelet aggregation by ninety percent, compared with thirty five percent for aspirin when used at 0.36 mM [90]. Again, no mechanism was advanced by Briggs and colleagues [90]. Although aspirin and allicin were compared in this study it seemed unlikely at this point that they were using the same mechanism of action since aspirin impairs TXA_2 formation [46]. TXA_2 is the first step in the pathway that allows a conformational change to occur in the platelet fibrinogen receptor integrin αIIbβ3 (glycoprotein IIbIIIa) and aggregation to occur [46].

4.1. Possible Mechanisms; Evidence from *In Vivo* Animal Models

Interestingly the last of the four studies reported that allicin possessed a novel method of inhibiting platelet aggregation, namely it directly affected the αIIbβ3 receptor itself [91]. Manaster and colleagues [91] compared the activity of allicin (40 μM) with that of the known thiol-blocking agent disulfiram (40 μM) in preventing human platelet aggregation initiated by the monoclonal antibody PT-25. They reported that at this concentration both agents inhibited αIIbβ3-fibrinogen binding to a similar degree and decreased P-selectin expression [91]. Allicin (20-40 μM) inhibited platelet aggregation induced by collagen (5 μg/ml), epinephrine (55 μM) or adenosine diphosphate (10 μM) [91].

Animal studies of garlic's anti-platelet effects have been relatively few but at least three are of note, all involving rabbit models [54, 58, 93]. Hyperlipidemic rabbits fed garlic oil (0.5 mg/kg for 12 weeks) reported an increase in fibrinolytic activity and a decrease in the platelet adhesive index [54]. A second rabbit study also correlated a rise in fbrinolytic activity after administration of garlic juice (0.25 g for 16 weeks) [58]. The third study involved pre-treatment of mixed breed rabbits (n =5) with an aqueous extract of garlic (500 mg/kg) for ten miunutes followed by a lethal injection of arachidonate or collagen (140 mg/kg) [93]. Ali and colleagues [93] observed no changes in serum TXB_2; results in keeping with the *in vitro* findings on allicin [87, 88]. This study also confirmed that the garlic treatment and impaired platelet aggregation, thereby preventing the lethal thrombosis produced by arachidonate or collagen [93].

A final recent study of interest appears to confirm allicin's effects on platelet recetors, this time inhibiting platelet endothelial cell adhesion molecule-1 (PECAM-1) [94]. Allicin (5, 10 or 20 mg/kg/day for 4 weeks) was able to impair the expression of PECAM-1 in Wistar rats (n = 10) that had undergone aortic ligation to produce a model of cardiac hypertrophy [94]. These studies are of note as they simultaneously reduced PECAM-1 expression and decreased the hypertension which the animals displayed [94]. Pilong and colleagues also reported that allicin at all doses prevented cardiomyopathy by decreasing the death of the endothelial cells that lined the vasculature of the rodents' hearts [94].

4.2. Effects of Allicin and Garlic on Platelet Activation; Human Studies

Ten DBRPCT human trials of garlic oil [95-97], powder [98-102], raw garlic [103] or stabilized allicin (Allicor) [104] have appeared in the literature of which eight reported positive findings [95-101, 103]. The design and findings of these studies are summarized in Table 4 below.

Table 4. Platelet effect DBRPCT studies of allicin-containing products

Study design	Results	Reference
Short term: 5 healthy volunteers (30-35 y) given garlic oil from garlic (1 g) for 5 days Long term: 5 healthy and 10 CAD patients (40-60 y) for 4 weeks	No effect on platelet activation after 5 days ↓ platelet activation after 4 weeks, garlic oil *in vitro* inhibited the production of TXB_2 and the uptake of AA by platelets	[95]
20 healthy volunteers (mean age 26 y) given garlic oil (18 mg, 4 weeks)	↓ platelet activation that correlated with improved lipid functions (fall in cholesterol and increased HDL) ↑ AA and phospholipids in the red blood cells	[96]
14 healthy volunteers (mean age 32 y) given garlic oil extract (9.9 g of garlic) as one dose	Four hours after garlic administration ↓ platelet aggregation by 12%	[97]
120 healthy subjects (mean age = 24 y) given garlic powder tablets (900 mg, 4 weeks)	Elimination of spontaneous thrombocyte aggregation and decrease in plasma viscosity ↓ diastolic blood pressure by ~ 10% and blood glucose concentration by ~ 12%	[98]
120 healthy volunteers (mean age 25 y) given garlic powder tablets (800 mg, 8 weeks)	10% ↓ in circulating platelet aggregates and > 50% ↓ in spontaneous platelet aggregation	[99]
12 healthy volunteers given garlic powder tablets (900 mg for 2 weeks)	After four or six hours ↑ plasminogen activator and ↓decrease fibrinolytic activity After one to two weeks ↓ platelet aggregation	[100]
280 atherosclerotic subjects (50-80 y) given garlic powder tablets (90 mg, for up to 48 months)	61 of the subjects in the garlic group were able to be compared with 91 in the placebo group for a full four years ↓ Platelet aggregation, plasma viscosity and a decrease in atherosclerotic plaque size ~ 20%)	[101]
Hypercholesterolemic patients (mean age not provided in paper) given dried garlic 34 (594 mg, 6 weeks) 51 (1,350 mg, 6 weeks)	No effect on platelet aggregation	[102]
18 healthy volunteers (mean age 29 y) given tsatsiki with or without garlic (4.2 g) for 1 week	No effect on platelet aggregation	[103]
29 atherosclerotic men (35-70 y) given Allicor (80 μg/ml for 2 weeks)	↓ ADP-induced platelet aggregation by 25% and ↑ fibrinolytic activity by ~ 20%	[104]

Abbreviations used: AA (arachidonic acid), ADP (adenosine diphosphate), HDL (high density lipoprotein), y (years)

These studies are of interest in that various subjects were investigated including healthy individuals [95-99, 100, 103] and those with atherosclerosis and or hyperlipidemia [95, 101, 102, 104]. One of the studies, by Sobenin and colleagues [104], extended the group's findings on Allicor's mediation of lipid profiles to anti-platelet activity. Interestingly, long-term (up to forty-eight month) administration of garlic powder (900 mg) correlated with decreased platelet aggregation, plasma viscosity and a decrease in atherosclerotic plaque size [104]. In one very long-term study, sixty-one of the subjects in the garlic group were able to be compared with ninety-one in the placebo group for a full four years [101]. The results of garlic treatment on atherosclerotic plaque persistence was particularly staggering with decreases of nearly twenty percent over this time period [101]. It is important to note that similar results were also reported in animal models and correlated with plasma lipid changes [54, 55, 58-60], again underlining the interrelated nature of these pathological changes. Three studies reported no effects on platelet aggregation [95, 102, 103]. One of these involved two studies, employing different doses of dried garlic and a duration of six weeks [102]. Why this produced no effects on platelets is unknown although "dried garlic" is known to be hypervariable in chemical consistency [74]. A second study involved healthy subjects and was for only one week [102]. Similar data were also reported by Bordia and colleagues [94] in their study of healthy subjects, which might go some way to explain the lack of changes.

Studies were variable in length (4 hours to 48 months), subject recruitment (healthy versus CVD patients) and garlic preparation, making overall analyses complex. Apart from three larger DBRPCT [98, 99, 101], the studies were small, involving between 5 and 51 patients [94-97, 100, 102-104]. It is also important to note at this point that although other human trials of garlic have been performed and reported positive anti-aggregation data, these were either unblinded or utilized garlic unlikely to contain allicin [66]. Despite the relatively few studies on garlic's effects on platelet aggregation its use remains contraindicated for patients on anticoagulant therapies such as warfarin [105] and is still considered to impact blood coagulation.

5. Allicin, Garlic and Hypertension

As blood pressure is an easy non-invasive way to monitor CVD, the effects of garlic and to some extent allicin have been monitored with some frequency [66]. In total over a hundred studies have been performed to investigate the effects of whole garlic preparations containing allicin on models of hypertension [50, 51, 106-111] and DBRCT of human patients [113-116]. Since not all garlic preparations contain allicin, data will only be analyzed from those studies in which this thiosulfinate is likely to be present namely garlic powder or garlic oil [74].

5.1. Effects of Allicin and Garlic on Hypertension; Animal Studies

At least eight well constructed animal studies have appeared in the literature [50, 51, 106-111], the details of which are summarized in Table 5 below.

Table 5. Allicin or garlic containing allicin and hypertension

Experimental Design	Result	Reference
Sprague Dawley rats (n = 90; 3 groups) fed fructose-rich diet (60%, 5 weeks); Allicin given for last 2 weeks (8 mg/kg/day, orally), compared with control and enalapril (20 mg/kg/day, orally)	Allicin ↓ blood pressure at 3 and 5 weeks; effects were especially evident on weeks 3-5. Comparable with enapralil	[50]
Male spontaneously hypertensive rats (n = 20; 2 groups) treated with or without allicin (80 mg/kg/ day orally) for 6 weeks	Allicin ↓ blood pressure to normal range after 6 weeks	[51]
Healthy dogs (n = 70) treated with or without garlic crushed extract (12.7-107.6 mg/kg I.V.). Cannulation of femoral vein and artery to obtain data	IC_{50} was 25.1 mg/kg to produce a 50% fall in blood pressure; unrelated to depression of cardiac output or stimulation of muscarinic receptors	[106]
Sprague Dawley rats (n = 40, 4 groups) hypertension artificially produced using 2 kidney 1 clip model. Treatment animals received garlic extract (500 mg/kg 0.5 ml aqueous I.V.) or garlic extract + L-NAME (0.5 mg/kg)	Garlic treatment had no effect on pressure in normotensive animal but significantly ↓ effects of L-NAME	[107]
In vivo and *Ex vivo* Sprague Dawley rats (n = 10) fed either gum arabic solution (5%) with or without garlic powder (100 mg/kg/day) for 5 days. Trachea removed, 5 rings cut per animal and studied.	Garlic inhibited acute hypoxic PV. No difference in mean arterial pressure or heart rate response to hypoxia was seen.	[108]
Ex vivo Sprague Dawley rats (n = 35) anesthetized and lungs removed and artificially aerated. Isolated lungs perfused and allicin (10-100 mg) injected into vascular bed.	Allicin reversed elevation of PV (U-46619 infusion) in a dose-dependent manner.	[109]
Hypertension induced in Wistar albino rats (n = 30) by streptozotocin (50 mg/kg, I.P.) infusion and allicin (8 mg/kg/ day oral) administered for 8 weeks	↓ BP of hypertensive rats *In vitro* studies suggested efficacy was produced by SUR-2 with SUR-1 potentiating allicin's effects	[110]
Hypertension induced in Wistar rats (n = 32, 8 per group) using 2 kidney 1 clip model. Test group received chopped garlic extract (50 mg/kg/day oral) for 4 weeks	↓ BP in garlic extract treated group and ACE activity	[111]

Abbreviations used: ACE (angiotensin-converting enzyme), BP (blood pressure), GME (garlic methanolic extract), IC_{50} (concentration used to produce a 50% decrease in function), I.V. (intravenous), L-NAME (L-nitroarginine methylester), PV (pulmonary vasoconstriction), SUR (sulphonurea receptor)

Three of the eight studies utilized pure allicin (8-100 mg/kg/day [50, 51, 109], All studies, excepting one [108] reported a significant fall in systemic blood pressure (BP) [50, 51, 106-111] with at least four suggesting mechanisms that could involve allicin [107-111].

5.1.1. Possible Mechanisms; Evidence from In Vivo Animal Models

Studies by Khaled and colleagues [107] reported that the efficacy of garlic extract in their model could be attributed to its ability to remove the block on NO production [107]. The observation that the effects of L-nitroarginine methylester (L-NAME), a known nitric oxidase inhibitor, were reversed by garlic was given as proof of these effects [107]. These results were duplicated in a second study with L-NAME [108] In contrast, a second study determined that allicin's effects were not impaired by inhibitors of NO, cyclooxygenase enzymes or inherent bronchomotor contraction indicating a separate mechanism of action [109]. Allicin has been previously shown to affect endothelial cell eNOS or iNOS [79, 81, 83] but is primarily considered to be an anti-oxidant and Nrf2 modulator [46]. Nrf2 inhibitors were not investigated in the latter study so it is difficult to determine if this might have been the mechanism involved. These inconsistencies underline the importance of using pure allicin as opposed to garlic, which is a mixture of moieties [74].

A second direct effect of allicin may be by acting as a sulfonurea receptor (SUR-2) opening agent [110]. SUR-2 receptors are present on cardiac tissues and when these potassium gated receptors open, they result in a decrease in blood pressure [110]. Several available therapeutics used in the treatment of angina are SUR-2 openers and this may add an additional property to allicin [110].

An indirect method by which garlic might affect hypertension is through its effects on the renin system [86, 87, 111]. Vasodilatation may also be mediated by the inhibitory effects of allicin on the renin-angiotensin system of the kidney [86, 87, 111]. One animal study by Sharifi and colleagues [111] suggested that garlic may mediate vasodilatation by directly inhibiting the angiotensin-converting enzyme (ACE). They further point to garlic extraction methods being important to retain hypotensive efficacy; ethanol extraction (destroys allicin) being ineffective on hypertension and aqueous (retains allicin) producing BP reduction [111]. When combined with the studies of Trejo and colleagues [86, 87], who demonstrated that allicin was equipotent to enalapril [87], suggest garlic may be the potential source of a new ACE inhibitor.

Another potential hypotensive mechanism for allicin may result from its rapid breakdown into sulfur containing compounds [112]. Red blood cells are able to utilize sulfur compounds to generate hydrogen sulfide (H_2S), which produces vasodilatation through potassium ion-induced hyperpolarization of vascular smooth muscle cells [112]. Which of these combinations of vasodilatory effects can be ascribed to allicin remains to be determined.

5.2. Effects of Allicin and Garlic on Hypertension; Human Studies Meta Analyses

Several clinical meta analyses of garlic and hypertension have appeared in the literature since the 1970s [66, 113-116], with the four most recent being analyzed in this chapter. All meta analyses only examined studies which were original (i.e., not duplicate publications), double blind randomized and placebo controlled design and extracted these using PubMed, EMBASE and Cochrane Library databases [113-]. Studies that did not report initial and final BP values or document changes were not evaluated [113-116]. A summary of their findings is shown in Table 6 below.

Only one of these DBRPCT directly involved administration of allicin (Allicor, 600 mg), Kwai garlic (900 mg) or placebo to eighty four hypertensive men for eight weeks [117]. Allicor and Kwai garlic (which contains allicin) produced comparable significant decreases in systolic and diastolic BP of approximately 10% [117]. Allicor and Kwai were equally effective for the enrolled subjects with both moderate and mild hypertension [117]. This trial was also the first suggesting that the anti-hypertension effects of garlic in humans could be attributed to allicin [117]

Table 6. Meta analyses of DBRPCT garlic efficacy on hypertension

Number of trials identified	Subjects in evaluated trials and study durations	Results	Reference
11/153 (#1)	Normotensive and hypertensive; 8-12 weeks	~ 10% ↓ in blood pressure	[113]
20 (#4)	Normotensive and hypertensive; 8-12 weeks	~ 14% ↓ in blood pressure	[114]
7/213 (#2)	Hypertensive; 8-12 weeks	~ 10% ↓ in blood pressure	[115]
17/245 (#4)	Normotensive and hypertensive; 8-12 weeks	~ 8% ↓ in blood pressure	[116]

= number of trials with aged garlic

Analyses of early DBRPCT by Reinhart and colleagues [118] reported that garlic only decreased elevated BP and had no effects on normotensive patients. Furthermore, Simons and colleagues [119] have critiqued the findings of Ried, stating that the positive findings should be interpreted with caution as many aspects of even these few trials were flawed. Poor documentation of how BP was taken, the angle of the arm during measurement and differing preparations ranging from garlic oil and powder to pure allicin (Allicor) were cited in Simon's publication [119]. Despite these issues it is important to note that an efficacy similar to conventional BP medications was reported by these studies [113-116]. It is however also clear that DBRPCT with standardized testing methods and garlic preparations are needed.

6. Allicin and Bacterial Dysregulation

Allicin is strongly antibacterial, as was previously discussed in detail in chapter 3. It is of note at this point that some *in vitro* [66, 120] and *in vivo* studies [120] have reported antibacterial efficacy against the primary oral and gut biome flora isolated from atherosclerotic plaques, namely *Streptococci*, *P. gingivalis* and *Fusarium* species [66, 120]. Studies by Wu and colleagues [120], also reported a signifiant ($p < .01$) decrease in TMAO levels in carnitine fed C57BL/6 mice that received allicin (10 mg/kg/day) for six weeks [121]. This antibacterial and regulatory capability could constitute wide-ranging benefits for allicin not only in the prevention of periodontal disease [120], but also in reducing the risk factors for initiating CVD [7, 8], as discussed earlier in this chapter.

7. Conclusion

Much of garlic's historical usage has been tied to reduction of cardiovascular effects as has the research into its efficacy [1-5, 66]. The majority of investigative studies, especially human DBRPCT, have focused on determining the utility of garlic as ameliorating blood lipid profiles [19, 47-63, 67, 68] or as hypotensive [50, 51, 106-116]. Interestingly, anti-hypertensive effects of garlic as a tincture were first observed by modern physicians Loeper and Debray in 1921 [122]. Their findings were one reason why garlic was used as a hypotensive agent by American physicians until the 1950s, when it was replaced by mainstream cardiovascular medicines [123].

Garlic is also already in use in the prevention and intervention of mild CVD in ten European countries where twenty separate formulations of the bulb are available [124]. A recent European Report on garlic as a whole [124] concluded that "*garlic supplementation might produce mild benefits on decreasing lipids, platelet activity and blood pressure*" [124]. This is in keeping with a 1999 World Health Organization Monograph [125] which concluded that there was support for garlic's use *"as an adjuvant to dietetic management in the treatment of hyperlipidaemia, and in the prevention of atherosclerotic (age-dependent) vascular changes. The drug may be useful in the treatment of mild hypertension."* In contrast the Federal Drug Administration (FDA) has not yet provided suggestions of garlic intake to prevent CVD, adhering instead to guidelines of low fat, low sodium and exercise [126]. It is likely therefore that allicin will need to prove itself through a variety of DBRPCT before being deemed acceptable in developed countries outside Europe.

Garlic has set some precedent for allicin but to be successful in the classical pharmaceutical market this derivative molecule will need to follow standard development strategies [127]. This is a twelve-step protocol beginning with target identification and validation (function and role of the medication in the disease), and molecular interactions of the putative medicine [127]. Most important is the identification of a drug like molecule that is sufficiently stable to be evaluated *in vitro*, pre-clinical and finally human studies [127]. Approximately $9.2 million U.S.D. is needed to propel a medication through to clinical proof and FDA approval so initial confidence in allicin would certainly be needed in order to proceed.

7.1. Allicin: Target Identification, Validation and Putative Molecular Mechanisms

Pure allicin has been shown independently *in vitro*, *in vivo* and in a few human DBRPCT to produce abrogation of blood lipid profiles [35, 40-42, 50, 51, 53, 56, 59, 60, 63, 71, 72], endothelial cell activation [75-82, 85, 86], atherosclerotic lesions [59, 60], platelet aggregation [88-91, 104] and is hypotensive through vasodilatation [50, 51, 109, 112, 117]. Allicin was reported as equipotent to the anti-hypertensive enapralil *in vivo* [50] and nearly three times as active as aspirin *in vitro* [90]. Potentially an ACE inhibitor [86], SUR-2 opener [110] or statin-like molecule [45]. Allicin may also possess unique effects on lipid metabolism through SREBP [41] or ABCA1 [64] activity and on platelet aggregation through αIIbβ3 receptor binding [91]. These various putative effects are summarized in Figure 1.

7.2. Allicin: Development of Drug-Like Molecule and Safety Considerations

Allicin has provided a significant challenge to researchers in this respect due to its instability [46] but several innovations are now facilitating its use [71, 72, 104, 117, 124-126]. Slow release stabilized allicin (Allicor) has been successfully used in four DBRPCT and demonstrated efficacy against hyperlipidemia [71, 72], platelet aggregation [104] and hypertension [117]. Other double layer, targeted release tablets are also under development [128]. New semi-synthetic allicin-like molecules have already been designed through combinatorial chemistry and may have superior potency and absorbtion profiles for various aspects of CVD intervention [129, 130].

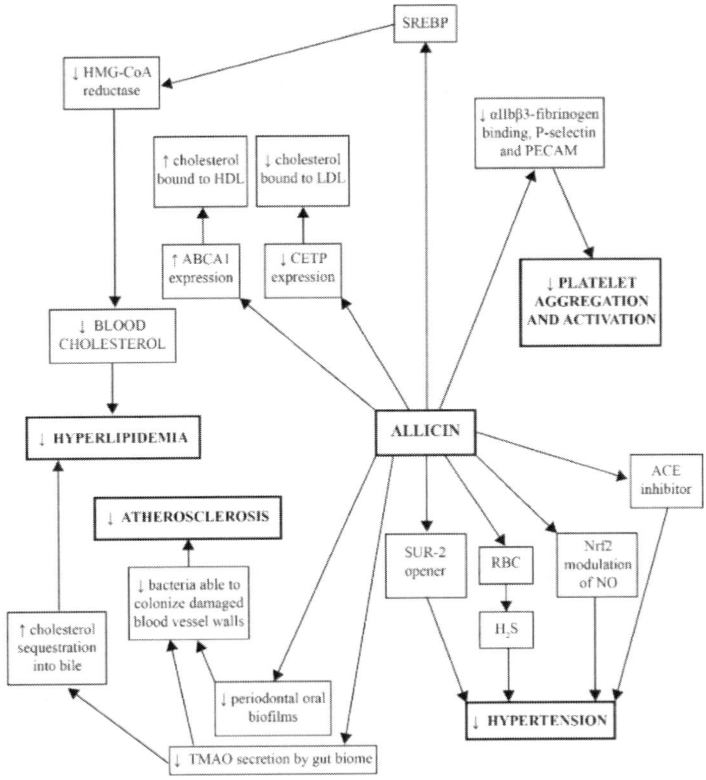

Legend: Allicin has interventional points on four cardinal dysfunctional events in CVD namely hyperlipidemia, platelet activation, oral and gut dysregulation and hypertension. Lipid lowering effects are potentially direct, by impairment of SREBP induced activation of cholesterol synthesis through HMG-CoA reductase, together with reduction of circulatory cholesterol by inceasing ABCA1 and decreasing CETP expression. Indirect reduction of blood lipids is mediated through decrease of gastrointestinal TMAO-secreting bacteria. Platelet activation and aggregation is decreased through inhibition of the αIIbβ3 receptor on platelets as well as impairment of P-selectin and PECAM-1 binding proteins. Allicin's modulation of hypertension, by increasing vasodilatation, can be achieved through several mechanisms including direct SUR-2 opening, inhibition of the renin angiotensin pathway (ACE inhibition) and nitric oxide secretion. Indirectly the breakdown of allicin may provide red cells with the sulfur components needed to secrete the vasodilator hydrogen sulfide. Finally, allicin's direct effects on oral and gut flora is believed to decrease their escape from the local milieu, colonization and aggravation of atherosclerotic plaque formation.

Abbreviations used in the figure: ACE (angiotensin-converting enzyme), αIIbβ3 (alpha 2 beta 3), CETP (cholesterol ester transfer protein), HMG CoA reductase (beta-hydroxy-beta-methylglutaryl coenzyme A), HDL (high density lipoprotein), H_2S (hydrogen sulfide), LDL (low density lipoprotein), NO (nitric oxide), PECAM (platelet endothelial cell adhesion molecule), RBC (red blood cells), SREBP (sterol regulatory element binding pathway), SUR-2 (sulfonurea receptor), TMAO (trimethylamine *N*-oxide)

References used to construct the figure: [41, 45, 50, 56, 64, 66, 81, 85, 86, 90, 91, 94, 110, 120].

Figure 1. Putative benefits of allicin on CVD.

While deemed safe as a nutraceutical [124, 125], the parent garlic has been shown to interact with several liver cytochromes (most notably P450 isoenzymes including CYP2C9) and either enhance or impair the metabolism of some medications including propranalol [124].

7.3. Allicin: Worth Developing for CVD

Nutraceuticals like allicin can provide relatively inexpensive and safe add on therapies for CVD patients with comorbitidies [131]. They are also useful for patients who either can not tolerate classic pharmaceuticals or who are unresponsive to them [131-133]. A prime example of the latter issue is resistance to the anti-coagulants aspirin or Plavix® (clopidogrel), which can affect from 0.4-83% depending on the population being treated [132]. Patients with resistance to these pharmaceuticals tend to be older as well as exhibiting a higher body mass i.e., many patients in developed countries [132]. These patients are also a population who are likely to advance to severe CVD more rapidly [132]. No DBRPCT on the effects of stabilized allicin on patients with "aspirin and/or clopidogrel resistance" have yet been performed. However, the positive preliminary anti-platelet data obtained on allicin to date are supportive of this being a direction that could provide much needed alternative for many at risk CVD patients. Statins have also been found to be ineffective in about one in three patients at reducing hyperlipidemia [133]. If allicin is affecting not just the HMG-CoA reductase enzyme (that is the statin target) but also SREBP, which modulates cholesterol synthesis, it might provide a new medication for this large group of patients.

Unlike the classical triad of CVD treatments of lipid lowering agents (statins), platelet aggregation inhibitors (aspirin, Plavix®) and beta blockers [14], allicin has the simultaneous potential to ameliorate all three (Figure 1) as well as reducing the primary risk factors of gut dysbiosis and periodontal disease [66, 120, 121]. Lowering a patient's risk factors for CVD also lowers their chance of developing type II diabetes [134] Patients with end stage renal disease are also more likely to develop or exacerbate their CVD [134]. CVD, hypertension and type II diabetes now affect millions around the world and their numbers continue to escalate [14, 134, 135]. Any intervention that reduces the risk of developing one or more of these conditions can effectively reduce the incidence of all and we can only hope that allicin can play a role in this endeavor.

REFERENCES

[1] Petrovska, Biljana B. & Svetlana, Cekovska. (2010). "Extracts from the history and medical properties of garlic". *Pharmacogn. Rev.*, *4*(7), 106-110.

[2] Bergner, Paul. (1996). "*The healing power of garlic*"., pp. 3-26. Rocklin, CA: Prima Publishing.

[3] Lawson, Larry D. (1998). "Garlic: a review of its medicinal effects and indicated active compounds". In: *Phytomedicines of Europe. Chemistry and Biological ACS Symposium Series 691* (Lawson L.D. & Bauer R eds.), pp. 176-209. American Chemical Society, Washington D.C.

[4] Moyers, Susan. (1996). "*Garlic in health, history and world cuisine*.," pp. 1-36. St. Petersberg, FL: Suncoast Press.

[5] Riddle, John M. (1996). "The medicines of Greco-Roman antiquity as a source for medicines today". In: *Prospecting for drugs in ancient and medieval European texts: A scientific approach* (Holland B.K. ed), pp. 7-17, Amsterdam, The Netherlands: Harwood Academic Publishers.

[6] Ambrose, John A. & Manmeet, Singh. (2015). "Pathophysiology of coronary artery disease leading to acute coronary syndromes." *F1000prime Reports*, *7*, 08. doi:10.12703/P7-08.

[7] Bu, Jin. & Zhaohui, Wang. (2018). "Cross-Talk between Gut Microbiota and Heart via the Routes of Metabolite and Immunity," *Gastroenterology Research and Practice*: Article ID 6458094. https://doi.org/10.1155/2018/6458094.

[8] Leishman, Shaneen J., Hong, L. Do. & Pauline, J. Ford. (2010). "Cardiovascular disease and the role of oral bacteria." *Journal of Oral Microbiology*, *2*, 10.3402/jom.v2i0.5781. doi: 10.3402/jom.v2i0.5781.

[9] Nowak, Witold N., Jiacheng, Deng., Xiong, Z. Ruan. & Quingbo, Xu. (2017). "Reactive oxygen species generation and atherosclerosis". *Arteriosclerosis, Thrombosis and Vascular Biology*, *37*, e41-e52. doi: 10.1161/ATVBAHA.117.309228.

[10] Schieber, Michael. & Navdeep, S. Chandel. (2014). "ROS Function in Redox Signaling and Oxidative Stress". *Current Biology: CB*, *24*(10), R453–R462. http://doi.org/10.1016/j.cub.2014.03.03

[11] Ahmed, S. M. U., Lin, Luo., Akhileshwar, Namani., Xiu, Jan Wang. & Xiuwen, Tang. (2016). "Nrf2 signaling pathway: Pivotal roles in inflammation". *Biochmimica et Biophysica Acta*, *1863*, 585-597. http://dx.doi.org/10.1016/j.badis.2016.11.005.

[12] Billingsley, Hayley E. & Salvatore, Carbone. (2018). "The antioxidant potential of the Mediterranean diet on patients at high cardiovascular risk: review of the PREDIMED. *Nutrition and Diabetes*, *8*, Article 13. https://www.nature.com/articles/s41387-018-0025-1.

[13] Giugliano, Dario., Antonio, Ceriello. & Katherine, Esposito. (2008). "Glucose metabolism and hyperglycemia." *The American Journal of Clinical Nutrition, 87*(1), 217S–222S. https://doi.org/10.1093/ajcn/87.1.217S.

[14] Stewart, Jack., Gavin, Manmathan. & Peter, Wilkinson. (2017). "Primary prevention of cardiovascular disease: A review of contemporary guidance and literature." *JRSM Cardiovascular Disease*. https://doi.org/10.1177/2048004016687211.

[15] Basilal, Sameer., José, M. Castellano. & Valentín, Fuster. (2015). "Global burder of CVD; focus on secondary prevention of cardiovascular disease. *Int. J Cardiology*, *201*, S1-S7.

[16] Celermajer, David S., Clara, K. Chow., Eloi, Marijon., Nicholas, M. Anstey. & Kam, S. Woo. (2012). "Cardiovascular disease in the developing world. Prevalences, patterns and the potential for early disease detection." *Journal of the American College of Cardiology*, *60*(13), 1207-1216. doi: 10.1016/j.jacc.2012.03.074.

[17] Cundell, Diana R. (2014). *Herbal phytochemicals as immunomodulators Current Immunology Reviews*, Volume 10, Issue 2, ISSN:1875-631X(Online), ISSN:1573-3955(Print). Accessed August 1, 2019. http://benthamscience.com/journal/index.php?journalID=cir.

[18] Qidwai, Waris. & Tabinda, Ashfaq. (2013). "Role of garlic usage in cardiovascular disease prevention: an evidence based approach." *Evidenc-Based Complementary and Alternative Medicine*, Article ID 125649, 9 pages. http://dx.doiorg/10.115/2013/125649.

[19] Sun, Yue-E., Weidong, Wang. & Jie, Qin. (2018). "Anti-hyperlipidemia of garlic by reducing the level of total cholesterol and low-density lipoprotein. A meta-analysis." *Medicine*, *97*, pe0255 doi: 10.1097/MD.0000000000010255.

[20] Wang, Hai-Peng., Jing, Yang., Li-Qiang, Qin. & Xiang-Jun, Yang. (2015). Effect of garlic on blood pressure: A meta analysis. *J Clin Hypertens (Greenwich).*, *17*, 223–231. doi: 10.1111/jch.12473.

[21] Galkina, Elena. & Klaus, Ley. (2009). "Immune and inflammatory mechanisms of atherosclerosis." *Annual Review of Immunology, 27*, 165-97. doi: 10.1146/annurev.immunol.021908.132620.

[22] Tompin, Gerald H. & Daphne, Owens. (2012). "LDL as a cause of atherosclerosis." *The Open Atherosclerosis and Thrombosis Journal, 5*, 13-21. https://benthamopen.com/contents/pdf/TOATHERTJ/TOATHERTJ-5-13.pdf.

[23] Liscum, Laura. (2002). "Chapter 15: Cholesterol biosynthesis." *In Biochemistry of Lipids, Lipoproteins and Membranes* 4th Ed, edited by D.E. Vance and J.E. Vance, 409-431. Amsterdam, NE: Elsevier Science Accessed on July 28, 2019. http://bio.ijs.si/~krizaj/group/Predavanja%202011/Biochemistry%20Lipids%20Lipoproteins%20and%20Membranes/15.pdf.

[24] Clayton, Peter T. (1998). "Disorders of cholesterol biosynthesis." *Arch. Dis. Child., 78*, 185-189. https://adc.bmj.com/content/archdischild/78/2/185.full.pdf.

[25] Shattat, G. F. (2014). "A review article on hyperlipidemia: types, treatments and new drug targets." *Biomed Pharmacol. J.*, *7*(2). Accessed on July 28, 2019. doi: http://dx.doi.org/10.13005/bpj/504.

[26] Lee, Ji-Young. & Timothy, P. Carr. (2004). "Dietary Fatty Acids Regulate Acyl-CoA:Cholesterol Acyltransferase and Cytosolic Cholesteryl Ester Hydrolase in Hamsters." *The Journal of Nutrition, 134*(12), 3239–3244, https://doi.org/10.1093/jn/134.12.3239.

[27] Wang, Xiadong., Ryuchiro, Sato., Michael, S. Brown., Xianxin, Hua. & Joseph, L. Goldstein. (1994). "SREBP-1, a membrane-bound transcription factor released by sterol regulated hydrolysis." *Cell, 177*(1), 53-62. doi: https://doi.org/10.1016/0092-8674(94)90234-8.

[28] Brown, Kirsty., Daniella, DeCoffe., Erin, Moican. & Deanna, L. Gibson. (2012). "Diet-induced dysbiosis of the intestinal microbiota and the effects on immunity and disease." *Nutrients*, *4*, 1095-1119.

[29] Libby, Peter., Paul, M. Ridker. & Attilio, Maseri. (2002). "Inflammation and atherosclerosis." *Circulation, 105*, 1135-1143. https://www.ahajournals.org/doi/full/10.1161/hc0902.104353.

[30] Shanshan, Zhou., Wanqing, Sun., Zhiguo, Zhang. & Yang, Zheng. (2014). "The Role of Nrf2-Mediated Pathway in Cardiac Remodeling and Heart Failure," *Oxidative Medicine and Cellular Longevity*, Article ID 260429. https://doi.org/10.1155/2014/260429.

[31] Tan, Yi., Tonogawa, Ichikawa., Jingqing, Li., Qiusheng, Si., Huaitao, Yang., Xiangbai, Chen., Curtis, S. Goldblatt., Colin, J. Mayer., Xioacun, Li., Lu, Cai. & Taixing, Cui. (2011). "Diabetic Downregulation of Nrf2 Activity via ERK Contributes to Oxidative Stress–Induced Insulin Resistance in Cardiac Cells *In Vitro* and *In Vivo*". *Diabetes*, *60*(2), 625–633. http://doi.org/10.2337/db10-1164.

[32] Kawashima, Seinosuke. & Mitsuhiro, Yokoyama. (2004). "Dysfunction of endothelial nitric oxide synthase and atherosclerosis". *Atherosclerosis, Thrombosis and Vascular Biology*, *24*, 998-1005.

[33] Fulton, David., John-Philippe, Gratton., Timothy, J. McCabe., Jason, Fontana. Yasushi, Fujio., Kenneth, Walsh., Thomas, F. Franke., Andreas, Papapetropoulos. & William, C. Sessa. (1999). "Regulation of endothelium-derived nitric oxide production by the protein kinase Akt." *Nature*, *399*(6736), 597–601. doi: 10.1038/21218.

[34] Jackson, S. P., Nesbitt, W. S. & Westein, E. (2009). "Dynamics of platelet thrombus formation." *Journal of Thrombosis and Hemostasis*, *7*(1), 17-20. Accessed November 6, 2018. https://onlinelibrary.wiley.com/doi/epdf/10.1111/j.1538-7836.2009.03401.x.

[35] Gebhardt, Rolf. (1993). "Multiple inhibitory effects of garlic extracts on cholesterol biosynthesis in hepatocytes." *Lipids*, *28*(6), 613-619. https://doi.org/10.1007/BF02536055.

[36] Gebhardt, R. (1995). "Amplification of palmitate-induced inhibition of cholesterol biosythesis in cultured rat hepatocytes by garlic derived organosulfur compounds." *Phytomedicine*., *2*, 29-34. https://www.sciencedirect.com/science/article/pii/S0944711311800450.

[37] Gebhardt, Rolf. & Halgund, Beck. (1996). "Differential inhibitory effects of garlic-derived organosulfur compounds on cholesterol biosynthesis in primary rat hepatocyte cultures." *Lipids*., *31*, 1269-1276. https://link.springer.com/article/10.1007%2FBF02587912.

[38] Gupta, Nisha. & Todd, D. Porter. (2001). "Garlic and garlic-derived compounds inhibit human squalene monooxygenase". *J. Nutr*., *131*, 1662–1666.

[39] Yeh, Yu-Yan. & Lijuan, Liu. (2001). "Cholesterol-Lowering Effect of Garlic Extracts and Organosulfur Compounds: Human and Animal Studies." *The Journal of Nutrition*, *131*(3), 989S–993S, https://doi.org/10.1093/jn/131.3.989S.

[40] Focke, Manfred., Andrea, Feld. & Harmut, K. Lichtenthaler. (1990). "Allicin, a naturally occurring antibiotic from garlic, specifically inhibits acetyl-CoA synthetase". *FEBS Lett*., *261*, 106–108.

[41] Lu, Jing., Bijun, cheng., Baochen, Fang., Zhuoqun, Meng., Yiying, Zheng., Xiaochen, Tian. & Shuang, Guan. (2017). "Protective effects of allicin on 1,3-DCP-induced lipid metabolism disorder in HepG2 cells," *Biomedicine & Pharmacotherapy*, *96*, 1411-1417. https://doi.org/10.1016/j.biopha.2017.10.125.

[42] Orekhov, Alexander N. & Vladimir, N. Tertov. (1997). "*In vitro* effect of garlic powder extract on lipid content in normal and atherosclerotic endothelial cells." *Lipids*, *32*(10), 1055-1060. https://doi.org/10.1007/s11745-997-0136-7.

[43] Qureshi, Asaf. A., Naji, Abiurmeileh., Zafir, Z. Din., Charles, E. Elson. & Warren, C. Buerger. (1983). "Inhibition of cholesterol and fatty acid biosynthesis in liver enzymes and chicken hepatocytes by polar fractions of garlic." *Lipids*., *18*, 343.-348. https://aocs.onlinelibrary.wiley.com/doi/abs/10.1007/BF02537229.

[44] Carroll, Richard G., Zbigniew, Zaslona., Silvia, Galvan-Pena., Emma, L. Koppe., Daniel, C. Sevin., Stefano, Angiari., Martha, Triantfilou., Kathy, Triantfilou., Louis, K. Modis. & Luke, A. O'Neill. (2018). "An unexpected link between fatty acid synthase and cholesterol synthesis in proinflammatory macrophage activation." *Journal of Biological Chemistry*, *293*, 5509-5521. doi.10.1074/jbc.RA1118.001921.

[45] Lestari, Sri R., Betty, Lukiati., Siti, N. Arifah., Alif, R. N. Alimah. & Abdul, Gofur. (2019). "Medicinal uses of single garlic in hyperlipidemia by fatty acid synthase enzyme inhibitory: molecular docking." *International Conference on Life Science and Technology*, *276*, 12008 doi:10.1088/1755-1315/276/1/012008.

[46] Borlinghaus, Jan., Frank, Albrecht., Martin, C. H. Grulke., Ifeanyi, D. Nwachukwu. & Alan, J. Slusarenko. (2014). "Allicin: Chemistry and biological properties". *Molecules*, *19*(8), 12591-12618.

[47] Chang, Mei Ling W. & Margaret, A. Johnson. (1980). "Effect of Garlic on Carbohydrate Metabolism and Lipid Synthesis in Rats." *The Journal of Nutrition, 110*(5), 931-936. https://doi.org/10.1093/jn/110.5.931.

[48] Chi, Myung S. (1982). "Effects of Garlic Products on Lipid Metabolism in Cholesterol-Fed Rats." *Proceedings of the Society for Experimental Biology and Medicine*, *171*(2), 174–178. https://doi.org/10.3181/00379727-171-41494.

[49] Chi, Myung S., Eunsook, T. Koh. & Troy, J. Stewart. (1982). "Effects of Garlic on Lipid Metabolism in Rats Fed Cholesterol or Lard." *The Journal of Nutrition, 112*(2), 241–248, https://doi.org/10.1093/jn/112.2.241.

[50] Elkayam, Amitai., David, Mirelman., Edna, Peleg., Meir, Wilcheck., Talia, Miron., Aharon, Rabinkov., Sigal, Sadetzki. & Talma, Rosenthal. (2001). "The Effects of allicin and enalapril in fructose-induced hyperlipidemic hypertensive rats." *American Journal of Hypertension*, *14*, 377-381.

[51] Elkayam, Almita., Edna, Peleg., Ehud, Grossman., Zehava, Shabtay. & Yehonatan, Sharabi. (2013). "Effects of allicin on cardiovascular risk factors in spontaneously hypertensive rats". *Israel Med. Assoc. J.*, *15*(3), 170-173. Accessed Sepember 25, 2018. https://www.ima.org.il/FilesUpload/IMAJ/0/52/26271.pdf.

[52] Kamanna, V. S. & Chandrasekhara, N. (1982). "Effect of garlic on serum lipoproteins cholesterol levels in albino rats rendered hypercholesteremic by feeding cholesterol." *Lipids*, *17*, 483–488.

[53] Ali, M., Al-Qattan, K., Al-Enezi, F., Khanafer, R. M. A. & Mustafa, T. (2000). "Effect of allicin from garlic powder on serum lipids and blood pressure in rats fed with a high cholesterol diet." *Prostaglandins, Leukotrienes and Essential Fatty Acids*, *62*(4), 253-259.

[54] Bordia, A. & Verma, S. K. (1980). "Effect of garlic feeding on regression of experimental atherosclerosis in rabbits." *Artery*, *7*, 428-437.

[55] Mand, J. K., Gupta, P. P., Soni, G. L. & Singh, R. (1985). "Effect of garlic on experimental atherosclerosis in rabbits." *Indian Heart Journal*, *37*(3), 183-188.

[56] Eilat, S., Oestraicher, Y., Rabinkov, A., Ohad, D., Mirelman, D., Battler, A., Eldar, M. & Vered, Z. (1995). "Alteration of lipid profile in hyperlipidemic rabbits by allicin, an active constituent of garlic." *Coronary Artery Disease*., *6*(12), 985-90.

[57] Kwon, Myung Ja., Young-Sun, Song., Myung-Sook, Choi., Sang-Joon, Park., Kyu-Shik, Jeong. & Yeong-Ok, Song. (2003). Cholesteryl ester transfer protein activity and atherogenic parameters in rabbits supplemented with cholesterol and garlic powder. *Life Sciences*, *72*(26), 2953-2964. https://doi.org/10.1016/S0024-3205(03)00234-0.

[58] Sainani, G. S., Desai, D. B., Natu, M. N., Katrodia, K. M., Valame, V. P. & Sainani, P. G. (1979). "Onion, garlic and experimental atherosclerosis." *Jpn Heart J*, *28*(3), 351-357.

[59] Abramovitz, Dana., Sagui, Gavri., Dror, Harats., Hanna, Levkovitz., David, Mirelman., Talia, Miron., Sigal, Eilat-Adar., Aharon, Rabinkov., Meir, Wilchek., Michael, Eldar. & Zvi, Vered. (1999). "Allicin-induced decrease in the formation of fatty streaks (atherosclerosis) in mice fed a cholesterol-rich diet." *Coronary Artery Disease*, *10*, 515-519.

[60] Gonen, Ayelet., Dror, Harats., Aharon, Rabinkov., Talia, Miron., David, Mirelman., Meir, Wilcheck., Lev, Weiner., Esfir, Ulman., Hana, Levkovitz., Dikla, Ben-Shushan.

& Aviv, Shaish. (2005). The antiatherogenic effect of allicin: possible mode of action. *Pathobiology*, *72*, 325-334.

[61] Espirito, Santo., Sonia, M. S., Bart, J. M. van Vlijmen., Rien, Buytenhek., Wim, van Duyvenvoorde., Louis, M. Havekes., Ingrid, Arnault., Jacques, Auger. & Hans, M. G. Princen. (2004). "Well-Characterized Garlic-Derived Materials Are Not Hypolipidemic in APOE*3-Leiden Transgenic Mice." *The Journal of Nutrition, 134*(6), 1500–1503, https://doi.org/10.1093/jn/134.6.1500.

[62] Qureshi, Asaf A. Z. Z. Din., Abuirmeileh, N., Burger, W. C., Ahmad, Y. & Elson, C. E. (1983). "Suppression of Avian Hepatic Lipid Metabolism by Solvent Extracts of Garlic: Impact on Serum Lipids." *The Journal of Nutrition, 113* (9), 1746–1755, https://doi.org/10.1093/jn/113.9.1746.

[63] Gong-chen, Wang Han Lu-lu., Wang, Jing., Lang, Wan-nan., Pan, Chuan-yi. & Li, Yan-fei. (2014). "Effects of Allicin on Lipid Metabolism and Antioxidant Activity in Chickens." *Journal of Northeast Agricultural University (English Edition)*., *21*(3), 46-49. https://doi.org/10.1016/S1006-8104(14)60068-4.

[64] Leong, Xin-Fang Chun-Yi Ng. & Kamsiah, Jaarin. (2015). "Animal Models in Cardiovascular Research: Hypertension and Atherosclerosis," *BioMed Research International*, *201*, Article ID 528757, 11 pages, 2015. https://doi.org/10.1155/2015/528757.

[65] Lin, Xiao-Lin., Hui-Jun, Hu., Yian-Bo, Liu., Xue-Mei, Hu., Xiao-Juan, Fan., Wei-Wen, Zou., Yong-Quan, Pan., Wen-Pan, Zhou., Min-Wen, Peng. & Cai-Hong, Gu. (2017). "Allicin induces the upregulation of ABCA1 expression via PPARγ/LXRα signaling in THP-1 macrophage-derived foam cells." *International Journal of Molecular Medicine*, *39*(6), 1452–1460. doi:10.3892/ijmm.2017.2949.

[66] Banerjee, Sanjay K. & Subir, K. Maulik. (2002). "Effect of garlic on cardiovascular disorders: a review." *Nutrition Journal*, *1*, 4 Accessed on July 30, 2019. https://nutritionj.biomedcentral.com/articles/10.1186/1475-2891-1-4.

[67] Khoo, Y. S. K. & Aziz, X. (2009). "Garlic supplementation and serum cholesterol : A meta analysis. " *Journal of Clinical Pharmacy and Therapeutics*, *34*(2), 133-145.

[68] Ried, Karin., Catherine, Toben. & Peter, Fakler. (2013). "Effect of garlic on serum lipids: an updated meta-analysis." *Nutrition Reviews*, *71*(5), 282–299, https://doi.org/10.1111/nure.12012.

[69] Shabani, Ehsan., Korosh, Sayemiri. & Mohammadtaghi, Mohammadpour. (2019). "The effect of garlic on lipid profile and glucose parameters in diabetic patients: A systematic review and meta analysis. " *Primary Care Diabetes*, *13*, 28-42.

[70] Gardner, Christopher D., Larry, D. Lawson., Eric, Block., Lorraine, M. Chatterjee., Alexandre, Kiazand., Raymond, R. Balise. & Helena, C. Kramer. (2007). "Effect of Raw Garlic vs Commercial Garlic Supplements on Plasma Lipid Concentrations in Adults With Moderate Hypercholesterolemia: A Randomized Clinical Trial." *Arch Intern Med.*, *167*(4), 346–353. doi:10.1001/archinte.167.4.346.

[71] Sobenin, Igor A., Irina, V. Andrianova., Olga, M. Demidova., Tatiana, V. Gorchakova. & Alexander, N. Orekhov (2008). "Lipid-lowering effects of time-released garlic powder tablets in double-blinded placebo-controlled randomized study." *Journal of Atherosclerosis and Thrombosis*, *15*(6), 334-338.

[72] Sobenin, Igor A., Valentin, V. Pryanishnikov., Lyudmilla, M. Kunnova., Yevgeny, A. Rabinovich., Danik, M. Martirosyan. & Alexander, N. Orekhov. (2010). "The effects of

time-released garlic powder tablets on multifunctional cardiovascular risk in patients with coronary artery disease." *Lipids in Health and Disease*, *9*, 119. doi: 10.1186/1476-511X-9-119.

[73] Kannar, David., Naiyana, Wattanapenpaiboon., Gayle, S. Savage. & Mark, L. Wahlqvist. (2001). "Hypercholesterolemic effect of an enteric-coated garlic supplement." *Journal of Nutrition*, *20*(3), 225-231. Accessed on July 30, 2019. http://apjcn.nhri.org.tw/ server../MarkWpapers/Papers/Papers%202001/P302.pdf.

[74] Lawson, Larry D. & Scott, M. Hunsaker. (2018). "Allicin Bioavailability and Bioequivalence from Garlic Supplements and Garlic Foods." *Nutrients*, *10*(7), 812. doi: 10.3390/nu10070812.

[75] Chen, Xiaoshu., Sunian, Pang., Jianfeng, Lin., Jianlian, Xia. & Yi, Wang. (2016). "Allicin prevents oxidized low density lipoprotein-induced cell injury by inhibiting apoptosis and oxidative stress pathway." *BMC Complementary and Alternative Medicine*, *16*, Article 133. https://bmccomplementalternmed.biomedcentral.com/ articles/10.1186/s12906-016-1126-9.

[76] Zhang, Min., Huichao, Pan., Yinjie, Xu., Xueting, Wang., Zhaohui, Qui. & Li, Jiang. (2018). "Allicin decreases lipopolysaccharide-induced oxidative stress and inflammation in human umbilical vein endothelial cells through suppression of mitochondrial dysfunction and activation of Nrf2". *Cell Physiol. Biochem.*, *41*, 2255-2267.

[77] Wang, Shu-Li., Di-Shan, Liu., Er-Shun, Liang., Yan-Hua, Gao., Ying, Cui., Yu-Zhao, Lui. & Wei, Gao. (2015). "Protective effect of allicin on high glucose/hypoxia-induced aortic endothelial cells via reduction of oxidative stress". *Experimental and Therapeutic Medicine*, *10*(4), 1394–1400. http://doi.org/10.3892/etm.2015.2708.

[78] Okada, Y., Tanaka, K., Fujita, I., Sato, E. & Okajima, H. (2005). "Antioxidant activity of thiosulfinates obtained from garlic." *Redox Report*, *10*(2), 96-102. https:// www.tandfonline.com/doi/pdf/10.1179/135100005X38851.

[79] Lina, Ma., Shangke, Chen., Shaochun, Li., Lijuan, Deng., Yikui, Li. & Hao, Li. (2018). "Effect of Allicin against Ischemia/Hypoxia-Induced H9c2 Myoblast Apoptosis via eNOS/NO Pathway-Mediated Antioxidant Activity." *Evidence-Based Complementary and Alternative Medicine*, Article ID 3207973. https://doi.org/10.1155/2018/ 3207973.

[80] Mo, Sung-Ji., Eun-Wha, Son., Dongquan, Rhee. & Sukhneung, Pyo. (2003). "Modulation of TNF-alpha induced ICAM-1 expression, NO and H_2O_2 production by alginate, allicin, and ascorbic acid in human endothelial cells." *Arch Pharm Res*, *26*, 244-251. https://doi.org/10.1007/BF02976837.

[81] Schwartz, Idit F., Rami, Hershkvitz, Adrian Iana., Ehud, Gnessin., Yoram, Wollman., Tamara, Chernichowski., Miriam, Blum., Yoram, Levo. & Doran, Schwartz. (2002). "Garlic attenuates nitric oxide production in rat cardiac myocytes through inhibition of nitric oxide synthase and the arginine transporter CAT-2 (cationic arginine transporter-2)." *Clinical Science*, *102*(5), 487-493. doi: 10.1042/cs1020487.

[82] Ba, Lina., Jingquan, Gao., Yunping, Chen., Hanping, Qi., Chonghui, Dong., Hao, Pan., Qianhui, Zhang., Pilong, Shi., Chao, Song., Xueying, Guan., Yonggang, Cao. & Hongli, Sun. (2019). "Allicin attenuates pathological cardiac hypertrophy by inhibiting autophagy via activation of PI3K/Akt/mTOR and MAPK/ERK/mTOR signaling pathways." *Phytomedicine*, *58*, 152765. https://doi.org/10.1016/j.phymed.2018.11.025.

[83] Ku, David D., Tarek, Abdel-Razek., Jarel, Dai., Sangae, Kim-Park., Michael, B. Fallon. & Gary, A. Abrams. (2002). "Garlic And Its Active Metabolite Allicin Produce Endothelium- And Nitric Oxide-Dependent Relaxation In Rat Pulmonary Arteries." *Clinical and Experimental Pharmacology and Physiology*, *29*, 84-91. doi:10.1046/j.1440-1681.2002.03596.x.

[84] Padiya, Raju., Debrabrata, Chowdhury., Roshan, Borkar., Srinivas, R., Manika, P. Bhadra. & Sanjay, K. Banerjee. (2014). "Garlic Attenuates Cardiac Oxidative Stress via Activation of PI3K/AKT/Nrf2-Keap1 Pathway in Fructose-Fed Diabetic Rat." *PLOS ONE*, *9*(5), e94228. https://doi.org/10.1371/journal.pone.0094228.

[85] Li, Xian-Hui., Chun-Yan, Li., Zhi-Gang, Xiang., Jian-Jun, Hu., Jian-Ming, Lu., Rong-Bo, Tian. & Wei, Jia. (2012). "Allicin ameliorates cardiac hypertrophy and fibrosis through enhancing Nrf2 antioxidant signaling pathways". *Cardiovascular Drugs and Therapy*, *26*(6), 457-465.

[86] García-Trejo, Ehécatl M. A., Abraham, S. Arellano-Buendía., Raúl, Argüello-García., María, L. Loredo-Menzoza., Fernando, E. García-Orroya., Moníca, G. Arrelano-Mendoza., María, C. Castillio-Hernández., Gustavo, Guevara-Balcázar., Edilia, Tapia., Laura, G. Sánchez-Lozada. & Horacio, Osorio-Alonso. (2016). "Effects of Allicin on Hypertension and Cardiac Function in Chronic Kidney Disease." *Oxidative Medicine and Cellular Longevity*, Article ID 3850402. https://doi.org/10.1155/2016/3850402.

[87] Xiao, Xu. & Bao-Liang, Song. (2013). "SREBP: a novel therapeutic target." *Acta Biochimica et Biophysica Sinica*, Volume *45*(1), 2–10. https://doi.org/10.1093/abbs/gms112.

[88] Mayeux, P. R., Agrawal, K. C., Tou, J. S. H., King, B. T., Lippton, H. L., Hyman, A. L., Kadowicz, P. J. & McNamara, D. B. (1988). "The pharmacological effects of allicin, a constituent of garlic oil." *Agents and Actions*, *25*, 182-190. https://doi.org/10.1007/ BF01969110.

[89] Makheja, A. N. & Bailey, J. M. (1990). "Antiplatelet constituents of garlic and onion." *Agents and Actions*, *29*(3-4), 360-363.

[90] Briggs, William H., Hang, Xiao., Kirk, L. Parkin., Cunxi, Shen. & Irwin, L. Goldman. (2000). "Differential inhibition of human platelet aggregation by selected Allium thiosulfinates." *J. Agric. Food Chem.*, *48*, 5731–5735.

[91] Manaster, Yoav., Boris, Shenkman., Nurit, Rosenberg. & Naphtali, Savion. (2009). "Allicin and diulfram enhance platelet inegrin αIIbβ3-binding." *Thrombosis Research*, *124*(4), 477-482. doi: 10.1016/j.thromres.2009.06.019.

[92] Apitz-Castro, R., Cabrera, S., Cruz, M. R., Ledezma, E. & Jain, M. K. (1983). Effects of garlic extract and of three pure components isolated from it on human platelet aggregation, arachidonate metabolism, release activity and platelet ultrastructure. *Thromb Res.*, *32*, 155–169.

[93] Ali, M., Thomson, M., Alnaqeeb, M. A., Al-Hassan, J. M., Khater, S. H. & Gomes, S. A. (1990). "Antithrombotic activity of garlic: its inhibition of the synthesis of thromboxane-B2 during infusion of arachidonic acid and collagen in rabbits." *Prostaglandins, Leukotrienes and Essential Fatty Acids*, *41*(2), 95-99. https://doi.org/10.1016/0952-3278(90)90060-X.

[94] Pilong, Shi., Yonggang, Cao., Jingquan, Gao., Bowen, Fu., Jing, Ren., Lina, Ba., Chao, Song., Hanping, Qi., Wei, Huang., Xueying, Guan. & Hongli, Sun. (2018). "Allicin improves the function of cardiac microvascular endothelial cells by increasing PECAM-

1 in rats with cardiac hypertrophy." *Phytomedicine*, *51*, 241-254. https://doi.org/10.1016/ j.phymed.2018.10.021.

[95] Bordia, A., Verma, S. K. & Srivastava, K. C. (1996). "Effect of garlic on platelet aggregation in humans: a study in healthy subjects and patients with coronary artery disease." *Prostaglandins, Leukotrienes and Essential Fatty Acids*, *55*(3), 201-205. https://doi.org/10.1016/S0952-3278(96)90099-X.

[96] Barrie, Steven A., Jonathan V. Wright, and Joseph E. Pizzorno. 1987. "Effects of garlic oil on platelet aggregation, serum lipids and blood pressure in humans." *Journal of Orthomolecular Medicine*, *2*(1), 1-20. Accessed on August 3, 2019. http://orthomolecular.org/library/jom/1987/pdf/1987-v02n01-p015.pdf.

[97] Wojcikowski, Ken., Stephen, Myers. & Lyndon, Brooks. (2009). "Effects of garlic oil on platelet aggregation: A double blind placebo-controlled crossover study." *Platelets*, *18*(1), 29-34.

[98] Kiesewetter, H., Jung, F., Pindur, G., Jung, E. M., Mrowietz, C. & Wenzel, E. (1991). Effect of garlic on thrombocyte aggregation, microcirculation, and other risk factors. *Int J. Clin Pharmacol Ther Toxicol*, *29*(4), 151-155.

[99] Kiesewetter, H., Jung, F., Jung, E. M., Mrowietz, C., Kosceilny, J. & Wenzel, E. (1993). "Effect of garlic on platelet aggregation on patients with increased risk of juvenile ischemic attack." *Eur J Clin Pharmacol*, *45*, 333-336. https://doi.org/ 10.1007/BF00265950.

[100] Legnani, C., Frascaro, M., Guazzaloca, G., Ludovici, S., Cesarano, G. & Coccheri, S. (1993). "Effects of a dried garlic preparation on fibrinolysis and platelet aggregation in healthy subjects." *Arzneimittelforschung*, *43*, 119–122.

[101] Koscielny, J., Klüßendorf, D., Latza, R., Schmitt, R., Radtke, H., Siegel, G. & Kiesewetter, H. (1999). "The antiatherosclerotic effect of Allium sativum." *Atherosclerosis*, *144*(1), 237-249. https://doi.org/10.1016/S0021-9150(99)00060-X.

[102] Luley, C., Lehmann-Leo, W., Moller, B., Martin, T. & Schwartzkopff, W. (1986). "Lack of efficacy of dried garlic in patients with hyperlipoproteinemia." *Arzneimittelforschung/Drug Res.*, *36*, 766–768.

[103] Scharbert, G., Kalb, M. L., Duris, M., Marschalek, C. & Kozek-Langenecker, S. A. (2007). "Garlic at dietary doses does not impair platelet function." *Anaesth. Analg.*, *105*(5), 1214-1218.

[104] Sobenin, Igor., Irina, Andrianova., Victoriya, Ionova., Vasily, Karagodin. & Aleander, Orekhov. (2012). "Anti-aggregatory and fibrinolytic effects of time-released garlic powder tablets." *Applied Technology and Technologies*, *7*(2), 40-45.

[105] Ge, Beikeng., Zhen, Zhang. & Zhong, Zuo. (2014). "Updates on the clinical evidenced herb-warfarin interactions." *Evidence-based Complementary and Alternative Medicine: eCAM*, 957362. doi:10.1155/2014/957362.

[106] Sial, A. Y. & Ahmed, S. J. (1982). "Study of the hypotensive action garlic extract in experimental animals." *J Pak Med Assoc.*, *32*, 237–239.

[107] Al-Qattan, Khaled K., Martha, Thomson., Sausan, Al-Mutawa'a., Dalal, Al-Hajeri., Hana, Drobiova. & Muslim, Ali. (2006). "Nitric Oxide Mediates the Blood-Pressure Lowering Effect of Garlic in the Rat Two-Kidney, One-Clip Model of Hypertension." *The Journal of Nutrition, 136*(3), 774S–776S, https://doi.org/ 10.1093/jn/136.3.774S.

[108] Fallon, Michael B., Gary, A. Abrams., Tarek, T. Abdel-Razek., Jun, Dai., Shi-Juan, Chen., Yui-Fai, Chen., Bao, Luo., Suzanne, Oprail. & David, D. Ku. (1998). "Garlic

prevents hypoxic pulmonary hypertension in rats." *Am. J. Physiol.*, *275*(2 pt 2), L283-287. https://doi.org/10.1152/ajplung.1998.275.2.L283.

[109] Kaye, Alan D., Bracken, J. De Witt., Muahmmad, Anwar., Donald, E. Smith., Chang, J. Feng., Philip, J. Kadowitz. & Bobby, D. Nossaman. (2000). Analysis of responses of garlic derivatives in the pulmonary vascular bed of the rat. *J. Appl. Physiol.*, *89*, 353-358. https://www.physiology.org/doi/pdf/10.1152/jappl.2000.89.1.353.

[110] Dubey, Harikesh., Anamika, Singh., Angad, M. Patole., Chandrashekhar, R. Tenpe. & Balu, V. Ghule. (2012). "Allicin, a SUR2 opener: possible mechanism for the treatment of diabetic hypertension in rats." *Revista Brasileira de Farmacognosia*, *22*(5), 1053-1059. https://dx.doi.org/10.1590/S0102-695X2012005000046.

[111] Sharifi, Ali M., Radbod, Darabi. & Nasrin, Akbarloo. (2003). Investigation of antihypertensive mechanism of garlic in 2K1C hypertensive rat. *Journal of Ethnopharmacology*, *86* (2–3), 219-224. https://doi.org/10.1016/S0378-8741(03) 00080-1.

[112] Benavides, Gloria A., Giuseppe, L. Squadrito., Robert, W. Mills., Hetal, D. Patel., Scott Isbell, T., Rakesh, P. Patel., Victor, M. Darley-Usmar., Jeannette, E. Doeller. & David, W. Kraus. (2007). "Hydrogen sulfide mediates the vasoactivity of garlic." *Proc Natl Acad Sci USA*, *104*, 17977-17982. doi: 10.1073/pnas.0705710104.

[113] Ried, Karin., Oliver, R. Franks., Nigel, P. Stocks., Peter, Fakler. & Thomas, Sullivan. (2008). "Effect of garlic on blood pressure: A systematic review and meta-analysis." *BMC Cardiovasc Disord.*, *8*, 13. doi: 10.1186/1471-2261-8-13.

[114] Ried, Karin. (2016). Garlic Lowers Blood Pressure in Hypertensive Individuals, Regulates Serum Cholesterol, and Stimulates Immunity: An Updated Meta-analysis and Review. *The Journal of Nutrition, 146*(2), 389S–396S. https://doi.org/10.3945/jn.114.202192.

[115] Xiong, X. J., Wang, P. Q., Li, S. J., Li, X. K., Zhang, Y. Q. & Wang, J. (2015). "Garlic for hypertension: A systematic review and meta-analysis of randomized controlled trials." *Phytomedicine*, *22*(3), 352-361. https://doi.org/10.1016/j.phymed.2014.12.013.

[116] Hai-Peng, Wang., Jin, Yan., Li-Qiang, Qin. & Xiang-Jun, Yang. (2015). "Effect of garlic on blood pressure a meta analysis." *J Clin Hypertens (Greenwich)*, *17*, 223–231. doi: 10.1111/jch.12473 https://doi.org/10.1111/jch.12473.

[117] Sobenin, Igor A., Irina, V. Andrianova., Igor, V. Fomchenkov., Tatiana, V. Gorchakova. & Alexander, N. Orekhov. (2009). "Time-released garlic powder tablets lower systolic and diastolic blood pressure in men with mild and moderate arterial hypertension. *Hypertension Research*, *32*, 433-437. Accessed on August 6, 2019. https://www.nature.
com/articles/hr200936.

[118] Reinhart, K. M., Coleman, C. I., Teevan, C., Vachhani, P. & White, C. M. (2008). "Effects of garlic on blood pressure in patients with and without systolic hypertension: A meta-analysis." *Ann Pharmacother.*, *42*, 1766–71.

[119] Simons, S., Wollersheim, H. & Thien, T. (2009). "A systematic review on the influence of trial quality on the effect of garlic on blood pressure." *The Journal of Medicine*, *67*(6), 212-219. Accessed on August 6, 2019 https://repository.ubn.ru.nl/bitstream/handle/2066/79686/79686.pdf.

[120] Guan, Xiaoxu., Yi, Zhou., Hui, Chen., Chaowei, Wang. & Huiming, Wang. (2018). Antibacterial, anti-inflammatory, and anti-osteoclastogenesis roles of allicin in periodontitis. *Int. J. Clin. Med., 11*(7), 6721-6730.

[121] Wei-Kai Wu, Wei-Kai., Suraphan, Panyod., Chi-Tang, Ho., Ching-Hua, Kuo., Ming-Shiang, Wu. & Lee-Yan, Sheen. (2015). "Dietary allicin reduces transformation of L-carnitine to TMAO through impact on gut microbiota." *Journal of Functional Foods, 15*, 408-417. https://doi.org/10.1016/j.jff.2015.04.001.

[122] Loeper, M. & DeBray, M. (1921). "Hypotensive effect of tincture of garlic." *Prog. Med., 36*, 391-392.

[123] Kemper, Kathy J. (2000). "Garlic." *Longwood Herbal Task Force*. Accessed on August 5, 2019. https://pdfs.semanticscholar.org/d3c9/2bcd9846141d5b7a645e5f858c16d6e80a27.pdf.

[124] Viguet Poupelloz, Jaqueline. (2016). "Assessment report on *Allium sativum* L. bulbus." *European Medicines Agency, Committee on Herbal Medicinal Products*. Accessed on August 6, 2019. https://www.ema.europa.eu/en/documents/herbal-report/draft-assessment-report-allium-sativum-l-bulbus_en.pdf.

[125] *WHO monographs on selected medicinal plants. Volume 1*. 1999. Geneva, Switzerland. ISBN 92 4 154517 8. Accessed on August 6, 2019 https://apps.who.int/ medicinedocs/pdf/s2200e/s2200e.pdf.

[126] Eilat-Adar, Sigal., Tali, Sinai., Chaim, Yosefy. & Yaakov, Henkin. (2013). "Nutritional recommendations for cardiovascular disease prevention." *Nutrients, 5*(9), 3646–3683. doi: 10.3390/nu5093646.

[127] Strovel, Jeffrey., Sitta, Sittampalam., Nathan, P. Coussens., Michael, Hughes., James, Inglese., Andrew, Kurtz., Ali, Andalibi., Lavonne, Patton., Chris, Austin., Michael, Baltezor., Michael, Beckloff., Michael, Weingarten. & Scott, Weir. (2012). "Early Drug Discovery and Development Guidelines: For Academic Researchers, Collaborators, and Start-up Companies.". In: Sittampalam GS, Grossman A, Brimacombe K, et al., editors. *Assay Guidance Manual [Internet]*. Bethesda (MD): Eli Lilly & Company and the National Center for Advancing Translational Sciences; 2004.Accessed on August 8, 2019. https://www.ncbi.nlm.nih.gov/books/NBK92015/.

[128] Liang, Yan., Jing-Jing, Zhang., Qi-Bing, Zhang., Zhong-Xia, Wang., Zong-Ning, Yin., Xin-Xia, Li., Jian, Chen. & Li-Ming, Ye. (2013). "Release test of alliin/alliinase double-layer tablet by HPLC—Allicin determination." *Journal of Pharmaceutical Analysis, 3*(3), 187-192. https://doi.org/10.1016/j.jpha.2012.08.001.

[129] Leontiev, Roman., Nils, Hohaus., Jacob, Claus., Martin, C. H. Gruhlke. & Alan, J. Slusarenko. (2018). "Comparison of the Antibacterial and Antifungal Activities of Thiosulfinate Analogues of Allicin." *Scientific Reports, 6763*, 8(1). Accessed on February 22, 2019 https://www.nature.com/articles/s41598-018-25154-9.

[130] Lubenets, Vira., Sofiya, Vasylyuk., Nataliya, Monka., Khrystina, Bolibrukh., Olena, Komarovska-Porokhnyavets., Diana, Baranovych., Rostyslav, Musyanovych., Ewa, Zaczynska., Anna, Czarny., Urszula, Nawrot. & Volodymyr, Novikov. (2016). "Synthesis and antimicrobial properties of 4-acylaminobenzenethiosulfoacid S-esters." *Saudi Pharmaceutical Journal: SPJ: The Official publication of the Saudi Pharmaceutical Society, 25*(2), 266-274. doi: 10.1016/j.jsps.2016.06.007.

[131] Joe, W. E. Moss., Joe, W. E. Jessica O. Williams. & Dipak, P. Ramji. (2018). "Nutraceuticals as therapeutic agents for atherosclerosis." *Biochimica et Biophysica*

Acta (BBA) - Molecular Basis of Disease, *1864*, (5 Part A), 1562-1572. https://doi.org/10.1016/j.bbadis.2018.02.006.

[132] Feher, Gergely., Andrea, Feher., Gabriella, Pusch., Katalin, Koltai., Antal, Tibold., Beata, Gasztonyi., Elod, Papp., Laszlo, Szapary., Gabor, Kesmarky. & Kalman, Toth. (2010). "Clinical importance of aspirin and clopidogrel resistance." *World Journal of Cardiology*, *2*(7), 171–186. doi: 10.4330/wjc.v2.i7.171.

[133] Trompet, S., Postmus, I., Slagboom, P. E., Heijmans, B. T., Smit, R. A., Maier, A. B., Buckley, B. M., Sattar, N., Stott, D. J., Ford, I., Westendorp, R. G., de Craen, A. J. & Jukema, J. W. (2016). "Non-response to (statin) therapy: the importance of distinguishing non-responders from non-adherers in pharmacogenetic studies." *Eur J Clin Pharmacol.*, *72*(4), 431-7. doi: 10.1007/s00228-015-1994-9. Epub 2015 Dec 19.

[134] Martín-Timón, Iciar., Christina, Sevillano-Collantes., Amparo, Segura-Galindo. & Francisco, J. Del Cañizo-Gómez. (2014). "Type 2 diabetes and cardiovascular disease: Have all risk factors the same strength?" *World Journal of Diabetes*, *5*(4), 444–470. doi:10.4239/wjd.v5.i4.444.

[135] Said, Sarmad. & German, T. Hernandez. (2014). "The link between chronic kidney disease and cardiovascular disease." *Journal of Nephropathology*, *3*(3), 99–104. doi:10.12860/jnp.2014.19.

In: Allicin
Editor: Diana R. Cundell
ISBN: 978-1-53617-339-0

Chapter 11

CARTILAGE AND BONE PROTECTING EFFECTS OF ALLICIN IN CHRONIC DISEASE

Diana R. Cundell*, PhD
College of Life Sciences, Jefferson University, Philadelphia, PA, US

ABSTRACT

Sustained damage to the chondrocytes that provide joint articulation results both in their demise and to changes in the ratios of osteoclast (bone destroying) and osteoblast (bone building cells) beneath. Maintenance of chondroblast health is therefore a key process in preventing common chronic inflammatory osteodegenerative diseases that include ankylosing spondylitis (AS), osteoarthritis (OA), osteoporosis (OP) and even advanced periodontal disease (PD). Since its discovery in 1944 allicin has been shown in a variety of models to be primarily anti-inflammatory through modulating the activation of nuclear factor kappa beta (NF-κβ) reactive oxygen species (ROS), nitric oxide (NO), NF-E2, p45related factor (Nrf2) and the mitogen activated kinase pathways (MAPKs). Recently allicin's effects been investigated on cartilage and bone degenerating diseases using nine animal and *in vitro* cellular models of AS, OA, OP and PD. The results are encouraging and appear to show allicin, promotes cartilage and bone health by affecting several major biochemical pathways including NF-κB, nuclear factor kappa beta ligand (RANKL), extracellular signal regulated kinase (ERK) and phosphoinositide-3-phosphate/ protein kinase B (P13K/Akt). Allicin was shown to downregulate ROS and inflammatory cytokine production in five separate studies. One animal study of AS, also reported that allicin was uniquely able to prevent the surface expression of the mis-folded HLA-B27, which is the target for cartilage and bone destroying immune-mediated mechanisms in that disease. In this chapter an explanation of the pathophysiology that triggers cartilage and/ or bone destruction in these conditions will be combined with an analysis of how allicin is able to improve symptoms in models of AS, OA, OP and PD. The chapter will also discuss allicin's future potential in acting as a complementary treatment in these and other related diseases.

Keywords: Ankylosing spondylitis, osteoarthritis, osteoporosis, periodontal disease

---

* Corresponding Author's Email: Diana.Cundell@jefferson.edu.

1. INTRODUCTION

Normal movement of the synovial joints requires both the continued production of lubricating synovial fluid, and the continued health of the chrondrocytes that secrete the thin layer of articular (hyaline) cartilage [1, 2]. Maintenance of articulating cartilage requires its relatively frequent remodeling throughout life, especially the surface layers [1, 2]. This remodeling is relatively slow, due to a lack of blood vessels within the cartilage, but is possible, as seen following minor joint trauma [1] Healthy chondrocyte activity in the surface layers is upregulated by two biochemical pathways; MAPK p38 and transforming growth factor-β/bone morphogenetic protein (TGF-β) [3, 4]. MAPK p38 stimulates chondrocyte proliferation and TGF-β is able to increase the repair of cartilage by upregulating matrix production [3, 4]. Activation of a second MAPK pathway, extracellular receptor kinase (ERK) decreases chondrocyte number [1]. Through crosstalk, chondrocytes also control the environment of the the active (osteoblast) and resting (osteocyte) bone-building cells that lie beneath the articulating surface [1].

This indicates that loss of chondrocytes during degenerative disease decreases the homogeneity of the bone beneath by decreasing the ability for osteoblast activation [1, 2]. Sclerosis of the bone in turn results in further death of cartilage cells [5]. Maintenance of cartilage therefore requires bone health and vice versa [5]. Cartilage and chondrocyte loss occurs for various reasons including genetic anomalies in cartilage collagen proteins, aging and estrogen loss post-menopause [1, 2, 6]. Cracks that form in degenerating cartilage also allow blood vessels to invade from the bone beneath [1]. Vascularization of the cartilage forces chondrocytes into terminal differentiation, apoptosis and death, with surviving cells rendered unable to maintain repairs [1]. This cycle of inflammation and damage removes functional cartilage since once lost the chondrocytes cannot be replaced [1]. Their demise plays a central role in the etiology and progression of osteoarthritis (OA) [1] and ankylosing spondylitis (AS) [6].

Further activation of bone-degrading/remodeling osteoclasts by inflammatory stimuli adds to the impaired activity of the bone-building osteoblasts [7]. External and exogenous inflammatory IL-1, IL-6 and IL-17 cytokine exposure [1] and osteoblast ERK activation [3] results in increased activity of these cells involving the upregulation of nuclear factor kappa beta ligand (RANKL) [1, 3, 7]. Disturbance of the osteoclasts also affects their ability to neutralize reactive oxygen species (ROS) through their normal glutathione (GpX) anti-oxidant enzyme systems [8]. Excessive ROS generation results and perturbs bone homeostasis still further [8]. The resulting osteoblast/osteoclast imbalance results in bone resorption seen in many conditions including AS [6], osteoporosis (OP) [8] and late stage osteoarthritis (OA) [1] and periodontal disease (PD) [9].

In developed countries, these conditions are typically managed with classical treatment regimens, namely anti-inflammatory medications for OA [1] and AS [6], osteoclast inhibitors for OP [10] and dental hygiene for PD [11]. In developing countries, where the need is greater especially for OA and OP, reliance is primarily on traditional plant-based healing methods [1, 12]. Many naturally available plants have been shown both *in vitro* and in animal studies to improve cartilage function [13] or decrease bone resorption [12]. Of these over ninety plants, only a few have been developed into effective pharmaceuticals medications, however, due to the complexities of the interactions of the multiple moieties within each plant and in some cases limited bioavailability [14].

Interestingly a single entity that has emerged as possessing both chondro *and* osteoprotective activity is *Allium satiivum* (garlic) and its extract diallyl sulfide, allicin [12, 13]. Since allicin was discovered in 1944, it has been described as possessing both antimicrobial and anti-inflammatory activity in a variety of body systems [15]. More recently, allicin's chondrocyte, osteoclast and osteoblast effects have been explored in eight models of four chronic degenerative conditions [16-23]. Using isolated cell or rodent models, allicin has been shown to be effective in ameliorating the damage of AS [16], osteoarthritis (OA) [17-21], osteoporosis (OP) [22, 23] and periodontal disease (PD) [24]. All the studies described only appeared within the last decade, with the individual studies of AS [16] and PD [24] being published within the past two years. A small, double blind, randomized placebo-controlled trial (DBRPCT) on patients with knee OA also observed improved mobility and lessened pain following garlic ingestion [25].

So why develop allicin or indeed any plant-based medicine further for any of these illnesses? The simple answer is that OA [1], OP [10, 26] and PD [27] are worldwide issues that still require well-researched, affordable and accessible interventions that either prevent or reverse disease progression. Patients with OA are mostly in developed countries, where they are offered a range of treatments that temporarily reduce pain and inflammation, but ultimately face joint replacement [1, 28, 29]. This lack of effective outcome for pharmaceutical interventions has already led to a decrease in patient compliance and a search for viable and safe alternatives for many OA patients [1]. For nearly half of all OA patients in developed countries [12] "safe" means a variety of herbal medicines. In developing countries over eighty percent of OA patients use locally sourced, often traditional plant-based therapies [1]. Clearly, it would not be a leap of faith to use allicin, its parent the garlic clove or another phytomedicine for these patients. Allicin, like many phytomedicines [14], shows simultaneous utility against several biochemical pathways and is able to "rebalance" the redox potential of cells in many organ systems [15].

In contrast to OA, OP is a major issue for developing countries, where malnutrition and thalassemia impair peak bone density, thereby accelerating the speed at which osteopenia occurs [26]. Many patients in developing nations are already exploring alternative therapies for OP, many of which are components of traditional Ayurvedic or Chinese medicines [12]. Plants of the *Epimedium* species have been well explored using *in vitro* and animal models and appear to be particularly beneficial in preventing post-menopausal OP, while others like *Dioscorea* appear to prevent the condition by decreasing osteoclast activity [12]. One older study demonstrated that garlic oil extract was able to prevent bone loss in an animal model of post-menopausal OP [23]. Garlic oil contains significant levels of allicin [30] and this study can be considered as supporting evidence for its efficacy. More recent studies of allicin itself, suggest that may be able to promote osteoblast activity when non-menopausal bone is utilized, as will be discussed later [22].

Affordability and access also hamper effective prevention of alveolar bone loss in PD [27]. Good dental hygiene prevents the development of periodontal disease [27]. A common problem in adulthood for individuals in developed nations, advanced PD is widespread in developing countries and tooth loss may be apparent in even young adults [26]. Allicin's extensive antibacterial activity includes targeting the major organism that cause plaque deposition, namely *Porphyromonas gingivalis* and was shown in a very recent study to also downregulate osteoclast RANKL [24]. Both these findings would support its development as an oral treatment, especially for those less well able to afford or access classical treatments. Finally the relatively rare disease of AS, is also known to involve dysregulation of the gut biome as an underlying contributory factor to disease development, particularly allowing the growth of *Klebsiella pneumoniae* [31]. AS has very specific inheritance patterns with the majority of patients expressing an altered HLA-B27 antigen that promotes the eventual sequelae of OA or OP [6]. Allicin's potential to act as both cartilage and bone protective agent could provide a novel approach to later disease but this agent has also recently been suggested to decrease the expression of the mis-folded HLA-B27 in a murine model of the disease [16].

2. Allicin as Antibacterial Agent for AS and PD Intervention

Since its discovery in 1944 allicin has been shown to be effective against a diversity of gram positive and negative bacteria, including multi-resistant organisms [15]. Most importantly, allicin possesses broad-spectrum antibacterial activity against the major agents related to the pathophysiology of AS and PD, namely *Klebsiella pneumoniae* [32-34] and *Porphyromonas ginigivalis* [24, 35, 36] respectively.

2.1. Ankylosing Spondylitis and *K. pneumoniae*

Overgrowth of the common gastrointestinal bacterium *Klebsiella pneumoniae* results from gastrointestinal dysbiosis also associated with chronic inflammation [6]. *K. pneumoniae* antibodies cross react with synovial tissues, thereby providing an initiating point for the autoimmune responses associated with AS [6]. Patients with active disease display elevated serum antibody titers, whereas anti-*K. pneumoniae* antibodies are low or absent in those with quiescent symptoms [6]. As many as one in ten patients with AS will develop full blown IBD and an estimated seventy percent have subclinical illness [31]. At least three studies have demonstrated garlic extracts or allicin to possess *in vitro* antibacterial activity against *K. pneumoniae* [33]. Different minimum inhibitory concentrations (MIC) against clinical isolates of *K. pneumoniae* were reported in these studies [32-34]. A purified sample of allicin possessed an MIC of 8 μg/ml [32] and a later study showed an aqueous extract of garlic to have an MIC of 24 mg/ml [33]. Most recently, allicin as a volatile vapor was reported to have an MIC of 128 μg/ml against two separate strains of *K. pneumoniae* [34].

2.2. Periodontal Disease and *P. gingivalis*

Altered oral flora composition in which biofilm-forming pathogens colonize the gingiva, is the precursor to PD [37]. Several bacteria have been recognized as pathogens in the disease, most notably *P. gingivalis* and to a lesser extent *Prevotella denticola* and *Fusobacterium* species [37]. Oral pathogens responsible for PD induce the expression of MMP enzymes in gingival epithelia [38]. Once activated, MMP can degrade type I collagen, thereby destroying the periodontal ligament, cement and underlying bone [39]. *P. gingivalis* induces local dendritic macrophage maturation and activation of both classic Th1 cells and Th17 cells [40]. Adaptive responses are then selectively made against the initiating bacterium e.g., *P. gingivalis* [41]. Controlling the pathogens of PD therefore prevents the later bone resoprtion phase of the disease [37].

At least three studies have demonstrated garlic extracts or allicin to possess *in vitro* antibacterial activity against *P. gingivalis* and other periodontal pathogens [24, 35, 36]. Different minimum inhibitory concentrations (MIC) against clinical isolates of *P. gingivalis* were reported in these studies [24, 35, 36]. A single comparative study of oral pathogens involved in initiating PD demonstrated that allicin was able to kill *Fusabacterium nucleatum* and *Aggregatibacter actinomycetecomitans* with an MIC of 300 μg/ml [36]. A higher MIC (2,400 μg/ml) was needed to kill *P. gingivalis* in two separate studies [24, 36]. A third study, which used aqueous extracts of garlic, reported a higher MIC of 62.5 mg/ml, although the exact allicin content was unclear [35]. One study also showed that allicin (32 mg/l) reduced the thickness of one day old *P. gingivalis* biofilms [24], making them easier to remove with a combination of classic debridement and antimicrobial techniques.

P. gingivalis secretes gingipains, which are involved in the ability of the organism to produce biofilms and initiate PD through acquisition of iron in the form of heme groups from red blood cells [42]. Studies with a gingipain mutant demonstrated a similar sensitivity to allicin (300 μg/ml) as other bacteria involved in oral biofilm formation [36]. Allicin may also be able to directly target gingipains, albeit when used at higher concentrations, which would make it a unique molecule in the treatment of PD [36]. Like most biofilms, those of *P. gingivalis* are upto five hundred times as resistant to antibiotics as planktonic i.e., unattached oral bacteria [42]. Antibiotic treatment of periodontal disease caused by these biofilms requires 1,000-2,500 mg/day, depending on the therapy used [43] i.e., an equivalent dosage as that of allicin [36]. Further extensive discussion of allicin's antibacterial activities can be seen in Chapter 5, but it is clear that its direct effects on the microbial triggers of AS and PD have the potential to delay the appearance of symptoms in susceptible individuals

3. Allicin's Possible Activity against HLA-B27 in Ankylosing Spondylitis

Only one literature study has appeared that investigated the effects of allicin on a murine model of AS [16] but it may represent the first ever description of an agent that can prevent the expression of the self antigen HLA-B27 [16]. Gu and colleagues [16] employed an HLA-B27 Kunming mouse model of AS. Oral dosing of the animals with high dose allicin (200 mg/kg) for two months resulted in a significant decrease in spinal damage as well as a reduction in expression of HLA-B27 protein (but not the gene itself) [16]. A significant reduction in levels of IL-6, IL-8 and TNF-α was also observed [16].

Animal models suggest there are two stages to AS disease, stemming from local macrophage activation [6]. The earliest involves macrophage activity, augmented by IL-6 and IL-8, which then activates Th1 cells [6]. Th1 cells generate IFN-γ, which feeds back to continue the macrophage activation as well as augmenting cytokine release [6]. The later stage involves further activation and recruitment of macrophages and neutrophils, through the combined effects of these cytokines [6].

The study of Gu and colleagues [6], if it translates into humans, is therefore important in that it suggests the ability of allicin to decrease the disease at the early phase in a two-fold manner; reduction in macrophage-induced cytokine secretion and HLA-B27 expression. Whether allicin affects IFN-γ in these animals was undocumented but garlic oil (which contains allicin [30], has been previously shown to suppress IFN-γ secretion from rodent lymph node macrophages [44]. In this study, garlic oil (10-200 mg/kg) given by gavage to rats for two weeks and their cervical lymph nodes examined [44]. The investigators reported that high doses of oil (>50 mg/kg) i.e., higher levels of allicin, were associated with the generation of an anti-inflammatory environment in which IFN-γ was suppressed [44]. This would be in keeping with the high dose allicin results (200 mg/ kg) seen by Gu and colleagues [3] and is suggestive for allicin providing immunosuppression at these doses.

HLA-B27, which is carried by around ninety percent of patients with AS and plays a central role in the pathophysiology of the condition AS have been suggested [6, 45]. HLA-B27 appears able to bind unique peptides including aggrecan and present these to $CD8^+$ T cytotoxic cells, which mediate tissue injury [6]. The self antigen does not always fold correctly and when displayed on cell surfaces may initiate autoimmune responses are a result [6]. Abnormally folded proteins of this type are particularly prone to recognition by NK cells, as well as Th1 cells, which promote attack of these target molecules [6]. HLA-B27 expression may also "autoactivate" the cells it is expressed on, creating inflammation by upregulating NF-κB [46]. Termed unfolded protein response (UPR), this results in activation of NK cells and macrophages, dendritic cell maturation and initiation of immune system inflammatory reactions [6].

So how is allicin effecting this change in HLA-B27 expression? Guo and colleagues [16] observed that allicin did not change the levels of the gene expression; rather, only the resulting protein was altered. This suggests that allicin may be targeting the ability of the HLA-B27 protein to fold into its final conformation, thereby preventing its expression. Similar effects were described by Cavallito [47], in his initial studies on the antibacterial effects of the thiosulfinate.

4. Allicin Improves Chrondrocyte/Cartilage Health in Models of Disease

Recent literature reports have suggested allicin has been shown to be effective in several *in vitro* [17-19, 21] and animal models of OA [17, 20, 21] and a single DBRPCT human trial [25]. The six studies, their design and findings are shown in Table 1.

The four *in vitro* studies of allicin employed similar micromolar dosages of allicin and efficacy times (24-36 hours) [17-19, 21, 22]. Although unblinded to the investigators, these investigations do provide a picture of allicin's potential for chondroprotection through increasing cartilage viability and ability to divide [18]. In addition, as well as several indices of cartilage function were noted to improve namely aggrecan and type II collagen content [19, 21]. Three separate *in vitro* studies using either interleukin-1 beta (IL-1β)-induced [19, 21] or urate-crystal-mediated OA [17] also showed allicin at micromolar levels (2.5-50 μM) ameliorated chondrocyte inflammatory markers [17, 19, 21]. These included metalloproteinase (MMP), NF-κB, MAPK, inducible nitric oxide synthase (iNOS) and prostaglandin E_2 (PGE_2) [17, 19, 21].

Although the MAPK pathway described as downregulated in allicin-treatment of IL-1β-stimulated OA human chondrocytes was not identified [19], it is likely to be ERK given the mitigation of damage. This is consistent with the effect of allicin on other chronic inflammatory disease models [15]. Allicin's ability to downregulate the phosphoinositide-3 kinase/protein kinase B (P13K/Akt) pathway *in vivo* is also of interest as this pathway is able to initiate new blood vessel growth (angiogenesis) [48]; an event which results in both chondrocyte death and advancing OA disease [1].

Table 1. Allicin's anti-inflammatory activity in models of OA

Study design	Results	Reference
In vitro OA assay; rabbit synovial cells (HIG-82), human knee OA chondrocytes and fibroblasts activated with urate crystals (2 mg/ml) or IL-1β (10 ng/ml) for 6 h and incubated in presence or absence of allicin (1-50 mM) for 6 h	Significant ($p < 0.01$) ↓ COX2 but not COX1 activation and PGE_2 production in presence of urate crystals using allicin at >10 mM ↓ COX2 activation production by IL-1β -stimulated OA chondrocytes and fibroblasts using allicin at >20 mM	[17]
In vitro OA assay; isolated healthy knee chondrocytes from Sprague-Dawley rats incubated in presence or absence of allicin (10-50 μM) for 36 h	Significant ($p < 0.01$) ↑ chondrocyte numbers and viability together with movement of cells into S phase (i.e., division) Allicin at all concentrations activated expression of division molecules (cell cyclin D1, CDK4 and CDK6)	[18]
In vitro OA assay: isolated human knee OA chondrocytes, activated by incubation with IL-1β and incubated in presence or absence of allicin (2.5, 5 and 10 μM) for 24 h	Significant ($p < 0.01$) ↓ IL-1β-induced PGE_2, iNOS, MAPK, MMP-3 and NF-κB activation ↑ type II collagen and aggrecan Allicin effective at all concentrations used	[19]
In vitro OA study; isolated murine chondrocytes, activated by incubation with IL-1β (10 ng/ml) in presence or absence of allicin (5 or 10 μM) for 24 h	Significant ($p < 0.05$) ↓ IL-1β-induced iNOS, NO, PGE_2, Il-6, TNF-α	[21]
In vivo OA study: Wistar rats inoculated with urate (2 mg) and 48.9 mg/kg of allicin into knee cavity and changes assessed at 16 h	Significant ($p < 0.01$) ↓ COX2 activation in harvested synovial tissue. Accompanied by ↓ in neutrophil infiltration of synovial space	[17]
In vivo OA study; 6 albino rats given 100 mg/kg of allicin or piroxicam by gavage. OA provoked by 0.01 ml turpentine oil injected into knee joint and changes assessed after 6 h.	Significant ($p < 0.05$) ↓ in knee swelling produced by both allicin and piroxicam (55-60% for each) Allicin believed to exert effects by ↓ROS through ↑ GpX and catalase	[20]
In vivo OA *study*; 30 C57BL/6 mice given OA by destabilization of knee meniscus, 15 received allicin (10 mg/kg/day in CMC by gavage) and 15 received CMC alone for 8 weeks	Significant ($p < 0.05$) ↓ P13K/Akt, MMP-13 activation in murine cartilage ↑ type II collagen and aggrecan	[21]
Human OA study; 76 obese/ overweight women with early OA in DBRPCT parallel trial, 1,000 mg garlic tablet# for 12 weeks	Overall WOMAC score was unchanged Pain, stiffness and physical function were significantly improved in garlic group ($p < 0.01$) compared with placebo	[25]

=expected to contain allicin but of an unknown strength.

Abbreviations used in the table: Akt (protein kinase B), CMC (carboxymethylcellulose), COX (cyclooxygenase), DBRPCT (double blind, randomized, placebo-controlled trial), ERK (extracellular signal redulated kinase), GpX (glutathione peroxidase), IL-1β (interleukin-1 beta), IL-6 (interleukin 6), iNOS (inducible nitric oxide synthase), MAPK (mitogen-activated protein kinase), MMP (metalloproteinase 3 and 13), NF-κB (nuclear factor kappa beta), NO (nitric oxide), OA (osteoarthritis), P13K (phosphoinositide-3 phosphate), PGE_2 (prostaglandin E_2), ROS (reactive oxygen species), TNF-α (tumor necrosis factor alpha), WOMAC (Western Ontario and McMaster Universities Osteoarthritis Index).

Allicin was able to suppress *in vivo* inflammation in three animal models of knee OA [17, 20, 21]. Activation of glutathione peroxidase (GpX) [20] and decrease of reactive oxygen species (ROS) [20] may result from the observed suppression of the NF-κB pathway [17]. OA cartilage damage is amplified by IL-1, IL-6 and TNF-α activated synovial macrophages (synoviocytes) as well as MMP activation [1]. MMP can further degrade type I collagen thereby damaging both cartilage and bone beneath [1]. Levels of joint-damaging MMP-3, are also highly expressed in AS patients and directly correlate with symptom levels [6]. Allicin was able to impair the expression of MMP-3 in one murine *in vivo* OA study [19] and the shared MMP-3 pathologies of OA [1] and AS [6] further point to the potential utility of the thiosulfinate in both osteodegenerative conditions.

In addition, the finding that allicin impaired *in vitro* OA chondrocyte generation of pro-inflammatory cytokines [21], MMP-3 and 13 [19, 21] is reflective of its downregulation of NF-κB [9, 21]. Further support for allicin's downregulation of NF-κB in OA chondrocytes was demonstrated in the *in vitro* study, which demonstrated a simultaneous reduction of prostaglandin E_2 (PGE_2) and the cyclooxygenase enzyme involved in their generation, (COX-2) [19, 21]. Activation of cyclooxygenase (COX-2) enzyme expression is associated with further OA damage through the production of large amounts of prostaglandin E_2 (PGE_2) [49]. PGE_2 reduces cartilage components as well as collagen levels within the cartilage matrix thereby weakening it [1, 4, 49]. More importantly PGE_2 upregulates the differentiation of Th17 helper cells, thereby facilitating the production of autoantibodies that are characteristic of the later stages of OA [50]. The ability of allicin to downregulate PGE_2 expression at micomolar concentrations *in vitro* may be as a result of its central effects on NF-κB or possibly a direct effect on the COX pathway itself. The mitigation of PGE_2 levels also correlates with the observation that the thiosulfinate increased levels of type II collagen both *in vitro* [19, 21] and *in* vivo [21]. Again, allicin's effects on pro-inflammatory cytokines, NF-κB and activation of thiol-sensitive ROS inhibitors like GpX are central to its abilities and well documented in other systems [15].

The single double blind, randomized placebo-controlled trial (DBRPCT) human study is the only one that differs from the others in that a 1,000 mg "garlic" tablet was administered [25]. Garlic powder contains between 0.64 and 4.64 mg/g of garlic [30] and the lowest recommended allicin doses for efficacy that have been used in clinical trials are somewhere between 3.6 and 7.8 mg [51]. This means that the 1,000 mg certainly has the potential to be effective but since allicin levels were not determined the study must be interpreted with caution. In addition, the WOMAC (Western Ontario and McMaster Universities Osteoarthritis Index) scale was the only criterion used for OA improvement in the study [25]. WOMAC is a self-administered scale that asks patients to report changes in stiffness, pain and mobility when walking, lying down and using stairs [52]. This reviewer would have preferred measurements of other parameters of OA, such as circulating inflammatory cytokine levels, as a more determinant method to assess the patients' improvement.

5. Allicin Improves Bone Health in Models of Disease

The *in vitro* model of OP reported that allicin at all concentrations (10-100 μg/ml) significantly improved the functionality of damaged osteoblast cells [22]. This was seen to proceed by activation of the P13K/Akt pathway, which is known to play a central role in the bone-building activity of these cells [53]. Maintenance of bone health is a delicate balance between the activities of the bone creators (osteoblasts) and bone remodelers/ destroyers (osteoclasts) [7, 8]. Since bone resorption is associated with excessive numbers or activation of osteoclasts, osteoblast activation would be expected to promote retention of bone density [7, 8]. Interestingly, increased bone density was reported in a single *in vivo* animal study, using a post-menopausal model of OP, after one month of oral administration of garlic oil (100 mg/kg/day) [23]. Taken together these results suggest allicin or garlic would be osteoprotective, especially for the post-menopausal women that account for the majority of cases [8-10].

Although allicin's effects on RANKL were not investigated in OA or OP, this has been investigated *in vitro* and *in vivo* on a related condition; periodontal disease (PD) [24]. Recent studies of a rodent model of PD reported that seven days of allicin (4 mg or 8 mg/L) injection was able to decrease gingivomucosal inflammation as well as prevent bone resorption [24]. Colorimetric kit analysis of the ginogivomucosa concentrations of allicin produced significant ($p < 0.05$) reductions in pro-inflammatory cytokines IL-1β, IL-6, IL-12, IFN-γ and TNF-α with a consequent increase in anti-inflammatory cytokines IL-4 and IL-10 [24]. Tibial bone marrow cells in the animals treated with allicin also demonstrated an over seventy percent decreased expression of inflammatory NF-κB p65, RANKL and macrophage colony stimulating factor (M-CSF) [24]. Guan and colleagues [24] also reported that this was reflected in a suppresson of tibial osteoclast activity [24]. Part of allicin's efficacy against RANKL may have been mediated by the impairment of *P. gingivalis* biofilm formation, as this is a major initiating factor of PD [24]. The effects on the local cytokines might have been partially abrogated through impairing *P. gingivalis* lipopolysaccharide (LPS)-induced inflammation although the direct effects on NF-κB inhibition are supported by other studies [15].

Table 2. Allicin and models of disease

Study design	Results	Reference
In vitro OP study: murine osteoblast MCT3T3-E1 cells damaged by incubation with H2O2 (200 μM) in presence or absence of allicin (10, 30 or 100 μg/ml)	At all concentrations allicin reduced oxidative stress ↑ P13K/Akt activation as well as the CRB/ERK pathway	[22]
In vivo OP study #: 6 albino rats underwent ovariectomy and were fed garlic oil (100 mg/kg/day) or saline vehicle for 30 days	No biochemical parameters of bone investigated. Ribs, thoracic and lumbar vertebrae all increased significantly in bone density ($p < 0.01$)	[23]
In vitro: tibia and fibial osteoblasts and osteoclast progenitor cells isolated from Sprague Dawley rat model of PD (see below) after 7 days of treatment. Cells co-cultured with either allicin (4 or 8 mg/L) or saline vehicle for 4 days	Significant ($p < 0.05$) ↓ in expression of NF-κB p65, RANKL and M-CSF Tibial osteoclast numbers analyzed by TRAP and significantly ($p < 0.05$) ↓in both 4 and 8 mg/L allicin-treated animals	[24]
In vivo: Sprague Dawley rat (n = 9) model of PD created by tying a wire ligature around molars and gingivomucosa. Animals injected in palate with allicin (4 or 8 mg/L) or saline vehicle for 7 days	Gingivomucosal tissues of allicin treated animals demonstrated significant ↓ in NF-κB and pro-inflammatory cytokines and ↑ in anti-inflammatory cytokines	[24]

Abbreviations used in the table: Akt (protein kinase B), COX (cyclooxygenase), CRB (cyclic monophosphate response element-binding protein), ERK (extracellular signal redulated kinase), H2O2 (hydrogen peroxide), M-CSF (macrophage colony stimulating factor), NF-κB (nuclear factor kappa beta), OP (osteoporosis), P13K (phosphoinositide-3 phosphate), PD (periodontal disease), RANKL (nuclear factor kappa beta ligand), TRAP (tartrate resistant acid phosphatase stain).

The single striking finding from Guan's study was the ability of allicin entering the mouth palate to decrease inflammation in the distant bone (tibia) through preventing osteoclast activation [24]. Currently no agents exist that are able to inhibit RANKL or translocation of the NF-κB subunit p65 [24]. Given the importance of RANKL overactivity in the alveolar bone loss of PD [24], as well as bone resorption in OA [1] allicin may be useful in reducing osteodegeneration for both conditions.

An overview of allicin's potential effects in the four conditions of AS, OA, OP and PD is summarized in Figure 1 below.

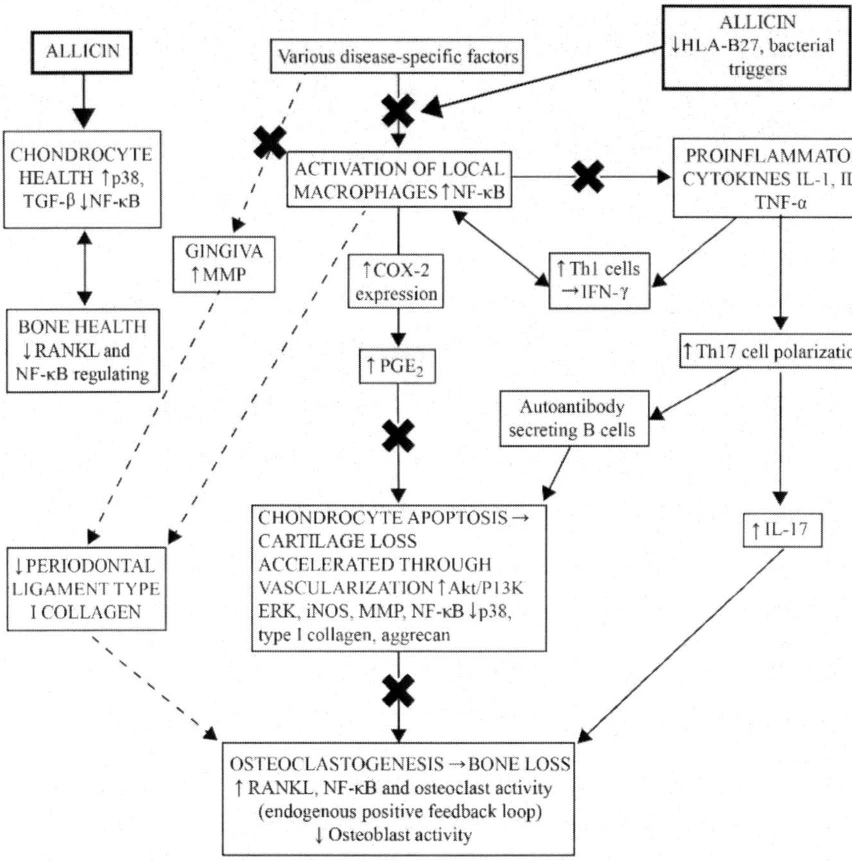

✖ Allicin's points of inhibition ◄──► crosstalk – – – ► periodontal disease only.

Legend: Maintenance of synovial bone health is dependent on cartilage integrity above and lack of inflammation of the surrounding tissues. Damage phenomena, including aging, trauma and bacterial dysbiosis can perturb this homeostasis resulting in the chronic inflammatory syndromes of AS, OA, OP and PD. Cartilage loss, accelerated through vascularization, then stimulates further bone loss by tipping the balance in favor of osteoclast (bone resorption cells). Allicin can "reset" this balance by decreasing initiation factors, improving chondrocyte health and simultaneously decreasing osteoclast activity while boosting osteoblast functions. Allicin's anti-inflammatory activies would decrease macrophage activation and reduce the chronic inflammation that is a hallmark of AS, OA, OP and PD.

Abbreviations: Akt, COX-2 (cyclooxygenase 2), ERK (extracellular receptor kinase), IL (interleukin), iNOS (inducible nitric oxide synthase), MMP (metalloproteinase), P13K, RANKL (nuclear factor kappa beta ligand), TNF-α (tumor necrosis factor alpha).

References: [3-5, 7, 8, 12, 21, 22, 34-38, 46, 52, 55, 59].

Figure 1. Allicin's impact on the pathophysiology of osteodegenerative disease.

CONCLUSION AND FUTURE DIRECTIONS

The literature on allicin or allicin-containing garlic products is supportive of its ability to maintain cartilage health and re-establish bone integrity through a diversity of mechanisms (Figure 1). First and foremost, allicin is antibacterial [15, 24, 32-36]. With reference to cartilage and bone protection, this capacity allows it to eliminate *K. pneumoniae* [31-33] and *P. gingivalis* [24, 34-36]; the microbial triggers of AS and PD, respectively. In AS patients, treatment is primarily with acetylsalicylic acid (ASA) to reduce inflammation during flares of the disease [6], rather than modifying the gut biome. Recent studies have suggested that ASA can promote various mutations leading to increased antibiotic resistant strains and have suggested alternatives should be used in these patients [54]. ASA become active when cleaved by gastrointestinal bacteria and are preferred by clinicians and patients due to their low incidence of side effects.

P. gingivalis is of particular import as its ability to form biofilms is central to the pathology of PD [11]. As a result, traditional treatment of PD seeks to remove these biofilms by painful debridement, antibiotic treatment and ultimately surgery if these methods fail [11]. Most patients in developed countries have some kind of dental access, which means that periodontitis generally does not emerge as a major issue until late adulthood [26]. In contrast, by their late teens somewhere between thirty five and seventy percent of residents in developing countries already display bleeding gums and plaque deposition [26]. Incorporation of allicin into mouthwash may also be effective [55]. Comparison of chlorhexidine mouthwash alone with that containing a five percent alcohol extract of garlic (containing allicin) demonstrated a decrease in oral flora count of approximately ninety-eight percent [55]. Presumably for patients the major issue might be an unpalatable taste but this might be rectified if a semi-synthetic or synthetic form of the thiosulfinate were used.

Allicin's efficacy against oral *P. gingivalis* may have additional benefits; the prevention of rheumatoid arthritis (RA) development [56-61]. The strong links between PD and RA have been provided by findings from several studies [56-62]. Several observations have connected infection with *P. gingivalis* with the precipitation and progression of RA [56 62]. Animals infected with *P. gingivalis* produce an RA syndrome of disease [56]. Treatment of PD reduces RA symptoms [57]. Patients with RA produce anti-*P. gingivalis* antibodies and their titer corresponds both to the classic anti-CCP (cyclic citrullinated peptide) and rheumatoid factor RA autoantibodies [58]. Antibodies against these proteins appear years before disease symptoms and are a specific pathology associated with RA [59]. *P. gingivalis* is able to produce citrullinated human fibrinogen and α-enolase proteins [60]. The bacterial α-enolase, shares over eighty percent homology with the human variant [61] and allows the bacteria to "confuse" the immune system to produce RA [61]. Finally, PG is able to directly induce early and late apoptosis of human chondrocytes, whch contributes to the cartilage loss in RA [62]. So why hasn't allicin been tested for its efficacy against RA? Interestingly, one of the animal studies of the effect of allicin on OA utilized a turpentine-induced arthritis which is also used to represent RA pathology [20]. The study found that allicin (100 mg/kg) was able to abrogate the swelling and ROS-induced inflammation in knee synovium within six hours of administration [20]. No additional studies have appeared in the literature that examine the effects of allicin and RA, either *in vitro* or *in vivo*.

Allicin's potential efficacy in maintaining healthy chondrocyte function and repair [17-19] as well as suppressing inflammatory pathways in damaged chondrocytes [18, 19, 21] would support its utility in the cartilage and fibrocartilage-eroding syndromes of OA and AS. Patient mangement involves non-steroidal anti-inflammatory agents (NSAIDs), to reduce pain and stiffness in both conditions [1, 63]. NSAIDs inhibit inflammation through down-regulating NF-κB, thereby preventing the generation of pro-inflammatory prostaglandins through the COX pathway [1]. Patients who take NSAIDs long term are prone to gatrointestinal ulcers and irritation [1], as well as an acceleration of underlying pathological changes in OA [1]. Most clinicians in this field agree that new therapies for AS and OA are urgently needed, especially those addressing molecular mechanisms contributing to the underlying pathologies [1, 6].

Allicin was reported to possess efficacy in several animal models of knee OA [17, 20, 21] as well as in a single DBRPCT human trial [25]. Current strategies for knee OA are to delay joint replacement by direct annual injections of lubricating hyaluronic acid into the synovial space [1]. Given that this treatment does not require oral absorption some groups are already exploring adding phytochemicals to the injectable, to produce an anti-inflammatory effect [64]. For example, a recent notable study was performed using a rodent model of knee OA and was able to demonstrate direct anti-inflammatory activity using the volatile, turmeric-derived injectable spice curcumin [64]. Injection would theoretically maximize the efficacy of allicin and its potential now needs to be investigated for corresponding human efficacy. Allicin's potentially unique ability to prevent HLA-B27 expression in AS patients [6] is one avenue that is worth exploring as no therapy has, to date, been able to intervene with the altered protein that is the hallmark of many patients with this condition.

Although much of allicin's beneficial effects on chrondrocyte function have been studied in OA these may also extend to other conditions. For example, fibrocartilage cells in AS (enthesophytes) invade the bone beneath, resulting in cracks and granulation tissue [6]. Blood vessels that infiltrate the bone from the internal marrow cause hollowing and later these "tunnels" fill with bone [6]. This weakened bone is then prone to developing either OA or OP [6]. Cells that generate fibrocartilage have characteristics of both chondrocytes and fibroblasts and appear to process proteins differently [54, 55]. At least one study reported allicin (48.9 mg/kg) was able to decrease both fibroblast and chondrocyte damage [17]. These data suggest that allicin should be effective against the enthesophytes that initiate early symptoms of AS, although this clearly remains to be proven. Allicin's ability to rebalance P13K/Akt expression in both chondrocyte [21] and osteoblasts [22] would reduce the initiation of angiogenesis and bone resorption common to AS, as well as OA and OP [1, 6, 26]. When allicin's ameliorating effects on the AS precipitating factors of HLA-B27 protein expression [16] and gut dysbiosis [32-34] are added to the equation, this suggests the thiosulfinate may also be of great future utility in preventing AS disease progression into either OP or OA.

As was previously mentioned, patients with OP acquire the condition either early in life due to precipitating factors of malnutrition, thalassemia, or AS or post-menopausally due to a drop in estrogen levels [26]. About five percent of the two hundred million worldwide OP sufferers live in the United States, where they are well managed with a variety of established osteoclast inhibitors, with relatively low side effects [26]. In contrast, patients in developing countries still suffer extensive morbidity [26]. For example, Asia has just under ten percent of all OP cases worldwide, but current estimates are that only one in five of these individuals are given effective bone density-promoting pharmaceuticals [26]. Cost and access are major barriers to access for OP patients in developing nations and clinicians there are already beginning to explore naturopathic, local plants as bone density boosting agents [26]. Over seventy plants have been identified, of which ten have been researched extensively [26]. Most important in this regard have been the *Psorylea cordilifolia* and *Pueraria lobata* (Kudzu) plants which are already used extensively in traditional Chinese and Ayurvedic medicine for many bone conditions [26]. *P. cordilifolia*'s isoflavone bavachalcone is able to inhibit osteoclastogenesis and upregulate osteoblast bone manufacture directly through P13K/Akt and ERK modulation [26]. Kudzu extract has estrogen-like properties and promotes bone building by upregulating osteoblast activity [26]. Allicin and the garlic clove from which it originates have not been well studied in this respect but their ability to increase bone density in post-menopausal models suggests they may have merit in further testing, particularly as the activity is restricted to an individual entity.

The thiol- and redox-targeting nature of allicin provides it with the ability to simultaneous modulate a series of cell pathways [15-24] rather than suppressing them like conventional drugs do [1, 6, 26]. This ability is not unique to phytochemicals as many are adaptogens for pathways like NF-κB i.e., dial up or dial down activation, and avoid producing unwanted effects on normal cell systems as a result [12, 13, 65].

Finally, allicin's potential ability to reduce triggers for OA and PD can not be undersold in managing these conditions [66-68]. The strong links between existing cardiovascular disease and type II diabetes as increased risk for OA and PD have been demonstrated in many clinical studies [66-68]. Allicin and the garlic clove from which it originates have been demonstrated in several studies to be cadioprotective by improving cholesterol metabolism [69-71] and reducing plasma cortisol [72] (see also Chapter 10 for details). A significant ($p < 0.001$) reduction in serum cholesterol was produced by oral administration of allicin (5-20 mg/kg) for twelve weeks in a hyperlipidemic murine model [69]. Allicin was also shown, *in vitro*, to impair two enzymes involved in cholesterol biosynthesis, namely squalene-monooxygenase [70] and acetyl coA synthase [71]. A fourth study reported that allicin (in 0.8 g/100 g garlic powder) was able to reduce plasma cortisol in a rodent model [72]. Cholesterol and cortisol dysfunction combine to produce a metabolic syndrome that produces insulin resistance [69-72]. Allicin's has the potential to simultaneously abrogate both conditions thereby reducing one major risk factor for both OA and PD.

So why have no human DBRPCT appeared in the literature for allicin (not the parent garlic) with the conditions discussed in this chapter? One obvious reason is that all the literature studies are very recent i.e., research is only just beginning [16-25]. A second issue is the stability of allicin, which has provided a very real challenge to a prolonged bioavailability in the body [15]. At least two stabilized forms of allicin exist [73, 74] and *in situ* generation of allicin attached to a McAb has been successful in animal models [75]. Two groups have also synthesized "allicin-like" molecules and compared their antimicrobial activity with that of the parent allicin [76, 77]. These substituted allicins are at least as effective and have a longer duration of potency so may be a good direction to drug development for the thiosulfinate [76, 77]. Finally, it is important to realize that the process of developing a new pharmaceutical is both long and expensive and will necessitate a number of human DBRPCT at the end [78]. This means that any treatment being developed, whether from natural or synthetic sources, must prove devoid of significant side effects as well as effective [78].

Allicin, like other phytochemicals, is likely to be well received as "safe and natural" by patients in most developed countries [1, 12, 13] as well as being an extension of traditional plant-based therapies in developing ones [14]. At least three of the conditions mentioned in this chapter, namely OA, OP and PD are expected to see a significant upward trend in numbers in developing countries [1, 26, 79]. OA is anticipated to affect 130 million people from middle age on by 2050, many of whom live in developing nations [1]. OP already affects 200 million people worldwide with the resulting fractures being associated with increased mortality rates [80]. Some suggest that by 2050, half of all fractures due to OP will occur in Asia, where the health systems are ill-equipped to deal with these patients [80]. Similarly poor oral hygiene and PD are major issues for individuals living in Africa and Asia, where the condition is associated with significant morbidity [79]. Just as the search for antimicrobial agents took us to natural products, recent studies are now suggesting a role for plant-derived phytochemicals [12, 13]. The literature of the past few years suggests allicin is poised to take a lead role due to its cartilage and bone protective abilities at the molecular level and the next steps should see a move from animal models to human clinical trials with this promising thiofulfinate.

References

[1] Cundell, Diana R., and Kathryn E. Mickle. 2018. "Osteoarthritis: potential for herbal medicines as therapies in the management of chronic inflammatory damage." *Current Immunology Reviews,* 14:68-80. E Pub ahead of print link. Accessed on September 25, 2018 http://www.eurekaselect.com/node/162555/article/osteoarthritis-potential-for-herbal-medicines-as-therapies-in-the-management-of-chronic-inflammatory-damage.

[2] Houard, Xavier, Mary B. Goldring, and Francis Berenbaum. 2013. Homeostatic mechanisms in articular cartilage and role of inflammation in osteoarthritis. *Current Rheumatology Reports* 15(11), 375. doi: 10.1007/s11926-013-0375-6.

[3] Oh, Chung-Doh, Sung-Hee Chang, Young-Mee Soon, Su-Jae Lee, Yun-Sil Lee, Shin-Sung Kang, and Jang-Soo Chun. 2000. "Opposing roles of mitogen-activated protein kinase subtypes, ERK-1/2 and p38 in the regulation of chondrogenesis of mesenchymes." *J. Biol. Chem.* 275: 5613-5619. doi: 10.1074/jbc.275.8.5613.

[4] Yang, Xiao, Li Chen, Xioaling Xu, Cuiling Li, Cuifen Huang, and Chu-Xia Deng. 2001. "TGF-beta/Smad3 signals repress chondrocyte hypertrophic differentiation and are required for maintaining articular cartilage." *The Journal of Cell Biology* 153(1): 35-46.

[5] Findlay, David M., and Julia S. Kuliwaba. 2016. "Bone-cartilage crosstalk: a conversation for understanding osteoarthritis." *Bone Research* 4:16028. doi:10.1038/boneres.2016.28.

[6] Shamji, Mohammed F., Mohammed Bafaquh, and Eve Tsai. 2008. "The pathogenesis of ankylosing spondylitis." *Neurosurg. Focus* 24(1): E3. Accessed October 25, 2018. https://thejns.org/focus/view/journals/neurosurg-focus/24/1/article-pE3.xml?rfr_dat=cr_pub=pubmed&rfr_id=ori:rid:crossref.org&url_ver=Z39.88-2003#container-4202-item-4200.

[7] Rinaldo Florencio-Silva, Gisela Rodrigues da Silva Sasso, Estela Sasso-Cerri, Manuel Jesus Simões, and Paulo Sérgio Cerri. 2015. "Biology of Bone Tissue: Structure, Function, and Factors That Influence Bone Cells," *BioMed Research International* 2015, Article ID 421746, 17 pages, 2015. https://doi.org/10.1155/2015/421746.

[8] Abdollabi, Mohammed, Bagher Larijani, Roja Rabini, and Pooneh Salar. 2005. "Role of oxidative stress in osteoporosis." *Therapy* 2(5):77-86. Accesssed on April 15, 2019.

https://www.openaccessjournals.com/articles/role-of-oxidative-stress-in-osteoporosis.pdf.

[9] Hienz, Stefan A., Sweta Paliwal, and Saso Ivanovski. 2015. "Mechanisms of Bone Resorption in Periodontitis." *Journal of Immunology Research* 2015: 615486. doi: 10.1155/2015/615486.

[10] Tu, Kristie N., Janette D. Lie, Chew K. V. Wan, Madison Cameron, Alaina G. Austel, Jenny K. Nguyen, Kevin Van, and Diana Hyun. 2018. "Osteoporosis: A Review of Treatment Options." *P & T: A Peer-reviewed Journal for Formulary Management* 43(2): 92–104. Accessed on April 15, 2019. https://www.ptcommunity.com/system/files/pdf/ptj4302092.pdf.

[11] Armitage, Gary C., and Paul B. Robertson. 2009. "The biology, prevention, diagnosis and treatment of periodontal disease." *J. A. D. A.* 140(1):36S-43S. doi: https://doi.org/10.14219/jada.archive.2009.0356.

[12] Jia, Min, Yang Nie, Da-Ping Cao, Yun-Yun Xue, Jie-Si Wang, Lu Zhao, Khalid Rahman, Qiao-Yan Zhang, and Lu-Ping Qin. 2012. "Potential antiosteoporotic agents from plants: a comprehensive review." *Evidence-based Complementary and Alternative Medicine: eCAM* 2012: 364604. doi: 10.1155/2012/364604.

[13] Leong, Daniel J., Marwa Choudhury, David M. Hirsh, John A. Hardin, Neil J. Cobelli, and Hui B. Sun. 2013. Nutraceuticals: potential for chondroprotection and molecular targeting of osteoarthritis. *International Journal of Molecular Sciences* 14(11):23063–23085. doi: 10.3390/ijms141123063.

[14] Cundell, Diana R. 2014. Herbal phytochemicals as immunomodulators *Current Immunology Reviews 2014*, Volume 10 Issue 2 ISSN:1875-631X(Online), ISSN:1573-3955(Print) Accessed September 10, 2018. http://benthamscience.com/journal/index.php?journalID=cir.

[15] Borlinghaus, Jan, Frank Albrecht, Martin C. H. Grulke, Ifeanyi D. Nwachukwu, and Alan J. Slusarenko. 2014. "Allicin: Chemistry and biological properties." *Molecules* 19(8): 12591-12618.

[16] Gu, Xin, Haishin Wu, and Fu Peilang. 2013. Allicin attenuates inflammation and suppresses HLA-B27 protein expression in ankylosing spondylitis mice. *BioMed Research international* 2013:171573 doi: 10.1155/2013/171573.

[17] Lee, H-S., C-H. Lee, H-S. Tsai, and D. M. Salter. 2009. "Inhibition of cyclooxygenase 2 expression by diallyl sulfide on joint inflammation induced by urate and IL-1β. "*Osteoarthritis and Cartilage* 90(1):91-99. doi: https://doi.org/10.1016/j.joca.2008.05.010.

[18] Li, Tao, Hong-Yan Shi, Yong-Xin Hua, Chen Gao, Qing Xia, Guang Yang, and Bin Li. 2015. "Effects of allicin on the proliferation and cell cycle of chondrocytes." *International Journal of Clinical and Experimental Pathology* 8(10): 12525-32.Accessed on March 12, 2019. https://www.ncbi.nlm.nih.gov/pmc/articles/ PMC4680385/.

[19] Wang, Lin, Hai-Tao Pan., Bing Wang, Yang Liu, Kai Fei, and Wei-Feng Han. 2016. "Allicin reduces IL-1β-induced inflammatory cytokines via attenuating the NF-κβ and MMP-3 activation in human osteoarthritis chondrocyte model." *Int. J. Clin. Exp. Pathol.,* 9(10): 10320-10326. Accessed March 21, 2019. http://www.ijcep.com/files/ijcep0034372.pdf.

[20] Jayanthi, K., Naidu Sushma, V. Pramod, and Sunil. 2017. "Antioxidant and antiarthritic activity of allicin in animal models." *International Journal of Pharmaceutical Sciences*

and Research 26:1150-1155. Accessed on October 25, 2018. http://ijpsr.com/bft-article/antioxidant-and-antiarthritic-activity-of-allicin-in-animal-models/?view=fulltext.

[21] Qian, Yu-Qin, Zhen-Hua Feng, Xiao-Bin Li, Zhi-Chao Hu, Jiang-Wei Xuan, Xiang-Yang Wang, Hai-Chao Xu, and Jiao-Xiang Chen. 2018. "Downregulating P13/Akt/NF-κB signaling with allicin for ameliorating the progression of osteoarthritis." *Food Funct.* 19;9(9):4865-4875. doi: 10.1039/c8fo01095a.

[22] Ding, Guoling, Jinguan Zhao, and Dianming Jiang. 2016. "Allicin inhibits oxidative stress-induced mitochondrial dysfunction and apoptosis by promoting P13K/Akt and CREB/ERK signaling in osteoblast cells."*Experimental and Therapeutic Medicine* 11:2553-2560. doi:10.3892/etm.2016.3179.

[23] Mukherjee, M., A. S. Das, S. Mitra, and C. Mitra. 2004. "Prevention of bone loss by oil extract of garlic (*Allium sativum* Linn.) in an ovariectomied model of osteoporosis." *Phytother. Res.* 18:389-394. doi: 10.1002/ptr.1448.

[24] Guan, Xiaoxu, Yi Zhou, Hui Chen, Chaowei Wang, and Huiming Wang. 2018. "Antibacterial, anti-inflammatory, and anti-osteoclastogenesis roles of allicin in periodontitis." *Int. J. Clin. Med.*, 11(7): 6721-6730. Accessed on March 13, 2019 http://www.ijcem.com/files/ijcem0066740.pdf.

[25] Salimzadeh, Ahmad, Elham Alipoor, Sahar Dehghani, Mehdi Yaseri, Mostafa Husseini, Christine Feinle-Bisset, and Mohammad J. Hosseinzadeh-Attar.2018. "The effect of 12-week garlic supplementation on symptom relief in overweight or obese women with knee osteoarthritis." *Int J Clin Pract:* e13208. https://doi.org/10.1111/ijcp.13208.

[26] Rijayakumar, Rajasree, Dietrich Bussellberg. 2016. "*Osteoporosis an under-recognized public health problem.*" 2016:2. Accessed on April 15, 2019. http://www.qscience.com/doi/pdf/10.5339/jlghs.2016.2.

[27] Nazir, Muhammad A. 2017. "Prevalence of periodontal disease, its association with systemic diseases and prevention." *International Journal of Health sciences* 11(2): 72–80. Accessed on April 16, 2019. https://www.ncbi.nlm.nih.gov/pmc/articles/PMC5426403/.

[28] Wu, Yin, En L. Goh, Dong Wang, and Shaocheng Ma. 2018. "Novel treatments for osteoarthritis: an update." *Open Access Rheumatology: Research and Reviews* 10: 135–140. doi: 10.2147/OARRR.S176666.

[29] Holmquist, Gregory L. 2009. "Opioid Metabolism and Effects of Cytochrome P450." *Pain Medicine* 109 (Suppl 1):S20–S29. https://doi.org/10.1111/j.1526-4637.2009.00596.x.

[30] Lawson, Larry D., and Scott M. Hunsaker. 2018. "Allicin Bioavailability and Bioequivalence from Garlic Supplements and Garlic Foods." *Nutrients* 10(7): 812. doi: 10.3390/nu10070812.

[31] Costello, Mary-Ellen, Dirk Elewaut, Tony J. Kenna, and Matthew A. Brown. 2013. "Microbes, the gut and ankylosing spondylitis." *Arthritis Research and Therapy* 15(3): 214. doi: 10.1186/ar4228.

[32] Ankri, Serge, and David Mirelman. 1999. "Antimicrobial properties of allicin from garlic." *Microbes and Infection* 2: 125-129.

[33] Dikasso, D., H. Lemma, K. Urga, A. Debella, G. Addis, A. Tadele, and K. Yirsaw. 2002. "Investigation on the antibacterial properties of garlic (*Allium sativum*) on pneumonia-causing bacteria." *Ethiopian Medical Journal* 40(3): 241-249.

[34] Reiter, Jan, Natalja Levina, Mark van der Linden, Martin Gruhlke, Christian Martin, and Alan J. Slusarenko. 2017. "Diallythiosulfinate (allicin), a volatile antimicrobial from garlic (*Allium sativum*), kills human lung pathogenic bacteria including MDR strains." *Molecules* 22:1711 doi:10.3390/molecules22101711.

[35] Shetty, Sunaina, Biju Thomas, Veena Shetty, Rahul Bhandary, and Raghavendra M Shetty RM. 2013. "An *in-vitro* evaluation of the efficacy of garlic extract as an antimicrobial agent on periodontal pathogens: A microbiological study. " *Ayu.* 34(4):445-51 doi: 10.4103/0974-8520.127732.

[36] Bachrach, Gilad, Areen Jamil, Ronit Naor, Golan Tal, Zvi Ludmer, and Doron Steinberg. 2011. "Garlic allicin as a potential agent for controlling oral pathogens." *Journal of Medicinal Food* 14(11):1338-1343. doi: 10.1089/jmf.2010.0165.

[37] Cekici, Ali, Alpdogan Kntarci, Hatice Hasturk, and Thomas E. Van Dyke. 2000. "Inflammatory and immune pathways in the pathogenesis of periodontal disease." *Periodontal* 64(1): 57-80. doi: 10.1111/prd.12002.

[38] Hou, Guo-Qing, Chun Guo, Guo-Hua Song, Na Fang, Wen-Juan Fan, Xu-Dong Chen, Lei Yuan, and Zhen-Quan Wang 2013."Lipopolysaccharide (LPS) promotes osteoclast differentiation and activation by enhancing the MAPK pathway and COX-2 expression in RAW264.7 cells." *International Journal of Molecular Medicine* 32: 503-510. https://doi.org/10.3892/ijmm.2013.1406.

[39] Franco, Cavalla, Hernández-Rios Patricia, Sorsa Timo, Biguetti Claudia, and Hernández Marcela, H. 2017. "Matrix Metalloproteinases as Regulators of Periodontal Inflammation." *International Journal of Molecular Sciences* 18(2): 440. doi:10.3390/ijms18020440.

[40] Ebersole, Jeffrey L., Dolphus R. Dawson, Lorri A. Morford, Rebecca Peyyala, Craig S. Miller, and Octavio A. Gonzaléz 2013. "Periodontal disease immunology: 'double indemnity' in protecting the host." *Periodontology 2000* 62(1), 163-202. doi: 10.1111/prd.12005.

[41] Röhner, Eric, Paula Hoff, Georg Matziolis, Carsten Perka, Brigit Riep, Frank C. Nichols, Andrej M. Kielbassa, Jacqueline Detert, Gerd R. Burmeister, Frank Buttergeit, Janine Zahlten Zahlten, and Nicole Pischon 2012. "The impact of *Porphyromonas gingivalis* lipids on apoptosis of human chondrocytes." *Connective Tissue Research* 4:327-333. https://doi.org/10.3109/03008207.2012.657308.

[42] Gerits, Evelien., Natalie Verstraeten, and Jan Michiels. 2017. "New approaches to combat *Porphyromonas gingivalis* biofilms." *Journal of Oral Microbiology*: *9*(1): 1300366. doi:10.1080/20002297.2017.1300366.

[43] Prakasam, Abinaya, S. Sugumari Elavarasu, and Ravi K. Natarajan. 2012. "Antibiotics in the management of aggressive periodontitis." *Journal of Pharmacy & Bioallied Sciences* 4(Suppl 2), S252-5. doi: 10.4103/0975-7406.100226.

[44] Liu, Cheg-Tzu, Hsing-Min Tzu, Chong-Kue Lii, and Lee-Yian Sheen. 2009. "Effect of supplementation with garlic oil on activity of Th1 and Th2 lymphocytes from rats." *Planta Med* 75(3):205-210. doi: 10.1055/s-0028-1088396.

[45] Shaikh, Saeed A. 2007. "Ankylosing spondylitis: recent breakthroughs in diagnosis and treatment." *The Journal of the Canadian Chiropractic Association* 51(4): 249-60.

[46] Turner, Matthew J., Dawn P. Sowders, Monica L. Delay, Rajashree Mohapatra, Shuzhen Bai, Judith A, Smith, Jaclyn R. Brandewie, Joel D. Taurog, and Robert A, Colbert. 2005. "HLA-B27 misfolding in transgenic rats is associated with activation of the unfolded

protein response." *J. Immunol.* 175: 2438-2448. doi. https://doi.org/10.4049/jimmunol.175.4.2438.

[47] Cavallito, Chester J. 1946. "Relationship of thiol groups to reactions with antibiotics. " *J. Biol. Chem.* 164:29-34. Accessed on March 19, 2019. http://www.jbc.org/content/164/1/29.full.pdf.

[48] Xie, Kun, Jianze Nian, Xingyang Zhu, Xiaoping Geng, and Fubao Liu. 2015. "Modulatory role of garlicin in migration and invasion of intrahepatic cholangiosarcoma via P13K/AKT pathway." *Int. J. Clin. Exp. Pathol.* 8(11): 14028-14033.

[49] Li, Xin, Michael Ellman, Prasuna Muddasani, James H-C. Wang, Gabriella Cs-Szabo, Andre van Wijnen, and Hee-Jong Im. 2009. "Prostaglandin E2 and its cognate EP receptors control human adult articular cartilage homeostasis and are linked to the pathophysiology of osteoarthritis." *Arthritis and Rheumatism* 60(2): 513-23. doi: 10.1002/art.24258.

[50] Boniface, Katia, Christian S. Bak-Jensen, Ying Li, Wendy M. Blumenschein, Mandy J. McGeachy, Terrill K. McClanahan, Brent S. McKenzie, Robert A. Kastelein, Daniel J. Cua, and Réne de Waal Malefyt. 2009. "Prostaglandin E2 regulates Th17 cell differentiation and function through cyclic AMP and EP2/EP4 receptor signaling." *The Journal of Experimental Medicine* 206(3): 535-48. doi: 10.1084/jem.20082293.

[51] Rahman, Mohammad S. 2007. "Allicin and other functional active components in garlic: health benefits and bioavailability." *Int J Food Properties* 10: 245-268. doi: 10.1080/10942910601113327.

[52] Woolacott, Nerys F. Mark S. Corbett, Stephen J. C. Rice. 2012. "The use and reporting of WOMAC in the assessment of the benefit of physical therapies for the pain of osteoarthritis of the knee: findings from a systematic review of clinical trials." *Rheumatology* 51(8): 1440–1446. https://doi.org/10.1093/rheumatology/kes043.

[53] Guntur, Anyonya R, and Clifford J. Rosen. 2011."The skeleton: a multi-functional complex organ: new insights into osteoblasts and their role in bone formation: the central role of PI3Kinase." *J Endocrinol.* 211(2):123-30. doi: 10.1530/JOE-11-0175.

[54] Zimmermann, Petra, and Nigel Curtis. 2018. "The effect of aspirin on antibiotic susceptibility." *Expert Opinion on Therapeutic Targets* 22(11): 967-972, doi: 10.1080/14728222.2018.1527314.

[55] Rao, H. T. Ajay, Sham S. Bhat, Sundeep Hegde, S., and Vikram B. Jhamb. 2014. "Efficacy of garlic extract and chlorhexidine mouthwash in reduction of oral salivary microorganisms, an in vitro study." *Ancient Science of Life* 34(2): 85-8. doi: 10.4103/0257-7941.153465.

[56] Okada, Moe, Tatsuo Kobayashi, Satoshi Ito, Tomoko Yokoyama, Asami Abe, Akira Murasawa, and Horomasa Yoshie. 2013. "Periodontal treatment decreases levels of antibodies to Porphyromonas gingivalis and citrulline in patients with rheumatoid arthritis. " *J. Periodontol.* 84(12): e74-e84. https://doi.org/10.1902/jop.2013.130079.

[57] Maresz, Katarzyna J., Annelie Hellvard, Aneta Sroka, Karina Adamowicz, Ewa Bielecka, Joanna Koziel, Katarzyna Gawron, Danuta Mizgalska, Katarzyna A. Marcinska, Malgorzata Benedyk, Krzystof Pyrc, Anne-Marie Quirke, Roland Jonsson, Saba Alzabin, Patrick J. Venables, Ky-Anh Nguyen, Piotr Mydel, and Jan Potempa. 2013. "Porphyromonas gingivalis facilitates the development and progression of destructive arthritis through its unique bacterial peptidylarginine deiminase (PAD)." *PLoS Pathogens* 9(9): e1003627. doi: 10.1371/journal.ppat.1003627.

[58] Mikuls, Ted R., Geoffrey M. Thiele, Kevin D. Deane, Jeffrey B. Payne, James R. O'Dell, Fang Yu, Harlan Sayles, Michael H. Weisman, Peter K. Gregersen, Jane H. Buckner, Richard M. Keating, Lezlie A. Derber, William H. Robinson, V. Michael Holers, and Jill M. Norris. 2012. "Porphyromonas gingivalis and disease-related autoantibodies in individuals at increased risk of rheumatoid arthritis." *Arthritis and Rheumatism* 64(11): 3522-30. doi: 10.1002/art.34595.

[59] van de Stadt, Lottie A., Margret H. M. T. de Konig, Rob J. van de Stadt, Gertjan Wolbink, Ben A. C. Dijkmans, Dörte Hamann, and Dirkan van Shaadenberg. 2011. "Development of the anti-citrullinated protein antibody repertoire prior to the onset of rheumatoid arthritis." *Arthritis Rheum.* 63: 3226-3233. https://doi.org/10.1002/art. 30537.

[60] Wegner, Natalia, Robin Wait, Aneta Sroka, Sigrun Eick, Ky-Anh Nguyen, Karin Lundberg, Andrew Kinloch, Shauna Culshaw, Jan Potempa, and Patrick J. Venables. 2010. "Peptidylarginine deiminase from Porphyromonas gingivalis citrullinates human fibrinogen and α-enolase: implications for autoimmunity in rheumatoid arthritis." *Arthritis and Rheumatism* 62(9): 2662-72. doi: 10.1002/art.27552.

[61] Lundberg, Karin, Andrew Kinloch, Benjamin A. Fisher, Natalia Wegner, Robin Wait, Peter Charles, Ted R. Mikuls, and Patrick J. Venables. 2008. "Antibodies to citrullinates alpha-enolase peptide 1 are specific for rheumatoid arthritis and cross-react with bacterial enolase." *Arthritis Rheum.* 58:3009-3019. https://doi.org/10.1002/ art.23936.

[62] Röhner, Eric, Paula Hoff, Georg Matziolis, Carsten Perka, Brigit Riep, Frank C. Nichols, Andrej M. Kielbassa, Jacqueline Detert, Gerd R. Burmeister, Frank Buttergeit, Janine Zahlten, and Nicole Pischon. 2012. "The impact of *Porphyromonas gingivalis* lipids on apoptosis of human chondrocytes." *Connective Tissue Research* 4:327-333. https://doi.org/10.3109/03008207.2012.657308.

[63] Moon, Kyoung-Ho, and Young-Tae Kim.2014. "Medical Treatment of Ankylosing Spondylitis." *Hip Pelvis.* 26(3):129-35. doi: 10.5371/hp.2014.26.3.129.

[64] Zhang, Zhuo, Daniel J. Leong, Lin Xu, Zhiyong He, Angela Wang, Mahantesh Navati, Sun J. Kim, David M. Hirsh, John A. Hardin, Neil J. Cobelli, Joel M. Friedman, and Hui B. Sun. 2016. "Curcumin slows osteoarthritis progression and relieves osteoarthritis-associated pain symptoms in a post-traumatic osteoarthritis mouse model." *Arthritis Research & Therapy* 18(1): 128. doi:10.1186/s13075-016-1025-y.

[65] Wilkinson, Frank, and Diana R. Cundell. 2014. "From test tube to clinical trial; promising herbs with NF-κB and COX-2 activity." Current Immunology Reviews 2014, Volume 10 Issue 2 ISSN: 1875-631X (Online), ISSN: 1573-3955(Print). Accessed September 25, 2018. http://benthamscience.com/journal/index.php?journalID=cir.

[66] Connaghan, P. G., H. Vanharanta, and P. A. Dieppe. 2005. "Is progressive osteoarthritis an atheromatous disease?" *Ann. Rheum. Dis.* 64: 1539-1541. doi: 10.1136/ard.2005. 039263.

[67] Dhadse, Prasad, Deepti Gattani, and Rohit Mishra. 2010. "The link between periodontal disease and cardiovascular disease: How far have we come ?" *J. Indian Soc. Periodontitis* 14(3): 148-154. doi: 10.4103/0972-124X.75908.

[68] Preshaw, P. M., A. L. Alba, D. Herrera, S. Jepsen, A. Konstantinidis, K. Makrilakis, K., and R. Taylor. 2011. "Periodontitis and diabetes: a two-way relationship." *Diabetologia* 55(1): 21-31. doi: 10.1007/s00125-011-2342-y.

[69] Yin, Lu, He Zhuojin, Shen Xiuying Shen, Xiaolu Xu, Jie Fan, Shaohu Wu, and Deyong Zhang. 2012. "Cholesterol-Lowering Effect of Allicin on Hypercholesterolemic ICR

Mice." *Oxidative Medicine and Cellular Longevity*: Article ID 489690 https://doi.org/10.1155/2012/489690.

[70] Gupta, Nisha, and Todd D. Porter 2001. "Garlic and garlic-derived compounds inhibit human squalene monooxygenase." *J. Nutr.* 131: 1662–1667.

[71] Focke, Manfred, Andrea Feld, and Harmut K. Lichtenthaler. 1990. "Allicin, a naturally occurring antibiotic from garlic, specifically inhibits acetyl-CoA synthetase." *FEBS Lett.* 261: 106–108.

[72] Oi, Yuriko, Mika Imafuku, Chiaki Shishido, Yutaka Kominato, Syoji Nishimura, and Kazuo Iwai. 2001. "Garlic Supplementation Increases Testicular Testosterone and Decreases Plasma Corticosterone in Rats Fed a High Protein Diet." *The Journal of Nutrition* 131(8): 2150–2156, https://doi.org/10.1093/jn/131.8.2150.

[73] Feng, Fang, Li Hong, Cui Wen, and Yongsui Dong. 1999. "Treatment of hepatitis caused by cytomegalovirus with allitridin injection – An experimental study." *Journal of Tongji Medical University* 19(4): 271-274. https://doi.org/10.1007/BF02886960.

[74] Suddek, Ghada M. 2014. "Allicin enhances chemotherapeutic response and ameliorates tamoxifen-induced liver injury." *Pharmaceutical Biology* 52(8): 1009-1014. Accessed November 22, 2018. https://www.tandfonline.com/doi/full/10.3109/13880209.2013.876053.

[75] Miron, Talia, Marina Mironchik, David Mirelman, Meir Wilchek, and Aharon Rabinkov. 2003. "Inhibition of tumor growth by a novel approach: *in situ* allicin generation using targeted alliinase delivery." *Molecular Cancer Therapeutics* 2 (12):1295-1301. http://mct.aacrjournals.org/content/molcanther/2/12/1295.full.pdf.

[76] Leontiev, Roman, Nils Hohaus, Jacob Claus, Martin C.H. Gruhlke, and Alan J. Slusarenko .2018."Comparison of the Antibacterial and Antifungal Activities of Thiosulfinate Analogues of Allicin." *Scientific Reports* 6763:8(1). Accessed on February 22, 2019 https://www.nature.com/articles/s41598-018-25154-9.

[77] Lubenets, Vira, Sofiya Vasylyuk, Nataliya Monka, Khrystina Bolibrukh, Olena Komarovska-Porokhnyavets, Diana Baranovych, Rostyslav Musyanovych, Ewa Zaczynska, Anna Czarny, Urszula Nawrot, and Volodymyr Novikov. 2016. "Synthesis and antimicrobial properties of 4-acylaminobenzenethiosulfoacid S-esters." *Saudi Pharmaceutical Journal: SPJ: The Official publication of the Saudi Pharmaceutical Society* 25(2), 266-274. doi: 10.1016/j.jsps.2016.06.007.

[78] Kaitin, K. I. 2010. "Deconstructing the drug development process: the new face of innovation." *Clinical Pharmacology and Therapeutics* 87(3): 356-61. doi: 10.1038/clpt.2009.293.

[79] Nazir, Muhammad A. 2017. "Prevalence of periodontal disease, its association with systemic diseases and prevention." *International Journal of Health Sciences* 11(2): 72-80. PMID: 28539867.

[80] Cauley, Jane A. 2013. "Public Health Impact of Osteoporosis. " *The Journals of Gerontology: Series A* 68(10): 1243–1251. https://doi.org/10.1093/gerona/glt093.

In: Allicin
Editor: Diana R. Cundell

ISBN: 978-1-53617-339-0

Chapter 12

NEUROPROTECTIVE EFFECTS OF ALLICIN

Diana R. Cundell*[*], *PhD
College of Life Sciences, Jefferson University, Philadelphia, PA, US

ABSTRACT

During the past decade, sixteen either *in vitro* or animal studies have reported that allicin can inhibit neuroinflammation in models of traumatic brain injury (TBI), acute spinal cord injury (ASCI), ischemic strokes (IS), subarachnoid hemorrhage (SAH), Alzheimer's (AD) and Parkinson's disease (PkD). Neuroinflammation and neuronal death in these conditions is associated with an upregulation of mitochondrial reactive oxygen species (ROS) in concert with decreased efficacy of the pathways removing these moieties, namely NF-E2, p45related factor (Nrf2) and its downstream targets glutathione peroxidase (GpH) and glutathione (GSH) together with constitutionally expressed endothelial NOS (eNOS). In these sixteen studies, allicin was reported to reduce brain inflammation by upregulating Nrf2, GSH, GpX and eNOS, consequently reducing ROS-induced damage. In three AD models of disease, animals treated with allicin demonstrated significantly improved cognitive abilities. These results are intriguing sinceTBI and IS currently have no effective management strategies either to control the inflammation or reduce the incidence of rapid demise in these patients. Similarly AD and PkD treatments do not reverse disease damage or halt ongoing neuronal loss. Cost and availability of AD and PkD medications has also been an issue, especially for patients in developing countries. These latter patients rely on traditional phytomedicines including garlic, ginko biloba and ginseng. Allicin, as the major active phytochemical of garlic, is a relative newcomer to the lineup of potential neuroprotective agents. Its actual effects on human disease are therefore unknown. This chapter will closely examine the data from the twelve literature studies, identifying the neuroprotective benefits of the thiosulfinate with reference to acute (TBI, SCI, IS, SAH) and chronic (AD, PkD) brain inflammation.

Keywords: acetylcholinesterase, Alzheimer's, amyloid protein (APP), eNOS, ischemic stroke, Nrf2, Parkinson's disease, ROS, traumatic brain injury

---

[*] Corresponding Author's Email: Diana.Cundell@jefferson.edu.

1. Introduction

Central nervous system (CNS) neurons are particularly sensitive to the effects of damaging stimuli and are more likely than other body cells to go into apoptosis and are not repopulated [1]. Neuronal damage results in either acute or chronic inflammation and may be induced by a variety of stimuli including direct physical trauma, loss of blood supply, infectious agents (such as viruses) or indirectly from the effects of cardiovascular disease or aging on a continued blood supply [1]. An understanding of the pathways that result in acute and chronic brain inflammation has been gained, primarily from animal models and human autopsy samples [1]. In both cases, neuroinflammation is associated with an uptick in the activation of glial support cells, particularly the macrophage-like microglia [1]. Together with two other types of glia, the astrocyte and myelin-producing oligodendrocyte, these cells release a diversity of proinflammatory cytokines, including interleukin-1 (IL-1) and tumor necrosis factor alpha (TNF-α) and activate local blood vessel-lining endothelial cells [1].

Brain inflammation is also associated with the production of protein aggregates termed inflammasomes [2]. Several proteins are involved in this process including systemically activated C-reactive protein (CRP) and local brain-derived alpha synuclein (α-Syn) [2]. These initiate inflammation by activating the proinflammatory cytokines interleukin 1 beta (IL-1β), IL-18 and IL-33 [2]. Proinflammatory cytokines in turn activate biochemical pathways in the brain's glial cells creating an oxidative stress-based environment [1, 2]. Damaging stimuli are then mediated through a combination of reactive oxygen species (ROS) and elevated levels of nitric oxide (NO) [1]. These molecules are directly neurotoxic [3] and can be exacerbated by a concommitant release of ROS and NO directly from the damaged neurons themselves [1]. Brain tissues utilize more oxygen than other body cells and their high metabolic activity results in rapid ROS generation and a similarly rapid removal by antioxidant enzymes, including those of the glutathione (GSH) pathway and superoxide dismutase (SOD) [3]. CNS damage results in decreased levels of these enzymes thereby allowing toxic ROS to accumulate [3]. The majority of brain NO is produced by two major separate nitric oxide synthase (NOS) brain pathways involving endothelial cells (eNOS) and neurons (nNOS) [4]. Unlike other body systems the inducible NOS pathway (iNOS) appears to play only a minor role in CNS tissues [4]. During acute inflammatory episodes, such as traumatic brain injury (TBI) and ischemic stroke, it is apparent that not just the degree of neuronal damage but also the imbalance between neuroprotective eNOS and damaging nNOS determines the degree of recovery [4]. The importance of optimal eNOS secretion by vascular endothelial cells is also important in the predisposition to chronic neurodegenerative illness [5]. For example, substantial animal research points to chronic underproduction of eNOS playing a primary role in the initiation of the amyloid plaques associated with Alzheimer's disease (AD) [5]. Both acute and chronic forms of CNS inflammation are now being studied in animal models, particularly rats and mice to determine both their underlying etiologies as well as the connections between them [1-5]. From this research it is already apparent that the secondary phase of TBI neuronal injury, which is associated with demise of nearly half of all patients, results from a combination of NO and ROS in concert with continued neuronal mitochondrial dysfunction and damage to the blood brain barrier [6]. That patients surviving TBI and associated ischemic brain damage often go on to develop AD-like dementias further connects these major forms of acute and chronic neuropathologies [7].

Since its discovery as the major phytochemical in garlic in 1944, allicin has been shown in many studies to possess a variety of anti-inflammatory activities primarily involving its ability to act as an antioxidant and "rebalance" the environment of cells towards health [8]. Allicin has been shown to be effective in several acute and chronic inflammatory conditions, most particularly tumors, cardiovascular health and infectious disease (see also Chapters 3-8 and 12 for more details) [8]. Numerous studies have reported that allicin achieves these effects by targeting several commonly used pathways of inflammation, namely GSH, NF-E2, p45related factor (Nrf2) and the cytokine-regulating nuclear factor kappa beta (NF-κB) [8]. Interestingly, perturbation of these redox pathways also plays a major role in the morbidity and mortality of patients suffering acute and chronic neurological syndromes [1-5]. This begs the question of why no studies have examined the effects of allicin on neuroinflammation until recently. The reason is relatively simple. Until the 1980s, the brain was considered a "privileged organ" where inflammation was controlled by local microglia and astrocyte-based responses [9].

With the realization, in the 1990s that uncontrolled neuroinflammation was a major contributory factor to the morbidity and mortality of patients with neurodegenerative diseases such as AD, the scene was set for a sea change in attitudes towards understanding the etiology of these conditions [9]. Traditional neuroprotective phytochemicals, such as those from ginko biloba, turmeric and ginseng began to be investigated around this time and showed early promise in animal models [10]. Some, such as phytostigmine from the castor oil plant *Phytostigmes venenosum* even acquired federal drug administration (FDA) approval for the treatment of mild AD [10]. In contrast, at that time the focus on garlic/ allicin remained on its anti-tumor and antimicrobial activities in other tissues [8]. Only during the past decade were allicin's neuroprotective activities finally investigated [11-26]. To date, published literature has explored the neuroprotective effects of allicin in sixteen isolated cell or animal models of the acute neuroinflammatory conditions of traumatic brain injury (TBI) [11, 12], spinal cord injury (ASCI) [13-16], ischemic stroke (IS) [17, 18] and subarachnoid hemorrhage (SAH)[19], the chronic inflammatory conditions of AD [20-24] and Parkinson's disease (PkD) [25, 26]. In the *in vivo* models of disease allicin was able to easily cross the blood brain barrier unassisted, when given by injection intraperitoneally (i.p.) [12-15, 19] or as a dietary supplement [14, 17, 18, 21, 23, 24]. The anti-inflammatory effects of allicin on the animals was also matched by a significant improvement in their cognitive abilities [13, 18, 20, 21, 23, 24].

So why consider the further development of allicin for any of these illnesses? For the acute neurological traumas of TBI [27], SCI [28], IS [29] and SAH [30] there is an urgent need for effective strategies to prevent the irreversble brain damage that occurs. TBI patients are managed with hyperbaric oxygen, head elevation, and surgery to remove fluid buildup in affected areas [27]. This has decreased the mortality rates but instead increased the numbers of patients living with permanent damage [27]. SCI intervention involves a combination of rapid (within twenty four hours) spinal decompression, surgical intervention and anticoagulant administration [28]. Prevention of the incidence of ischemic stroke relies on pharmaceutical and dietary prevention of hemostasis in cardiovascular atherosclerotic disease [29]. Unfortunately, a stroke begins there is only a narrow window of less than five hours to dissaggregate the clot and prevent the demise or permanent damage that occurs in the survivors [29]. Similarly, SAH patients need a rapid identification and ligation of the bleed to prevent rapid demise [30]. None of the conditions currently uses interventions that address the underlying inflammation that occurs [27-30] although these agents are being explored in phase I and II trials [31, 32].

A second issue revolves around therapeutics for the chronic neurodegenerative illnesses AD and PkD. Like their acute inflammatory counterparts, AD [33] and PkD [34] produce long-term morbidity and suffering for millions around the world, both in developing and developed countries. AD and PkD are especially an issue in cultures with aging populations [35, 36]. Worldwde, AD affects about one-third of adults over eight-five and is estimated to increase rapidly over the next four decades [36]. PkD has a much lower incidence rate of less than 1% of the population but given risk factors of trauma (including concussions) and toxin exposure (including lead) this condition may also be on the increase, given also its association with CVD [35]. These patients are maintained on nootropic therapies directed at increasing the availability of the neurotransmitter acetylcholine in AD [34] and dopamine [35]. These medications are replaced by other interventional strategies as AD and PkD progress, but none reverse the course of the disease [33, 34].

Added to this AD medications currently cost around $5 per day, placing them well out of reach for sufferers in developing nations [37]. Concern over the lack of affordable, available, effective medications is already encouraging developing nations to explore plant-based therapies, particularly for the treatment of AD [38]. Viable and sustainable solutions are particularly presssing issue as for developing nations given that the fear of disclosure of the condition as well as poor access to healthcare means a severely truncated lifespan for AD patients [38]. As new strategies are being explored and phytomedicines again begin to be examined this chapter will explore the potential contribution allicin might make to this field. A close scrutiny of the literature reports on models of six neurological conditions will be used to reveal the underlying molecular targets of the thiosulfinate. Comparing these, mechanistically, with extant medications will also be used to elucidate potentially novel strategies for allicin.

2. Neuroprotective Effects of Allicin on Acute Neuroinflammation

Eight studies have appeared in the literature to suggest that allicin has efficacy against *in vitro* or *in vivo* models of TBI [11, 12], ASCI [13-16], ischemic stroke [17, 18] or subarachnoid hemorrhage [18, 19]. A description of the experimental design and results of these studies is shown in Table 1.

Seven of the eight studies of acute brain inflammation utilized animal models of illness and similar dosages of allicin (2-70 mg/kg) [12-15, 18, 19]. Two major routes of administration were used for the allicin; oral [12, 13, 15, 18] and intraperitoneally [14, 17, 19]. That each produced efficacy supports the concept that allicin can cross the blood-brain barrier [12-15, 17]. Brain swelling was measured in two studies as a gross assessment of inflammation and found to be significantly reduced ($p < 0.05$) in both cases [12, 15]. In all but two studies, the animals were sacrificed to assess biochemical alterations produced by allicin, so it is unknown whether any of the pre-trauma functionality was restored [12, 14, 15, 17]. Lv and colleagues [13] evaluated rat motor function after spinal cord damage and observed that it was significantly increased in animals ($p < 0.05$) with the highest dose of allicin fourteen days after laminectomy. Twenty-one days post trauma, allicin treated rats (50 mg/kg) obtained motor function, assessed by walking and limb motion, that was approximately three quarters of that of the control rats [13]. Shao and colleagues [19] evaluated rats 24 hours after inducing a SAH for their ability to eat, walk and demonstrate a steady gait. They reported that rats that received 70 mg/ kg allicin i.p. thirty minutes after injury demonstrated neurological functionality significantly ($p < 0.05$) greater than those animals with either no treatment or who were given a lower dose of allicin (30 mg/kg) [19]. Looking at the data of Shao and colleagues [17], the 70 mg/ kg dose of allicin improved the neurological functions of the rats by of the order of sixty percent. If reproducible, these data are staggering and support the earlier study of Lv [13] in suggesting allicin could be both neuroprotective and allow retention of cognitive functions post acute inflammatory trauma.

Continued functionality of neurons relies on allicin both reducing neural inflammation and preventing neuronal death. In two animal studies allicin reduced neuronal apoptosis as assessed by direct microscopic examination [12, 15], as well as cleaving of caspases [12], poly (ADP) ribose polymerase (PARPs)[12] and decrease of Bax (Bcl-2 associated x protein), Bcl-2 (B-cell lymphoma 2) ratio [12]. Similarly, the activation of the protein kinase B (Akt) pathway, assessed by *in vitro* [11] and *in vivo* phosphorylation [12] would prevent neuronal apoptosis [39]. The time frame for the animal studies is important as in TBI patients as the first month represents the window after which for many patients no further recovery of function occurs [6]. The ability of allicin to restore much of the motor function to the animals in this one study [13] is of note as it has not seen in any current interventional strategies for acute inflammatory neurological damage [6, 7].

Analysis of the underlying biochemical pathways affected by allicin in these models provides a good insight into its potential mechanisms [12-19] additional to prevention of neuronal death [11, 12]. The first is a regulation of oxidative stress [12-14, 16-19]. Oxidative stress was assessed in five of the six animal studies of acute neuroinflammation studies [12-14, 17-19]. Allicin significantly increased CNS levels of both enzymes that directly decreased ROS levels, namely superoxide dismutase (SOD) [12-14, 17-19] and catalase [12, 14] as well as those generating glutathione (GSH) [13], including glutathione peroxidase (GpX) [14, 17, 19] and glutathione transferase (GST)[12, 14, 17]. Allicin-induced activation of the NF-E2, p45 related factor (Nrf2) pathway in both brain astrocytes and neural cells was also seen in one rat study of ASCI [13]. Lv and colleagues [13] also reported that simultaenously injection of allicin (2, 10 or 50 mg/kg) with a small interfering (siRNA) Nrf2 inhibitor eliminated the neuroprotective effects in an ASCI rat model [13]. Nrf2 also directly inhibits ROS [40]. As previously stated, chronic oxidative stress is the primary issue for neuroinflammatory damage [1-3].

The second major focus for allicin appears to be its differential effects on nitric oxide synthase (NOS) activity in the brains of animal with acute inflammation [11, 12]. A single *in vitro* TBI study of isolated rat cortical neurons demonstrated allicin (1-200 μM) phosphorylated (activated) endoethelial-derived (eNOS) but not inducible NOS (iNOS) [11]. This finding was reproduced in an animal model of TBI [12]. As was previously stated eNOS is neuroprotective [4] and is activated by Akt phosphorylation [12]. Akt-induced eNOS activation was confirmed as a second central mechanism of neuroprotection by allicin [12] through the finding that antagonists of only Akt (LY294002) but not eNOS (L-NIO) inhibited a TBI animal model [12]. Three of the studies administered allicin after the acute inflammatory episode, namely TBI [12] and ASCI [13, 15]. A single *in vitro* study of a gluatamate model of ASCI [16] reported that allicin was able to decrease iNOS by activating the heat shock 70 protein pathway. Two studies also suggested allicin has effects on the extracellular regulated kinase pathway (ERK) [11, 18] although with differential effects, possibly due to differential activation versus expression of the pathway [11]. The *in vivo* study reported that allicin's upregulation of ERK was also associated with a decrease in caspase activation i.e., neuroprotection [18]. ERK activation, at least transiently, is widely believed to prevent neuronal death [41]. These are interesting findings suggesting that if allicin is given early after a neurological event it will be able to resolve several aspects of proinflammatory biochemical activation. A summary of these activities is shown in Figure 1.

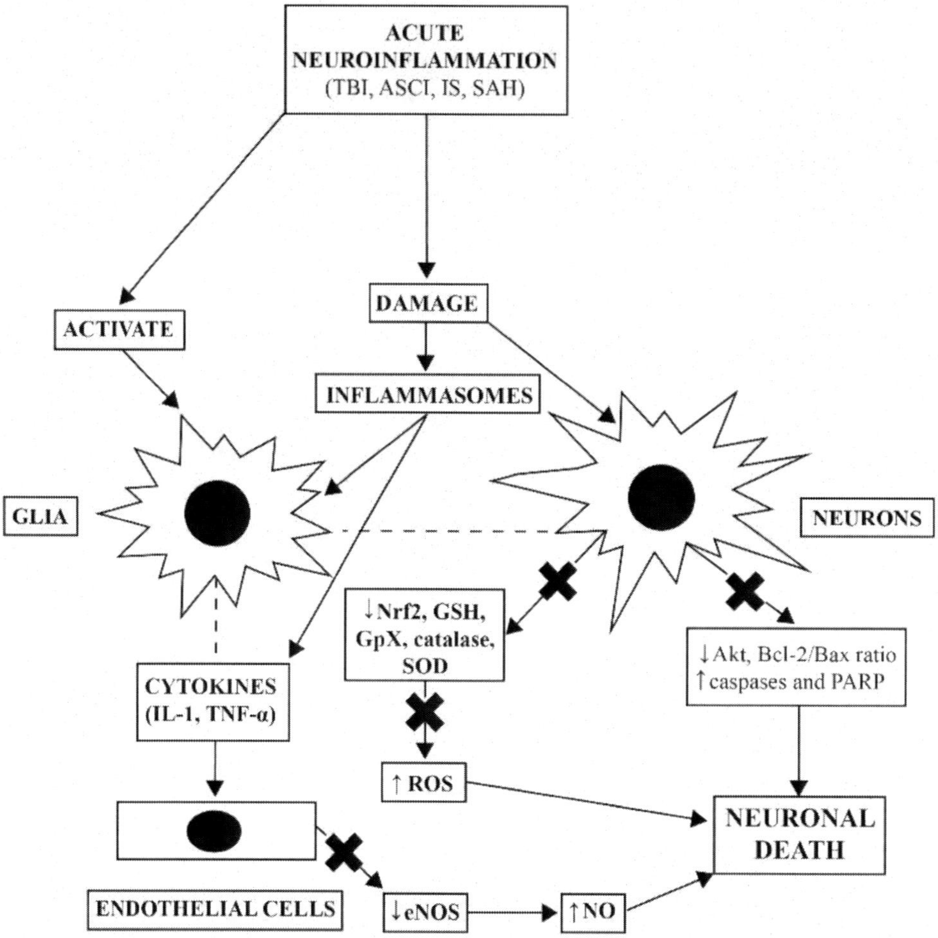

✖ Allicin's points of inhibition ▬ ▬ ▬ crosstalk.

Legend: Damage and inflammasomes induce activation of glia and consequent release of inflammatory cytokines. Neuronal damage results in activation of apoptosis cascases via PARP, caspase and Akt modulation. Oxidative stress is induced by neuronal failure to inactivate ROS further fueling neuronal death. Allicin inhibits cytokine release, prevents aooptosis by inhibiting caspase and PARP activation and enhances eNOS activation. This combined to maintain neuronal health and decrease inflammation.

Abbreviations used: Akt (protein kinase B), ASCI (acute spinal cord injury), Bax (apoptosis regulator Bax), Bcl-2 (B-cell lymphoma 2), eNOS (endothelial nitric oxide synthase), GpX (glutathione peroxidase), GSH (glutathione), IL-1 (interleukin-1), IS (ischemic stroke), NO (nitric oxide), PARP (poly(ADP)-ribose), ROS (reactive oxygen species), SOD (superoxide dismutase), TBI (traumatic brain injury), SAH (subarachnoid hemorrhage), TNF-α (tumor necrosis factor alpha).

References used: [1, 2, 11-19].

Figure 1. Neuroprotective mechanisms of allicin in models of acute neuroinflammation.

Table 1. Neuroprotective effects of allicin in acute inflammation

Disease	Model used	Results	Reference
TBI	*In vitro* isolated embryonic rat cortical neurons pretreated with allicin (1, 10, 50, 100 or 200 μM) 1 h before injury and assessed for 6-48 h after	↑phosphorylation of Akt and ↓ERK expression but not total protein levels ↑ phosphorylated eNOS but not iNOS. Inhibitor studies determined allicin directly affected Akt and ERK pathways	[11]
TBI	Rats (two groups of 18) treated with allicin (10 or 50 mg/kg i.p.) immediately after craniotomy and up to 8 h after. Changes assessed for 7 days.	Allicin at both doses able to protect from damage up to 8 h after craniotomy and optimal 2-4 h later. ↓ water accumulation in brain cortex and neuronal apoptosis (no activation caspase 3 or PARPs, ↑ Bcl-2/Bax ratio) ↑ oxidative enzymes (SOD, catalase, GST), phosphorylation of Akt and eNOS ↓proinflammatory cytokines IL-1β, IL-10, TGF-β and TNF-α	[12]
ASCI	Sprague Dawley rats (n = 18, 3 groups) treated with allicin (2, 10 or 50 mg/kg i.p.) immediately after undergoing laminectomy and having rod-damage spinal cord. Changes assessed at 7, 14, and 21 days post trauma.	Motor function significantly increased in animals ($p < 0.05$) with 10 and 50 mg at day 21 and in the 50 mg/kg group at both day 14 and day 21. ↑ oxidative enzymes (SOD, GHS) and expression of Nrf2 (astrocyte and neuronal); blocking Nrf2 with specific inhibitors ↓ allicin protection ↓proinflammatory cytokines IL-1β, IL-6 and TNF-α	[13]
ASCI	Male New Zealand white rabbits (n = 8 per group) pretreated with allicin (1, 10 or 50 mg/kg oral) for 14 days then given aortic occlusion spinal injury. Changes evaluated 4 and 24 h after reperfusion.	↑ oxidative enzymes (SOD, catalase, GpX and GST) ↓ ROS	[14]
	Sprague Dawley rats (n = 20) blocked right middle cerebral artery and allicin given (50 mg/kg i.p.) 3 h after and daily for 5 days	Allicin ↓ neural defect, brain swelling, infarct size and apoptosis of neurons. ↓ MPO and serum TNF-α	[15]
	In vitro model: rat spinal cord neurons pretreated with allicin (5 μM 30 minutes) and then activated with glutamate (5 mM) for 24 h	↑ CAT and SOD, ↓iNOS but had no effects on nNOS; effects through activation of heat shock protein 70 ↓ caspase 3 activation	[16]
IS	C57BL/6 mice (n −15) pretreated with allicin (50 mg/kg oral) for 14 days and middle cerebral artery occluded. Changes evaluated after 1 and 24 h.	↑ oxidative enzymes (SOD, GpX and GST)	[17]
	Mongolian Gerbils (n = 9) and bilateral common carotid arteries occluded (7 minutes) and administered allicin (20, 40 or 80 mg/kg, intragastric) for 7 days	↑ neurological function (↓ seizures, ptosis and hunched posture) all doses. ↑SOD (40 or 80 mg/kg allicin) ↑ ERK 1/2 (80 mg/kg allicin)	[18]
SAH	Sprague Dawley rats (n = 15) treated with allicin (70 mg/kg i.p.) 30 minutes after injection of blood into pre-chiasmatic cistern	↑ oxidative enzymes (SOD, GSH) and ↓ caspase cleavage	[19]

Abbreviations used: Akt (protein kinase B), Bax (Bcl-2 associated x protein), ASCI (acute spinal cord injury), Bcl-2 (B-cell lymphoma 2), eNOS (endothelial nitric oxide synthase), ERK (extracellular signal-regulated kinase), GpX (glutathione peroxidase), GSH (glutathione), GST (glutathione S transferase), h (hour), IL (interleukin), iNOS (inducible nitric oxide synthase), i.p. (intraperitoneally), IS (ischemic stroke), MPO (myeloperoxidase), Nrf2 (NF-E2, p45 related factor), PARP (poly (ADP) ribose polymerase), ROS (reactive oxygen species), SAH (subarachnoid hemorrhage), SOD (superoxide dismutase), TBI (traumatic brain injury), TNF-α (tumor necrosis factor alpha).

3. Neuroprotective Effects of Allicin on Chronic Neurodegenerative Disease

Seven studies have appeared in the literature to suggest that allicin has efficacy against *in vitro* or *in vivo* models of AD [20-24] or PkD [25, 26]. A description of the experimental design and results of these studies is shown in Table 2.

Table 2. Neuroprotective effects of allicin in AD and PkD models of disease

Disease	Model used	Results	Reference
AD	In vitro assay; AChE and BuChE from bovine erythrocytes incubated with allicin (0.003-0.1 mg/ml) 6 minutes	Dose dependent ↓ in both AChE and BuChE activity induced by allicin Strong inhibitor of AChE, weaker inhibitor of BuChE	[22]
AD	20 Kunming mice AD model (Aβ injected into brains); allicin (180 mg/kg/ day for 14 days injected i.p.) and compared with PBS	↓Aβ and MDA levels ↓ p38 activation ↑ SOD activity Significant ↑ cognitive abilities ($p < 0.001$)	[20]
	6APP/PS1 4-month old Mice; allicin (10 mg/kg/ day by gavage) compared with corn oil controls for 3 months	↓APP lyase levels ↓Aβ levels ↓JNK levels (preventing apoptosis) Significant ↑ cognitive abilities ($p < 0.001$)	[23]
	Test groups of 16; 20-month old male C57BL/6 mice received allicin (180 mg/kg/day, oral) for 8 weeks. Compared with 3-month old and 20-month old C57BL/6 mice	↑ GPx, GSH levels and total antioxidant capacity in hippocampus, ↓ ROS ↑ Nrf2 activity and of downstream targets NQ01 and γ-GCS Significant ↑ cognitive abilities ($p < 0.001$)	[21]
	Sprague Dawley rats (n = 12, 4 groups) treated with allicin (180 mg/kg oral) or sulforaphane (12 mg/kg oral) for 16 weeks Tunicamycin (TM) (5 μl) injected into lateral ventricle	Allicin and sulforaphane ↑ Nrf2 and PERK activity and of downstream targets NQ01 and γ-GCS Significant ($p < 0.05$) ↑ GpX and GSH in hippocampus and cognitive abilities	[24]
PkD	In vitro assay rat PC12 cells incubated with allicin (0.01, 0.1 or 1 μg/ml) and exposed to H2O2 for 2 h	Dose dependent ↓ apoptosis by ↓caspase 3 activation and Bcl-2 ↑ Bax and mitochondrial cytochrome C ↓ ROS	[25]
	In vitro assay rat PC12 cells incubated with allicin (50 μM) for 2 h then exposed to 6-OHDA for 24 h	↓ apoptosis by ↑ GPx, GSH levels. Mitochondrial preservation (evidenced by ↑ cytochrome C levels and maintenance of NRF-1)	[26]

Abbreviations used: AChE (acetylcholinesterase), Aβ (amyloid proteins), AD (Alzheimer's disease), APP (amyloid precursor protein), Bax (Bcl-2 associated X protein), Bcl-2 (B cell lymphoma-2 protein), BuChE (butyrylcholinesterase), γ-GCS (γ-glutamylcysteine synthetase), GPx (glutathione peroxidase), GSH (glutathione), h (hour), H2O2 (hydrogen peroxide), i.p. (intraparenterally), JNK (Jun amino-terminal kinase), MDA (malondialdehyde), NRF-1 (nuclear respiratory factor 1), Nrf2 (NF-E2, p45-related factor 2), NQO1 (NAD(P)H:quinone oxoreductase 1), 6-OHDA (oxidopamine), PC-12 (pheochromocytoma cells), PERK (protein kinase endoplasmic reticulum like kinase), PkD (Parkinson's disease), PBS (phosphate buffered saline), PS1 (presenilin 1), ROS (reactive oxygen species).

3.1. Allicin and AD

The four rodent studies on AD utilized well recognized animal models of the disease but two very different dosages of allicin as well as time frames [20, 21, 23, 24]. It is also important to point out that an achievable physiological concentration of allicin, would be of the order of 37 mg/g, which is comparable to levels in freshly chopped cloves [42]. The two studies, by the same group, that employed dosages of 180 mg/ kg stated that this was chosen "*based on the report by others*" [20, 21]. Allicin is unlikely to reach toxic levels until 5-30 g/kg is reached [43] so the data themselves for all three murine studies are still likely to be sound.

All four animal models demonstrated an improvement of cognitive symptoms when allicin was given for between two and twelve weeks [20, 21, 23, 24]. These changes were very profound [20, 21, 23, 24]. One investigator noted that during the water platform test (in which mice had to locate and climb onto a platform next to a shallow pool of water) that those not given the thiosfulfinate "*frequently swam randomly without any purpose, and away from the corresponding position of platform position* " [23]. Mechanistically, these animal changes were associated with biochemical shifts that revolved around a direct decrease in neuronal death, through impairment of Jun amino-terminal kinase (JNK) activation [23], combined with a reduction in inflammatory reactive oxygen species (ROS) through activation of NF-E2, p45-related factor 2 (Nrf2) [21, 24], superoxide dismutase (SOD) [20] and glutathione peroxidase/ glutathione (GpX/GSH) levels [21, 24]. Allicin's ability to affect redox levels in cells has been well documented [8]. Primarily this involves a thiol-based interaction directly on GpX/GSH [8, 44]. Allicin's activity on Nrf2 has been shown in a yeast cell model to target the redox sensitive signaling protein YAP1 [44]. This corresponds to Kelch-like ECH-associated protein 1 (Keap1) in mammalian cells [44] and is a major target for sulfur-containing phytomedicines including sulforaphanes from crucifers [45]. Zhu and colleagues [24] reported that an approximately ten-fold higher oral dose of allicin than sulforaphane (180 mg versus 12.5 mg/kg) was able to significantly increase Nrf2 and protein kinase A like endoplasmic reticulum kinase (PERK) activity in a tunicamycin model of AD [24]. Nrf2 activation would decrease neuronal death by ameliorating the level of ROS in the cells [40] and this property may underpin allicin's neuroprotective nature.

Allicin's anti-inflammatory effects on brain chemistry were also supported by the reduction in p38 activation seen in mice injected intraparenterally with 180 mg/kg of allicin per day for fourteen days [20]. Activation of the p38 pathway occurs following cytokine exposure and results in NF-κB upregulation [46]. Although NF-κB levels were not assessed in these animals it is reasonable to assume that they were simultaneously reduced given the thiosulfinate's effects on p38. The elevated cytokines seen in AD are believed to originate from activation of local macrophage-like microglial cells by plaque-producing Aβ proteins [47, 48]. Activated microglia also perpetuate the chronic inflammatory environment seen in AD by being the primary source of ROS [47, 48]. Three separate studies suggested allicin may also uniquely affect the deposition of amyloid plaques after administration for either two [20], twelve [23] or sixteen [24] weeks. One study observed these effects were directly correlated to a significant decrease in activity of the lyase enzymes that generate the amyloid precursor proteins (APP) [23]. Much of the damage in AD results from deposition of these amyloid (senile) plaques and neurofibrillarly tangles in the hippocampus, thereby impairing memory and learning processes [47, 48]. Senile plaques consist of aggregations of (β amyloid peptides or Aβ) [47, 48]. These accumulations are neurotoxic and the primary cause of brain inflammation in AD [47, 48].

Amyloid plaques are generated through amyloid precursor protein (APP) being acted upon by two sets of lyase enzymes; the β secretases (BACE) and γ secretases [47, 48]. The γ secretase is a quartet of proteins consisting of anterior pharynx defective (APH-1), nicastrin (NCT), preselinin (PS1 or PS2) and preselinin enhancer (PEN-2)[22]. The most recent AD animal study reported that allicin (10 mg/kg/day) impaired the activity of BACE, PS1, PS2 and NCT lyases, as assessed by Western blot methodology [23]. Currently it is unclear whether allicin directly inihibits these enzymes by interfering with thiols in their makeup or just prevents their activation by providing a reduction in their being triggered as a result of elevated inflammation. Allicin does appear to directly inhibit the brain acetylcholinesterase (AChE) and butyrylcholinesterase (BuChE) [22]. AChE consists of two dimers connected by a cysteine linkage [49], which would provide an excellent target for allicin. If reproducible these studies would provide novel mechanisms to prevent and possibly reverse AD progression. A synopsis of the potential targets for allicin in AD is shown in Figure 2.

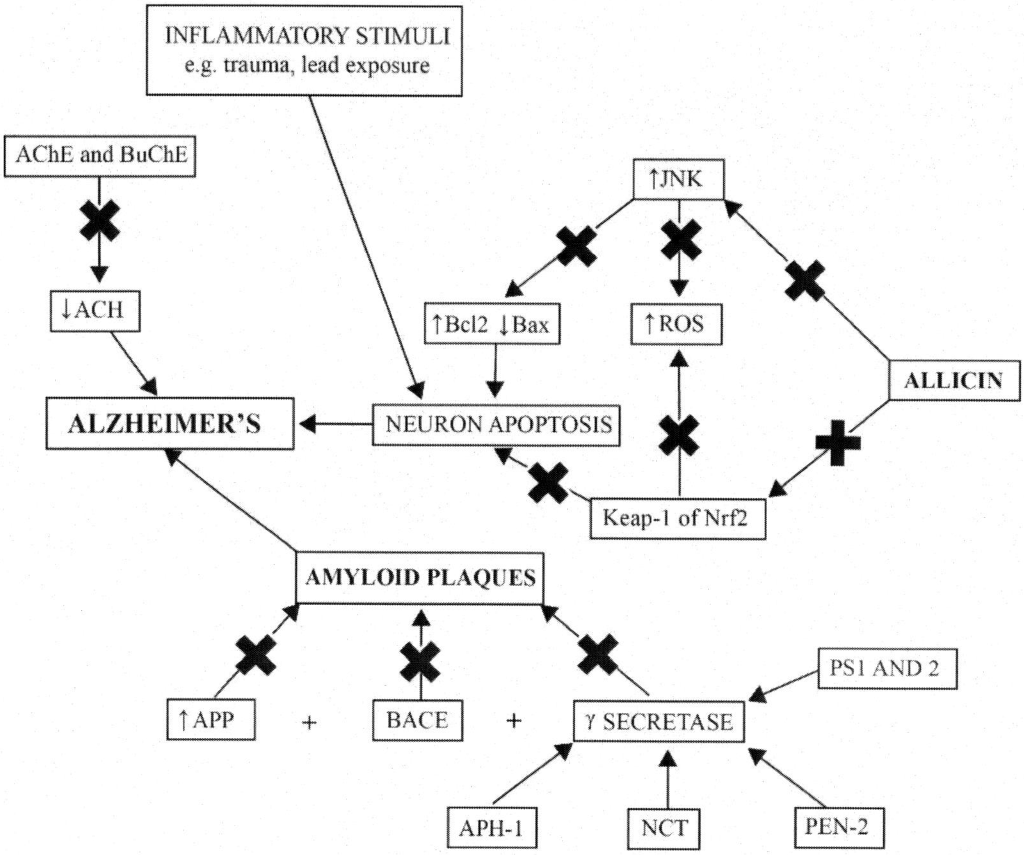

✖ Allicin's points of inhibition (animal neurodegenerative models/ cell lines) ✚ enhanced activity.

Legend: inflammatory stimuli induce neuronal apoptosis and the overexpression of enzymes generating amyloid plaques as well as ROS in AD brains. Chronic neuroinflammation also affects the neurotransmitter metaboliing enzymes AChE and to a lesser extent BuChE reducing acetylcholine secretion. Allicin is able to increse neuronal expression of anti-apoptotic proteins (Bcl-2) by decreasing JNK expression. Allicin also reestablishes a normal redox environment by upregulating Nrf2 and the antioxidant enzyme GpX. Allicin can reduce APP plaques, through impairing amyloid enzymes, increase acetylcholine secretion and increase animal cognitive abilities in models of AD as a result.

Abbreviations used: Aβ-1-40 and 1-42 (β peptides), ACH (acetylcholine), AChE (acetylcholinesterase), APH-1 (anterior pharynx defective), APP (amyloid precursor protein), BACE (β secretase), Bax (apoptosis regulator Bax), Bcl-2 (B-cell lymphoma 2), BuChE (butyrylcholinesterase), JNK (c-Jun N terminal kinase pathway), (NCT (nicastrin), PEN-2 (preselenin enhancer), PS1 and 2 (preselenin 1 and 2) and ROS (reactive oxygen species).

References used to construct diagram: [1-4, 20-24].

Figure 2. Allicin's impact on the pathophysiology of AD models.

3.2. Allicin and PkD

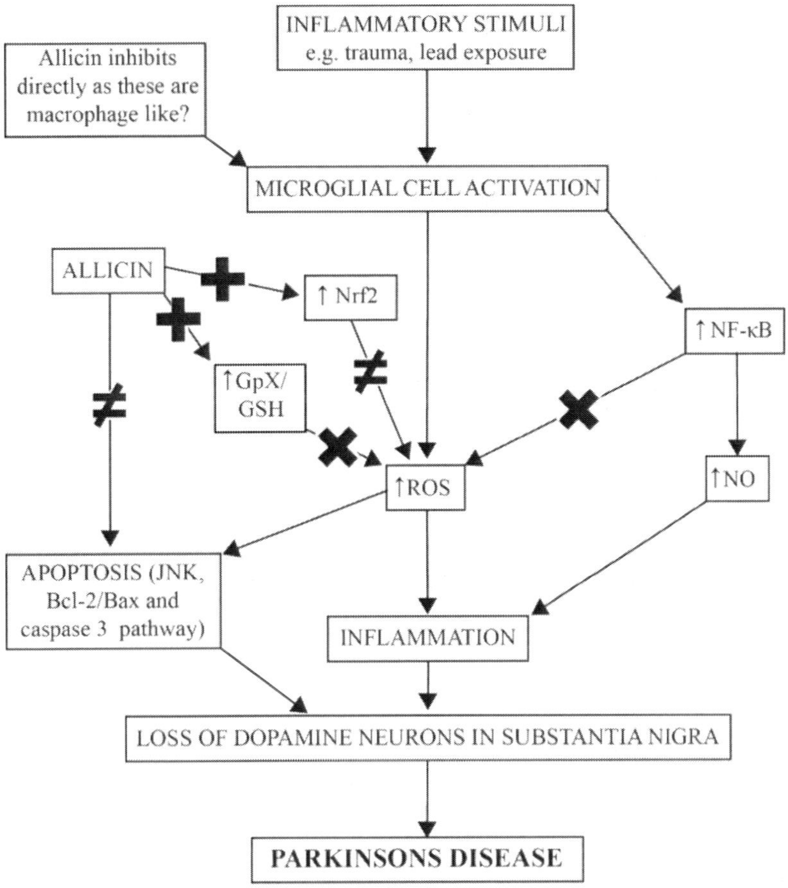

✖ Allicin's points of inhibition (animal neurodegenerative models/cell lines).
Allicin's potential effects based on AD models ✚ Enhanced activity.

Legend: Microglial activation through various stimuli activates proinflammatory pathways in substantia nigra neurons of PkD patients. Resulting oxidative damage through unchecked ROS generation and activation of neuronal apoptotic pathways leads to loss of neurons and the dopamine they secrete. *In* vitro studies have shown allicin is able to impair apoptosis by impairing JNK, Bcl-2/Bax and caspase 3 pathways and inflammation by reducing ROS generation. Allicin may also be able to directly impair microglial activation due to the macrophage-like nature of these cells.

Abbreviations used: Bax (apoptosis regulator Bax), Bcl-2 (B-cell lymphoma 2), GPx (glutathione peroxidase), GSH (glutathione), JNK (Jun amino-terminal kinase), NF-κB (nuclear factor kappa beta), NO (nitric oxide), Nrf2 (NF-E2, p45-related factor 2), ROS (reactive oxygen species).

References used to construct diagram: [8, 12, 25, 26, 50, 51, 53, 54].

Figure 3. Allicin's potential impact on the pathophysiology of PkD models.

Using the classical *in vitro* cellular model of PkD, rat pheochromocytochroma (PC12) cells, allicin at low doses (0.1-1 µg/ml) has been shown in two separate studies to protect the cells from hydrogen peroxide [25] or oxidopamine-induced damage [26] (Table 2). Allicin was reported to inhibit apoptosis well as decreased levels of ROS, [25, 26]. As in the AD studies [20, 21, 24], allicin exerted much of its neuroprotective activity by affecting the redox level in the cells through interacting with GpX and GSH [50]. Oxidative stress is widely believed to be central to the damaging effects seen in PkD, which are concentrated on dopamine-secreting neurons in the substantia nigra [50-52]. In a murine model of the disease agonists activating the

Nrf2 pathway in astrocytes spared dopamine-secreting neurons [50]. Put simply, current evidence suggests an inverse correlation exists between Nrf2 activation and neuronal death in PkD [52]. Patients with PkD display elevated inducible nitric oxide synthase (iNOS) levels in the substantia nigra, adding to the inflammatory environment [51, 52]. Activation of Nrf2 directly inhibits NO as well as decreasing NF-κB activity through crosstalk [50]. Allicin's ablity to activate Nrf2 in other cell systems has been documented [4, 8, 53] and in PkD models it would be anticipated to be of great merit in directly preventing neuronal oxidative stress.

Allicin may exert neuroprotective effects through preventing mitochondrial damage [25]. Mitochondria are the major source of ROS and are in turn sensitive to their actions [25]. Elevated ROS results in mitochondrial damage and demise and in turn activation of neuronal apoptosis [25]. Allicin was able to prevent the hydrogen peroxide-induced apoptosis of PC-12 cells as seen by a decrease in caspase 3 and Bcl-2 expression [25]. Damage to mitochondria can also induce their division (biogenesis) to produce replacements [25]. Mitochondrial biogenesis involves activation of nuclear respiratory factor (NRF1) and mitochondrial transcription factor A (TFAM), both of which were suppressed in the presence of 50 μM allicin [26]. Allicin treatment protected PC12 cell mitochondria sufficiently to maintain their normal production of ATP [26].

PkD pathology is also tied to chronically activated microglial cells, which then upregulate NF-κB and consequently increase the levels of inflammatory cytokines including interleukin beta (IL-1β) and tumor necrosis factor alpha (TNF-α) [47]. Microglial cells are the brain's versions of monocyte-macrophages and share much of their origins and physiology with those populating the rest of the body [46]. Allicin has been previously shown to down-regulate peripheral blood monocyte attachment to endothelial cells [54] as well as prevent their proliferation in response to mitogens [55]. It is reasonable to suggest that allicin would possess similar activities against microglial activation and proliferation, thereby directly inhibiting the central conributor to brain inflammation seen in PkD. A synopsis of the potential targets for allicin in PkD is shown in Figure 3.

4. Indirect Neuroprotective Activities for Allicin

Although AD and PkD have separate risk factors and underlying pathophysiologies they share one feature in common; the irreperable destruction of central nervous system neurons [35, 36]. Neuronal damage can occur in a number of ways including CVD, aging, physical trauma, and exposure to environmental toxins [35, 36]. Taken together this means that any reduction in neuroinflammation would need to target as many of these risk factors as possible. Literature reports of animal models have suggested allicin is able to impair blood cortisol in CVD [56] and decrease neural toxicity following acute high level lead exposure [57-59]. Both chronic elevated blood cortisol [60, 61] and lead [62-64] exposure have strong correlations with the development of both AD and PkD. PkD has been shown to be triggered by herpes or influenza A exposure [65]. Allicin has been shown in several studies to impair the growth of these viruses both *in* vitro, in animal models and in human DBRPCT [66-70]. Finally, although not yet explored allicin may have additional effects on inflammasome formation, possibly through its effects on redox-sensitive enzymes that generate α-Syn [71-74]. A description of the published data on these indirect effects of allicin on neuroinflammation will now follow.

4.1. Allicin and Elevated Cortisol

Local inflammation also triggers the expression of GC recetptors in the brain and a subsequent rise in plasma cortisol through activation of the hypothalamic-pituitary adrenal axis (HPA)[36]. The hippocampus, which is the seat of memory and learning, is particularly vulnerable in this respect since it has the greatest distribution of GCR [60]. Elevated circulating cortisol levels have been reported for both AD and PkD patients, suggesting a role for GCR in the progression of these neurological conditions [60, 61]. Studies by Oi and colleagues [56], have shown that injection of allicin (10, 20 or 30 mmol) into male rats with high plasma cortisone and testosterone concentrations was able to increase luteinizing hormone (LH) levels within thirty minutes. LH, from the pituitary, stimulates an increase in testosterone secretion from the testis and a consequent decrease in plasma cortisol [56]. Steroid hormones, like testosterone, are generated from cholesterol [56] and a $C_{17,20}$-enzyme determines whether cortisol or sex steroids are made [75].

These data suggest several possibilities for how allicin could be affecting plasma cortisol. First, since the animals in the study were on a fat-free diet, allicin could be impairing endogenous cholesterol manufacture. Allicin has been shown to reduce serum cholesterol in a hyperlipidemic murine model [76]. The thiosulfinate has been shown to impair two enzymes involved in cholesterol biosynthesis, namely squalene-monooxygenase [77] and acetyl coA synthase [78]. Second, since allicin boosted testosterone and decreased cortisol, it might be affecting the activity of the $C_{17,20}$-enzyme [75]. When $C_{17,20}$-cooperates with the electron carrier P-450 reductase lyase activity increases relative to hydroxylase i.e., steroids are made at the expense of cortisol [75]. P450 reductase is redox sensitive [79] and allicin is known to affect the redox potential of cells by virtue of its ability to directly bind to thiols in proteins or stimulate GpX to reduce ROS levels in cells [8]. Further studies will be needed to identify which of these mechanisms allicin employs and if they translate into being effective in managing AD and PkD.

4.2. Allicin and Elevated Lead

Allicin may therefore be able to help with the management of AD and PkD, but are there any ways it could prevent the conditions from occurring? One mechanism is by preventing absorption of the damaging stimuli [61-63]. Strong evidence now links AD and PkD with chronic elevated lead exposure [61-63]. The heavy metal may also be involved in the etiology of amytrophic lateral sclerosis (ALS) [62]. Results of the Veteran's Affair's Normative Aging Study, which examined a cohort of one hundred and forty one middle aged men over a period of thirty years directly correlated continuous high lead blood and bone levels with reduced pattern memory and visual spatial skills [62]. This AD-related deficit was greater than could be expected by aging alone [62]. Weisskopf and colleagues [63] performed a magnetic resonance spectroscopy (MRI) hippocampal study on the fifteen men with the thinnest patella bone from the VA study. They observed that the brain target of high, prolonged lead exposure was the hippocampus, which underwent damage and glial repair (gliosis) as a result [63]. Similar results have also been seen when correlating PkD with bone (tibial) associated lead [64]. Having elevated lead in the long bones can increase the risk of developing PkD in susceptible individuals two-fold [64].

A single murine study demonstrated that allicin (12, 24 and 48 μg/kg, orally, twice daily for two weeks) was able to significantly reduce the absorption of high doses of lead (1,000 ppm) [57]. Although only a short term investigation, allicin decreased lead absorption to the brain (45%), kidney (45%) and liver (74%) of the animals in a dose-dependent fashion [57]. Since the liver is primarily responsible for the removal of lead from the circulation this is likely to also correlate with a decrease in lead becoming bone-associated [57]. A small randomized double-blind placebo-controlled trial (DBRPCT) of one hundred and seventeen car battery workers reported allicin (1,200 mg/ day for four weeks) significantly decreased ($p < 0.05$) blood lead concentration [58]. The drop was of a similar magnitude to that induced by the standard lead chelating agent D-penicillamine [58]. Finally an *in vitro* study also documented the ability of allicin to behave as a chelating (binding out) agent for several heavy metals including lead [59]. Taken together these studies suggest that allicin might be useful in preventing acute lead exposure. Daily use of allicin also holds promise as a preventative and longer term DBRPCT investigations are needed to confirm or refute these early findings.

4.3. Allicin Could Minimize Herpes and Influenza A Infections; Reducing PkD Risk

PkD may also be initiated following aberrant activation of microglia by herpes simplex-1 (HSV) and influenza A viruses [65]. Allicin has been found to be effective on HSV-1 proliferation in two separate *in vitro* studies [66, 67] as well as against influenza A in a single study [54]. One human DBRPCT found that allicin (180 mg/day) could decrease the number of "colds" three fold in human volunteers over a three month time period [69]. A single Russian human randomized double-blind placebo-controlled trial (DBRPCT) also reported that the incidence of "colds" was decreased nearly two fold in subjects who took stabilized allicin (Allicor) for five months [70]. Since influenza is one of the main causative agents of colds [79], it is possible that the thiosulfinate also works *in vivo* to prevent influenza infection.

4.4. Possible Effects for Allicin against Alpha Synuclein (α-Syn) Synthesis

Recent studies have suggested that both AD and PkD are connected by an abnormal reactivity to the protein α-Syn [70]. Monomers of α-Syn are expressed on neurons and support survivial of glia in various parts of the brain including hippocampus and substantia nigra [72]. Cell death allows the protein to be released and it then assembles into inflammasome tangles that closely resemble the plaques found in AD and are central to the pathology of PD, since these aggregates are the predominant protein in Lewy bodies [71]. Aggregation of α-Syn is produced by Polo-like kinases (PLK) and is redox sensitive [73]. Allicin's effects on PLK have not been investigated but it may inhibit the aggregation of α-Syn through affecting the brain redox environment. PLK activity seems to be regulated through mitogen activated kinases (MAPK) [74] that include JNK and p38 so allicin may also directly interact with these enzymes through a similar thiol-dependent mechanism.

CONCLUSION AND FUTURE DIRECTIONS

Allicin has a variety of anti-inflammatory and anti-oxidant targets [8, 12-26], which would help prevent the underlying inflammation that is the hallmark of many neuroinflammatory diseases including TBI, ASCI, IS, SAH, AD and PkD [12-26] These include activation of Nrf2 [13, 20, 23] and SOD/GpX/GSH [12-14, 16-21, 24, 26] to decrease damaging ROS and activation of eNOS [11, 12, 16] to prevent neuronal death. This reduction of inflammatory stimuli in turn lessens the release of proinflammatory cytokines from glial cells and feeds in to the maintenance of neuronal integrity. Allicin also inhibits a number of specific brain enzyme systems including those metabolizing acetylocholine (AChE, BuChE)[21] and the overstimulated lyases that generate amyloid plaques [20, 23, 24]. These effects have been shown to maintain cognitive function in animal models [13, 20, 21, 23, 24].

Levels of acute neuroinflammation directly correlate to permanent changes in functionality [1, 2]. In contrast, none of the acute neurological conditions discussed in this chapter uses interventions that address the underlying inflammation that occurs [27-31]. For TPI one therapy currently being explored is N-actyl cysteine, which acts by re-regulating the brain's oxidative enzymes [31]. Phase I and phase II clinical trials are also ongoing to develop three neuroprotective anti-inflammatory medications [31]. One is a cytokine-blocking agent (cutamesine), the second reduces oxidative stress (edaravone) and the third is a repurposed diabetic medication (Glyburide), anticipated to block the neural sulfonylurea receptor [32]. Overactivation of the SUR-1 receptor occurs on astroglia and microglial cells during cerebral edema and infarction and increase levels of oxidative stress [32, 81]. Combinatorial chemistry docking studies recently demonstrated that allicin possessed an affinity to bind to the isolated SUR-1 receptor [81]. Allicin is of a lower affinity than the pharmaceutical glyburide, its added potency as an antioxidant may also make it worthy of further investigation [81].

Management of IS [29] and SAH [30] involves rapid restoration of blood flow after the traumatic event. Despite advances in treatment strategies, which include clot dissolution within five hours for IS [29] and stabilization of the patient to prevent re-bleeding, which typically occurs within seventy-two hours [30]. One recent animal study administered allicin (80 mg/kg) for seven days after IS [18] and observed a significant cognitive improvement in the animals. Two other studies demonstrated allicin was effective if the animals were pre-treated with allicin before experimental IS [17] or given allicin within thirty minutes of experimental SAH [19] If any of these studies translate into human efficacy it may well extend the window of opportunity to reverse these acute inflammatory syndromes.

Although decreasing underlying brain inflammation and consequent neurodegeneration is a treatment goal for AD and PkD patients [82, 83], current strategies revolve solely around maintaining bioavailability of neutrotransmitters for the surviving neural networks [33, 34, 37]. AD is considered to involve a cholinergic deficit and memory loss during the mild to moderate disease stages is managed by well tolerated cholinesterase inhibitors [8]. Allicin can impair *in* vitro generation of AChE and BuChE, although it is difficult to determine whether this would correspond with a similar mole-to-mole dosage of between five and 10 mg/ day, which is that recommended for the classic cholinesterase inhibitors [34].

N-methyl D-aspartate receptor (NMDA) antagonists are already used for moderate to severe AD and reduce neural NO secretion due to glutamate-mediated excitation [31]. One *in* vitro study suggests allicin may utilize a similar mechanism, namely the down-redulation of iNOS secretion by glutamate-stimulated neurons [16]. The ability of Nrf2 agonists to decrease inflammation through reducing both NO and ROS release has also been proposed as an intervention for several chronic neurodegenerative conditions including Huntington's disease [84]. Allicin has been shown to be able to impair NO through increasing eNOS activity [11, 12] and reduce Nrf2 levels in three animal models of ASCI [13] or AD [21, 24]. Allicin might therefore offer a potential combination nootropic therapy that could be used throughout AD.

Neither cholinesterase inhibitors or NMDA decrease the speed of progression of AD or reverse the hippocampal damage that wipes memories [33, 34]. One small pilot DBRCT showed that visual memory and attention-based tasks increased significantly ($p < 0.05$) in young volunteers (ages 20-23, n = 10) who fresh garlic capsules (800 mg/twice daily) for five weeks than in a comparative placebo group [85]. No difference was seen between the groups in verbal memory or executive function tasks [85]. Recent studies of nine-week old C57BL/6 mice documented that those given oral allicin (garlic oil 10 mg/kg for twenty days) demonstrated improved novel object recognition compared with control mice [86] Histochemical analyses correlated these changes with neural proliferation and upregulated AChE activity in the dentate gyrus [86]. These mice would correspond to young adults [87].

In contrast, allicin has been proven to be able to improve cognition in murine models of AD [20, 21, 23, 24]. In these cases the researchers attributed the benefits to the reduction of senile plaques and underlying inflammation [20, 21, 23, 24]. Finally, to improve cognition in AD, β-secretase (BACE1) inhibitors are also under development but to date are of limited therapeutic potential because of high molecular weights likely to restrict transfer across the blood-brain barrier. [33]. In contrast allicin easily crosses the blood-brain barrier and was able to effectively inhibit these enzymes in a single, recent study [23].

Early PkD symptoms are managed by maintaining dopamine levels through a combination of the agonist L-dopa (levodopamine) and L-dopa deccarboxylase inhibitors (LDDI) [34]. Later, other therapies are added including NMDA) [34]. None of the medications reverse the condition or halt its progress [34]. Unlike AD, current evidence for allicin and PkD is not yet strong as it has not progressed past *in vitro* models [25, 26]. In contrast, alliin (S-acetyl cysteine), which is the precursor molecule for allicin, has been shown to be protective in a murine 1-methyl-4-phenyl-1,2,3,6-tetrahydropiridinium (MPTP) model of PkD [88]. García and colleagues [88] reported that the efficacy of this sulfur compound involved activation of the Nrf2 pathways and was associated in amelioration of dopamine secretion. Since all these reports are relatively recent [25, 26, 88] it is possible that groups may already be working on determining if allicin is similarly effective *in vivo* using the available PkD models [89].

More exciting even than allicin's potential interventions for extant AD or PkD [20-26] are the idea that it can decrease the risk of the disease even beginning [56-59, 64-70, 76-78]. Allicin's ability to decrease circulating factors like cholesterol [76-78], cortisol [56] and lead [57-59], that impair brain chemistry could decrease important disease triggers common to both AD and PkD [35, 36, 60-64]. Allicin's antiviral activities [62-66] may reduce some of the infectious etiologies of PkD [65]. Given that patients with AD and PkD are likely to be elderly and have other comorbidities, particularly osteoarthritis or CVD [34, 35], a more general anti-inflammatory agent devoid of side effects might be more appropriate for these individuals.

Much of the issue with any new medication is that in the early stages development costs are felt by the patient [33]. Estimates are that developing a new medication from *in vitro* models through DBRCT is approximately three billion dollars [90]. This means obtaining strong evidence that the potential therapeutic has extended availability i.e., it doesn't need to be taken frequently as well as possessing an optimal safety profile [91]. Allicin may be safe, but until the recent development of stabilized allicin derivatives including the injectible Allitridium [92] and orally absorbed Allimax [93], the rapid clearance of the thiosulfinate provided a major barrier to its use [8]. New synthetic or semi-synthetic allicin-like molecules designed through combinatorial chemistry may also provide superior potency and absorbtion profiles [94, 95].

In developed countries reliance and confidence of the consumer is based on a series of phase 1, 2 and 3 clinical trial methodologies [89, 90]. In contrast, around eighty percent of the population in developing countries rely on traditional, mostly plant-based medicines for their management of health conditions [95]. For example, in the Ayurvedic Indian system of medicines garlic is used for AD treatment [95]. Phytochemicals have the added benefits of usually being safer, with fewer side effects, as well as being able to intervene with multiple targets simulataneously [96]. Naturally-sourced molecules in medications also provide an added cost-saving advantage [96]. Garlic is tolerant to a wide variety of climates and is relatively easy to grow, thereby creating consistent source material [97]. Finally, ingestion of allicin would be of particular benefit in reducing the high lead exposure risk factor for AD and PkD risk in developing countries [98, 99]. Allicin would thereby provide a two-fold long term and acute exposure neuroprotection management strategy. Like the search for antimicrobial agents took us to natural products, plant-derived phytochemicals are likely to take us to future neuroprotective agents [96]. The literature of the past decade suggests allicin is poised to take a lead role and the next steps should see a move from animal models to human clinical trials with this thiofulfinate.

REFERENCES

[1] Allan, Stuart M., and Nancy J. Rothwell. 2003. "Inflammation in central nervous system injury." *Philosophical Transactions of the Royal Society of London. Series B Biological sciences* 358(1438): 1669–1677. doi: 10.1098/rstb.2003.1358.

[2] Gaurav, Singhal, Emily J. Jaehne, Frances Corrigan, Catherine Toben, and Baune Bernhard T. 2014. "Inflammasomes in neuroinflammation and changes in brain function: a focused review." *Frontiers in Neuroscience* 8: Article 315. doi: 10.3389/fnins.2014.00315.

[3] Angelova, Plamina R., and Andrey Y. Abramov. 2018. "Role of mitochondrial ROS in the brain: from physiology to neurodegeneration. *FEBS Letters* 582: 692-702. Accessed April 2, 2019. https://febs.onlinelibrary.wiley.com/doi/pdf/10.1002/1873-3468.12964.

[4] Parathath, Susana R., Iordanis Gravanis, and Stella E. Tsirka. 2007. "Nitric oxide synthase isoforms undertake unique roles during excitotoxicity." *Stroke* 38: 1938-1945. https://www.ahajournals.org/doi/pdf/10.1161/STROKEAHA.106.478826.

[5] Katusic, Zvonimir S., and Susan A. Austin. 2014. Endothelial nitric oxide: protector of a healthy mind. *European Heart Journal* 35(14): 888–894. doi: 10.1093/eurheartj/ eht544.

[6] Park, Eugene, Joshua T. Bell, and Andrew J. Baker. 2008. "Traumatic brain injury: can the consequences be stopped?" *CMAJ* 178(9):1163-1170. doi: https://doi.org/10.1503/cmaj.080282.

[7] Washington, Patricia M., Sonia Villapol, and Mark P. Burns. 2015. "Polypathology and dementia after brain trauma: Does brain injury trigger distinct neurodegenerative

diseases, or should they be classified together as traumatic encephalopathy?" *Experimental Neurology* 275(30:03): 381–388 doi: 10.1016/j.expneurol.2015.06.015.

[8] Borlinghaus, Jan, Frank Albrecht, Martin C. H. Grulke, Ifeanyi D. Nwachukwu, and Alan J. Slusarenko. 2014. "Allicin: Chemistry and biological properties." *Molecules* 19(8): 12591-12618.

[9] Kinney, Jefferson W., Shane M. Bemiller, Andrew S. Murtishaw, Amanda M. Leisgang, Arnold M. Salazar, and Bruce T. Lamb. 2018. "Inflammation as a central mechanism in Alzheimer's disease." *Alzheimer's & Dementia: Translational Research & Clinical Interventions* 4:575-590. https://doi.org/10.1016/j.trci.2018.06.014.

[10] Natarajan, Suganthy, Karutha Pandian Shunmugiah, and Pandima Devi Kasi. 2013. "Plants traditionally used in age-related brain disorders (dementia): an ethanopharmacological survey." *Pharmaceutical Biology* 51(4): 492-523, doi: 10.3109/13880209.2012.738423.

[11] Zhou, Yui-fei, Wen-tao Li, Hong-chen Han, Da-kuan Guo, Xiao-sheng He, Liang Li, Jin-ning Song, and Zhou Fei. 2014. "Allicin protects rat cortical neurons against mechanical trauma injury by regulating nitric oxide synthase pathways." *Brain Research Bulletin* 100:14-21. http://dx.doi.org/10.016/j.brainresbull.2013.10.013.

[12] Chen, Wei, Jun Qi, Feng Feng, Mao-de Wang, Gang Bao, Tuo Wang, Mu Xiang, and Wang-fu Xie. 2014. "Neuroprotective effect of allicin against traumatic brain injury via Akt/ endothelial nitric oxide synthase pathway-mediated anti-inflammatory and anti-oxidative mechanisms." *Neurochemistry International* 68:28-37. http://dx/doi.org/10.016/j.neurint.2014.01.015.

[13] Lv, Runxiao, Ningfang Mao, Jinhui Wu, Chunwen Lu, Muchen Ding, and Xiaochuan Gu. 2015. "Neuroprotective effect of allicin in a rat model of acute spinal cord injury." *Life Sciences* 143: 114-123. http://dx.doi.org/10.016/j.lfs.2015.11.001.

[14] Zhu, Jin-Wen, Tao Chen, Jianzhong Guan, Wen-bo Liu, and Jian Liu. 2012. "Neuroprotective effect of allicin on spinal cord ischemia-reperfusion injury via improvement of mitochondrial function in rabbits." *Neurochemistry International* 61(5):640-648. https://doi.org/10.1016/j.neuint.2012.06.021.

[15] Zhang, Benping, Feng Li, Weijiang Zhao, Jiebing Li, Quinsong Li, and Weizhi Wang. 2015. "Protective effects of allicin against ischemic stroke in a rat model of middle cerebral artery occlusion." *Molecular Medicine Reports* 12: 3734-3738. https://doi.org/10.3892/mmr.2015.3883.

[16] Liu, Shu-Guang, Peng-Yu Ren, Guo-Yu Wang, Shu-Xin Yao, and Xi-Jing He. 2015. "Allicin protects spinal cord neurons from glutamate-induced oxidative stress through regulating the heat shock protein 70/inducible nitric oxide synthase pathway." *Food Function* 6:320-329. doi: 10.1039/C4FO00761A.

[17] Kong, Xiangyi, Shun Gong, Lijuan Su, Chen Li, and Yanguo Kong. 2017. "Neuroprotective effects of allicin on ischemia-reperfusion brain injury." *Oncotarget* 8(61):104492–104507. doi:10.18632/oncotarget.22355.

[18] Yu, Juan, Ru-Xia Lu, Pen Yang, Yong-Gan Cao, Qian-Long Zhang, Hui Qiao, Qian Luo, Shu-Zhi Li, Chang-Lin Jiang, Li-Hui Qu. 2016. "Allicin attenuates global cerebral ischemia/ reperfusion injury in gerbils via anti-oxidative and apoptotic pathway." *Int J. Clin. Exp. Med.* 9(2): 2375-2382. http://www.ijcem.com/files/ijcem0017226.pdf.

[19] Shao, Jing, Qi Wu, Sheng-yin Lv, Xiao-ming Zhou, Xiang-sheng Zhang, Li-li Wen, Xin Xue, and Xin Zhang. 2019. 2019. "Allicin attenuates early brain injury after experimental

subarachnoid hemorrhage in rats." *J. Clin. Neurosci.* 63:202-208. https://www.sciencedirect.com/science/article/pii/S0967586818314103.

[20] Li, Xian-Hui, Chun-Yan Li, Zhi-Gang Xiang, Fei Chong, Zheng-Ying Chen, and Jiang-Ming Lu. 2010. "Allicin can reduce neuronal death and ameliorate the spatial memory impairment in Alzheimer's disease models." *Neurosciences (Riyadh)* 15(4): 237-243. Accessed on March 13, 2019. http://www.nsj.org.sa/PDFFILES/Oct10/Allicin 20100060.pdf.

[21] Li, Xian-Hui, Chun-Yan Li, Jiang-Ming Lu, Rong-Bo Tian, and Jia Wei. 2012. "Allicin ameliorates cognitive deficits ageing-induced memory and learning deficits through enhancing of Nrf2 antioxidant signaling pathways. "*Neuroscience Letters* 514: 46-50. doi: 10.1016/j.neulet.2012.02.054. http://gxy.hunnu.edu.cn/ResearchManagementSystem/tmp/2014%E4%B8%8A%E4%BC%A0%E9%99%84%E4%BB%B6/Allicin%20ameliorates%20cognitive%20deficits%20ageing-induced%20learning%20and%20memory%20deficits%20through%20enhancing%20of%20Nrf2%20antioxidant%20signaling%20pathways.pdf.

[22] Kumar, Suresh. 2015. "Dual inhibition of acetylcholinesterase and butyrylcholinesterase enzymes by allicin." *Indian J. Pharmacol.* 47(4): 444-446. doi: 10.4103/0253-7613.161274.

[23] Zhang, Hao, Ping Wang, Yixue Xue, Libo Liu., Zhen Li, and Yunhui Liu. 2018. "Allicin ameliorates cognitive impairment in APP/PS1 mice via suppressing oxidative stress by blocking JNK signaling pathways." *Tissue and Cell*, 50:89-95. doi:10.3389/fnana.2015.00032.

[24] Zhu, Yao-Feng, Xian-Hui Li, Zhi-Peng Yuan, Chun-Yan Li, Rong-Bo Tian, Wei Jia, and Zhu-Ping Zhao. 2015. "Allicin improves endoplasmic reticulum related stress-related cognitive deficits via PERK/Nrf2 antioxidative signaling pathway." *Eur. J. Pharmacol.* 762: 239-246. https://doi.org/10.1016/j.ejphar.2015.06.002.

[25] Lv, Runxiao, Lili Du, Chunwen Lu, Jinhui Wu, Muchen Ding, Chao Wang, Ningfang Mao, and Zhicai Shi. 2017. "Allicin protects against H_2O_2-induced apoptosis of PC12 cells via the mitochondrial pathway." *Experimental and Therapeutic Medicine* 14: 2053-2059. Accessed on October 25, 2018. https://pdfs.semanticscholar.org/5002/1b252deb67a05b78d3e188f562e452645396.pdf.

[26] Liu, Hao, Ping Mao, Jia Wang, Tuo Wang, and Chang-Hou Xie. 2015. "Allicin protects PC12 cells against 6-OHDA-induced oxidative stress and mitochondrial dysfunction via regulating mitochondrial dynamics." *Cellular Physiology and Biochemistry* 36:966-979. Accessed on October 25, 2018. https://www.karger.com/Article/PDF/430271.

[27] Galgano, Michael, Gentian Toshkezi, Xuecheng Qiu, Thomas Russell, Lawrence Chin, and Li-Ru Zhao.2017. "Traumatic Brain Injury: Current Treatment Strategies and Future Endeavors." *Cell Transplantation* 26(7):1118–30. doi:10.1177/0963689717 714102.

[28] Fehlings, Martin G., Lindsay A. Tetreault, Jefferson R. Wilson, Brian K. Kwon, Anthony S. Burns, Allan R. Martin, Gregory Hawryluk, and James S. Harrop. 2017. "A Clinical Practice Guideline for the Management of Acute Spinal Cord Injury: Introduction, Rationale, and Scope." *Global Spine Journal* 7(3 Suppl): 84S–94S. doi: 10.1177/2192568217703387.

[29] Musuka, Tapuwa D., Stephen B. Wilton, Mouhieddin Traboulsi., and Michael D. Hill. 2015. "Diagnosis and management of acute ischemic stroke: speed is critical." *CMAJ:*

Canadian Medical Association journal = Journal de l'Association Medicale Canadienne 187(12): 887–893. doi: 10.1503/cmaj.140355.

[30] Luoma, Astry, and Ugan Remy. 2012. Acute management of aneurysmal subarachnoid hemorrhage. *Continuing Education in Anasthesia Critical Care and Pain* 13(2):52-58. https://doi.org/10.1093/bjaceaccp/mks054.

[31] Hoffer, Barry J., Chaim G. Pick, Michael E. Hoffer, Robert E. Becker, Yung-Hsiao Chang, and Nigel H. Greig. 2017. "Repositioning drugs for traumatic brain injury – N-acetyl cysteine and phenserine." *Journal of Biomedical Science* 24:71. https://doi.org/10.1186/s12929-017-0377-1.

[32] Reis, Cesar, Onat Akyol, Wing Mann Ho, Camila Araujo, Lei Huang, Richard Applegate II, and John H. Zhang. 2017. "Phase I and Phase II Therapies for Acute Ischemic Stroke: An Update on Currently Studied Drugs in Clinical Research." *BioMed Research International* 2017: Article ID 4863079, 14 pages. https://doi.org/10.1155/2017/4863079.

[33] Mendiola-Precoma, J., L.C. Berumen, K. Padilla, K., and G. Garcia-Alcocer. 2016. "Therapies for Prevention and Treatment of Alzheimer's Disease." *BioMed Research International:* 2589276. doi: 10.1155/2016/2589276.

[34] Konta, Brigittte, and Wilhelm Frank. 2008. "The treatment of Parkinson's disease with dopamine agonists."*GMS Health Technology Assessment* 4: Doc05. PMID: 21289911.

[35] Santos, Cláudia, Peter J. Snyder, Wen-Chih Wu, Mia Zhang, Ana Echeverriá. 2017. "Pathophysiologic relationship between Alzheimer's disease, cerebrovascular disease, and cardiovascular risk: A review and synthesis." *Alzheimer's and Dementia Diagnosis, Assessment and Disease Monitoring* 7: 69-87. https://dx.doi.org/10.1016/j.adn.2017.01.005.

[36] Herrero, Maria T., Christina Estrada, Layal Maatouk, and Sheena Vyas. 2015. "Inflammation in Parkinson's disease: role of glucocorticoids." *Frontiers in Neuroanatomy* 9: 32.

[37] Casey, David A., Demetra Antimisiaris, and James O'Brien, J. 2010. "Drugs for Alzheimer's disease: are they effective?" *P & T: A Peer-reviewed Journal for Formulary Management* 35(4), 208-11. Accessed on March 15, 2019 https://www.ncbi.nlm.nih.gov/pmc/articles/PMC2873716/.

[38] Kalaria, Raj N., Gladys E. Maestre, Raul Arizaga, Robert P. Friedland, Doug Galasko, Kathleen Hall, Jose A. Luchsinger, Adesola Ogunniyi, Elaine K. Perry, Felix Potocnik, Martin Prince, Robert Stewart, Anders Wimo, Zhen-Xin Zhang, and Piero Antuono. World Federation of Neurology Dementia Research Group. 2008. "Alzheimer's disease and vascular dementia in developing countries: prevalence, management, and risk factors." *The Lancet. Neurology* 7(9): 812-26. doi: 10.1016/S1474-4422(08)70169-8.

[39] Zhu, Guo, and Suzanne B. Baker. 2016. "Detecting PTEN and PI3K Signaling in Brain." *Methods in Molecular Biology (Clifton, N.J.)* 1388: 53–62. doi: 10.1007/978-1-4939-3299-3_5.

[40] Ahmed, S.M.U., Lin Luo, Akhileshwar Namani, Xiu Jan Wang, and Xiuwen Tang. 2016. "Nrf2 signaling pathway: Pivotal roles in inflammation." *Biochmimica et Biophysica Acta* 1863: 585-597. http://dx.doi.org/10.1016/j.badis.2016.11.005.

[41] Subramaniam, Srinivasa, and Klaus Unsicker. 2010. "ERK and cell death: ERK1/2 in neuronal death." *The FEBS Journal* 277: 22-29. doi:10.1111/j.1742-4658.2009. 07367.x.

[42] Rahman, Mohammad S. 2007. "Allicin and other functional active components in garlic: health benefits and bioavailability." *Int J Food Properties* 10: 245-268.

[43] Kovalkovičová, Natália, Irena Sutiaková, Juraj Pistl, and Vaclav Šutiak 2009. "Some food toxic for pets." *Interdisciplinary Toxicology* 2(3), 169-76. doi: 10.2478/v10102-009-0012-4.

[44] Yu, Lu, Na Guo, Rizeng M. Meng, Bin Liu, Xudong Tang, Jing Jin, Yumei Cui, and Xuming Deng. 2010. "Allicin -induced global gene expression profile of *Saccharomyces cerevisiae*."Appl *Microbiol Biotechnol* 88: 219-229. https://doi.org/10.1007/s00253-010-2709-x.

[45] Milcovic, Lidija, Neven Zarcovic, and Luciano Saso. 2017. "Controversy about pharmacological modulation of Nrf2 for cancer therapy." *Redox Biology* 12: 727-732. https://doi.org/10.1016/j.redox.2017.04.013.

[46] Saccani, Simona, Serafina Pantano, and Gioacchino Natoli. 2002. "p38- dependent marking of inflammatory genes for increased NF-κB recruitment." *Nature Immunology* 3: 69-75.

[47] Kreutzberg, Georg W. 1996. "Microglia: A sensor for pathological events in the CNS." *Trends Neurosci.* 19: 312-318.

[48] Yu, Yang, and Richard D. Ye. 2017. "Microglial Aβ receptors in Alzheimer's disease." *Cell. Mol. Neurobiol.* 35: 71-83.

[49] Dvir, Hay, Israel Silman, Michal Harel, Terrone Rosenberry, and Joel L. Sussman. 2010. "Acetylcholinesterase: from 3D structure to function." *Chemico-Biological interactions* 187(1-3), 10-22. doi: 10.1016/j.cbi.2010.01.042.

[50] Chen, Pei-Chun, Marcelo R. Vargas, Amar K. Pani, Richard J. Smeyne, Delind A. Johnson, Yuet Wai Kan, and Jeffrey A. Johnson. 2009. "Nrf2-mediated neuroprotection in the MPTP mouse model of Parkinson's disease: Critical role for the astrocyte." *Proceedings of the National Academy of Sciences of the United States of America* 106(8): 2933-8.

[51] Whitton, P.S. 2007. "Inflammation as a causative factor in the aetiology of Parkinson's disease." *British Journal of Pharmacology* 150(8): 963-76.

[52] Ahmed, S. M. U., Lin Luo, Akhileshwar Namani, Xiu Jan Wang, and Xiuwen Tang. 2016. "Nrf2 signaling pathway: Pivotal roles in inflammation." *Biochmimica et Biophysica Acta* 1863: 585-597. http://dx.doi.org/10.1016/j.badis.2016.11.005.

[53] Zhang, Min, Huichao Pan, Yinjie Xu, Xueting Wang, Zhaohui Qui, and Li Jiang. 2018. "Allicin decreases lipopolysaccharide-induced oxidative stress and inflammation in human umbilical vein endothelial cells through suppression of mitochondrial dysfunction and activation of Nrf2." *Cell Physiol. Biochem.* 41: 2255-2267.

[54] Kang, N.S., E.Y. Moon, C.G. Cho, and S. Pyo. 2001. "Imunomodulating effect of garlic component, allicin, on murine peritoneal macrophages." *Nutrition Res* 4: 617-626. Accessed October 16, 2018. https://eurekamag.com/pdf/003/003469471.pdf.

[55] Salman, Hertzel, Michael Bergman, Hanna Bessler, Igor Punsky, and Meir Djaldetti. 1999. "Effect of a garlic derivative (alliin) on peripheral blood cell responses." *International J Immunopharmacol.* 21: 589-597.

[56] Oi, Yuriko, Mika Imafuku, Chiaki Shishido, Yutaka Kominato, Syoji Nishimura, and Kazuo Iwai. 2001. "Garlic Supplementation Increases Testicular Testosterone and Decreases Plasma Corticosterone in Rats Fed a High Protein Diet." *The Journal of Nutrition* 131(8): 2150–2156, https://doi.org/10.1093/jn/131.8.2150.

[57] Aslani, Mohammad R., V. Najarnezhad, M. Mohri, and M. Azad. 2011. "The effect of allicin on blood and tissue lead content in mice. " *Comparative Clinical Pathology* 20(2): 121-125. Accessed on March 18, 2019 https://link.springer.com/article/10.1007%2Fs00580-010-0964-y.

[58] Kianoush, Sina, Mahdi Balali-Mood, Sayed R. Mousavi, Valliola Moradi, Mahmoud Sadeghi, Bita Dadpour, Ohmed Rajabi, and Mohammed T. Shakeri. 2012. "Comparison of Therapeutic Effects of Garlic and D-Penicillamine in Patients with Chronic Occupational Lead Poisoning." *Basic & Clinical Pharmacology & Toxicology* 110: 476-481. doi:10.1111/j.1742-7843.2011.00841.x.

[59] Songsunkgan, J, and S. Chanthai. 2014. "Study of allicin extract chelated with some heavy metals (Cu, Co and Pb) by fluoerescence quenching and its antioxidant activity." *Asian J Chemistry* 26(1): 132-136. http://dx.doi.org/10.14233/ajchem.2014.15349.

[60] Ros-Bernal, Francisco, Stephåne Hunot, MariaT. Hererro, Sebastien Parnadeu, Jean-Christophe Corvol, Lixia Liu, Daniel A. Fischer, Maria A. Carillio-de Sauvage, Françoise Saurini, Christiane Coussieu, Kiyoka Kinugawa, Annick Prigent, Günter Höglinger, Michel Hamon, François Tronche, Etienne, and Sheela Vyas. 2011. "Microglial glucocorticoid receptors play a pivotal role in regulating dopaminergic neurodegeneration in parkinsonism." *Proc. Natl. Acad. Sci. U.S.A.* 108: 6632-6637. doi: 10.1073/pnas.1017820108.

[61] Huang, Chi-Wei., Chun-Chung Lui, Weng-Neng Chang, Cheng-Hsien Lu, Ya-Ling. Wang, and Chung-Chi Chang. 2009. "Elevated basal cortisol level predicts lower hippocampal volume and cognitive decline in Alzheimer's disease." *J. Clin. Neurosci.* 16:1283-1286. doi: 10.1016/j.jocn.2008.12.026.

[62] Marinelle Payton, Karen M Riggs, Avron Spiro, Scott T Weiss, and Howard Hu. 1998. "Relations of Bone and Blood Lead to Cognitive Function: The VA Normative Aging Study." *Neurotoxicology and Teratology* 20(1): 19-27. https://doi.org/10.1016/S0892-0362(97)00075-5.

[63] Weisskopf, Marc G., Howard Hu, David E. Sparrow, Robert E. Lenkinski, and Robert O. Wright. 2007. "Proton magnetic resonance spectroscopic evidence of glial effects of cumulative lead exposure in the adult human hippocampus." *Environ Health Perspect.* 2007 115(4) 519-523. doi:10.1289/ehp.9645.

[64] Weisskopf, Marc G., Jennifer Weuve, Huiling Ne, Marie-Helene Saint-Hilaire, Lewis Sudarsky, David K. Simon, Bonnie Hersch, Joel Schwartz, Robert O. Wright, and Howard Hu. 2010. "Association of cumulative lead exposure with Parkinson's disease. " *Environ. Health Perpect.* 118(11): 1609-1613. doi: 10.1289/ehp.1002339.

[65] Olsen, Laura K., Ellis Dowd, and Declan P. McKernan. 2018. "A role for viruses in Parkinson's etiology." *Neuronal Signaling* 2(2): NS20170166. doi: 10.1042/NS20170166. Accessed October, 25 2018. http://www.neuronalsignaling.org/content/2/2/NS20170166.

[66] Tsai, Yen, Linda L. Cole, Larry E. Davis, Steven J. Lockwood, Victoria Simmons, and Gaynor C. Wild. 1985. "Antiviral properties of garlic: *In vitro* effects on influenza B, herpes simplex and cocksackie viruses." *Planta Medica* 5:460-461. DOI: 10.1055/s-2007-969553.

[67] Weber, Norbert D., Douglas O. Andersen, James A. North, Byron K. Murray, Larry D. Lawson, and Bronwyn G. Hughes. 1992. "*In vitro* virucidal effects of *Allium sativum*

garlic extracts and compounds." *Planta Med* 58(5): 417-423. doi: 10.1055/s-2006-961504.

[68] Mehrbod, P. E. Amini, and M. Tavassoti-Kheiri. 2009. "Antiviral activity of garlic extract on influenza virus." *Iranian Journal of Virology* 3(1): 19-23. Accessed November 16, 2018. https://www.sid.ir/en/journal/ViewPaper.aspx?ID=168987.

[69] Josling, Peter. 2001. "Preventing the common cold with a garlic supplement: a double-blind, placebo-controlled study." *Advances in Therapy* 18(4):189-193. Accessed November 21, 2018 http://www.bravacorp.com/garlic%20and%20the%20common %20cold.pdf.

[70] Andrianova, I. V., I. A. Sobenin, E. V. Sereda, L. I. Bodina, and M. I. Studenkin. 2003. "Effect of long acting tablets "allicor" on the incidence of acute respiratory viral infections in children." *Ter. Arkh.* 75(3): 53-56. PMID:12718222.

[71] Roodveldt, Cintia, John Christodoulou, and Christopher M. Dobson. 2008. "Immunological features of alpha-synuclein in Parkinson's disease." *Journal of Cellular and Molecular medicine* 12(5B): 1820-9. doi: 10.1111/j.1582-4934.2008. 00450.x.

[72] Xu, Shengli, and Pu Chan. 2015. "Interaction between Neuromelanin and Alpha-Synuclein in Parkinson's Disease." *Biomolecules* 5(2): 1122-42. doi: 10.3390/biom 5021122.

[73] Li, Ji, Wenzhe Ma, Ping-yuan Wang, Paula J. Hurley, Fred Bunz, and Paul M. Hwang. 2014. "Polo-like kinase 2 activates an antioxidant pathway to promote the survival of cells with mitochondrial dysfunction." *Free Radical Biology & Medicine* 73: 270-7. doi: 10.1016/j.freeradbiomed.2014.05.022.

[74] Jalili, Ahmad, Anna Moser, Mikhail Pashenkov, Christine Wagner, Gaurav Pathria, Viola Borgdorff, Melanie Gschaider, Georg Stingl, Sridhar Ramaswamy, and Stephan N. Wagner. 2011. "Polo-Like Kinase 1 Is a Potential Therapeutic Target in Human Melanoma." *Journal of Investigative Dermatology* 131(9): 1886-1895. https://doi.org/10.1038/jid.2011.136.

[75] Hall, Peter F. 1991. Cytochrome P-450 C_{21SCC}: One enzyme with two actions hydroxylase and lyase. *J. Steroid Biochem. Molec. Biol.* 40(4-6):527-532.

[76] Yin, Lu, He Zhuojin, Shen Xiuying Shen, Xiaolu Xu, Jie Fan, Shaohu Wu, and Deyong Zhang. 2012. "Cholesterol-Lowering Effect of Allicin on Hypercholesterolemic ICR Mice." *Oxidative Medicine and Cellular Longevity*: Article ID 489690 https://doi.org/10.1155/2012/489690.

[77] Gupta, Nisha, and Todd D. Porter 2001. "Garlic and garlic-derived compounds inhibit human squalene monooxygenase." *J. Nutr.* 131: 1662–1667.

[78] Focke, Manfred, Andrea Feld, and Harmut K. Lichtenthaler. 1990. "Allicin, a naturally occurring antibiotic from garlic, specifically inhibits acetyl-CoA synthetase." *FEBS Lett.* 261: 106–108.

[79] Huang, Wei-Cheng, Jacqueline Ellis, Peter C. E. Moody, Emma L. Raven, and Gordon C.K. Roberts. 2013. Redox-Linked Domain Movements in the Catalytic Cycle of Cytochrome P450 Reductase. *Structure* 21(9): 1581-1589. https://doi.org/10.1016/j.str.2013.06.022.

[80] Mäkelä, Mika J., Tuomo Puhakka, Olli Ruuskanen, Maja Leinonen, Pekka Saikku, Marko Kimpimäki, Soile Blomqvist, Timo Hyypiä, and Perrti Arstila. 1998. "Viruses and bacteria in the etiology of the common cold." *Journal of Clinical Microbiology*

36(2):539-42. Accessed November 16, 2018. https://www.ncbi.nlm.nih.gov/pmc/articles/PMC104573/.

[81] Reynaldi, Muhammad A., Hafrizal Riza, and Sri Luliana. 2018. "Docking study of allicin with the sulfonylurea receptor 1, complex 1 and PPARγ receptor on insulin resistance." *International Journal of Pharmacy and Pharmaceutical Sciences* 10(10): 130-138. doi: https://doi.org/10.22159/ijpps.2018v10i10.28105.

[82] Rees, Karen, Rebecca Stowe, Smitaa Patel, Natalie Ives, Kieran Breen, Carl E. Clarke, and Yoav Ben-Shlomo. 2011. "Non-steroidal anti-Inflammatory drugs as disease-modifying agents for Parkinson's disease: evidence from observational studies." *Cochrane Database Syst. Rev.* 9:CD008454. doi: 10.1002/14651858.CD008454.

[83] McGeer, Patrick L., Joseph Rogers, and Edith G. McGeer. 2016. "Inflammation, anti-inflammatory agents and Alzheimer's Disease: The last 22 years." *Journal of Alzheimer's Disease* 54(3):853-857. doi: 10.3233/JAD-160488.

[84] Escartin, Carole, and Emmanuel Brouillet. 2016. "The Nrf2 pathway as a potential therapeutic target for Huntington disease A commentary on "Triterpenoids CDDO ethyl amide and CDDO trifluorylethyl amide improve the behavioral phenotype and brain pathology in a transgenic mouse model of Huntington disease." *Free Radical Biol. Med.* 49:144-146.

[85] Tasnim, Sara, Parsa S. Haque, Md. Sazzadul Bari, Md. Monir Hossain, Sardar M. A. Islam, Mohammad Shahriar, Mohiuddin Bhuiyan, and Mohammad S. Bin Sayeed. 2015. "Allium sativum L. Improves Visual Memory and Attention in Healthy Human Volunteers." *Evidence-based Complementary and Alternative Medicine: eCAM, 2015*, 103416. doi:10.1155/2015/103416.

[86] Jung, Hyo Y., Kwon Y. Lee, Dae Y. Yoo, Jong W. Kim, Miyoung Yoo, Sanghee Lee, Ki-Yeon Yoo, Yeo S. Yoon, Jung H. Choi, and In H. Hwang. 2016. "Essential oils from two *Allium* species exert effects on cell proliferation and neuroblast differentiation in the mouse dentate gyrus by modulating brain-derived neurotrophic factor and acetylcholinesterase." *BMC Complementary and Alternative Medicine* 16:431. https://doi.org/10.1186/s12906-016-1384-6.

[87] Dulatta, Sulagna, and Pallev Sengupta. 2016. "Men and mice: relating their ages." *Life Sciences* 152:244-248. https://doi.org/10.1016/j.lfs.2015.10.025.

[88] García, Esperanza, Ricardo Santana-Martínez, Carlos A. Silva-Islas, Ana L. Colín-González, Sonia Galván-Arzate, Yessica Heras, Perla D. Maldonado, Julio Sotelo, and Abel Santamaría. 2014. "S-allyl cysteine protects against MPTP-induced striatal and nigral oxidative neurotoxicity in mice: participation of Nrf2." *Free Radic. Res.* 48(2): 159-167. doi: 10.3109/10715762.2013.857019.

[89] Lee, E, J, H. H. Yoon, E. S. Park, J. Min, and S. R. Jeon. 2018. "A Novel Animal Model of Parkinson's Disease Using Optogenetics: Representation of Various Disease Stages by Modulating the Illumination Parameter." *Stereotact Funct Neurosurg* 96: 22-32. doi: 10.1159/000486644.

[90] Dana, Kaitlyn N., John B. Hertig, and Robert J. Weber. 2017. "Drug Pricing Transparency: The New Retail Revolution." *Hospital Pharmacy* 52(2), 155-159. doi: 10.1310/hpj5202-155.

[91] Kaitin, K. I. 2010. "Deconstructing the drug development process: the new face of innovation." *Clinical Pharmacology and Therapeutics* 87(3): 356-61. doi: 10.1038/clpt.2009.293.

[92] Feng, Fang, Li Hong, Cui Wen, and Yongsui Dong. 1999. "Treatment of hepatitis caused by cytomegalovirus with allitridin injection – An experimental study." *Journal of Tongji Medical University* 19(4): 271-274. https://doi.org/10.1007/BF02886960.

[93] Suddek, Ghada M. 2014. "Allicin enhances chemotherapeutic response and ameliorates tamoxifen-induced liver injury." *Pharmaceutical Biology* 52(8): 1009-1014. Accessed November 22, 2018. https://www.tandfonline.com/doi/full/10.3109/13880209.2013.876053.

[94] Leontiev, Roman, Nils Hohaus, Jacob Claus, Martin C. H. Gruhlke, and Alan J. Slusarenko. 2018. "Comparison of the Antibacterial and Antifungal Activities of Thiosulfinate Analogues of Allicin." *Scientific Reports* 6763:8(1). Accessed on February 22, 2019 https://www.nature.com/articles/s41598-018-25154-9.

[95] Lubenets, Vira, Sofiya Vasylyuk, Nataliya Monka, Khrystina Bolibrukh, Olena Komarovska-Porokhnyavets, Diana Baranovych, Rostyslav Musyanovych, Ewa Zaczynska, Anna Czarny, Urszula Nawrot, and Volodymyr Novikov. 2016. "Synthesis and antimicrobial properties of 4-acylaminobenzenethiosulfoacid S-esters." *Saudi Pharmaceutical Journal: SPJ: The Official publication of the Saudi Pharmaceutical Society* 25(2), 266-274. doi: 10.1016/j.jsps.2016.06.007.

[96] Kumar, G. Phani, and Farhath Khanum. 2012. "Neuroprotective potential of phytochemicals." *Pharmacognosy Reviews* 6(12): 81-90. doi: 10.4103/0973-7847.99898.

[97] Bayan, Leila, Peir H. Koulivand, and Ali Gorji.2014. "Garlic: a review of potential therapeutic effects." *Avicenna Journal of Phytomedicine* 4(1): 1-14.

[98] Wani, Ab L., Anjum Ara, and Jawed A. Usmani. 2015. "Lead toxicity: a review." *Interdisciplinary Toxicology* 8(2), 55-64. doi: 10.1515/intox-2015-0009.

[99] Tong, Shilu, Yasmin E. von Shirnding, and Tippawan Prapamtonolol. 2000. "Environmental lead exposure: a problem of global proportions." *Bulletin of the World Health Organization* 78(9): 1068-1077. Accessed on March 19, 2019 https://www.ncbi.nlm.nih.gov/pmc/articles/PMC2560844/pdf/11019456.pdf.

In: Allicin
Editor: Diana R. Cundell

ISBN: 978-1-53617-339-0

Chapter 13

TUMORICIDAL ACTIVITIES OF ALLICIN

Diana R. Cundell, PhD*
College of Life Sciences, Jefferson University, Philadelphia, PA

ABSTRACT

Garlic has been used throughout history as a remedy for the treatment of "abnormal growths", which were later to be termed tumors. Sixty years after allicin was first isolated from garlic cloves it was found to induce apoptosis in gastric cancer cells *in vitro*. Since that time, the thiosulfinate has been suggested to kill tumors of at least sixteen kinds, in both *in vitro* and *in vivo* models. The tumor microenvironment is a very unique one, able to both evade and coopt the immune system and enable both proliferation and metastasis. Several genetic and environmental factors have been demonstrated to enable neoplasia; these include the downstream consequences of inherited and acquired mutations, as well as oncogenic viral infection. Neoplastic cells avoid immune recognition and ignore the normal signals for programmed cell death. Thus, despite our understanding of how and why they develop from healthy cells, tumor cells still represent a significant therapeutic challenge. In this chapter, an evaluation of the tumors allicin is able to eliminate will be combined with the known mechanisms of the thiosulfinate's activity, including those shared with extant anti-tumor medications. Given the benign and multi-faceted effects of allicin, it may well provide an option as a directed or complementary medicine in the treatment of some viral diseases, including cancers. Limitations of fully comprehending this potential, based on literature review of the available studies, will also be discussed. Finally, future strategies for allicin, including effective delivery, will also be considered.

Keywords: angiogenesis, apoptosis, ERK, JNK, oncogenic, Nrf2, ROS

* Corresponding author: Room 320, Search Hall, Jefferson University, 4201, Henry Avenue, Philadelphia, PA 19144, E-mail: Diana.Cundell@jefferson.edu.

1. Introduction

The first recorded use of garlic in the treatment of tumors was in the Ancient Egyptian text the *Codex Ebers*, published around 1600 B.C. [1, 2]. The tumors first described were those affecting the breast and were given the name *karkinos* by the Greek physician Hippocrates around 1400 B.C. [3]. The influence of Hippocrates and his incorporation of garlic into his *armamentarium* for treating abdominal growths most likely supported the continued usage of this bulb well into modern times for naturopathic healing of "growths" and particularly of gastrointestinal ailments [1, 2]. At this point in history, an understanding of the active products in garlic was not available and the discovery of allicin as the major anti-microbial and anti-inflammatory phytochemical was hundreds of years in the future [1-3]. What is apparent, though, is that Hippocrates reported that maximum efficacy came from either eating the entire garlic bulb, or preparing it as a broth or "tea" [1-3]. We now know that either of these treatments would activate the thiosulfinate allicin from its inactive alliin form and preserve its activity [1-3]. As the studies of tumors advanced, they were believed to develop from an imbalance in the body's humors, trauma, and even parasitic disease [3]. Surgeons in the ancient world did remove the abnormal growths and although there was an understanding that they would recur [3] no effective treatment strategies were available at the time other than phytomedicines [1, 2].

As with most medical disciplines, the 19th century saw the beginnings of the field of oncology [3]. In 1846 the surgeons Bilroth, Handley, and Halstead first prevented spread and tumor growth by removing not only the neoplasia itself but also local lymph nodes [3]. Another surgeon of this period, Dr. Paget, noted that some tumors seeded into other organs [3]. The discovery of what was termed metastasis explained why simply removing tumors was not a completely effective treatment modality, but an understanding of the process of metastasis would require nearly another two hundred years of research [3]. A second weapon against cancer came with the discovery of X-rays by Roentgen in 1896 [3]. Within three years, radiation therapy in the form of X-rays were used to treat cancer and this method has continued to the current day [3].

Chemotherapy, which began in 1939 with the discovery that estrogen could be used to treat prostate cancer [4], has now become the classical method to treat tumors, both before removal and in preventing their recurrence [3-5]. Interestingly, the spur for chemotherapeutic drug development came from the discovery in the 1950s of natural alkaloids from the plant *Vinca rosea*, later to be refined into vincristine [4]. Again, modern scientists (as had the ancient people before them) looked towards naturally-derived products as weapons in their fight against cancer.

Effective tumor cell line models and animal models that could pattern human disease were available by the late 1990s and allowed the development of more targeted monoclonal antibody (mAb) therapies [3, 5]. These models were also used to develop a second group of "natural products"; the secondary fungal metabolite angiogenesis inhibitors [3, 6]. Angiogenesis inhibitors began to be used in 2004 to prevent aggressive tumors from metastasizing by preventing new blood vessel development, thus limiting the spread and growth of neoplastic cells [3, 6]. Tumors were now understood to represent normal cells that had gone wildly out of control, dividing rapidly, and producing a chronic inflammatory environment that beget and perpetuate their persistence [3, 5]. Accordingly, looking at the natural products that had been identified by this time as anti-inflammatory led some researchers to examine allicin as an anti-tumor agent [7-10].

The first four literature reports of allicin's *in vitro* tumoricidal activities appeared at the end of 2003 [7] and during 2004 [8-10]. Allicin was shown to be effective against cell lines of gastric [7], bladder [8], cervical [9], colon [9, fibrosarcoma [9, 10], and melanoma [10] tumors. Two of these reports also suggested allicin had *in vivo* activity in murine models of bladder [8], fibrosarcoma [10], and melanoma [10] tumors. Since this date, three more *in vitro* studies have demonstrated the *in vitro* efficacy of allicin against colon tumor lines [11-13] and six more against gastric cancers [14-18]. Research reports also demonstrate that allicin has reproducible *in vitro* efficacy against breast [11, 19], fibrosarcoma [9, 10, 11], and liver [20-22] tumors. There are also isolated reports of allicin being effective *in vitro* against six other tumor cell lines including the brain (glioblastoma) [25], kidney [26], lung [23], ovarian [27], thyroid [28], and B cell leukemia [29]. In addition, seven individual literature reports employing *in vivo* murine models of neoplasia have reported that intravenously injected allicin decreased the size of bladder [8], fibrosarcoma [10], B cell leukemia [28], liver [22], melanoma [10], neuroblastoma [29], osteosarcoma [30], and pancreatic [31] tumors.

Despite all of the pre-clinical evidence, however, the tumoricidal activity of allicin has not yet been explored using any human clinical trials, and a reviewer at this point must wonder why. Allicin's unstable nature, discussed in Chapter 1 and throughout this book, has definitely hampered any delivery vehicles being developed [32], but it is also most apparent that to be developed as a therapy an understanding of its mechanisms against the tumors needs to be fully delineated. Sifting through the literature, it is clear that the solutions to both of these problems are only just emerging, with sixteen of the twenty-five papers reviewed in the construction of this chapter only appearing in the past five years [11, 15-23, 25-27, 29-31]. The costs of completely developing a new medication from *in vitro* screenings through to double-blind, randomized, placebo-controlled trials (DBRPCT) is approximately three billion dollars [33]. While this may seem cost-prohibitive, a great need remains for new, accessible, and minimally toxic (or non-toxic) anti-tumor medications.

Worldwide, tumor deaths now number over eight million, and although survival rates are improving there is still considerable morbidity associated with most tumor-bearing patients [34]. Several tumor types (e.g., lung, pancreas, and brain) have poor prognoses, with five-year survival rates of less than ten percent [34-36]. Even in patients with survivable tumors (i.e., those diagnosed early or that are slow-growing), longtime survival and quality-of-life are limited due to heart disease or infections resulting from damage or compromise related to the toxicities inherent in modern anti-cancer treatment regimens, such as immunosuppressive chemotherapeutic and anti-angiogenesis drugs [34, 35]. And those are the figures for developed countries. In developing nations, the statistics are far worse [37]. Lack of early diagnosis and access to treatment continue to account for high levels of mortality from breast, stomach, and liver cancer in developing nations [37]. Less expensive, potentially locally-sourced treatment alternatives would provide desperately-needed options, particularly for these nations. It is of interest, in this regard, that twenty-two of the twenty-five papers on allicin were published by researchers residing in developing countries [7-9, 12-27, 29-31].

As mentioned, a major issue with current anti-cancer treatment is that standard pharmaceutical interventions result in significant, often debilitating, side effects [4, 6, 38]. Chemotherapeutic agents are associated with nausea, hair loss, digestive tract inflammation, and immunosuppression [38]. Angiogenesis inhibitors are associated with hemorrhage, blood clot formation, and high blood pressure [6]. For many patients, financial burden, lack of positive outcomes, and undesirable side effects have led to an exploration of complementary and alternative therapies (CAM) that may ease the unappealing process of chemotherapy and possibly increase their chance of survival [39]. Studies have suggested that as many as one in three cancer patients resort to CAM, including acupuncture and herbal (phytomedicinal) agents [39]. Phytochemicals are attractive as therapeutic agents in that they have a long history of use in both traditional Chinese and Ayurvedic medicines and are relatively devoid of side effects [39, 40]. Many patients who have used them successfully for other conditions (e.g., managing arthritis or menopausal syndromes) continue to do so when they develop cancer [39, 40]. Antiviral phytomedicines are particularly important in this respect since at least one in five tumors has a viral cause [41].

As will be seen in this chapter, allicin has much to recommend its further development into human use. There are now stabilized forms of the thiosulfinate [42, 43] and a deliverable methodology [28]. Allicin also possesses antiviral activity against at least two oncogenic viruses (see Chapter 8 for details). Finally, the thiosulfinate targets multiple viruses, which currently each require a cocktail of medications and individualized interventions [44-46]. All these activities have at their core the ability of allicin to rebalance the tumor microenvironment, both at the immunological [8, 10] and biochemical level [12, 13, 19, 23-27].

2. Antitumor Activities of Allicin: *In Vitro* Studies

Twenty-three independent literature studies have examined the effects of allicin against fifteen tumors, *in vitro* [7-28, 30]. A brief description of the experimental details and findings is provided in Table 1.

Examining the *in vitro* literature further reveals that the research studies for allicin were employed over thirty different cell lines, with at least five being murine [7-11]. Although, murine tumor cells have long been considered to behave differently than those derived from human clinical specimens [47], fibrosarcoma was the only tumor investigated solely using murine cell lines and the data from the three studies was remarkably consistent with respect to the effective dosage of allicin needed to kill these cells (1-20 μg/ml) [9-11]. In comparison, the human neoplastic cell studies utilized wildly varying dosages of allicin ranging from 0.1 ng/ml [19] to as high as 15 mg/ml [30]. Do these reported differences mean that breast tumors are very sensitive to allicin [19] and those of osteosarcoma [30] or bladder [8] are resistant? It might, but even when human cell lines for a specific cancer type are used they appear to show differential responsiveness to allicin [9, 11-13]. A prime example are the studies of allicin on seven human colon cancer lines which reported efficacies at levels ranging from 0.2 μg/ml [9] to as much as 150 μg/ml [13]. At first glance, this might be ascribed to allicin's instability, but studies of tumor cell lines may point to another issue [48]. Medico and colleagues [48] examined one hundred and fifty-one common colon cancer cell lines and reported they had differential expression of tyrosine kinases, oncogenic mutations, and gene translocations. The gene alterations influenced many features of the cell lines including their levels of sensitivity to the mAb cetuximab, which is currently used in treatment of colon cancers in patients [48]. For example, cell lines such as HCT-116 were found to be more resistant to this agent than the very sensitive HT-29 strain or intermediate SW and Caco strains [48]. Interestingly, this pattern of sensitivity and resistance was replicated in the responsiveness of the colon cancer cell lines to allicin, suggesting it is an inherent component of the cell lines themselves [9, 11-13], adding an additional layer of complexity to understanding and defining the potential role of allicin as part of a standardized CAM regimen.

All but three of the *in vitro* studies on allicin [8, 11, 28] identified a potential biochemical pathway or molecular target for allicin. Most prominent in this regard were fourteen studies that identified allicin as able to activate cell apoptosis through either a caspase-dependent [9, 12, 14-17, 20, 30] or -independent fashion [10, 12-16, 22, 24-26, 29]. The latter can involve several pathways that influence expression of the pro-apoptotic Bax (Bcl-2 associated X) proteins [12-16, 22, 25], including NF-E2 (nuclear factor, erythroid-derived 2), p45-related factor 2 (Nrf2) [13], extracellular regulated kinase (ERK 1/2) [10, 19, 24], Jun amino-terminal kinase (JNK) [26], and protein signal transducer and activation of transcription-3 (STAT-3) [22]. Furthermore, allicin's ability to increase apoptosis may be combined with autophagy via induction of the Akt-mTOR pathway, resulting in a decrease in tumor size [27].

One study suggested allicin could simultaneously decrease the activation of NF-κB (nuclear factor kappa beta), Nrf2, and inducible nitric oxide synthetase (iNOS) [12]. iNOS expression occurs following co-activation of both NF-κB and the p38 mitogen activated pathway and results in nitric oxide (NO) production [49]. In healthy cells, elevated NO signals cell death, but for cancer cells elevated NO is simply a byproduct of their increased metabolism so they develop an insensitivity to it [49]. Another side effect of this increased biochemical activity is elevated levels of reactive oxygen species (ROS) [8, 50]. Normally, ROS elevation induces apoptosis [32, 51] so tumor cells must typically upregulate Nrf2 to inactivate the ROS and prevent their apoptosis [52]. Allicin's ability to downregulate NF-κB and iNOS simultaneously would therefore be expected to decrease the tumor "block" on apoptosis and allow these immortal cells to die. This was indeed what occurred in the human colon cancer cell lines HCT-116 and SW620 [12].

The main driver for tumor development is that cancer cells are essentially unreceptive to both external and internal death signals [54]. Because of these nuances, teasing out allicin's role in the context of mechanistic cross-talk of pathways seems to be contigent upon the model. As an example of this point, Nrf2:NF-κB cross-talk is complex to describe because depending on the tumor, Nrf2 either enhances or inhibits NF-κB [13, 32]. Referred to as "*the Janus Face of Nrf2*" by one researcher [13, 32], this means that Nrf2 may be either activated or downregulated depending on which tumor is being investigated. In the case of the HCT-116 colon cancer cell line, for example, Nrf2 is downregulated and its activation by allicin induces cellular apoptosis [13]. Allicin has been shown to increase expression of the Nrf2 pathway in several *in vitro* models of both normal and transformed cells [32] so this observation is in keeping with allicin's "anti-inflammatory" nature. But how then does allicin affect tumors in which the Nrf2 pathway is already upregulated? An answer to this question may be provided by how allicin interacts with the mutated form of the Nrf2 initiating protein Keap 1 (Kelch-like ECH-associated protein 1) [53].

Table 1. Allicin cell line tumor studies

Tumor	Model used*	Results	Reference
Bladder	MBT-2 murine line; allicin 100 μg/ml-2.5 mg/ml	↑ cell death; allicin was immediately directly cytotoxic to 50% of cells at 100 μg/ml and to > 90% using allicin at 500 μg/ml or greater	[8]
Breast	MCF-7 human line; allicin 0.042-1.2 mM [11]; allicin 0.1-10 ng/ml [19]	↓ metastasis ↑ apoptosis ↓ activation of NF-κB, ERK1/2 expression of VCAM ↑ interaction between ER-α and p65	[11, 19] [19] [19]
Cervical	SiHa and HeLa human lines; allicin 0.1-10 mg/ml	↑ apoptosis through caspase (3, 8, 9) activation and DNA fragmentation	[17]
Colon	HT-29 human line; allicin 0.042-1.2 mM	↓ proliferation and ↑ apoptosis	[11]
Colon	SW480 human line; allicin 1-100 μM	↑ apoptosis through caspase (3, 8, 9) activation and DNA fragmentation	[9]
	HCT-116 and SW620 human lines; allicin 30-150 μg/ml	↑ apoptosis by ↓ NF-κB, iNOS and Bcl-2 expression and ↑ Bax, caspase C and PARP	[12]
	Caco-2, HCT-116, HT-29 and LS174T human lines; allicin 6.2-310 μM	↓ Bcl-2 and ↑ Bax, expression Apoptosis initiated through Nrf2 expression	[13]
Fibrosarcoma	3T3 murine line; 0.042-1.2 nM	↓ proliferation and ↑ apoptosis	[11]
	L929 murine line; allicin 1-100 μM	↑ apoptosis through caspase (3, 8, 9) activation and DNA fragmentation	[9]
	MCA-105 murine line; allicin 1-5 μg/ml	Allicin (maximal at 0.5-1 μg/ml) oxidizes $p21^{ras}$ and stimulates T lymphocyte activation through ERK1/2 →↓ tumor	[10]
Gastric	SGC-7901 human line; allicin 0-20 μg/ml [14]; allicin 15-120 μg/ml [15]; 72 hours allicin 0-20 μg/ml [16]; 3-12 mg/ml	↓ proliferation, telomerase activity; allicin 0.16-1 mg/ml	[7]
		↑ apoptosis ↓ Bcl-2 and ↑ Bax expression, DNA fragmentation and caspase (3, 8, 9) activation	[14-16]
Gastric	MGC-803 human line; allicin 0.1-10 mg/ml	↑ apoptosis, p38 activation of caspase 3	[17]
	GCC human line; allicin10-50 μg/ml for 36 hours	↓ expression of ZNF703 (reduces cell proliferation)	[18]
Glioblastoma	U87MG human line; allicin 0-150 μM	↑ ERK and apoptosis	[24]
Kidney	*In vitro* excised human RCC tissues; allicin 0.05 mg/ml	↑ apoptosis by ↓ HIF, Bcl-2 and VEGF	[25]
Leukemia (B cell)	B-CLL, EBV-transformed, and MCL human lines; generation of allicin *in situ* using alliin precursor (100 mg/ml) -mAb rituximab conjugate	Allicin generated *in situ* B-CLL numbers ↓ 81% EBV numbers ↓80% MCL numbers ↓80%	[28]
Liver	HCC Hep G2 human line; allicin 35 μM	↑ apoptosis by caspase-dependent pathway (3,8 and 9), p53 and independent (Bcl-2) pathway	[20]
	HCCC-9810 human line; Garlicin®# 0-5 μM	↓P13K/Akt pathway →↓ migration and invasion	[21]
	HuCCT-1 and QBC 939 human line; allicin 0-20 μM	↑SHP-1 ↓STAT-3 expression ↓ migration and angiogenesis ↑ apoptosis → ↓ Bcl-2	[22]
Lung	Human H1299 and murine 3LL lines; allicin 0-20 μM	↓proliferation and ↑ H1299 apoptosis ↓P13K/Akt pathway	[23]
Melanoma	B16 murine cell line; allicin 1-5 μg/ml	Allicin (maximal at 0.5-1 μg/ml) oxidizes $p21^{ras}$ and stimulates T lymphocyte activation through ERK1/2 →↓ tumor	[10]
Osteosarcoma	MG-63 and U20S human lines; allicin 15 mg/ml for up to 72 hours	Tumor cell division through a caspase 3 mechanism	[30]
Ovarian	SKOV3 human line; allicin 0-100 μg/ml	↑ JNK activation and apoptosis; 12.5 μg/ml for most experiments	[26]
Thyroid	HTh-7 and SW1736 human lines; allicin 10 μM +/- 10 μM cisplatin/ carboplatin/ rapamycin	↓Akt/ mTOR pathway → autophagy; Allicin alone was effective and had an additive effect with all three chemotherapies	[27]

* = all studies observed cell changes for 48-hours and used MTT assay unless otherwise stated, #Garlicin® = stabilized allicin

Abbreviations used: Akt (protein kinase B), Bax (Bcl-2 associated X protein), Bcl-2 (B cell lymphoma-2 protein), B-CLL (B cell chronic lymphocytic leukemia), ER-α (estrogen receptor alpha), EBV (Epstein-Barr virus), ERK1/2 (extracellular regulated kinase), IL-2 (interleukin-2), HCC (hepatocellular carcinoma), HIF (hypoxia inducible factor), iNOS (inducible nitric oxide synthase), JNK (Jun amino-terminal kinase), MCL (mantle cell lymphoma), mTOR (mechanistic target of rapamycin), NF-κB (nuclear factor kappa beta), Nrf2 (NF-E2, p45-related factor 2), PARP (poly(ADP)ribose polymerase), P13K (phosphatidyl inositol 3 kinase), RCC (renal clear cell carcinoma), SHP-1 SHP-1 (Src homology region containing phosphatase 1), STAT-3 (signal transducer and activation of transcription-3), VCAM (vascular cell adhesion molecule) and VEGF (vascular endothelial growth factor), ZNF703 (zinc finger protein 703).

Tumor cells that possess an altered Keap-1 may or may not be associated with upregulation of other proteins such as the IKB-kinase (IKK) (which allows NF-κB activation) or anti-apoptotic Bcl-2 (B cell lymphoma-2 protein) [53]. If an agent binds to Keap-1, thereby increasing Nrf2, and simultaneously suppresses IKK and Bcl-2 proteins, tumor apoptosis occurs [53]. This has been shown to be a mechanism for other sulfur-containing phytomedicines, including those occurring in broccoli, and is likely how allicin works [53]. Thus, allicin's ability to rectify the intracellular environment in the tumor cell results from it simultaneously acting on multiple apoptosis-inducing targets [9, 10, 12-17, 19, 20, 22, 24, 26, 29], directly reducing tumor cell numbers. In addition, rapid tumor cell division is also believed to result in telomere shortening with tumor cells making more telomerase enzymes to countreract the effect [7]. One study suggests that allicin can prevent telomerase activity in gastric cells, which may constitute another novel activity of the thiosulfinate [7] that can result in inhibition of tumor cell growth.

A second putative target for allicin is the prevention of tumor spread through metastasis [21, 22, 25]. In the *in vitro* studies this was demonstrated by lack of migration of the tumor cells [21, 22, 25]. Tumor spread is associated with the creation of a low oxygen environment that then promotes the growth of new blood vessels (angiogenesis) that supply the cells with the nutrients they need to proliferate and migrate [25]. Angiogenesis is activated by the protein kinase B-phosphatidyl inositol 3 kinase (P13K/Akt) pathway, which contains the Ras proteins detailed below, and increases secretion of vascular endothelial growth factor (VEGF) [55]. Activation of STAT-3 also increases VEGF secretion [22]. Allicin's ability to impair VEGF levels [25] probably stems from targeting both the P13K/Akt pathway directly [21, 23] and STAT-3 through activation of the regulator tyrosine phosphatase Src homology region 2 containing phosphatase 1 (SHP-1) [22]. Angiogenesis also involves an alteration in the expression of vascular endothelial adhesion molecule (VCAM) on the endothelial cell surface, which may result from stimulation by VEGF [56]. No medications currently exist against VCAM, but researchers have suggested this may be another means to combat tumors that highly express this target molecule [56].

To create the low oxygen environment to stimulate angiogenesis, tumors secrete hypoxia initiation factors (HIF/HIFs) [25]. If proven to follow through into *in vivo* studies, allicin would become the first moiety in existence that is reported to be able to inhibit the secretion of tumor HIF [25]. The mechanism by which allicin decreases HIF, however, remains to be elucidated and requires more studies of the *in vitro* blockade of HIF expression in excised human kidney tumor cells [25] among others. Given that the production of HIF was blocked in a true human tumor, and not just a cell line, this potentially unique property of allicin may be promising to develop as a future interventional strategy. This, combined with allicin's ability to affect VCAM levels through impairing VEGF, would make it a very unique molecule indeed.

In addition, allicin was shown (at least *in vitro* [12, 18, 19, 21, 23]) to affect molecules important in metastatic tumors, namely poly(ADP-ribose) polymerase proteins (PARPs) [57] and estrogen receptor alpha (ER-α) [58]. Brain, colon, lung, and pancreatic tumors overexpressing PARPs are typically aggressive and able to rapidly metastasize as they weaken junctions between local blood vessel endothelial cells [57]. Allicin appears to demonstrate *in vitro* activity in cleaving colon tumor PARPs [12]. This may be via the activation of caspases [12] but still adds an extra tumoricidal activity to the thiosulfinate.

In the case of breast cancer, around seventy percent of aggressive breast tumors express ER-α and this molecule is a major target for the chemotherapeutic tamoxifen as a result [58].

Allicin may directly [19] or indirectly [18, 21, 23] affect the expression of ER-α. One study suggested allicin decreased the expression of ER-α receptors through increasing their interaction wth p65, the protein subunit that prevents NF-κB activation [19]. In a different study, indirect suppression of ER-α receptor expression was mediated by inhibition of the oncogene ZNF703 (zinc finger protein 703) [18]. ZNF703 is overexpressed in breast tumors where it plays a major role in tamoxifen resistance through activation of the Akt/MTOR pathway and downregulation of ER-α [58]. Allicin can also decrease P13K/Akt [21, 23] activity, which in turn impairs ER-α expression in breast cancer tissue [58]. If this translates to *in vivo* efficacy, the thiosulfinate could provide at least an alternative to tamoxifen in preventing breast cancer metastases.

3. Antitumor Activities of Allicin: Animal Studies

Seven independent literature studies have examined the effects of allicin against eight tumors [8, 10, 22, 28-31]. A brief description of the experimental detail and findings is provided in Table 2.

Each of the studies [8, 10, 22, 28-31] being discussed here has not yet been replicated by another research group but have used the same animal (mouse), route of administration (injection), and similar dosage of allicin (2.5-20 mg/kg), so are worthy of examination. It is also important to point out that this is an achievable physiological concentration of allicin in humans, as the thiosulfinate is estimated at 37 mg/g of freshly chopped garlic cloves [59]. Two of the studies were performed only on *in vivo* xenogeneic tumors of neuroblastoma [29] and pancreas [31], so the direct effects on the tumors without immune system support cannot be gauged. The remaining five studies were also supported by *in vitro* data on the direct effects of the thiosulfinate on tumor cells [8, 10, 22, 28, 30, 31]. Four of these studies suggested that shrinkage of the tumors was due to apoptosis via STAT-3 inhibition [22], caspase 3 initiation [30], or T-lymphocyte stimulation through ERK [10]. The neuroblastoma study also supported allicin's inhibition of tumor metastasis (i.e., angiogenesis impairment) through decreased circulating levels of VEGF in the animals [29]. Although not measured in the study, this would also connect with a decrease in STAT-3 or P13K/Akt activation, as these pathways are interconnected [21-23, 55].

The effectiveness of allicin on recruitment of T cells to the tumor site was recorded in four studies [8, 10, 29, 31]. Three studies further identified the subsets of T cells as T cytotoxic and T helper (Th1) cells [10, 29, 31]. Two studies also reported a significant uptick in tumor-associated levels of NK cells [31] and/or macrophages [8, 31] in the presence of the thiosulfinate. This is notable given that NK cells and T cytotoxic cells play a primary role in the rapid elimination of early tumors [60, 61]. Whilst NK cells do not require previous tumor exposure [60], the specificity of T cytotoxic cells involves their "priming" by Th1 cells [61]. NK cells activate apoptosis in the tumor and this recruits T cytotoxic cells to the tissue [60], as well as phagocytic macrophages that are attracted by apoptotic debris [62].

Table 2. Allicin animal model tumor studies

Tumor	Model used	Results	Reference
Bladder	30 C3H/HeJ mice inoculated with MBT-2 cells; allicin 12.5-25 mg injected near inoculation site assessment of tumor at 21 days	↓ tumor size in animals and ↑ macrophage and lymphocyte infiltration after 21 days	[8]
Fibrosarcoma	42 C57BL/6 mice inoculated with MCA-105 murine line; 28 received allicin 12.5 -5 mg/kg, 4 i.p. injections assessment of tumor at 25 days	Allicin oxidizes $p21^{ras}$ and stimulates T lymphocyte activation through ERK1/2 →↓ tumor Maximal efficacy of allicin at 12.5 mg/kg	[10]
Leukemia (B cell)	18 BALB/c mice inoculated with B-CLL, EBV-transformed and MCL human lines; 12 received i.p. generation of allicin *in situ* 3 mg alliin precursor-McAb rituximab conjugate injected b.i.d for three days	Allicin generated *in situ* ↓tumor size B-CLL number ↓ 81% EBV numbers ↓80% MCL numbers ↓75%	[28]
Liver	18 BALB/c mice inoculated with HuCCT-1 and QBC 939 human lines; 6 mice each received 10 or 20 mg/kg i.p. daily for 28 days then tumor assessed	↓ migration and angiogenesis ↑ apoptosis → ↓ Bcl-2	[22]
Melanoma	42 C57BL/6 mice inoculated with B16 murine cell line; 28 received allicin 12.5- 5 mg/kg 4 i.p. injections assessment of tumor at 25 days	Allicin oxidizes $p21^{ras}$ and stimulates T lymphocyte activation through ERK1/2 →↓ tumor Maximal efficacy of allicin at 12.5 mg/kg	[10]
Neuroblastoma	50 BALB/c mice; allicin 10 mg/ kg gastric perfusion and cyclophosphamide 60/mg/kg via injection. Assessment of tumor at 29 days	Allicin + cyclophosphamide ↓ murine tumors and circulating VEGF ↑ proportions of available T cytotoxic cells and T helper cells	[29]
Osteosarcoma	20 BALB/c mice inoculated with MG-63 human line; allicin 5 mg/kg with or without artesunate (injected?) for 50 days	Allicin + artesunate, ↓ murine tumors by 50% through a caspase 3 mechanism	[30]
Pancreatic	60 C57BL/6 mice; 15 allicin 10 mg/kg alone and 15 allicin 10 mg/kg + 20 µg IL-2 i.v. for 28 days	↓ tumor size of mice treated with allicin alone (70%) or in combination with IL-2 (90%) ↑ survival when treated with both treatments of > 10 days past controls ↑ T cytotoxic, NK and T helper cells	[31]

Abbreviations used: Bcl-2 (B cell lymphoma-2 protein), B-CLL (B cell chronic lymphocytic leukemia), b.i.d (twice a day), ERK1/2 (extracellular initiated kinase), IL-2 (interleukin-2), i.p. (intraperitoneal injection), i.v. (intravenous), mAb (monoclonal antibody), MCL (mantle cell lymphoma), NK (natural killer)

Is all this likely to translate to humans? Mice have NK cells and macrophages that behave similarly to our own, but their circulation contains primarily lymphocytes and fewer neutrophils [63]. This may make them a difficult study for acute inflammatory reactions but an excellent model for chronic inflammation and tumors, where neutrophils play a subordinate role [63]. The ability of allicin to increase the presence of all three antitumor immune cells [8, 10, 29, 31] therefore appears to add a second effective layer to its potential human tumoricidal abilities.

4. Piecing Things Together: How Does Allicin Inhibit Tumors?

Allicin's effects on tumors has been investigated using models of sixteen tumor types of over twenty human and animal cell lines, as well as xenogeneic murine models [7-31] (Tables 1 and 2). Analysis of the findings from these studies suggests allicin targets several common biochemical pathways to increase tumor cell apoptosis primarily through caspase, JNK, ERK, and Bax activation (or Bcl-2 reduction) [9, 10, 12-17, 19, 20, 22, 24, 2, 29]. Caspases play an essential role in apoptosis as they both begin the process (caspases 2, 8, 9, and 10), as well as act as the "executioner" for the cell (caspases 3, 6, and 7) [54]. Determination of whether death will occur is also associated with activation of an internal pathway gated by the Bcl-2 family of proteins, which contains both anti-apoptotic (Bcl-2) and pro-apoptotic members (Bax) [54]. The main issue for tumors is that they essentially either ignore these signals to die or have suppressed them through mutations [54, 64, 65]. Ignoring caspase signals probably occurs through tumor expression of a protein called survivin, which binds to caspases 3 and 9 and prevents the process of cell apoptosis [65]. Lung tumor cells with Ras-mutations display an altered form of one of the JNK isoforms: JNK-1 [64]. At least three separate variants of JNK (JNK1-JNK3) exist and are encoded by either separate genes or splice isoforms of these genes [64]. Mutated JNK-1 (and to a lesser extent JNK-2) have been demonstrated to be involved in the etiology of gastric, hepatic, and glioma tumors [64]. Specifically, one Ras protein, $p21^{ras}$, is upstream of ERK 1/2 and induces its activation [66], and upregulation of $p21^{ras}$ expression is seen in leukemia, breast, and prostate cancer and is associated with a poor clinical outcome [66]. In another feedback loop, ERK1/2 also functions to inhibit Nrf2, thereby promoting the tumor microenvironment [66], as described above. At least one *in vitro* study reported that allicin could impair the expression of ERK 1/2 in the human breast tumor line MCF-7 [19]. Allicin was also able to activate expression of ERK 1/2 in healthy T lymphocytes, enabling them to reduce the size of murine melanoma and fibrosarcoma tumors *in vivo* [10]. If this translates to humans, these data suggest that allicin could simultaneously decrease tumor cell function while boosting lysis via enhanced T lymphocyte function, thus making it a unique agent for cancer treatment.

As was stated earlier, the creation of an oxygen-poor environment through the secretion of HIF is the signal for angiogenesis to occur [25] and the P13K/Akt pathway then controls the process of new vessel growth [21, 23]. Activation of the P13K/Akt pathway can also induce HIFs (i.e., there is cross-talk occurring here), and the secretion of HIFs is associated with aggressive tumors [67]. Metastatic tumor cells also need to downregulate their cell-cell communication integrins to allow them to replicate while traveling through the circulation [51]. Integrin expression also feeds back into the JNK pathway and regulation of apoptosis [51, 68]. In addition, chronic activation of NF-κB indirectly supports the tumor microenvironment through promotion of gene transcription stimulating angiogenesis (HIFs and VEGF), tumor growth (cyclin proteins), and contributing to apoptotic suppression of tumor cells (Bcl-2 and survivin proteins) [70]. Several *in vitro* studies have suggested that allicin can decrease angiogenesis and metastasis through interaction with the HIF [25] and P13K/Akt [21, 23] pathways. Allicin has also been reported to decrease the expression of the signaling molecules VEGF [25] and VCAM [19], possibly also through the P13K/Akt pathway although this is not yet clear. For the *in vivo* animal models, allicin's ability to impair one or more of these pathways was associated with a decrease in primary tumor size after between 21 and 50 days of administration (injection or gavage) [8, 10, 22, 28-31].

So how is allicin managing to interact with all of these pathways? The thiosulfinate has, as its basic property, the ability to affect the redox potential of a cell through oxidizing glutathione and cysteine (thiol) protein residues [32]. Further biochemical investigation reveals that transcriptional regulation of HIF, NF-κB, ER-α, p53, and Nrf2 are all mediated by redox-sensitive transcription factors [69]. Their point of intersection is through the protein thioredoxin, which regulates the redox levels of both eukaryotic and microbial cells through "mopping up" secreted ROS and NO [69]. Thioredoxin also controls the expression of the apoptosis signaling kinase (ASK-1) protein, which is the initiating step for both the JNK and p38 apoptosis pathways [69]. The protein can also regulate the P13K/Akt pathway by interacting with the tumor suppressor protein phosphatase and tensin homolog (PTEN) [69], and dysregulation of PTEN stimulates tumor growth [69]. Mutated forms of thioredoxin are also common in tumors but these retain an active site containing two cysteines; a conformation which can be inactivated by thiosulfinates, including allicin [68].

As mentioned, allicin targets thiol sidechains on cysteines, and it has been shown in at least one study to inactivate thioredoxin as well as other thiol-containing enzymes such as cysteine proteases [71]. This latter target includes tumor caspases, which have also been shown to be targeted by allicin in several *in vitro* studies [9, 12, 14-17, 20, 30]. This proved a conundrum for explanation because if allicin directly bound to the cysteines in caspase enzymes it would inactivate them and *prevent* apoptosis. There are two possible explanations for this discrepancy: mutations [72], or allicin preferentially binding to the tumor caspase-suppressor molecule (survivin) [65].

Some tumors, such as those of the lung and kidney, are associated with caspase 3 mutations, whereas gastric and colon tumors show no such mutations [72]. Tumors that have no known caspase alteration are believed to impair the pathways that signal their expression [72]. Allicin was able to upregulate caspase 3, 8, and 9 expression in gastric [14-16] and colon tumors [9] (i.e., those with potential to contain caspase 3 mutations), as well as those affecting the cervix [17], fibroblasts [9], liver [20], and bone [30]. Whether these findings point towards efficacy in the context of mutated caspases remains to be determined.

The ability of allicin to inhibit the tumor protein survivin has not yet been assessed in the literature but seems a more likely target as inhibition of survivin would "unblock" the caspase pathway and allow apoptosis [65]. Survivin prevents apoptosis by selectively targeting caspase 3, thereby preventing pathway initiation [65]. The studies of allicin's effects have described either an upregulating effect on caspase 3 only [17, 30], or caspase 3 in concert with caspases 8 and 9 [9, 14-17, 20]. Survivin contains a "zinc finger" cysteine motif [65], which would make a good target for allicin. Interestingly, a closely similar "zinc finger" motif is also present in another tumor molecule, ZNF703 [18]. Allicin was able to inhibit ZNF703 expression *in vitro* in a gastric cell line [18], so it is not unreasonable to propose that it can also inhibit survivin. Since survivin is overexpressed in metastatic tumors found in breast, colon, gastric, lung, and thyroid cancers [65], this is another potentially exciting and novel target for allicin. A schematic diagram of allicin's two central targets and the biochemical pathways this would impair in tumor cells is shown in Figure 1.

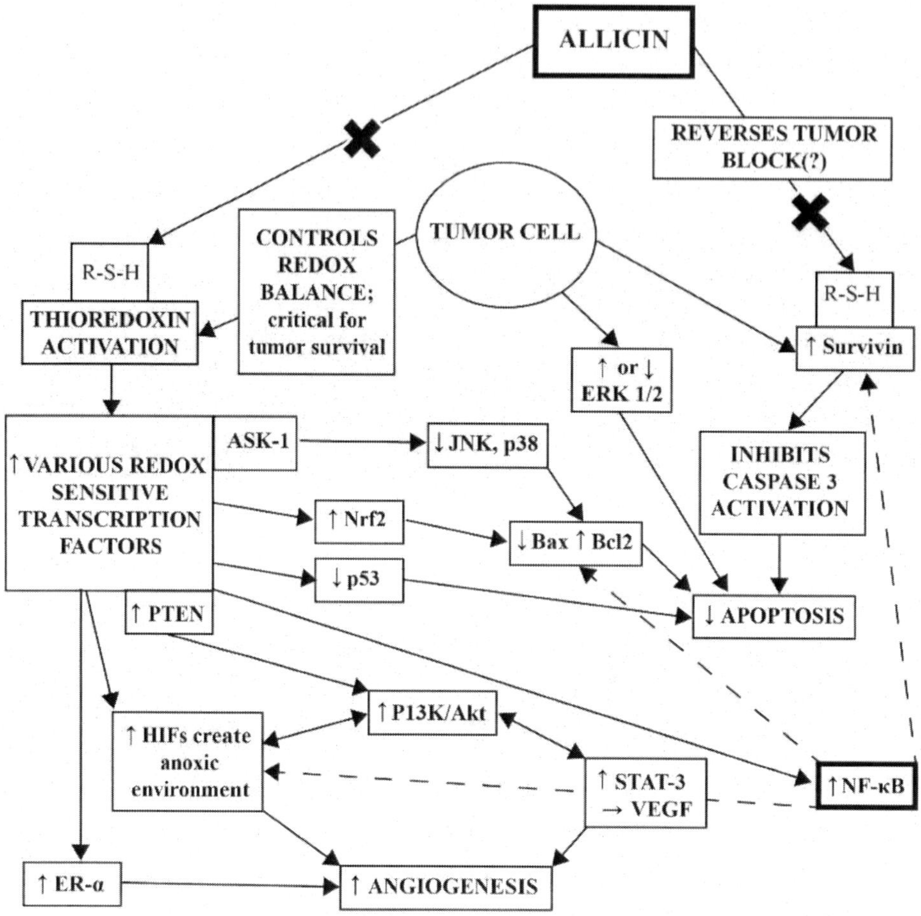

✖ = biochemical pathway points blocked by allicin

⟷ = crosstalk – – → = promotes transcription

Legend: Tumor cells need to control the redox balance of their survival and block caspases inducing cell death. High metabolic activity of the tumor equates to high levels of redox enzymes to inactivate the ROS generated. Survival is therefore a delicate balance of making and inactivating ROS through diverse biochemical pathways, including Nrf2. Tumor growth also creates an anaerobic environment with the production of HIF, which stimulates angiogenesis and facilitates tumor proliferation and escape. Allicin has been shown to act on several pathways including Nrf2, survivin, P13K/Akt, ERK, JNK, and caspases. These pathways have two major intersection points: thioredoxin and survivin. Thioredoxin controls the redox potential of the cell and possesses a thiol (RSH) group sensitive to allicin. Allicin's effects on thioredoxin would control PTEN and ASK-1 transcription factors and in turn allow tumor apoptosis to occur and prevent angiogenesis. This would also decrease tumor growth by inhibiting HIF formaton. Survivin binds to caspases preventing cell death and contains a vulnerable thiol group. Allicin binding to survivin would remove the tumor-induced caspase block and reinstate apoptosis.

Abbreviations used: Akt (protein kinase B), ASK-1 (apoptosis signaling kinase 1), Bax (Bcl-2 associated X protein), Bcl-2 (B cell lymphoma-2 protein), ER-α (estrogen receptor alpha), ERK 1/2 (extracellular initiated kinase), HIF (hypoxia inducing factors), JNK (Jun amino-terminal kinase), NF-κB (nuclear factor kappa beta), Nrf2 (NF-E2, p45-related factor 2), P13K (phosphatidyl inositol 3 kinase), PTEN (tumor suppressor protein phosphatase and tensin homolog), R-S-H (thiol group), STAT-3 (signal transducer and activation of transcription-3), and VEGF (vascular endothelial growth factor)

References used to construct diagram: - [21-23, 58, 65, 67, 69, 70]

Figure 1. Possible central mechanisms of antitumor activity of allicin.

Allicin also creates a harsh environment for tumor persistence by activating immune cells to attack a variety of tumors [8, 10, 29, 31], as detailed in Chapter 4. However, the tumor microenvironment is, by its very nature, immunosuppressive, which inherently prevents attack by tumoricidal T cytotoxic, NK, and macrophage/monocyte cells [73-75]. Specifically, tumors prevent terminal macrophage differentiation, in addition to coopting existing macrophages into becoming M2 or tumor-associated (TAMs) [73, 74]. TAMs in turn prevent the generation of tumoricidal T cytotoxic cells and the immature myeloid-derived suppressor macrophages (MDSC) prevent NK cell activation [75]. Allicin's activities against P13K/Akt extends to reversing the tumor impairment of B cell, T cell, macrophage, neutrophil, and endothelial cell activation stimulated by this pathway [55]. The finding that allicin can lift this immunosuppressive block by inhibiting P13K/Akt signaling [21, 23] and thus activating monocytes [8], NK cells [31], and T lymphocytes [8, 10, 29, 31] adds another level of therapeutic utility to its activities.

Conclusion

Tumors are a major health issue globally and remain the second leading cause of death in the United States alone [76]. Current statistics indicate there were just under two million new diagnoses of cancer, and just over six-hundred thousand cancer-related deaths occurred, in the United States in 2018 [76]. Although surgical techniques have been optimized for tumor removal procedures, there continues to be significant activity in the search for new, targeted therapies that can minimize side effects and the development of anti-cancer drug resistance [77-79]. In addition, most of future cancer treatment needs are also likely to come from developing nations [37]. Currently, two of every three new cancer cases occurs in countries such as India, Pakistan, and China, where diagnosis and treatment strategies are not widely available [37]. These nations have a long history of phytomedicinal use [40], and thus are likely to be receptive to formulations involving herbal medicines. Plants have already proven useful in the generation of potent chemotherapics, with taxanes coming from the Pacific yew (*Taxus brevifolia*) [80], and the alkaloids vincristine and vinblastine from the Madagascar periwinkle (*Catharanthus roseus*) [81]. As a natural molecule, allicin would be very appealing as a tumor therapy due to its lack of side effects and public perception of safety [32]. For example, at least one study points to its specificity in inducing apoptosis only in gastric cancer cells, and not in their healthy counterparts [82]. Given its early *in vitro* and pre-clinical promise, it is not an enormous leap to therefore suggest allicin be investigated for its potential as either an individual or complementary therapy in cancer treatment.

Current chemotherapies are associated with significant side effects, apart from nausea and hair loss [77]. Patients receiving platinum, taxane, or alkaloid drugs frequently experience long-term peripheral neuropathies and wound-healing issues [77]. Several medications, including tamoxifen, are also associated with liver injury [77, 78]. Allicin administration has been shown in at least one study to result in no side effects at doses of 25 and 50g/kg [83] and is considered safe for all patients, excepting those on warfarin [84], or the small percentage with garlic allergies [85].

Another major issue for modern chemotherapeutic agents used for patient treatment is the development of tumor resistance or insensitivity to the therapy [44, 45, 58, 79]. To avoid this, most patients receive a cocktail of drugs, which is modified as the disease progresses [78]. Allicin may represent a combination therapy in its own right since it can activate apoptosis through several pathways [9, 11-17, 19, 20, 22-26, 30]. The thiosulfinate can also prevent angiogenesis by several means [21, 22, 25], most notable of which is the P13K/Akt pathway [21, 23]. The lack of effective medications blocking P13K/Akt and its centrality to angiogenesis [55] places allicin in a unique position in this respect. Other novel molecular tumor targets for allicin include HIF [25], VCAM [19], ZNF703 [18], and thioredoxin [69]. None of these molecules are currently targeted with medications but all have been already suggested as having potential for future drug development [58, 86-88]. Chemotherapies that simultaneously activate several biochemical pathways do exist and include the taxane paclitaxel [80]. Paclitaxel prevents tumor cell division by attaching to tubulin, and initiates apoptosis by phosphorylating Bcl-2 and activating p53 and caspases [80]. This type of approach is extremely important against tumors that evade early diagnosis, including ovarian and lung cancers [62, 79]. Allicin has similar effects on apoptotic proteins [12-16, 22, 25] and also prevents tumor cell division [7, 11, 18]. Both allicin and paclitaxel are phytomedicines and it has been suggested that the ability to target multiple cellular pathways is a common feature of these agents [89].

Allicin could also be useful as an adjunct therapy. The thiosulfinate has been proven effective in reversing hepatic injury produced by tamoxifen, at least in rodent models [43]. Allicin has also been shown to potentiate the effects of artesunate [30], cyclophosphamide [29], and 5-fluorouracil [90] in killing osteosarcoma, neuroblastoma, and hepatocellular tumors in animal models. An *in vitro* model of thyroid cancer demonstrated that allicin enhanced the tumor-specific toxicity of the standard chemotherapeutics cisplatin, carboplatin, or rapamycin [27]. In these models, allicin was found to be either synergistic [30] or at least additive in nature, although the exact mechanisms involved are unclear [27, 29, 90]. The ability of allicin, at least *in vitro*, to affect expression of ER-α [19] may also allow it to be used for resistant forms of breast cancer.

Until recently, delivery of allicin to cell targets was hampered by its instability [28, 91, 92]. Miron and colleagues [90] were able to create allicin *in situ* and reduce the size of a mutated ErbB2-bearing gastric carcinoma in a murine xenograft tumor model. Alliinase, the enzyme responsible for metabolizing alliin to allicin, was chemically conjugated to an ErbB2 mAb and injected intravenously five times a day into the mice at three to four day intervals [90]. These N87 human tumor xenograft nude mice were then injected intraperitoneally with alliin twice a day [90]. Miron and colleagues reported that the murine tumors stopped growing after two weeks of treatment and failed to grow even after treatment was discontinued at eighteen days [90]. They were able to directly attribute these effects to allicin generation as a tumor that did not express the ErbB2 mutation showed no reduction in size [90]. Notably, ErbB2 mutations are present in a wide variety of tumors including those of the bladder, bowel, and cervix and increased expression of ErbB2 occurs in around 10% of solid tumors [93]. Thus, the ability to both bypass allicin's inherent lability by *in situ* targeting of the thiosulfinate and directly target tumor molecules via mAb coupling clearly has great future potential for clinical application. A second study by the same group utilized the standard mAb (rituximab) treatment for B-cell leukemia and used the same protocol to create allicin *in situ* using a human xenograft murine model [28]. In both cases, the locally producd allicin resulted in rapid shrinkage and death of the tumor via apoptosis [28, 90].

The utilization of mAbs, in the context of immune-based therapies for cancer treatment, have already represented a significant breakthrough in treatment regimens for various types of tumors [3]. Exploiting the highly specific capabilities of mAb to target only mutated cells and thereby direct alliinase (and ultimately, allicin) to a specific *in situ* location could provide at least a complementary or additive benefit for tumor therapies by using them to load tumors with the alliinase enzyme. In a different approach, nanoparticles of locust bean gum containing functionalized allicin were also recently created and found to be non-toxic and able to retain activity both *in vitro* and in an animal model [92]. Finally, chemically modified forms of allicin might provide additional molecular stability and bioavailability for the thiosulfinate, potentially matching or even improving the toxicity profile in relation to tumor cell targets [94]. In this vein, Leontiev and colleagues [94] synthesized four analogs of allicin (diethyl-, dimethyl-, dipropany- and dibenzyl-thiosulfinates) and compared them with the parent molecule for *in vitro* tumoricidal activity. All of the analogs tested caused apoptosis of human lung adenocarcinoma cells and were found to be more stable than the parent compound (allicin) [94]. Continued employment of these types of strategies is expected to ensure a stable and consistent product which will allow the realistic testing of allicin using the gold standard of DBRPCT moving forward.

REFERENCES

[1] Moyers, Susan. (1996). "*Garlic in health, history and world cuisine.*," pp 1-36. St. Petersberg, FL: Suncoast Press.

[2] Petrovska, Biljana B. & Svetlana, Cekovska. (2010). "Extracts from the history and medical properties of garlic". *Pharmacogn. Rev.*, *4*(7), 106-110.

[3] Sudhakar Akulapalli. (2009). "History of Cancer, Ancient and Modern Treatment Methods." *Journal of Cancer Science & Therapy*, *1*(2), 1-4. doi: 10.4172/1948-5956.100000e2.

[4] Devita, Vincent T. & Edward, Chu. (2008). "A History of Cancer Chemotherapy." *Cancer Research*, *68*(21), 8643-8653. doi: 10.1158/0008-5472.CAN-07-6611.

[5] Baudino, Troy A. (2015). "Targeted cancer therapy: the next generation of cancer treatment." *Current Drug Discovery Technologies*, *12*, 3-20. Accessed December 5, 2018. http://www.eurekaselect.com/131876/article.

[6] Maj, Ewa., Diana, Papiernik. & Joanna, Wietrzyk. (2016). "Antiangiogenic cancer treatment: The great discovery and greater complexity (Review)." *International Journal of Oncology*, *49*(5), 1773-1784. doi:10.3892/ijo.2016.3709.

[7] Sun, Li. & Xu, Wang. (2003). Effects of allicin on both telomerase activity and apoptosis in gastric cancer SGC-7901 cells." *World Journal of Gastroenterology*, *9*(9), 1930-4. doi: 10.3748/wjg.v9.i9.1930.

[8] Jian, Wang., Hui-Juan, He., Cheng-wei, He., Wu, Ping. & Jan-jun, Lu. (2004). "Effect of allicin in antagonizing mice's bladder cancer *in vitro* and *in vivo*." *Chinese Journal of Integrated Medicine*, *10*(3), 208-212. Accessed on January 4, 2019. https://link.springer.com/article/10.1007/BF02836409.

[9] Ooommen, Suby., Ruby, J. Anto., Gopal, Srinivas. & Devarajan, Karunagaran. (2004). "Allicin (from garlic) induces caspase-mediated apoptosis in cancer cells". *Eur. J. Pharmacol.*, *485*, 97-103. Accessed January 4, 2019. https://pdfs.semanticscholar.org/5193/eeeda4e2d9d812b2409edc012c13f7171a0f.pdf.

[10] Patya, Miriam., Muayad, A. Zahalka., Alexey, Vanichkin., Aharon, Rabinkov., Talia, Miron., David, Mirelman., Meir, Wilchek., Harry, M. Lander. & Abraham, Novogrodsky. (2004). "Allicin stimulates lymphocytes and elicits an antitumor effect: a possible role of $p21^{ras}$." *International Immunology*, *16*(2), 275-281. https://doi.org/10.1093/intimm/dxh038.

[11] Gruhlke, Martin C. H., Carole, Nicco., Frederic, Batteux. & Alan, J. Slusarenko. (2017). "The Effects of Allicin, a Reactive Sulfur Species from Garlic, on a Selection of Mammalian Cell Lines". *Antioxidants*, *6*(1). Accessed September 25, 2018. http://doi.org/10.3390/antiox6010001.

[12] Ban, Jun OK., Dong, Yeun Yuk., Koan, Sik Woo., Tae, Myoung Kim., Ung, Soo Lee., Heon-Sang, Jeong., Dae, Joong Kim., Yeun, Bok Chung., Bang, Yeon Hwang., Ki, Wan Oh. & Jin, Tae Hong. (2007). "Inhibition of cell growth and induction of apoptosis via inactivation of NF-κB by a sulfur compound isolated from garlic in human colon cancer cells". *J. Pharmacol. Sci.*, *104*, 374-383. Accessed January 4, 2019. https://www.jstage.jst.go.jp/article/jphs/104/4/104_4_374/_article.

[13] Bat-Chen, Wolf., Tal, Golan., Irena, Peri., Zvi, Ludmer. & Betty, Schwartz. (2010). "Allicin purified from fresh garlic cloves induces apoptosis in colon cancer cells via Nrf2". *Nutr. Cancer*, *60*, 1-3. https://doi.org/10.1080/01635581.2010.509837.

[14] Park, Sook-Young., Seong-Jun, Cho., Hak-chul, Kwon., Kang-Ro, Lee., Dong-Kwon, Rhee. & Suhkneung, Pyo. (2005). "Caspase-independent cell death by allicin in human epithelial carcinoma cells: Involvement of PKA". *Cancer Letters*, *224*, 123-132.

[15] Zhang, Wenlu., Minwen, Ha., Yuehua Gong, Y., Yin, Xu., Nannan, Dong. & Yuan Yuan, Y. (2010). "Allicin induces apoptosis in gastric cancer cells through activation of both extrinsic and intrinsic pathways." *Oncology Reports*, *24*(6), 1585-1592. https://doi.org/10.3892/or_00001021.

[16] Tao, Ming., Linghan, Gao., Jie, Pan. & Xiaoye, Wang. (2013). Study on the inhibitory effect of allicin on human gastric cancer cell line SGC-7901 and its mechanism. *African Journal of Traditional, Complementary, and Alternative Medicines AJTCAM*, *11*(1), 176-9. Accessed on January 1, 2019. https://www.ncbi.nlm.nih.gov/pmc/articles/PMC3957262/.

[17] Zhang, Xuecheng., Yong, Zhu., Hue, Duan., Chen, Feng. & Xuan, He. (2015). Allicin induces apoptosis of the MGC-803 human gastric carcinoma cell line through the p38 mitogen-activated protein kinase/caspase 3 signaling pathway." *Mol. Med. Rep.*, *11*, 2755-2760. https://doi.org/10.3892/mmr.2014.3109.

[18] Ganjipoor, Naji., Eghbalnia, S., Khodabakshsh, P., Daustany, M. & Tahereh, Naji. (2016). "The effect of allicin on ZNF703 gene expression in GCC lines." *Proceedings of 2016 International Conference on Cellular and Molecular Biology and Medical Sciences.* ISBN 978-93-84468-71-2. https://doi. org/10.17758/URUAE.AE0916405.

[19] Lee, Chung Gi., Hee-Weon, Lee., Byung-Oh, Kim., Dong-Kwon, Rhee. & Suknneung, Pyo. (2015). "Allicin inhibits invasion and migration of breast cancer cells through the inhibition of VCAM-1: Regulation of association between p65 and ER-α." *Journal of Functional Foods*, *15*, 172-185.doi https://doi.org/10.1016/j.jff.2015.03.017.

[20] Chu, Yung-Lin., Ch-Tang, Ho., Jing-Gung, Chung., Rajasekharan, Raghu., Yi-Chen, Lo. & Lee-Yan, Sheen. (2013). "Allicin induces anti human liver cancer cells through p53 gene mediating apoposis and autophagy." *J. Agric. Food Chem.*, *61* (41), 9839–9848. DOI: 10.1021/jf403241s. https://pubs.acs.org/doi/10.1021/jf403241s.

[21] Xie, Kun., Jianze, Nian., Xingyang, Zhu., Xiaoping, Geng. & Fubao, Liu. (2015). "Modulatory role of garlicin in migration and invasion of intrahepatic cholangiosarcoma via P13K/AKT pathway." *Int. J. Clin. Exp. Pathol.*, *8*(11), 14028-14033.

[22] Chen, Huinan., Biquiang, Zhu., Lei, Zhao., Yang, Liu., Fuya, Zhao., Jing, Feng., Ye, Jin., Jiayu, Sun., Rui, Geng. & Yunwei, Wei. (2018). "Allicin inhibits proliferation and invasion *in vitro* and *in vivo* via SHP-1 mediated STAT3 signaling in cholangiosarcoma." *Cell Physiol. Biochem.*, *47*, 641-653. Accessed on October 18, 2018 https://www.karger.com/Article/FullText/490019.

[23] Huang, Ling., Yuanhong, Song., Jianping, Lian. & Zhiwei, Wang. (2017). "Allicin inhibits the invasion of lung adenocarcinoma cells by altering tissue inhibitor of metalloproteinase/matrix metalloproteinase balance via reducing the activity of phosphoinositide 3-kinase/AKT signaling." *Oncology Letters*, *14*(1), 468-474. doi: 10.3892/ol.2017.6129.

[24] Cha, Jae Hun., Yoon, Ji Choi., Seung, Heon Cha., Chang, Hwa Choi. & Won, Ho Cho. (2012). "Allicin inhibits cell growth and induces apoptosis in U87MG human glioblastoma cells through an ERK-dependent pathway. *Oncology Reports*, *28*, 41-48. doi: 10.3892/or.2012.1772.

[25] Song, Bin., Shu, Ying., Cui, Tianlei. & Fu, Ping. (2015). "Allicin inhibits human renal clear cell carcinoma progression vi suppressing HIF pathway." *Int. J. Clin. Exp. Med.*, *8*(11), 20573-20580. Accessed on January 1, 2019. http://www.ijcem.com/files/ijcem0015487.pdf.

[26] Xu, Ling., Jin, Yu., Dongxia, Zhai., Danying, Zhang., Wei, Shen., Lingling, Bai., Zailong, Cai. & Chaoqin, Yu. (2014). "Role of JNK activation and mitochondrial Bax translocation in allicin-induced apoptosis in human ovarian cancer SKOV3 cells." *Evidence-Based Complementary and Alternative Medicine*: Article ID 378684. https://doi.org/10.1155/2014/378684.

[27] Xiang, Yangfeng., Jonquang, Zhao., Ming, Zhao. & Kejing, Wang. (2018). "Allicin activates autophagic cell death to alleviate the malignant development of thyroid cancer." *Experimental and Therapeutic Medicine*, *15*, 3537-3543. doi: 10.3892/ etm.2018.5828.

[28] Arditti, Fabian D., Aharon, Rabinkov., Talia, Miron., Yair, Reisner., Alain, Berrebi., Meir, Wilchek. & David, Mirelman. (2005). "Apoptotic killing of B-chronic lymphocytic leukemia cells by allicin generated *in situ* using a rituximab-alliinase conjugate." *Mol. Cancer Ther.*, *4*(2), 325-331.

[29] Gou, Yiang-Yang., Xian-Je, Geng., Wen-Long, Zhai., Xian-Wei, Zhang., Yuan, Wei. & Guang-Jun, Hou. (2015). "Effect of combined treatment with cyclophosphamidium and allicin on neuroblastoma-bearing mice." *Asian Pacific Journal of Tropical Medicine*, *8*(2), 137-141. https://doi.org/10.1016/S1995-7645(14)60304-7.

[30] Jiang, Wei., Yong, Huang., Jing-Peng, Wang., Xiao-Yun, Yu. & Lin-Yi, Zhang. (2013). "The synergistic effect of artesunate combined with allicin in osteosarcoma cell line *in vitro* and *in vivo*." *Asian Pacific Journal of Cancer Prevention*, *14*(8), 4615-4619. doi: http://dx.doi.org/10.7314/APJCP.2013.14.8.4615.

[31] Wang, Con-Jun., Chao, Wang., Jiang, Han., Yong-Kun, Wang., Lin, Tang., Dong-Wei, Shen., Yi, Zhao., Rong-Hua, Xu. & Hui, Xiang. (2013). "Effect of combined treatment with interleukin-2 and allicin on pancreatic cancer." *Mol. Bio. Reports*, *40*(12), 6579-6585.

[32] Borlinghaus, Jan., Frank, Albrecht., Martin, C. H. Grulke., Ifeanyi, D. Nwachukwu. & Alan, J. Slusarenko. (2014). "Allicin: Chemistry and biological properties". *Molecules, 19*(8), 12591-12618.

[33] Dana, Kaitlyn N., John, B. Hertig. & Robert, J. Weber. (2017). "Drug Pricing Transparency: The New Retail Revolution." *Hospital Pharmacy, 52*(2), 155-159. doi: 10.1310/hpj5202-155.

[34] Zaorsky, N. G., Churilla, T. M., Egleston, B. L., Fisher, S. G., Ridge, J. A., Horwitz, E. M. & Meyer, J. E. (2017). "Causes of death among cancer patients." *Annals of Oncology, 28*(2), 400-407. https://doi.org/10.1093/annonc/mdw604.

[35] Holmes, Jordan A. & Ronald, C. Chen. (2018). "Racial Disparities in Time From Diagnosis to Treatment for Stage I Non–Small Cell Lung Cancer." *JNCI Cancer Spectrum, 2*(1) pky007. https://doi.org/10.1093/jncics/pky007.

[36] Oberstein, Paul E. & Kenneth, P. Olive. (2013). "Pancreatic cancer: why is it so hard to treat?" *Therapeutic Advances in Gastroenterology, 6*(4), 321-37. doi: 10.1177/1756283X13478680.

[37] Torre, Lindsey A., Freddie, Bray., Rebecca, L. Siegel., Jacques, Ferlay., Joannie, Lortet-Tieulent. & Ahmedin, Jemal. (2015). "Global cancer statistics 2012." *CA: A Cancer Journal for Clinicians, 65*, 87-108. doi: 10.3322/caac.21262.

[38] Alam, Afroze., Farooq, U., Ruchi, Singh., Dubey, V. B., Shailendra, Kumar., Rashmi, Kumari., Kamlesh, K. Naik., Tripathi, B. D. & Dhar, K. L. (2018). "Chemotherapy treatment and strategy schemes: A review." *Open Access Journal of Toxicology, 2*(5), March 2018. doi: 10.19080/OAJT.2018.02.555600. Accessed December 5, 2018 https://juniperpublishers.com/oajt/pdf/OAJT.MS.ID.555600.pdf.

[39] Rossi, Elio., Mariella, Di Stefano., Fabio, Firenzuoli., Maria, V. Monechi. & Sonia, Baccetti. (2017). "Add-On Complementary Medicine in Cancer Care: Evidence in Literature and Experiences of Integration." *Medicines (Basel, Switzerland), 4*(1), 5. doi: 10.3390/medicines4010005.

[40] Cundell, Diana R. (2014). *Herbal phytochemicals as immunomodulators Current Immunology Reviews*, Volume *10*, Issue 2, ISSN:1875-631X(Online), ISSN:1573-3955(Print) Accessed September 10, 2018. http://benthamscience.com/journal/index.php?journalID=cir.

[41] Chang, Yuan., Patrick, S. Moore. & Robin, A. Weiss. (2017). "Human oncogenic viruses: nature and discovery." *Philosophical transactions of the Royal Society of London. Series B, Biological Sciences, 372*(1732). doi: 10.1098/rstb.2016.0264.

[42] Feng, Fang., Li, Hong., Cui, Wen. & Yongsui, Dong. (1999). "Treatment of hepatitis caused by cytomegalovirus with allitridin injection – An experimental study." *Journal of Tongji Medical University, 19*(4), 271-274. https://doi.org/10.1007/BF02886960.

[43] Suddek, Ghada M. (2014). "Allicin enhances chemotherapeutic response and ameliorates tamoxifen-induced liver injury." *Pharmaceutical Biology, 52*(8), 1009-1014. Accessed November 22, 2018. https://www.tandfonline.com/doi/full/10.3109/13880209.2013.876053.

[44] Cortez, Alexander J., Patrycja, Tudrej., Katarzyna, A. Kujawa. & Katarzyna, M. Lisowska. (2017). "Advances in ovarian cancer therapy." *Cancer Chemotherapy and Pharmacology, 81*(1), 17-38. doi: 10.1007/s00280-017-3501-8.

[45] Malhotra, Vikas. & Michael, C. Perry. (2003). "Models of anti-cancer therapy. Classical chemotherapy mechanisms, toxicities and the chemotherapy window." *Cancer*

Biology Therapy, *2*(4, Suppl. 1), S2-S4. Accessed on December 30, 2018. https://www.tandfonline.com/doi/pdf/10.4161/cbt.199.

[46] Huang, Chih-Yang., Da-Tong, Ju., Chih-Fen, Chang., Muralidhar Reddy, P. & Bharath, K. Velmurugan. (2017). "A review on the effects of current chemotherapy drugs and natural agents in treating non-small cell lung cancer." *BioMedicine*, *7*(4), 23. doi: 10.1051/bmdcn/2017070423.

[47] Balmain, Allan. & Curtis, C. Harris. (2000). "Carcinogenesis in mouse and human cells: parallels and paradoxes." *Carcinogenesis*, *21*(3), 371–377, https://doi.org/10.1093/carcin/21.3.371.

[48] Medico, Enzo., Mariaangelo, Russo., Gabriele, Picco., Carlotta, Canciliere., Emanuele, Valtorta., Georgio, Corti., Michela, Buscarino., Claudio, Isella., Simona, Lamba., Barbara, Martinoglio., Silvio, Veronese., Salvatore, Siena., Andrea, Sartore-Bianchi., Marco, Beccuti., Marcello, Mottelese., Michael, Linnebacher., Francesca, Cordero., Federica, Di Nicolantonio. & Alberto, Bardelli. (2015). "The molecular landscape of colorectal cancer lines unveils clinically actionable kinase targets." *Nature Communications*, *6*, Article Number 7002. Accessed on February 28, 2019. https://www.nature.com/articles/ncomms8002#f2.

[49] Vannini, Federica., Khosrow, Kashfi. & Naharika, Nath. (2015). "The dual role of iNOS in cancer". *Redox Biology*, *6*, 334–343. http://doi.org/10.1016/ j.redox.2015.08.009.

[50] DeBerardinis, Ralph J. & Navdeep, S. Chandel. (2016). "Fundamentals of cancer metabolism." *Science Advances*, *2*(5), e1600200. doi: 10.1126/sciadv.1600200.

[51] Hanahan, Douglas. & Robert, A. Weinberg. (2000). "The Hallmarks of Cancer." *Cell*, *100*(1), 57-80. https://doi.org/10.1016/S0092-8674(00)81683-9.

[52] Lau, Alexandria., Nicole, F. Villeneuve., Zheng Sun, Z., Pak, K. Wong. & Donna, D. Zhang. (2008). "Dual Roles of Nrf2 in Cancer". *Pharmacological Research: The Official Journal of the Italian Pharmacological Society*, *58*(5-6), 262–270. http://doi.org/10.1016/j.phrs.2008.09.003.

[53] Milcovic, Lidija., Neven, Zarcovic. & Luciano, Saso. (2017). "Controversy about pharmacological modulation of Nrf2 for cancer therapy." *Redox Biology*, *12*, 727-732. https://doi.org/10.1016/j.redox.2017.04.013.

[54] Pfeffer, Claire M. & Amareshwar, T. Singh. (2018). "Apoptosis: A Target for Anticancer Therapy." *International Journal of Molecular Sciences*, *19*(2), 448. doi: 10.3390/ijms19020448.

[55] Soler, Adriana., Ana, Angulo-Urarte. & Mariana, Graupera. (2015). "PI3K at the crossroads of tumor angiogenesis signaling pathways." *Molecular & Cellular Oncology*, *2*(2), e975624. doi:10.4161/23723556.2014.975624.

[56] Kong, Deok-Hoon., Young, K. Kim., Mi, R. Kim., Ji, H. Jang. & Sookmook, Lee. (2018). "Emerging Roles of Vascular Cell Adhesion Molecule-1 (VCAM-1) in Immunological Disorders and Cancer." *International Journal of Molecular Sciences*, *19*(4), 1057. doi: 10.3390/ijms19041057.

[57] Bai, Peter. (2014). "Biology of ADP ribose polymerases: The factotums of cell maintenance." *Molecular Cell*, *58*, 947-958. Accessed on December 31, 2018. https://www.cell.com/molecular-cell/pdf/S1097-2765(15)00057-X.pdf.

[58] Zhang, Xi., Xin, Mu X., Ou, Huang., Zuouquan, Xie., Min, Jiang., Miyou, Geng. & Kunwei, Shen. (2013). "Luminal Breast Cancer Cell Lines Overexpressing ZNF703 Are

Resistant to Tamoxifen through Activation of Akt/mTOR Signaling." *PLoS ONE*, *8*(8), e72053. https://doi.org/10.1371/journal.pone.0072053.

[59] Rahman, Mohammad S. (2007). "Allicin and other functional active components in garlic : health benefits and bioavailability". *Int J Food Properties*, *10*, 245-268.

[60] Vivier, Eric., David, H. Raulet., Alissandro, Moretta., Michael, U. Caligiuri., Lawrence, Zitvogel., Lewis, L. Lanier., Waynde, M. Yokoyama. & Sophie, Ugolini. (2011). "Innate or Adaptive Immunity? The Example of Natural Killer Cells". *Science (New York, N.Y.)*, *331*(6013), 44–49. http://doi.org/10.1126/science.1198687.

[61] Andersen, Mads H., David, Schrama., Per, T. Straten. & Jürgen, C. Becker. (2006). "Cytotoxic T cells." *Journal of Investigative Dermatology*, *126*(1), 32-41. doi: https://doi.org/10.1038/sj.jid.5700001.

[62] Chaplin, David D. (2010). "Overview of the Immune Response". *The Journal of Allergy and Clinical Immunology*, *125*(2 Suppl 2), S3–23. Accessed September 25, 2018. http://doi.org/10.1016/j.jaci.2009.12.980.

[63] Javier Mestas, Javier. & Christopher, C. W. Hughes. (2004). "Of mice and not men: Differences between mouse and not human immunology." *The Journal of Immunology*, *172* (5), 2731-2738. doi: 10.4049/jimmunol.172.5.2731.

[64] Zeke, András., Mariya, Misheva., Attila, Reményi. & Marie, A. Bogoyevitch. (2016). "JNK signaling: Regulation and functions based on complex protein-protein partnerships". *Microbiology and Molecular Biology Reviews*, *80*(3), 793-835. doi: 10.1128/MMBR.00043-14.

[65] Altieri, David C. (2015). "Survivin - The inconvenient IAP." *Seminars in Cell & Developmental Biology*, *39*, 91-6.doi: 10.1016/j.semcdb.2014.12.007.

[66] McCubrey, James A., Linda, S. Steelman., William, H. Chappell., Steven, L. Abrams., Ellis, W. T. Wong., Fuhmin, Chang., Brian, Lehmann., David, M. Terrian., Michele, Milella., Agostino, Tafuri., Franca, Stivala., Massimo, Libra., Jorg, Basecke., Camilla, Evangelisti., Alberto, M. Martelli. & Richard, A. Franklin. (2007). "Roles of the RAF/MEK/ERK pathway in cell growth, malignant transformation and drug resistance". *Biochimica et Biophysica Acta*, *1773*(8), 1263–1284. http://doi.org/10.1016/j.bbamcr. 2006.10.001.

[67] Gordon, Michael S., David, S. Mendelson. & Gerry, Kato. (2010). "Tumor angiogenesis and novel anti-angiogenic strategies." *International Journal of Cancer*, *126*(8), 1777-1787. Accessed on December 31, 2018. https://onlinelibrary.wiley.com/doi/full/ 10.1002/ijc.25026.

[68] Schwartz, Martin A. (1997). "Integrins, oncogenes, and anchorage independence." *The Journal of Cell Biology*, *139*(3), 575-8.

[69] Lee, Samuel., Soo, M. Kim. & Richard, T. Lee. (2013). "Thioredoxin and thioredoxin target proteins: from molecular mechanisms to functional significance." *Antioxidants & Redox Signaling*, *18*(10), 1165-207. doi: 10.1089/ars.2011.4322.

[70] Park, Mi H. & Jin, T. Hong. (2016). "Roles of NF-κB in Cancer and Inflammatory Diseases and Their Therapeutic Approaches." *Cells*, *5*(2), 15. doi:10.3390/ cells5020015.

[71] Kim, Young-Sun., Kyung, S. Kim., Ihn, Han I., Mi-Hyun, Kim., Min, H. Jung. & Hun-Kuk, Park. (2012). "Quantitative and Qualitative Analysis of the Antifungal Activity of Allicin Alone and in Combination with Antifungal Drugs." *PLOS ONE*, *7*(6), e38242. https://doi.org/10.1371/journal.pone.0038242.

[72] McIlwain, David R., Thorsten, Berger. & Tak, W. Mak. (2012). "Caspases functions in cell death and disease." *Cold Spring Harb. Perspect. Biol.* doi: 10.1101/cshperspect.a008656. Accessed March 5, 2019. https://cshperspectives.cshlp.org/content/5/4/a008656.full.

[73] Disis, Mary L. (2010). "Immune regulation of cancer." *Journal of Clinical Oncology*, *28*(29), 4531-4538. doi: 10.1200/JCO.2009.27.2146.

[74] Sica, Antonio., Paola, Larghi., Alessandra, Mancino., Luca, Rubino., Chiara, Porta., Maria, G. Totaro., Monica, Rimoldi., Subra, K. Biswas., Paola, Allavena. & Alberto, Montovani. (2008). "Macrophage polarization in tumour progression". *Semin Cancer Biol.*, *18*, 349-355.

[75] Banchereau, Jacques., Francine, Briere., Christophe, Caux., Jean, Davoust., Serge, Lebecque., Yong-Jun, Liu., Bali, Pulendran. & Karolina, Palucka. (2000). "Immunobiology of dendritic cells". *Annu. Rev. Immunol.*, *18*, 767-811.

[76] Siegel, Rebecca L., Kimberley, D. Miller. & Ahmedin, Jamal. (2018). "Cancer Statistics 2018." *CA: A Cancer Journal for Clinicians.*, *68*(1), 7-30. Accessed on January 16, 2019. https://onlinelibrary.wiley.com/doi/full/10.3322/caac.21442.

[77] Nurgali, Kulmira., Thomas Jagoe, R. & Raquel, Abalo. (2018). "Editorial: Adverse Effects of Cancer Chemotherapy: Anything New to Improve Tolerance and Reduce Sequelae?" *Frontiers in Pharmacology*, *9*, 245. doi: 10.3389/fphar.2018.00245.

[78] Suddek, Ghada M. (2014). "Allicin enhances chemotherapeutic response and ameliorates tamoxifen-induced liver injury." *Pharmaceutical Biology*, *52*(8), 1009-1014. Accessed November 22, 2018. https://www.tandfonline.com/doi/full/10.3109/13880209.2013.876053.

[79] Alfarouk, Khalid O., Christian-Martin, Stock., Sophie, Taylor., Megan, Walsh., Abdel, K. Muddathir., Daniel, Verduzco., Adil, H. H. Bashir., Osama, Y. Mohammed., Gamal, O. Elhassan., Salvador, Harguindey., Stephan, J. Reshkin., Muntaser, E. Ibrahim. & Cyril, Rauch. (2015). "Resistance to cancer chemotherapy: failure in drug response from ADME to P-gp." *Cancer Cell International*, *15*, 71. doi: 10.1186/s12935-015-0221-1.

[80] Kampan, Nirmala C., Mutsa, T. Madondo., Orla, M. McNally., Michael, Quinn. & Magdalena, Plebanski. (2015). Paclitaxel and Its Evolving Role in the Management of Ovarian Cancer. *BioMed Research International*, 413076. doi: 10.1155/2015/413076.

[81] Moudi, Maryam., Rusea, Go., Christina, Y. Yien. & Mohd, Nazre. (2013). "Vinca alkaloids." *International Journal of Preventive Medicine*, *4*(11), 1231-5. Accessed on January 16, 2019. https://www.ncbi.nlm.nih.gov/pmc/articles/PMC3883245/.

[82] Mansingh, Debjani P., Dalpati, Nibedita., Sali, Veeresh Kumar. & Hannah, A. R. Vasanthi. (2018). "Alliin the precursor of allicin in garlic extract mitigates proliferation of gastric adenocarcinoma cells by modulating apoptosis." *Pharmacognosy Magazine*, *14*(55), 85-91. doi: 10.4103/pm.pm_342_17.

[83] Rao, R. R. & Natarajan, S. (1949). "Toxicity of ptergospermin and allicin." *Proceedings of the Indian Academy of Sciences - Section B*, *29*, 148. https://doi.org/10.1007/BF03049967.

[84] Tachjian, Argar., Vigar, Maria. & Arshad, Jahangir. (2010). "Use of herbal products and potential interactions in patients with cardiovascular diseases." *Journal of the American College of Cardiology*, *55*(6), 515-25. doi: 10.1016/j.jacc.2009.07.074.

[85] Moneret-Vautrin, Anne D., Martine, Morisset., Lemerdy, P. H., Croizier, A. & Gisele, Kanny. (2002). "Food allergy and IgE sensitization caused by spices: CICBAA data

(based on 589 cases of food allergy).” *Allerg. Immunol., 34*, 135–140. Accessed on February 15, 2019. https://europepmc.org/abstract/med/12078423.

[86] Zhang, Junmin., Xingmin, Lee., Xiao, Han., Ruijuan, Liu. & Jianguo, Fang. (2017). “Targeting the thioredoxin system for cancer therapy.” *Trends in Pharmacological Sciences, 38*(9), 794-808. doi: 10.1016/j.tips.2017.06.001.

[87] Yu, Tianchu., Bo, Tang. & Xueying, Sun. (2017). “Development of Inhibitors Targeting Hypoxia-Inducible Factor 1 and 2 for Cancer Therapy.” *Yonsei Medical Journal, 58*(3), 489-496. doi: 10.3349/ymj.2017.58.3.489.

[88] Chen, Qing. & Joan, Massagué. (2012). “Molecular pathways: VCAM-1 as a potential therapeutic target in metastasis.” *Clinical Cancer Research: An official journal of the American Association for Cancer Research, 18*(20), 5520-5. doi: 10.1158/1078-0432. CCR-11-2904.

[89] Cheng, Yu-Ting., Chun-Chi, Yang. & Li-Fen, Shyur. (2016). “Phytomedicine – modulating oxidative stresss and the cancer microenvironment for therapy.” *Pharmacological Research, 114*, 128-143. doi: 10.1016/j.phrs.2016.10.022.

[90] Zou, Xuejing., Jiyun, Liang., Jingyuan, Sun., Xiaoyun, Hu., Ling, Lei. & Dehua, Wu. (2016). “Allicin sensitizes hepatocellular cancer cells to anti-tumor pathway of 5-fluoracil through ROS-mediated mitochondrial pathway.” *Journal of Pharmacological Sciences, 131*, 233-240.

[91] Miron, Talia., Marina, Mironchik., David, Mirelman., Meir, Wilchek. & Aharon, Rabinkov. (2003). “Inhibition of tumor growth by a novel approach: *in situ* allicin generation using targeted alliinase delivery.” *Molecular Cancer Therapeutics, 2*(12), 1295-1301. http://mct.aacrjournals.org/content/molcanther/2/12/1295.full.pdf.

[92] Soumya, R. S., Sherin, S., Raghu, K. G. & Annie, Abraham. (2018). “Allicin functionalized locust bean gum nanoparticles for improved therapeutic efficacy: An *in silico, in vitro* and *in vivo* approach.” *International Journal of Biological Macromolecules, 109*(1), 740-747. https://doi.org/10.1016/j.ijbiomac.2017.11.065.

[93] Cousin, Sophie., Emmanuel, Khalifa., Amandine, Crombe., Yech’an, Laizet., Carlo, Lucchesi., Maud, Toulmonde., Sylvestre, Le Moulec., Céline, Auzanneau., Isabelle, Soubeyran. & Antoine, Italiano. (2018). “Targeting ERBB2 mutations in solid tumors: biological and clinical implications.” *Journal of Hematology and Oncology, 11*, 86 doi: 10.1186/s13045-018-0630-4.

[94] Leontiev, Roman., Nils, Hohaus., Jacob, Claus., Martin, C. H. Gruhlke. & Alan, J. Slusarenko. (2018). “Comparison of the Antibacterial and Antifungal Activities of Thiosulfinate Analogues of Allicin.” *Scientific Reports, 6763*, 8(1). Accessed on February 22, 2019. https://www.nature.com/articles/s41598-018-25154-9.

In: Allicin
Editor: Diana R. Cundell
ISBN: 978-1-53617-339-0

Chapter 14

ALLICIN AND OUR CHANGING WORLD

Diana R. Cundell*, PhD
College of Life Sciences, Jefferson University, Philadelphia, PA

ABSTRACT

Allicin has been demonstrated to possess antimicrobial, insecticidal, biochemical and immunomodulatory activities. An understanding of both the chemistry and stabilization strategies for the thiosulfinate are nearing completion. This should finally allow double blind randomized placebo controlled trials to narrow down which of the myriad of uses for which allicin would be effective. To identify where it can fit in future health and agricultural considerations requires us to also project how these will alter as our planet changes Apart from its other roles, allicin has potential application as an alternative phytomedicine for organic farming. Global climate change is expected to produce inreased surface temperatures which will requre new, effective approaches to agriculture as well as aquaculture to feed the world's inhabitants. Climate change also augurs the selection of more virulent microbes. Vectors for these microbes, such as mosquitoes, will also survive longer and be able to increase their range of activity to spread disease. Much of the deleterious effects of these changes will be felt in developing nations and require solutions that are both inexpensive as well as relatively simple to put into practice. Potential future strategies for allicin, including effective delivery, and optimal human testing will be considered for all these projections.

Keywords: aquaculture, climate change, organic farming, vector, virulence

1. INTRODUCTION

The chapters in this book have explored the diverse potential for allicin's use as antimicrobial (Chapters 5-8), insecticide (Chapter 9) and as at least adjunct therapies for chronic inflammatory diseases that include diabetes and cardiovascular disease (Chapter 10),

* Corresponding author: Room 320, Search Hall, Jefferson University, 4201, Henry Avenue, Philadelphia, PA 19144, E-mail: Diana.Cundell@jefferson.edu.

cancer (Chapter 13) and even osteoarthritis (Chapter 11) and Alzheimer's (Chapter 12). Much of allicin's diversity comes from its combination of direct modulation of leukocyte activation (Chapter 4) as well as indirectly through the targeting of biochemical pathways (Chapter 3). The thiosulfinate is appealing as its chemical structure allows it to be lipid permeable, thus entering cells with relative ease (Chapter 2). Until recently the Achilles heel of allicin had been its short half life (Chapter 2). Since its metabolite ajoene is equally effective (Chapter 2) and stable forms of allicin are now available (Chapters 11-13) this seems to represent a good point at which to determine optimal usage strategies for the thiosulfinate.

Lack of allicin standardization due, at least in part to its instability, has been an issue in preparing the phytochemical for either nutraceutical or pharmaceutical usage [1]. Because allicin is not regarded as a pharmaceutical it is not required to meet a consistent global standard in terms of the preparations being sold [2]. In the United States, for example, herbal preparations are considered dietary supplements under the Dietary Supplement, Health and Education Act (DSHEA) of 1994 and do not require extensive Federal Drug Administration (FDA) testing as a result [2]. In Europe, where herbal medicines are more often utilized, the European Directive of 2004 states that there must be protocols for herbal preparation, inspection of facilities as well as documentation of efficacy for at least thirty years within Europe [2]. Allicin's stability is also important here so that any extract or preparation needs to have both a standard amount of the thiosulfinate and a reasonable shelf life [1]. Ingestion of raw garlic may be optimal for allicin as a nutraceutical, but not appealing to most individuals [5]. Studies have shown that preparing an acidified paste of the garlic allows it to retain allicin activity for as much as six months at room temperature whereas boiling or frying results in significant loss of activity [3]. In contrast, two commercially stabilized forms of allicin AlliMax [4] and garlicin [5] are stable to ingestion and have shown to have efficacy in animal models.

In terms of allicin as a pharmaceutical, animal models and *in vitro* cellular assays are good beginnings but must eventually result in several gold standard double blind randomized placebo controlled (DBRCT) human trials to provide data allowing any product to enter mainsteam pharmaceutical preparation [6]. At this point, formulations must be standardized and stable and might include nanoparticle technology [7]. Nanoparticles are used in various processes and have the added benefit of protecting the internal constituents from degradation [7]. Whether incorporated into ointments [8] or bonded to nitrocellulose to produce wrapping materials [9] such functionalization of native allicin would allow it to retain efficacy until required for use. Pharmaceuticals, especially for tumors, are now becoming more targeted therapies involving monoclonal antibodies [10]. The patented methodology that allows allicin to be delivered using extant monoclonals should allow for their use in combination therapy in a variety of conditions, particularly tumor treatments [10] Time and cost investment in any such ventures is staggering, even for a natural product such as allicin, and can be expected to take around ten years and more than eight hundred million dollars to complete [11]. As a result, it is important to determine whether it is worth sending allicin down this road based on the potential roles it might play in the future. To assess this requires an understanding of the changes our world is facing and where products can establish new, underexplored niche markets.

Two such pressing issues are global climate change combined with a world population that is expected to number around ten billion by the year 2050 [12]. To feed such a growth in human beings will require new agricultural strategies to provide adequate nutrients to all corners of the globe. Experts in the field have suggested that we still have the capability to meet nutritional needs of the world's population but that this will require a change in agricultural methods as well as human diets [13].

So the reader may be asking themselves how allicin could fit in to all this? The benefits to human health and disease have been extensively discussed throughout this book but what of agriculture and aquaculture? Organic farming and a plant-based diet is already a reality for developing nations and is considered to be the predicted scenario for our future food production [13]. This will require a change in approaches and methodology to farming of terrestrial and aquatic crops in order to naturally manage or control disease-causing bacteria and fungi that attack food supplies [13]. Natural biological control methods are beginning to be used in both developing as well as European countries to both control insect and microbial attack of crops, but have yet to include phytomedicines as extracts [14]. In contrast, garlic sprays are readily available to control fungal diseases on plants (see Chapter 6 for details) and have already been shown to impair the reproduction of insect storage pests (see Chapter 9 for details). Given that allicin is the major bioactive agent available in garlic, this spectrum of activity is more likely to reflect this single moiety as opposed to the entire garlic bulb. This chapter will discuss the salient features of global climate change as they relate to human health and nutrition as well as providing ways in which allicin, in particular, might improve our future changing world. Areas where allicin may be impactful are discussed and the reader is provided with a complete picture of these issues.

2. Global Climate Change Issues

Driven by current rising greenhouse gases from human industrialization, forest destruction, aggressive agricultural practices and fossil fuel combustion, global climate change is likely to result in significant impacts on biodiversity, infection rates and spread, as well as agricultural yields as outlined in Figure 1.

2.1. Effect of Temperature on Vectors and Microbial Virulence

Current projections of temperature increase are believed to range between 1 and 4°C by the end of the next century [16]. When many people think of climate change they consider only the few degrees projected, but fail to consider that by 2030 around sixty percent of the world's population will be urban residents [17]. Cities demonstrate what is termed an urban heat island effect and can raise air temperatures by up to 10°C [17]. They also release trapped heat at night [17]. Elevated heat levels affect human health by promoting mortality (especially of the elderly) [13], as well as increasing microbial virulence [18], vector spread [17] and zoonotic illness [17].

Studies on an urban population in India, observed that infections with methicillin-resistant *Staphylococcus aureus* (MRSA), for example, were more prevalent in conditions of high humidity (55-78%) combined with higher temperatures (> 33°C)[18]. Small increments in temperature, such as those projected to occur, increase the biting frequency and maturation of mosquitoes such as the malaria carrying mosquito *Anopheles* [16]. The malaria parasite correspondingly reproduces and reaches maturity more rapidly [16]. Studies have shown that if the temperature is increased from 20°C to 25°C this halves the maturation time of malaria parasites [16]. In addition to transporting disease animals repeatedly bitten demonstrate reduced quality milk and meat production [16].

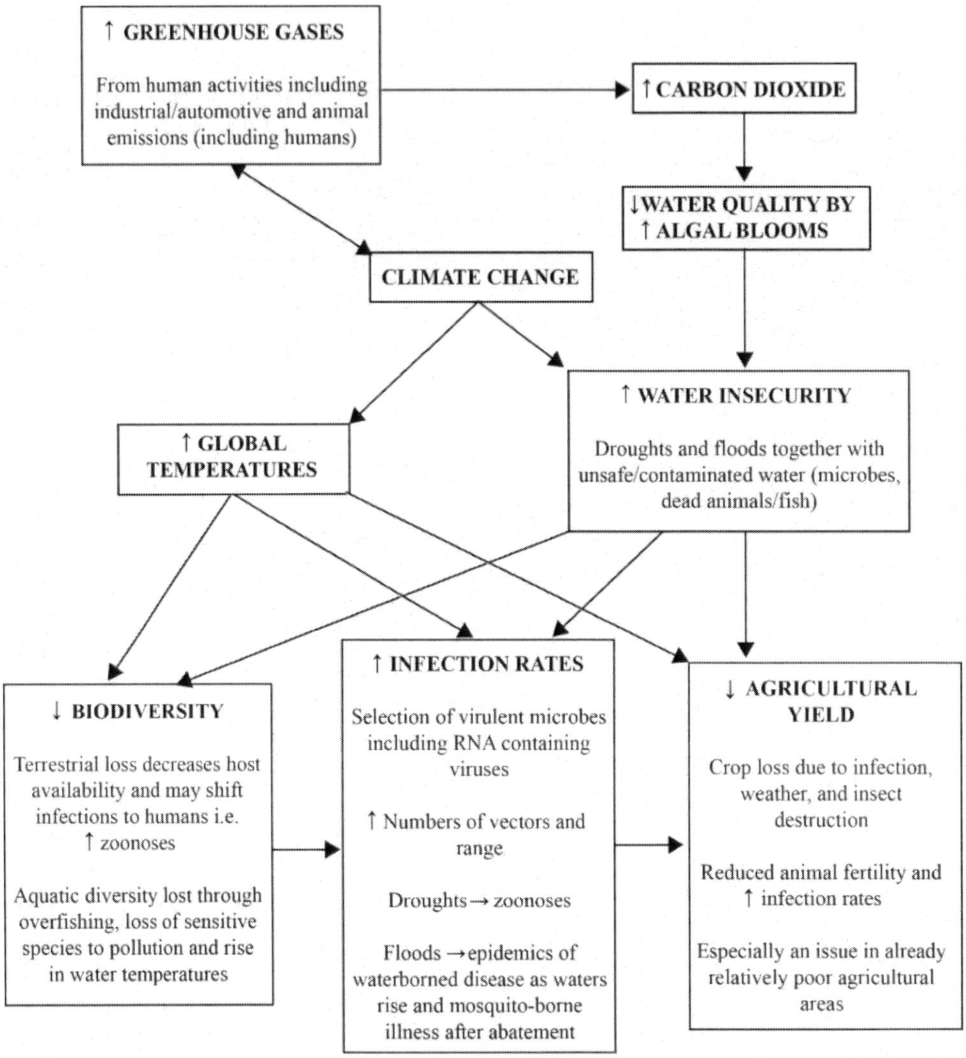

Legend: Rising greenhouse gases directly link to climate change and raise the atmospheric carbon dioxide. Carbon dioxide directly increases the replication of aquatic algae, decreasing water quality and feeding into water insecurity. The twin major issues of water insecurity and global temperature changes that ensue result in a loss of biodiversity, increased infection rates and decrease in agricultural yields.
See reference for a more detailed discussion of climate change [15].

Figure 1. Human issues stemming from climate change.

1.1.1. Allicin, Vectors and Microbial Virulence

Global climate change is already selecting out the more virulent pathogens, including multi-resistant microbes as well as vectors of zoonotic diseases. Allicin's broad antimicrobial activities, which include being bactericidal for MRSA, have been extensively discussed in Chapters 5-8. Clearly, if DBRCT of deliverable forms of allicin can be developed these will be invaluable especially among populations where locally sourced medicines are urgently needed. Apart from using allicin independently coupled to McAb [10] and in nanoparticle form [9], the thiosulfinate can also be combined with existing medications [8]. In a murine model of MRSA skin infection, a salve combination of silver and allicin was found to speed healing as well as decrease the minimum inhibitory concentration (MIC) needed to kill the bacterium ten fold [8]. Animal models have also shown similar synergistic effects of allicin at potentiating the effects of tumor medications (see Chapter 13 for details).

Allicin has also been demonstrated to be effective in the control of insect vectors of disease, particularly mosquitoes [19]. An important study performed in Israeli wetlands demonstrated that over a six week period, *Anopheles* mosquitoes that consumed sugar bait supplemented with garlic both decreased their biting frequency and were significantly ($p < 0.05$) reduced in numbers [19]. Those mosquitoes that had ingested the bait appeared to be unable to metabolize sugar and were more likely to be older insects i.e., likely to carry malaria [19]. The mosquito is attracted to the sugar in the bait and is therefore unlikely to become resistant to it, adding to the appeal. Allicin's abilities to prevent microbes from reproducing are both varied and not able to be overcome by mutations (see Chapters 5-8 for details). Allicin is also able to impair antibiotic multi-resistant organisms including MRSA

2.2. Effect of Temperature on Animals

Heat also affects farm animal reproduction [20]. Studies of artificially inseminated cows demonstrated that conception rates could be lower than thirty percent in hot summers compared with nearly fifty percent in winter months [20]. This has further implications for milk production for the sixty percent of farms that are currently located in tropical and subtropical climates [20]. As well as affecting the quantity of milk produced there is evidence that its nutritional quality i.e., protein and fat content are also inferior [20]. Meat and milk sources are also likely to change in tropical climates during periods of excessive heat [21]. Studies of African farming practices demonstrate a shift to heat tolerant goats, which are more able to forage on a wide variety of food sources [21]. Farmers are also switching from animals to crops when rainfall increases, due to a consequent uptick in animal infections [21]. Warming of the world's oceans is also affecting the number and distribution of mammals, fish and bird life [22]. Rapid decreases have been seen in fish such as cod, herring and haddock and in turn the animals feeding on them, which include the grey seal [22]. When combined with overfishing these species, including their predator, may disappear from our oceans entirely by 2090 [22]. These issues have also fueled the concept of our future nutrition coming from organically obtained plant-based diets [13, 15] with a move towards fish-derived proteins that are organically farmed as opposed to wild caught [23].

1.2.1. Allicin's Potential Impact on the Thriving of Pregnant Farmed Animals

Clearly garlic and allicin can have no influence on temperature-induced breeding issues, but they may have an impact on the health of reproducing animals, according to one study [24]. Administration of freshly ground garlic (100 mg/kg), to hypercholesteremic pregnant rats, both prior to and during gestation, decreased serum lipids, trigycerides and cholesterol and improved myocardial functionality [24]. The pups born to these animals were also found to have normal body weight and bone ossification, in contrast to those animals whose mothers did not receive garlic [124. El-Sayyad and colleagues [24] concluded that the decrease in atherosclerosis produced by garlic resulted in improved circulation and thereby development of the unborn pups.

2.3. Water Insecurity

Climate change is also typically associated with drought, which both creates food insecurity and crop loss as well as increasing the spread of zoonotic diseases such as the Ebola virus [17, 25]. Some areas will not see drought, but instead extreme rainfall, creating conditions for water-borne illness to be spread [17]. Although such floods may initially destroy the habitats of some vectors, such as mosquitoes, studies have shown that as groundwater recedes it provides new areas of immobile water for them to breed [26]. Finally, climate change is coupled with rising carbon dioxide levels which in turn facilitate the growth of algae in rivers and lakes [17]. Exacerbated by excessive usage of fertilizer, this eutrophication is both deadly to fish that inhabit the water and can produce illness in those that consume them [17]. Given that nearly three quarters of the world's water is being used for agricultural purposes [13] water insecurity is directly related to food insecurity.

2.3.1. Allicin's Potential Impact on the Consequences of Water Insecurity

In addition to garlic/ allicin's effects on mosquito species (see section 1.11), at least one article has suggested that the breakdown product of allicin, diallyl trisulide (DATS), or the crushed parent garlic may be used as an algaecide [27]. Studies by Zhou and colleagues [27] reported that garlic or DATS (0.08%) inhibited the growth of six species of algal bloom and red tide producing organisms *in vitro*. Growth of *Alexandrium tamarense*, *A. catanella*, *A. minutum*, *A. satoanum*, *Scrippsiella trochoidea* and *Chaetocerus* species was strongly inhibited after three days of incubation with the *Alexandrium* species being most sensitive [27].

2.4. Biodiversity

Biodiversity of the species on this planet has at no time been more threatened than by human encroachment on previously wild areas due to need for products, arable land and can both feed into and be directly impacted by climate change [28]. Ectothermic species, both terrestrial and aquatic, are in general expected to decline as they are able to adapt to cold but not heat thereby decreasing their diversity as well as any predators that rely on them for existence [28]. Loss of such diversity affects human beings in a number of ways [13, 17, 26].

Zoonotic diseases such as Ebola and Lyme disease are diluted in their effects on the human population due to carriage by a number of hosts [17]. As these reservoirs are lost, virulent illness more commonly infects human beings [17]. Studies suggest many of these are likely to be RNA-containing viruses (see Chapter 8) and that rather than adapting to their hosts a series of "waves" or mini epidemics is likely to occur [30]. Virulent viruses are transorted by arthropod vectors including mosquitoes and ticks, which are either not impacted by heat or are able to increase their range and reproduction capabilities [31]. Increased temperatures, especially at high altitudes or middle altitudes negatively impact more benign insects such as leaf rollers thereby shifting the variation of food sources for insectivorous animals [29].

A second issue is that the loss of biodiversity can directly impact human food sources [13]. The fifteen crops grown around the world that provide nearly all the caloric intake for many individuals are very low in diversity [13]. Inbreeding focused on output rather than resistance to pests, and climatic factors and future use of wild relatives, especially those locally sourced, is likely to provide the basis for new world crops [13]. Loss of crops to insect damage, weeds and pathogens such as mold at either the seed or plant stage currently account for somewhere between 20 and 40% of all harvests [32]. This is unlikely to decrease as temperatures rise, especially favoring these pests [32]. As mentioned earlier, marine biodiversity is also declining as the surface temperatures rise [21]. These types of impacts are likely to be keenly felt in poorer countries that rely on food sources involving native plants and animals as well as wild caught fish [33].

2.4.1. Allicin's Potential Impact on the Consequences of Biodiversity Loss

Allicin has been shown to be effective against several RNA-containing viruses, including those with unstable genomes that belong to the orthomyxovirus and retrovirus classes (see Chapter 8). Garlic is also an effective weapon against mosquitoes [19] and was recently reported to control ticks as a repellent spray [34]. Bharadwaj and colleagues [34] were able to signficantly ($p < 0.01$) reduce nymphal tick densities of *Ixodes scapularis* by nearly fifty percent after an eighteen day spraying period. Given that these ticks carry Lyme disease, anaplasmosis and babesiosis this observation provides a low cost, safe and effective solution to tick infestation. When garlic extract (containing allicin) was added to sugar bait, the investigators reported that this was preferentially ingested by most mosquitoes and less than one percent of beneficial insects, indicating it is environmentally friendly [19]. Using this type of approach is clearly better than classic insecticides which remove all insects including necessary pollinators [19].

Food shortages from both yield and harvest loss are already an issue [13, 32] and require simple and effective solutions. Allicin's ability to remove several fungi associated with significant world crop losses has already been demonstrated (see Chapter 7 for details). Miron and colleagues [35] already hold a patent in this area for *"(a) protecting agricultural crops, particularly fruits and vegetables, against insects, by treating the crops with allicin prior to harvesting; (b) protecting fruits and vegetables from decay and extending the shelf life thereof by treating the fruits and vegetables with allicin after harvesting; and (c) repelling insects such as ants or insects that attack agricultural crops from an object or an area, which comprises treating the object or area with a repelling effective amount of allicin."*

3. The Rising Global Population

With food insecurity already an issue in 2019 it is not anticipated to improve by 2050 unless changes are made to feed the additional two million expected to join the human population [12]. Analysts are predicting continued increases in rural birth rates with those of cities likely to remain relatively constant [12]. India is likely to be the most densely populated of all countries with the largest increase in numbers occurring in Asia as a whole [12]. China is the other major contributor to the growth in the Asian population, but it is expected that an intensive female educational program will ultimately result in adult women having less children [12]. In contrast literacy and schooling of females is low in both India and many African countries, which has implications not just for population but also an understanding of hygiene and health as well as avoidance of food insecurity during climatic shifts [12]. Any strategies being put into practice must therefore be relatively easy to follow and communicate [12]. Even in 2050 Asia and Africa are likely to have somewhere between forty and fifty percent of their population occupying rural areas, adding to issues in implementation of new strategies [36]. This is in stark contrast to less than twenty five percent in Europe and America [36].

Another issue is that the percentage of the global population that will be over the age of sixty five is expected to double to nearly twenty percent [12]. Elderly are particularly susceptible to the stresses of heat and exposure to virulent microbes [12]. They are also likely to suffer from the classic "diseases of aging" namely osteoarthritis, tumors and Alzheimer's among others [12]. Athough the percentages of elderly will vary between different global communities they can still be expected to provide a significant burden in terms of health management [12].

4. Future Needs for Food: How will This Impact Farming, Fishing and Crops?

Current methods of intensive farming, overfishing and even crop growth are becoming both unsustainable and unlikely to be able to support the world's population even in the near future [13]. Many point to the intensive rearing of animals (factory farming) as both significant contributors to climate change [13, 16] as well as rising antibiotic resistance [13]. Factory farming of cows for meat and milk is a particular issue in this regard as the unhygienic conditions of close quartering allow rapid spread of contagious infections are quickly spread between the animals [37, 38]. A prime example in this regard is mastitis, which is typically managed by quickly separating the infected animal and injecting the udders with antibiotics [37]. Apart from the loss in revenue from unusable, contaminated milk, which is an estimated fifteen percent of productivity in an affected area [38], there is also a loss of animals due to early culling of those with repeat infections [37, 38]. Although the mastitis bacteria have not yet demonstrated significant upticks in antibiotic resistance the same cannot be said for the limited numbers of antihelminthics used to treat sheep and goats [39]. The negatives of intensive farming are often cited as demonstrating that organic farming is the way forward in that it would provide healthier animals that would in turn produce nutritious milk and meat [40].

4.1. Organic Livestock Farming

Organic farming has been shown to reduce infections rates (including mastitis) through allowing the animals to be free range [37], raising indigenous rather than crossbred stock [37] and keeping the calf for longer with the heifer [41]. Indeed, organic farming is widely believed to be the way forward in providing food for the growing world's population, especially in the developing world. Currently, organic does still allow for a limited number of times that classic pharmaceuticals can be used for treatment, particularly of livestock [39], but truly organic means moving beyond this. As will be seen, in the sections to follow, we are at the beginning of an exploration into the use of plant-based therapies and food scientists are learning these may be as effective, if not more so, than the commercial pharmaceuticals used until now [39].

4.1.1. Organic Livestock Farming and Allicin

Countries in the European Union are already using various phytomedicines in organic farming, including garlic [39]. Allicin functions as a broad spectrum antimicrobial in its own right and could be incorporated into lotions, pastes and salves relatively easily for topical infections [1]. In Europe, garlic is already used topically to treat mite infestations [39]. Allicin is also effective, at least *in vitro* against the main causes of mastititis; *Staphylococcus aureus* and *agalacticae* (see Chapter 5). The thiosulfinate easily penetrates skin [1] and could be developed into a lotion-based treatment for this condition. Allicin has demonstrated activity against at least some gastrointestinal animal trematode and schistosomulan parasites (see Chapter 7 for details) and is tolerated when added to the feed of Murrah Buffalo calves [42], piglets [43] and broiler chickens [44].

The latter study was made more remarkable as it demonstrated that garlic could reverse choline deficiency in these fowl [44]. Choline deficiencies are an issue for both human and animal development of cellular membranes and the neurotransmitter acetylcholine [45]. Deficiencies are more common in developing countries and result in liver damage [45]. Since the only current method to reverse choline deficiency is to increase its consumption [45] this finding is important to both the livestock being raised and humans that consume them. Addition of fresh garlic to feed has also been shown to increase food intake and growth in these livestock [42-44]. To date, no veterinary DBRCT studies have been performed on either allicin or garlic and these are definitely needed to identify new formulations.

4.2. Organic Aquaculture

When the burden of feeding all these animals on either forage or feed is added into the equation, it is apparent that humans will need to seek a more plant-based diet supplemented with fish rather than meat i.e., piscatarian [13]. But can we live on the ocean's fish? Climate change to the fish species (see section 1.2 Water Insecurity), compounded with overfishing has already resulted in limits on natural, wild caught fish [46] and a concern that without intervention nearly ninety percent of fish stocks will be endangered (red listed) by 2050 [47]. Some species such as the tiger shrimp (*Peneus monodon)* and Pacific white shrimp (*Litopenaeus vannamei*) are already on the IUCN Red List of Threatened Species, which indicates they are close to becoming extinct [46]. African and most Asian sources of fish still remain primarily wild caught, using cultural traditions of net and line [33]. These areas are also some of the primary producers of the fish products that both provide local food as well as exports [36].

Given dwindling wild caught fish, there is a growing trend in Asia particularly but also worldwide to develop aquaculture [27]. Aquaculture faces similar issues as agriculture in that areas must be created to hold the fish i.e., artificial ponds and this keeps them in close proximity with each other [27]. Overuse of antibiotics has had similar consequences as factory farmed animal meat with fish containing resistant bacterial strains that were transmissable to humans [48]. Current concepts of farmed fish are also an issue is that they are considered less healthy than their wild caught relatives, although this may actually be a myth since contaminants exist in both [49]. Farmed raised often contain antimicrobials, chiefly used to treat fungal and bacterial consequences of overstocking [49]. Disease can be a major result of loss in farmed fish [50]. For example, one particularly huge epidemic of the parasitic flatworm *Neobenedenia girallae* in Australia was responsible for the deaths of twenty thousand farmed barramundi in 2001 [50]. Farmed fish can also contain mercury from the ingestion of ocean fish made into feed, although this trend may be changing as soymeal is used [49]. Fresh caught fish, especially apex varieties such as swordfish and bottom feeders, are often contaminated with heavy metals including mercury [49]. Seafood consumption rates continue to rise and aquaculture of some form will clearly be required that is able to meet the need of a growing world population [48].

4.2.1. Organic Aquaculture and Allicin

Organic aquaculture is in its infancy by comparison to the five billion tonnes of farmed fish produced every year but this is expected to rise at least ten times over the next few decades [51]. Like organic animal products, fish grown this way still need to be treated for infections if the fishery is overstocked [49]. For many organic aquaculturists they are using techniques such as multi-species culture systems to reduce the fish waste that promotes disease establishment as well as not overfeeding or overstocking [49]. Food sources are natural-based organics such as soymeal and are administered to produce normal growth development [51].

Allicin has already been investigated in several aquaculture models [52-65]. There have been at least thirteen well constructed, accessible studies on the effects of garlic feed supplementation on eight fish and two shrimp species (Table 1).

With the exception of tilapia fingerlings and rice eel, for which it has been reported to be toxic [48, 66], allicin was able to promote growth [48, 53, 54, 56, 58, 61, 62, 64] and improve overall fish flavor [39] in the species investigated. Garlic contaning allicin appears to reduce the lipid content of the fish and increase protein levels [39, 56]. Allicin is also able to kill several microbes toxic to fish including the bacteria *Aeromonas hydrophila* [56, 58, 60, 65], *Pseudomonas fluorescens* [56, 65] and *Edwardsiella tarda* [65], the toxic flatworm *Neobenedenia* [50] as well as gregarines [60]. Allicin is able to increase innate immune system function in several fish species [53-55, 59, 60, 62], particularly phagocytic activity [53-55, 59, 62]. Aquaculture using garlic/allicin results in fish that improves their viability on ice as well as decreasing the speed of mold spoilage [46]. Given the future growing need for safe and inexpensive ways to ensure protein reaches all areas of the globe, allicin can clearly be of great beneft [46]. Fish flakes containing garlic are already commercially available for home fish tanks. Asian countries have local access to products like soybeans, algae and garlic allows which would allow inexpensive formulations for aquaculture supplements [46]. As these are the growth areas of the future full investigations of the range of fish species whose growth and yield could be optimized by such strategies.

Table 1. Benefits of allicin* as aquaculture supplement

Species	Mode of administration	Effect	Reference
Barramundi (fish)	Allicin added for 10 and 30 days	After 30 days ↓ mortality by 70% from *Neobenedenia* helminths	[52]
Carp; Grass (fish)	Allicin and *pericarpum citri reticulatae* (Eucommia) for 50 days	↑ Growth by 31% ↓ infection rates and ↑ phagocytic activity	[53, 54]
Carp; Rohu (fish)	Garlic (0.1, 05 and 1%) for 60 days	↑ innate immune system function and ↓ mortality due to *Aeromonas hydrophilus* by 85%	[55]
Grey mullet (larvae)	Garlic extract (3%) for 30 days	Increased protein acquisition. Feed conversion of nearly 2x control was reported	[56]
Nile tilapia (fingerlings)	1% and 3% garlic or 1.5% Biogen® for 3 months in summer and 6 months in winter	Fresh garlic was 2x better than Biogen® (commercial allicin preparation) at ↓ *Pseudomonas fluorescens* mortality but both reduced fish death (↓40 and 63% respectively) ↑ weight for both treatments	[57]
Nile tilapia (fish)	Freeze dried 3% garlic for 90 days	Garlic produced similar increases in weight gain as chloramphenicol treatment ↓ *A. hydrophilus* and coliform infection rates	[58]
Nile tilapia (fish)	3% garlic for 3 months in summer	↑ in immune system functions (neutrophil adherence and leukocyte counts) ↓ mortality due to *A. hydrophilus* by 85%	[59]
Rainbow trout (fish)	Allimed in feed for 14 days	↓ mortality in *A. hydrophilus* from 80 to 8%, ↑ innate immunity	[60]
	Garlic (1-2%) for 120 days	dose-dependent ↑ in weight gain and beneficial bacterial intestinal flora	[61]
Shrimp; Black tiger (Kuruma)	Garlic paste (10g per 1 kg feed) for 4 weeks	↑ expression of innate immunity genes and ↓ infection with gregarines by 100%	[62]
Shrimp; Pacific white leg (fry)	Garlic (2-6%) for 60 days	↑ survival rates (90%) weight gain and feed conversion	[63]
Sterlet sturgeon (fingerlings)	Garlic powder for 12 weeks	Sturgeon increased in protein acquisition and weight gain was ~2% more than those without the non-toxic supplement	[64]
Thai silver barb (fish)	Garlic (bulb extract 2-8 mg/ml) for 10 days	90% ↓ in mortality from experimental infection with *A. hydrophilus*, *P. fluorescens* and *Edwardsiella tarda*	[65]

* only garlic preparations containing allicin have been included in this table

4.3. Organic Crop Farming

Plant-based diets of the future will also need to evolve crops that withstand climatic variability in rainfall and accompanying disease and insect damage [13]. Experts suggest that seed usage will need to complement regional needs and insect/ microbial infection issues rather than be optimized for productivity [13]. Countermeasures to pests in developed countries have resulted in overuse and resistance to a whole series of insecticides and fungicides [67, 68]. In contrast, the pesticides available in developing countries are the cheap, outdated, inefffective and toxic solutions that developed countries have abandoned [69]. Fortunately, many of the current over one and a half million organic farmers live in developing countries such as Argentina, China and Brazil and this is a trend that is set to continue [70, 71].

Organic farming of crops requires an initial intensive labor input involving the incorporation of organic matter and reduction of aggressive soil tilling methods [70]. An understanding of the natural ecology is also needed, so there is an education component [70]. In spite of this there is a noticeable benefit in that soils farmed this way hold more water and retain nitrogen-based nutrients better [70]. This latter finding is important as runoff from organically-farmed land is less likely to produce river eutrophication and its associated health and environmental problems [70] (see Section 1.2 Water Insecurity).

An absence of pesticides and fungicides also allows persistence of native ecosystems [70, 71]. Finally a lack of water loss also means the soils are more stable in areas subject to drought [70, 71]. Organic crop yields are the same as conventional farming methods for rice, soybeans and corn; all traditional staples for developing countries adding to their appeal [71]. Studies have also shown that organic produce is healthier as it lacks potential carcinogenic pesticides together with containing much higher nutrient levels and antioxidants [70]. If livestock rearing, aquaculture and crop production are to be performed organically to maximize health and nutrient value then measures must be taken to minimize loss through microbial and insect pests. For many, this has already meant examining natural phytomedicines for their benefits [39].

4.3.1. Organic Crop Pest Control and Allicin

Crops being raised organically need management to prevent fungal destruction of seeds and plants [72, 73]. Seeds and young seedlings are particularly prone to attack by pathogens that include rust (*Botrytis cinerea*) and leaf spot (*Aspergillus* species) (see Section 1.21 Chapter 1). To avoid what is termed "damping off" most commercial growers ensure they are first planting healthy seed, but may also use some type of seed treatment involving steam or hot water immersion of the seeds [73]. Non-organic farmers may also treat with the same fungicides later used to treat any disease in the plants [73]. All fungicides currently available are designed to attack thiol groups in the fungi [72]; a target shared by allicin [1]. Seed treatment with allicin has been shown by several authors to both improve germination of seedlings and prevent fungal infection (see Chapter 6 for details). Although fungicide resistance is increasing [72], allicin's multiple microbial targets would allow its continued use and garlic's ease of growth would allow local availability [1]. Organic crops are also lost due to damage by insects such as aphids [74] and post harvest from storage pests (see Chapter 9 for details). Allicin has been shown to be effective in controlling aphid contamination of brassica plants [75] and can protect soybean and groundnut crops from the cutworm moth [76]. Nanoparticles containing allicin have recently been coupled to methyl cellulose and would further reduce storage pests when used in packaging [9]. These benefits suggest eco-friendly allicin is a good fit for organic farming use.

5. Future Human Health Issues; More Places for Allicin

Allicin could play a role in alleviating health concerns in two very diferent populations: children and the elderly. The previous section of this chapter has discussed mechanisms to prevent malnutrition in the light of an exploding world population. Current estimates are that malnutrition affects around just under a billion people, primarily residents of developing countries [77]. The connection between malnutrition and infection is a strong one [77]. Just over half of all childhood deaths from infectious diseases are seen in children with some degree of malnutrition [77]. In severe malnutrition (at least two standard deviations under normal weight for age) children often don't present symptoms of infection [77]. This is due to poor migration of phagocytic cells and depressed levels of antibacterial complement proteins [77].

Malnutrition is compounded by a combination of poor food intake, worm infestations and has its root causes in poverty and lack of education [77]. As well as children, elderly people are also more prone to infectious diseases and tumors due to a decrease in immune system potency [78]. As the world experiences a doubling of the number of those over sixty five health concerns will also involve those of aging and immunosenescence [78]. Malnourishment, together with locally prevalent inherited diseases such as thalassemia, is also expected to increase the rates of osteoporosis (OP); already at epidemic proportions in developing countries [79].

Programs to improve nutrient sources, food preparation, sanitation, avoidance of disease and management of "aging-associated diseases" need to be relatively straight forward to reach all individuals as well as inexpensive to maintain [77]. Clearly, the "human side" of illness would be best approached by using locally sourced materials either individually or in combination with classic pharmaceuticals [11]. Allicin's diverse effects make it an ideal subject for study and its points of entry will be discussed in the following sections.

5.1. Allicin and Non-Infectious Diseases of Younger Individuals

In developed countries the conditions of OP and periodontal disease (PD) affect younger individuals due to a combination of malnutrition and poor oral health care [79, 80]. Reduction in malnutrition including vitamin D-based bone loss would help reduce the risk of OP but for the post-menopausal, estrogen-related form allicin has already been shown to be of benefit (see Chapter 11 for details). Oral health programs continue to be established in developing nations but are unlikely to meet the needs of the rapid population growth that continues there [81]. Poor oral health for children results in periodontal disease by teenage years, tooth loss and a higher incidence of other later issues such as miscarriages, cardiovascular disease and diabetes [81]. Allicin as a mouthwash would reduce the pathogen-forming biofilm bacteria that initiate PD as well as potentially being effective to reverse bone resorption as an injectable for later stage disease (discussed in Chapter 11).

5.2. Allicin and Non-Infectious Diseases of Aging

Since being confirmed as antibacterial in 1944, the majority of work on allicin's activities has focused on its tumoricidal capabilities [1]. Targeting many of the biochemical pathways that play a role in driving tumorigenesis (see Chapter 2 for details) allicin has already shown great potential in animal models of at least sixteen different tumors (see Chapter 13 for details). Since the world of 2050 will contain twice as many older individuals than today there will be an uptick in diseases such as osteoarthritis (OA), neurological conditions such as Alzheimer's disease (AD), cardiovascular illness (CVD) and type II diabetes [78]. Allicin has demonstrated efficacy against all four conditions, which are both incurable and currently not able to be effectively managed (see Chapters 10-12 for details).

All these conditions are likely to reach epidemic proportions in the next few decades [2, 82, 83]. OA cases are set to affect over one hundred million worldwide by 2030 [2] and will be especially problematic to manage in developing nations where the number of sufferers is likely to double [82]. A similar pattern in also being projected for the number of AD cases, which are expected to double to over eighty million in 2040 [82]. Hardest hit will be the countries of China and India that are expected to have both the greatest population growth and number of elderly individuals [83]. Co-morbidities of AD such as diabetes and CVD now affect just under one in ten of the world's population [84]. The conditions are more common in developed nations but still constitute a significant cause of demise for those over sixty in developing countries including India and China [84].

CONCLUSION

Our society is facing some of the greatest challenges to its integrity due to climate change and population expansion. As this forces us to seek out new strategies in obtaining and distributing food and medical care, it is clear that local sourcing of inexpensive and easily produced agents will be necessary. Studies by the World Health Organization have predicted that three-quarters of the over sixties population will be resident in developing nations by 2025 [83], which is going to require a shift in strategy to care for and manage all these conditions inexpensively. Developing nations have a strong adherence to ethnopharmacology [2] and it can be anticipated that this will spur studies to identify easily cultivated, inexpensive, local phytomedicines for the effective treatment of disease. Allicin's biochemical targets provide many potential interventions as summarized in Figure 2.

Currently the main obstacles that are faced in using the thiosulfinate are its relative instability (see Chapter 2) and lack of effective DBRPCT. The new stabilized forms of allicin have appeared in the last decade and have begun to be investigated as to efficacy for the treatment of the common cold (see Chapter 8 for details). Mistrust of herbal preparations in general is finally waning even in developed countries as more establishment of government legislated standardization [2]. Approximately five percent of children and eight percent of adults show reactive skin sensitivity to garlic [85], and reactivity to allicin alone is unknown. This may limit its use in certain individuals but does not provide a formidable barrier to therapeutic development. Instead, the final hurdle for this phytomedicine will be, as for other plants, continued source material [2].

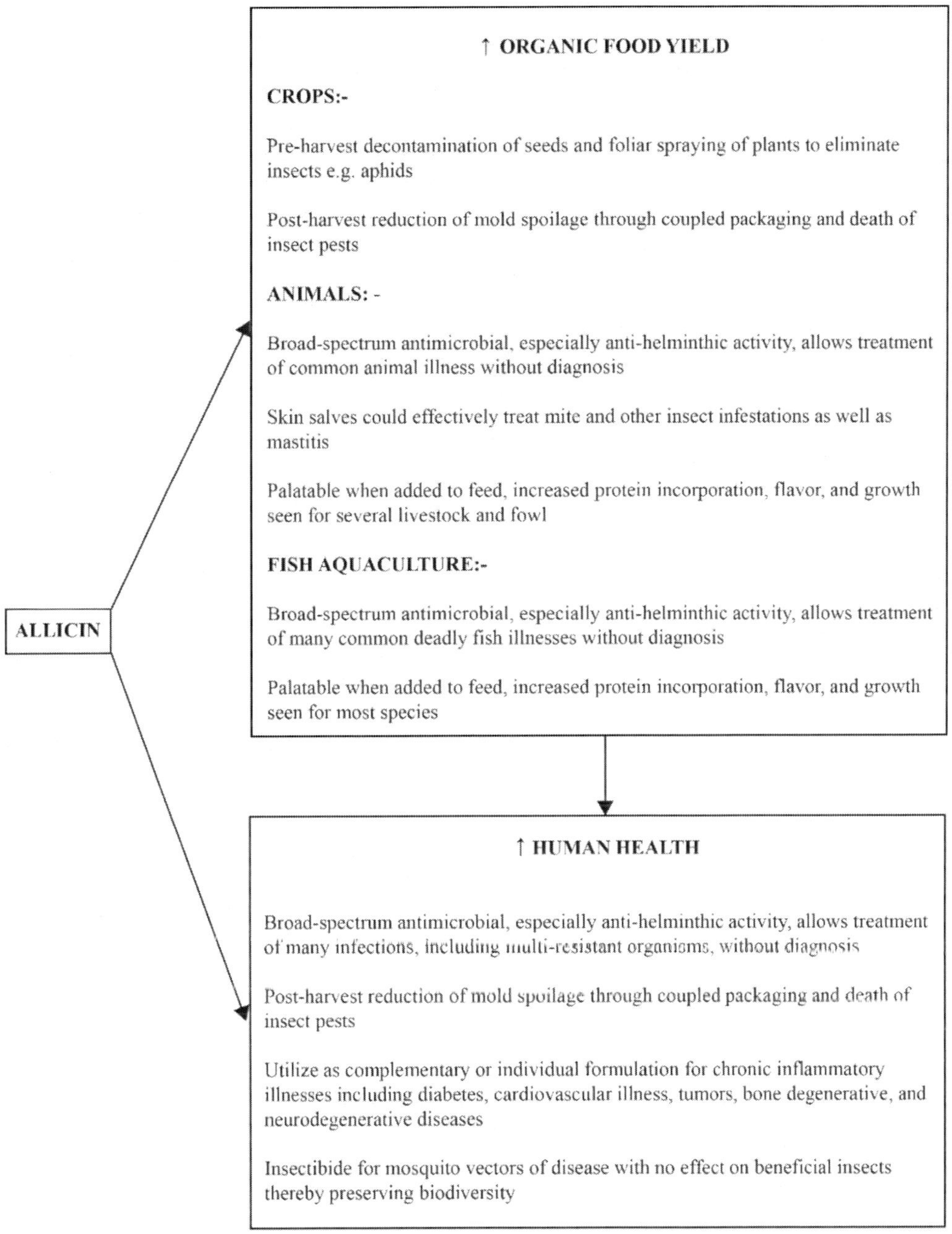

Legend: Allicin's broad spectrum antimicrobial, insecticidal, neuroprotective, cardioprotective, cartilage and osteoprotective and tumoricidal activities could be utilized in various optimizable delivery systems to increase organic food yield and improve human health.

Figure 2. Allicin's potential roles in organic agriculture and human health.

For some plants this is an issue as their cultivation is restricted to certain areas but garlic grows easily throughout most of the world (as does its wild allicin-containing *Allium* relatives) (see Chapter 1,for details). Concerns have been raised about garlic propagation as, unlike other plants, this is completely reliant on humans as the commercial varieties are sterile [86, 87] The resultant loss in diversity of garlic's genome is significant and this could eventually herald species loss [86, 87]. Cultivated garlic shows high levels of single nucleotide polymorphisms (SNPs) in nearly 80% of the markers measured in the genome [84]. Progeny carrying two copies of these types of genes typically either die or fail to produce effective crops [86]. As a result cross-breeding of cultivated garlic with its wild relatives is now being recommended [86].

So, just as this book began with the story of allicin as told through the garlic clove, scientists are looking to the still fertile male sources of this bulb from the Tien Shen mountains to provide a potential solution [85, 86]. Unlike their cultivated counterparts, wild fertile clones of garlic are typically inferior bulb producers as they both flower and set seed [85, 87]. In 2005, scientists sequenced the genome of garlic and are now establishing a germoplasm reserve of the different varieties available for future genetic assortment [88]. It is anticipated that future optimization of the allicin-producing capabilities will be incorporated into new, cross bred, hardier and possibly self-fertile varieties. We can but hope that by 2050 DBRPCT will have established several of the multiple potentials of allicin the natural sulfur compound from garlic with many uses.

REFERENCES

[1] Borlinghaus, Jan., Frank, Albrecht., Martin, C. H. Grulke., Ifeanyi, D. Nwachukwu. & Alan, J. Slusarenko. (2014). "Allicin: Chemistry and biological properties". *Molecules*, *19*(8), 12591-12618. Accessed February 1, 2019. https://www.mdpi.com/1420-3049/19/8/12591/htm.

[2] Cundell, Diana R. (2014). *Herbal phytochemicals as immunomodulators Current Immunology Reviews*, Volume *10*, Issue 2, ISSN:1875-631X(Online),ISSN:1573-3955(Print) Accessed February 1, 2019 https://www.researchgate.net/profile/Diana_Cundell/publication/273333150_Herbal_Phytochemicals_as_Immunomodulators/links/563b9ec808ae405111a76fd8/Herbal-Phytochemicals-as-Immunomodulators.pdf.

[3] Prati, Patricia., Celina, M. Henrique., Aparecida, S. de Souza., Vera, S. N. da Silva. & Maria, T. B. Pacheco. (2014). "Evaluation of allicin stability in processed garlic of different cultures." *Food Science and Technology Campinas*, *34*(3), 623-628. doi: http://dx.doi.org/10.1590/1678-457X.6397.

[4] Suddek, Ghada M. (2014). "Allicin enhances chemotherapeutic response and ameliorates tamoxifen-induced liver injury in experimental animals." *Pharmaceutical Biology*, *52*(8), 1009-1014, doi: 10.3109/13880209.2013.876053.

[5] Xie, Kun., Jianze, Nian., Xingyang, Zhu., Xiaoping, Geng. & Fubao, Liu. (2015). "Modulatory role of garlicin in migration and invasion of intrahepatic cholangiosarcoma via P13K/AKT pathway." *Int. J. Clin. Exp. Pathol.*, *8*(11), 14028-14033.

[6] Kaptchuk, Ted J. (2001). "The double-blind, randomized placebo-controlled trial : Gold standard or golden calf?" *Journal of Clinical Epidemiology*, *54*(6), 541-549. Accessed February 1, 2019. https://www.sciencedirect.com/science/article/pii/ S0895435600003474?via%3Dihub.

[7] Kondo, Tamotsu. (2001). "Microcapsules: Their science and technology Part III. Industrial, medical and pharmaceutical applications." *J. Oleo Sci.*, *50*(3), 143-152. Accessed February 1, 2019. https://www.jstage.jst.go.jp/article/jos/50/3/50_3_143/_pdf.

[8] Sharifi-Rad, J., Hoseini-Alfatemi, S. M., Sharifi-Rad, M. & Iriti, M. (2014). "Antimicrobial synergic effect of silver nanoparticles on skin infection caused by methicillin-resistant *Staphylococcus aureus* spp." *Annals of Medical and Health Sciences Research*, *4*(6), 863-868 Accessed on February 1, 2019. https://pdfs.semanticscholar.org/b884/47b4a5f4e5e7a723349e541f96974688a9d5.pdf.

[9] Jebali, Ali., Seyedhossein, Hekmatimoghaddam., Aliasghar, Behzadi., Iraj, Rezapor., Bahador, H. Mohammadi., Tahereh, Jasemizad., Seyed, A. Yasini., Morteza, Javadzadeh., Asiye, Amiri., Mansoure, Soltani., Zeynab, Rezaei., Najme, Sedighi., Mina, Seyfi., Mohammad, Rezaei. & Mehran, Sayadi. (2013). "Antimicrobial activity of nanocellulose conjugated with allicin and lysozyme". *Cellulose*, *20*, 2897-2907. doi: 10.1007/s10570-013-0084-3. Accessed on February 1, 2019. https://www.researchgate.net/profile/Mohammad_Rezaei47/publication/258162262_Antimicrobial_activity_of_nanocellulose_conjugated_with_allicin_and_lysozyme/links/0f31753c8ca618fafc000000/Antimicrobial-activity-of-nanocellulose-conjugated-with-allicin-and-lysozyme.pdf.

[10] Chhabria, Sagar V., Mohammad, A. Akbarsha., Albert, P. Li., Prashant, S. Kharkar. & Krutika, B. Desai. (2015). "*In situ* allicin generation using targeted alliinase delivery for inhibition of MIA PaCa-2 cells via epigenetic changes, oxidative stress and cyclin dependent kinase inhibitor (CDKI) expression. *Apoptosis*, *20*, 1388-1409. https://doi.org/10.1007/s10495-015-1159-4.

[11] Balunas, Mercy J. & Douglas Kinghorn. (2005). "Drug discovery from medicinal plants." *Life Sciences*, *78*(5), 431-441. https://doi.org/10.1016/j.lfs.2005.09.012.

[12] Lutz, Wolfgang. & Samir, K. C. (2010). "Dimensions of global population projections: what do we know about future population trends and structures?" *Philosophical Transactions of the Royal Society of London. Series B, Biological Xciences*, *365*(1554), 2779-91. doi: 10.1098/rstb.2010.0133.

[13] Green, Hilary., Pierre, Broun., Douglas, Cook., Karen, Cooper., Adam, Drewnowski., Duncan, Pollard., Gary, Sweeney. & Anne, Roulin. (2018). "Healthy and sustainable diets for future generations." *Journal of the Science of Food and Agriculture*, *98*(9), 3219-3224. doi: 10.1002/jsfa.8953.

[14] Bale, J. S., van Lenteren, J. C. & Bigler, F. (2008). "Biological control and sustainable food production." *Philosophical Transactions of the Royal Society of London. Series B, Biological sciences*, *363*(1492), 761–776. doi:10.1098/rstb.2007.2182.

[15] *The Intergovermental Panel on Climate Change*. 2019. Accessed on August 12, 2019 https://www.ipcc.ch/.

[16] Yi, Hoonbok., Bijaya, R. Devkota., Jaesoong, Yu., Kicheol, Oh., Jinhong, Kim. & Hyung-Jun, Kim. (2014). "Effects of global warming on mosquitoes and mosquito-borne diseases and the new strategies for mosquito control." *Entomological Research*, *44*, 215-235. Accessed on February 7, 2019. https://onlinelibrary.wiley.com/doi/pdf/10.1111/1748-5967.12084.

[17] Luber, George. & Natasha, Prudent. (2009). "Climate change and human health." *Transactions of the American Clinical and Climatological Association*, *120*, 113-7.

[18] Sahoo, Krushna C., Soumayakanta, Sahoo., Gaetano, Marrone., Ashish, Pathak., Cecilia, S. Lundborg. & Ashok, J. Tamhankar. (2014). "Climatic factors and community - associated methicillin-resistant Staphylococcus aureus skin and soft-tissue infections - a time-series analysis study." *International Journal of Environmental Research and Public Health*, *11*(9), 8996-9007. doi: 10.3390/ijerph110908996.

[19] Revay, Edita E., Yosef, Schlein., Onie, Tsabari., Vasiliy, Kravchenko., Whitney, Qualls., Rui, De-Xue., John, C. Beier., Sekou, F. Traore., Seydou, Doumbia., Axel, Hausmann. & Günter, C. Müller. (2015). "Formulation of attractive toxic sugar bait (ATSB) with safe EPA-exempt substance significantly diminishes the *Anopheles sergentii* population in a desert oasis." *Acta Trop*, *150*, 29-34. doi: 10.1016/j.actatropica.2015.06.018.

[20] Prathap, Pragna., Archana, P. R., Joy, Aleena., Veerasamy, Sejian., Govindan, Krishnan., Madiajagan, Bagath., Manimaran, A., Beena, V., Kurien, E. K., Girish, Varma. & Raghavendra, Bhatta. (2017). "Heat Stress and Dairy Cow: Impact on Both Milk Yield and Composition." *International Journal of Dairy Science.*, *12*, 1-11.doi: 10.3923/ijds.2017.1.11.

[21] Rust, J. M. & Rust, T. (2013). "Climate change and livestock production: A review with emphasis on Africa." *South African Journal of Animal Science*, *43*(3), 256-267. Accessed February 05, 2019, from http://www.scielo.org.za/scielo.php?script=sci_arttext&pid=S0375-15892013000300004&lng=en&tlng=en.

[22] Serpetti, N., Baudron, A. R., Burrows, M. T., Payne, B. L., Helaouët, P., Fernandes, P. G. & Heymans, J. J. (2017). "Impact of ocean warming on sustainable fisheries management informs the Ecosystem Approach to Fisheries." *Scientific Reports*, *7*(1), 13438. doi: 10.1038/s41598-017-13220-7.

[23] Diana, James S. (2009). "Aquaculture Production and Biodiversity Conservation." *BioScience*, *59*(1), 27–38. Accessed on February 7, 2019. https://doi.org/10.1525/bio.2009.59.1.7.

[24] El-Sayyed, Hassan I., Amoura, M. Abou-El-Naga., Abdelalim, A. Gadallah. & Imam, H. Bakr. (2010). "Protective effects of *Alium sativum* against defects of hypocholesterolemia on pregnant rats and their offspring. " *Int. J. Clin. Exp. Med.*, *3*(2), 152-163. http://www.ijcem.com/files/IJCEM1001002.pdf.

[25] Barros, Ceres., Wilfried, Thuiller. & Tamara, Münkemüller. (2018). "Drought effects on the stability of forest-grassland ecotones under gradual climate change." *PLoS One*, *13*(10), e0206138. https://doi.org/10.1371/journal.pone.0206138.

[26] Tjaden, Nils B., Cyril, Caminade., Carl, Beierkuhnlein. & Stephanie, M. Thomas. (2018). "Mosquito-borne diseases: Advances in modeling climate change impacts." *Trends in Parasitology*, *34*(3), 227-245. doi: https://doi.org/10.1016/j.pt.2017.11.006.

[27] Zhou, L. H., Zheng, T. L., Chen, X. H., Wang, X., Chen, S. B., Tiang, Y. & Hong, H. S. (2008). "The inhibitory effects of garlic (*Allium sativum*) and diallyl trisulfide on *Alexandrium tamarense* and other harmful algal species." *J. Appl. Phycol.*, *20*, 349-358. Accessed on August 12, 2019. https://core.ac.uk/download/pdf/41349359.pdf.

[28] Hoban, Sean. & Christano, Vernesi. (2012). "Challenges in global biodiversity conservation and solutions that cross sociology, politics, economics and ecology." *Biology Letters*, *8*(6), 897-9. doi: 10.1098/rsbl.2012.0596.

[29] García-Robledo, Carlos., Erin, K. Kuprewicz., Charles, L. Staines., Terry, L. Erwin. & John Kress, W. (2016). "Limited tolerance by insects to high temperatures across tropical

elevational gradients and the implications of global warming for extinction." *PNAS*, *113* (3), 680-68 doi: 10.1073/pnas.1507681113.

[30] Casadevall, Arturo., Ferric, F. Fang. & Liise-anne, Pirofski. (2011). "Microbial virulence as emergent property: Consequences and opportunities." *PLos Pathog*, *7*(7), e1002136. doi: 10.1371/journal.ppat.1002136.

[31] Githeko, A. K., Lindsay, S. W., Confalonieri, U. E. & Patz, J. A. (2000). "Climate change and vector-borne diseases: a regional analysis." *Bulletin of the World Health Organization*, *78*, 1136–1147. Accessed on February 7, 2019. https://www.ncbi.nlm.nih.gov/ pmc/articles/PMC2560843/pdf/11019462.pdf.

[32] Ficke, Andrea., Jean-Nöel, Aubertot. & Clayton, Hollier. (2012). "Crop losses due to disease and their implications for global food production losses and food security." *Food Security*, *4*(4), 519-537. Accessed on February 7, 2019. https://doi.org/10.1007/s12571-012-0200-5.

[33] Allison, Edward H. & David, J. Mills. (2018). "Counting the fish eaten rather than the fish caught." *PNAS* 115(29): 7459-7461. https://doi.org/10.1073/pnas.1808755115.

[34] Bharadwaj, Anuja., Laura, E. Hayes. & Kirby, C. Stafford. (2015). "Effectiveness of Garlic for the Control of *Ixodes scapularis* (Acari: Ixodidae) on Residential Properties in Western Connecticut." *Journal of Medical Entomology*., *52*(4), 722-725. https://doi.org/10.1093/jme/tjv044.

[35] U.S. Patent US20060110472A1. Miron, Talia., Aharon, Rabinkov., Meir, Wilchek., David, Mirelman. & Talila, Volk. (2002). "Use of allicin as insect repellant and insecticide in agricultural crops." Accessed August 12, 2019. https:// patents.google.com/patent/ US20060110472A1/en.

[36] Leeson, George W. (2018). "The growth, ageing and urbanization of our world." *Journal of Population Ageing*, *11*(2), 107-115. https://doi.org/10.1007/s12062-018-9225-7.

[37] Sarba, E. J. & Getachew, K. Tola. (2017). "Cross-sectional study on bovine mastitis and its associated risk factors in Ambo district of West Shewa zone, Oromia, Ethiopia." *Veterinary World*, *10*(4), 398-402. doi: 10.14202/vetworld.2017.398 402.

[38] Pyörälä S. (2009). "Treatment of mastitis during lactation. *Irish Veterinary Journal*, *62*(Suppl 4), S40-44. doi: 10.1186/2046-0481-62-S4-S40. Accessed on Feruary 7, 2019. https://www.ncbi.nlm.nih.gov/pmc/articles/PMC3339349/#B33.

[39] Mayer, Maria., Christian, R. Vogl., Michele, Amorena., Matthias, Hamburger. & Michael, Walknhorst. (2014). "Treatment of organic livestock with medicinal plants: A systematic review of ethnoveterinary research." *Forsch. Komplementmed*, *21*, 375-386. doi: 10.1159/000370216.

[40] Regangold, John P. & Jonathan, M. Wachter. (2016). "Organic agriculture in the 21st Century." *Nature Plants*, Article Number 15221. Accessed on February 7, 2019. doi: 10.1038/NPLANTS.2015.221. https://www.researchgate.net/publication/293014068_Organic_agriculture_in_the_twenty-first_century.

[41] Føske, Johnsen., Julie, Katharina A. Zipp., Tasia, Kälber., Anne, Marie de Passalé., Ute, Knierim., Kerstin, Barth. & Cecilie, M. Mejdell. (2016). "Is rearing calves with the dam a feasible option for dairy farms?" Current and future research". *Applied Animal Behavior Science*, *181*, 1-11. https://www.sciencedirect.com/science/article/pii/ S0168159115003159.

[42] Duvvu, Mohan V., Ananda Rao, K., Venkata Seshiah, Ch. & Srinivas Kumar, D. (2018). "Effect of garlic supplementation on the growth performance and body condition score

of Murrah Buffalo Calves." *Int. J. Curr. Microbiol. App. Sci., 7*(2), 2972-2977. Accessed on February 12, 2019. https://www.ijcmas.com/7-2-2018/ Mohan%20Vamsi%20Duvvu, %20et%20al.pdf.

[43] Cullen, S. P., Monahan, F. J., Callaghan, J. J. & O'Doherty, J. V. (2005). "The Effect of Dietary Garlic and Rosemary on Grower-Finisher Pig Performance and Sensory Characteristics of Pork." *Irish Journal of Agricultural and Food Research*, vol. *44*(1), 57–67. *JSTOR*, www.jstor.org/stable/25562532.

[44] Navidshad, Bahman., Zeinab, Maghsoodi., Saeid, Nikbin., Vahid, Vahedi., Masoud, Adibmoradi., Farzad, Mirzaei Aghjehgheshlagh. & Hamidreza, Moradi. (2018). "The compensation effect of dietary garlic on chicken consuming a minimal level of choline." *Italian Journal of Animal Science, 17*(1), 175-179, doi: 10.1080/1828051X. 2017.1338537.

[45] Mehedint, Mihai G. & Steven, H. Zeisel. (2013). "Choline's role in maintaining liver function: new evidence for epigenetic mechanisms." *Current Opinion in Clinical Nutrition and Metabolic Care, 16*(3), 339-45. doi: 10.1097/MCO.0b013e3283600d46.

[46] Chakravartty, D. (2015). "Natural nutritional ingredients hold the key to a sustainable future in aquaculture: Awakening the Indian sundarbans for self preservation." *IJAPBC, 4*(1), 60-70 http://www.ijapbc.com/files/08-34192.pdf.

[47] Worm, Boris. (2016). "Averting a global fisheries disaster." *PNAS, 113*(18), 4895-4897. Accessed on February 7, 2019. https://www.pnas.org/content/113/18/4895.

[48] Erguig, Marwane., Ahmed, Yahyaoui., Mohamed, Fekhaoui. & Mohammed, Dakki. (2015). "The use of garlic in aquaculture." *European Journal of Biotechnology and Bioscience, 3*(8), 28-33. http://www.biosciencejournals.com/vol3/issue8/pdf/15.1.pdf.

[49] Gormaz, Juan G., Jillian, P. Fry., Marcia, Erazo. & David, C. Love. (2014). "Public Health Perspectives on Aquaculture." *Current Environmental Health Reports, 1*(3), 227-238. doi: 10.1007/s40572-014-0018-8.

[50] Brazenor, Alexander K., Terry, Bertozzi., Terrence, L. Miller., Ian, D. Whittington & Kate, S. Hutson. (2018). "DNA profiling reveals Neobenedenia girallae as the primary culprit in global fisheries and aquaculture." *Molecular Phylogenetics and Evolution, 129*, 130-137. doi: https://doi.org/10.1101/304261.

[51] Perdikaris, Costas. & Ioannis, Paschos. (2010). "Organic aquaculture in Greece: a brief review." *Reviews in Aquaculture, 2*, 102-105. doi:10.1111/j.1753-5131.2010.01025.x.

[52] Militz, Thane A. Paul C. Southgate., Alexander, G. Carton. & Kate, S. Hutson. (2013). "Dietary supplementation of garlic (*Allium sativum*) to prevent monogenean infection in aquaculture." *Aquaculture, 408-409*, 95-99. Accessed on February 8, 2019. https://www.sciencedirect.com/science/article/abs/pii/S0044848613002615#

[53] Pu, Hongyu., Xiaoyu, Li., Qingbo, Du., Hao, Cui. & Yongping, Xu. (2017). "Research progress in the application of Chinese herbal medicines in aquaculture: A review." *Engineering, 3*(5), 731-737. https://www.sciencedirect.com/science/article/pii/ S2095809917307269#bib39.

[54] Luo, Q. H. (2008). *Masters Thesis. "Effect of the combined food additive of Eucommia extract and allicin on the immunity and performance of grass carp."* Accessed on February 8, 2019. https://www.globethesis.com/?t=2143360218954062.

[55] Sahu, S., Das, B. K., Mishra, B. K., Pradhan, J. & Sarangi, N. (2007). "Effect of *Allium sativum* on the immunity and survival of *Labeo rohita* infected with *Aeromonas*

hydrophila." *Journal of Applied Ichthyology*, *23*, 80-86. doi: 10.1111/j.1439-0426. 2006.00785.x.

[56] Akbary, P., Negahdari Jafarbeigi, Y. & Sondakzeihi, A. (2016). "Effects of garlic (*Allium sativum* L) extract on growth, feed utilization and carcass composition in *Mugil cephalus* (Linneus 1758) larvae. " *Iranian Journal of Fisheries Sciences*, *15*(1), 552-557. Accessed on February 12, 2019. http://aquaticcommons.org/22888/1/IFRO-v15n1p552-en.pdf.

[57] Diab, Ahmed S., Salah, M. Aly., George, John., Yasser, Abde-Hadi. & Mohamed, F. Mohammed. (2008). "Effect of garlic, black seed and Biogen as immunostimulants on the growth of Nile Tilapia (*Oreochromis niloticus*) (Tilosei:Cichlidae) and their response to artificial infection by *Pseudomonas fluorescens*." *African Journal of Aquatic Science*, *33*(1), 63-68. doi:10.2989/AJAS.2007.33.1.7.391.

[58] Shalaby, Y. M., Kattab, Y. A. & Abdel Rahman, A. M. (2006). "Effect of garlic (*Allium sativum* L) and chloramphenicol on growth parameters, physiological performance and survival of Nile tilapia (*Oreochromis niloticus*)." *Journal of Venomous Animals and Toxins*, *12*(2), 172-201. Accessed on February 12, 2019. http://www.scielo.br/scielo.php?script=sci_arttext&pid=S1678-91992006000200003.

[59] Aly, S. M. & Mohamed, M. F. (2010). "*Echinacea purpurea* and *Allium sativum* as immunostimulants in fish culture using Nile tilapia (*Oreochromis niloticus*)." *Journal of Animal Physiology and Animal Nutrition*, *94*, e31-e39. doi: 10.1111/j.1439-0396. 2009.00971.x.

[60] Nya, E. J., Dawood, Z. & Austin, B. (2010). "The garlic component, allicin, prevents disease caused by *Aeromonas hydrophila* in rainbow trout, *Oncorhynchus mykiss* (Walbaum)." *Journal of Fish Diseases*, *33*(4), 293-300. Accessed on February 8, 2019. https://onlinelibrary.wiley.com/doi/abs/10.1111/j.1365-2761.2009.01121.x.

[61] Miray, Etyemez Büyükdeveci., José, L. Balcázar., İbrahim, Demirkale. & Suat, Dikel. (2018). "Effects of garlic-supplemented diet on growth performance and intestinal microbiota of rainbow trout (*Oncorhynchus mykiss*)." *Aquaculture*, *486*, 170-174. https://doi.org/10.1016/j.aquaculture.2017.12.022.

[62] Tanekhy, M. & Fall, J. (2015). "Expression of innate immunity genes in kuruma shrimp *Marsupenaeus japonicus* after *in vivo* stimulation with garlic extract (allicin)." *Veterinarni Medicina*, *60*(1), 39 7. https://www.agriculturejournals.cz/publicFiles/143005.pdf.

[63] Labrador, Jack R. P., Recamar, C. Guiñares., Gaily, Jubie S. Hontiveros. & Pedro, González-Redondo (Reviewing Editor). (2016). "Effect of garlic powder-supplemented diets on the growth and survival of Pacific white leg shrimp (*Litopenaeus vannamei*)." *Cogent Food & Agriculture*, *2*, 1, doi: 10.1080/23311932.2016.1210066.

[64] Lee, Dong-Hoon., Seong-Ryul, Lim., Jung-Jo, Han., Sang-Woo, Lee., Chang-Six, Ra. & Jeong-Dae, Kim. (2014). "Effects of Dietary Garlic Powder on Growth, Feed Utilization and Whole Body Composition Changes in Fingerling Sterlet Sturgeon," Acipenser ruthenus. *Asian-Australasian Journal of Animal Sciences*, *27*(9), 1303-10. doi: 10.5713/ajas.2014.14087.

[65] Rahman, T., Akanda, M. M. R. & Rahman, M. M. (2009). "Evaluation of the efficacies of selected antibiotics and medicinal plants on fish pathogens." *Journal of the Bangladesh Agricultural University*, *7*, 163-168.

[66] Hussein, Mortada M. A. H., Abdel-Hamid, Hussein., Walid, H. Hassan. & Ihab, H. I. Moussa. (2013). "Potential use of allicin (garlic, *Alllium sativum* Linn. Essential oil)

against fish pathogenic bacteria and its safety for monosex Nile tilapia (*Oreochromis niloticus*)." *Journal of Food, Agriculture and Environment, 11*(1), 696-699. http://citeseerx.ist.psu.edu/viewdoc/download?doi=10.1.1.659.622&rep=rep1&type=pdf.

[67] Stratonovitch, Pierre., Jan, Elias., Ian, Denholm., Russell, Slater. & Mikhail, A. Semenov. (2014). "An Individual-Based Model of the Evolution of Pesticide Resistance in Heterogeneous Environments: Control of *Meligethes aeneus* Population in Oilseed Rape Crops." *PLoS ONE, 9*(12), e115631. https://doi.org/10.1371/ journal.pone.0115631.

[68] Deising, Holger B., Sven, Reimann. & Sergo, F. Pascholati. (2008). "Mechanisms and significance of fungicide resistance." *Brazilian Journal of Microbiology, 39*(2), 286-95. doi: 10.1590/S1517-838220080002000017.

[69] Ecobichon, Donald J. (2001). "Pesticide use in developing countries." *Toxicology, 160*(1-3), 27-33. https://doi.org/10.1016/S0300-483X(00)00452-2.

[70] Regangold, John P. & Jonathan, M. Wachter. (2016). "Organic agriculture in the 21st Century." *Nature Plants, 2016*, Article Number 15221. doi: 10.1038/NPLANTS.2015.221. Accessed on February 7, 2019.

[71] Schoonbeek, Sanne., Hossein, Azadi., Hossein, Mahmoudi., Ben, Derudder., Philippe, De Maeyer. & Frank, Witlox. (2013). "Organic agriculture and undernourishment in developing countries: Main potentials and challenges." *Critical Reviews in Food Sciences and Nutrition, 53*(9), 917-928. doi: 10.1080/10408398.2011.573886.

[72] Hahn, Matthias. (2014). "The rising threat of fungicide resistance in plant pathogenic fungi: Botrytis as a case study." *Journal of Chemical Biology, 7*(4), 133-41. doi: 10.1007/s12154-014-0113-1.

[73] Mancini, Valeria. & Gianfranco, Romanazzi. (2014). "Seed treatments to control seedborne fungal pathogens of vegetable crops." *Pest. Manag. Sci., 70*, 860-868. doi: 10.1002/ps.3693.

[74] Bahlai, Christine A., Yingen, Xue., Cara, M. McCreary., Arthur, W. Schaafsma. & Rebecca, H. Hallett. (2010). "Choosing organic pesticides over synthetic pesticides may not effectively mitigate environmental risk in soybeans." *PloS One, 5*(6), e11250. doi: 10.1371/journal.pone.0011250.

[75] Baidoo, P. K. & Mochiah, M. B. (2016). "Comparing the effectiveness of garlic (*Allium sativum* L.) and hot pepper (*Capsicum frutescens* L.) in the management of major pests of cabbage *Brassica olaracea* (L.)" *Sustainable Agricultural Research, 5*(2), 83-91. Accessed on February 13, 2019. https://ageconsearch.umn.edu/bitstream/234995/2/P7-p83-91.pdf.

[76] Fand, Babasaheb B. N., Nitin, T. Sul., Santanu, K. Bal. & Minhas, P. S. (2015). "Temperature Impacts the Development and Survival of Common Cutworm (*Spodoptera litura*): Simulation and Visualization of Potential Population Growth in India under Warmer Temperatures through Life Cycle Modelling and Spatial Mapping". *PLoS ONE, 10*(4), e0124682. Accessed September 20, 2018. http:// doi.org/10.1371/journal.pone.0124682.

[77] Müller, Olaf. & Michael, Krawinkel. (2005). "Malnutrition and health in developing countries." *CMAJ: Canadian Medical Association Journal = Journal de l'Association Medicale Canadienne, 173*(3), 279-86. doi: 10.1503/cmaj.050342.

[78] Montecino-Rodriguez, Enacarnacion., Beata, Berent-Maoz. & Kenneth, Dorshkind. (2013). Causes, consequences, and reversal of immune system aging. *The Journal of Clinical Investigation*, *123*(3), 958-65. doi: 10.1172/JCI64096.

[79] Rijayakumar, Rajasree. & Dietrich, Bussellberg. (2016). "*Osteoporosis an under-recognized public health problem.*," *2*. Accessed on April 15, 2019. http://www.qscience.com/doi/pdf/10.5339/jlghs.2016.2.

[80] Nazir, Muhammad A. (2017). "Prevalence of periodontal disease, its association with systemic diseases and prevention." *International Journal of Health sciences*, *11*(2), 72–80. Accessed on April 16, 2019. https://www.ncbi.nlm.nih.gov/pmc/articles/PMC5426403/.

[81] Macnab, Andrew J. (2015). "Children's Oral Health: The Opportunity for Improvement Using the WHO Health Promoting School Model, Advances in Public Health." Article ID 651836. https://doi.org/10.1155/2015/651836.

[82] Cundell, Diana R. & Kathryn, E. Mickle. (2018). "Osteoarthritis: potential for herbal medicines as therapies in the management of chronic inflammatory damage". *Current Immunology Reviews*, *14*, 68-80. E Pub ahead of print link. Accessed on February 13, 2019. http://www.eurekaselect.com/node/162555/article/osteoarthritis-potential-for-herbal-medicines-as-therapies-in-the-management-of-chronic-inflammatory-damage.

[83] Rizzi, Liana., Idiane, Rosset. & Mattheus, Roriz-Cruz. (2014). "Global epidemiology of dementia: Alzheimer's and vascular types." *BioMed Research International*, *204*, 908915. doi: 10.1155/2014/908915.

[84] Einarson, Thomas R., Annabel, Acs., Craig, Ludwig. & Ulrig, H. Panton. (2018). "Prevalence of cardiovascular disease in type 2 diabetes: a systematic literature review of scientific evidence from across the world in 2007-2017." *Cardiovascular Diabetology*, *17*(1), 83. doi: 10.1186/s12933-018-0728-6.

[85] Moneret-Vautrin, Anne D., Martine, Morisset., Lemerdy, P. H., Croizier, A. & Gisele, Kanny. (2002). "Food allergy and IgE sensitization caused by spices: CICBAA data (based on 589 cases of food allergy)."*Allerg. Immunol.*, *34*, 135–140. Accessed on February 15, 2019. https://europepmc.org/abstract/med/12078423.

[86] Shemesh-Meyer, Einat., Tomer, Ben-Michael., Neta, Rotem., Haim, D. Rabinowitch., Adi, Doron-Fagenboim., Arkadiusz, Kosmala., Dawid, Kerlikowski., Amir, Sherman. & Rina, Kamenetsky. (2015). "Garlic (Allium sativum L.) fertility: transcriptome and proteome analyses provide insight into flower and pollen development." *Frontiers in Plant Science*, *6*, 271. doi: 10.3389/fpls.2015.00271.

[87] Zewdie, Yayeh., James, P. Prince. & Maria, M. Jenderek. (2005). "The first genetic linkages among expressed regions of the garlic genome." *J. Amer. Soc. Hort. Sci.*, *130*(4), 569-574. doi: https://doi.org/10.21273/JASHS.130.4.569.

[88] Egea, Leticia A., Rosa, Mérida-García., Andrzej, Kilian., Pilar, Hernandez. & Gabriel, Dorado. (2017). "Assessment of Genetic Diversity and Structure of Large Garlic (*Allium sativum*) Germplasm Bank, by Diversity Arrays Technology "Genotyping-by-Sequencing" Platform (DArTseq)." *Frontiers in Genetics*, *8*, 98. doi: 10.3389/fgene.2017.00098.

ABOUT THE EDITOR

Dr. Diana R. Cundell received her Ph.D. in medicine from The Royal Postgraduate Medical Federation, London, U.K. in 1993 and is currently a Professor of Biology and the Pre-Medical Studies Program Director at Jefferson University. Her research spans over thirty years and during the past decade has focused on herbal medicines as antimicrobial and immunomodulatory agents. Dr. Cundell has published research on several phytomedicines including curcumin (turmeric) and their utility in safely managing chronic inflammatory disease. She is the author of over 60 articles and holds 4 process patents associated with breathing wall systems. Dr. Cundell sits on the Editorial Board of Plant Biology and Phytomedicine and has acted as a guest editor for Current Immunology Reviews.

Email: Diana.Cundell@jefferson.edu.

INDEX

A

B

C

D

E

F

G

H

I

J

K

L

M

N

O

P

R

S

T

U

V

W

Y

Z

Related Nova Publications

Nutrition: Infants, Children and Adults

Editor: Sven Schulz

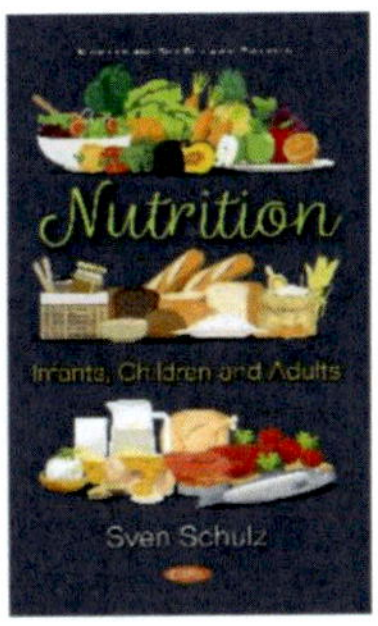

Series: Nutrition and Diet Research Progress

Book Description: Every day, the United States Department of Agriculture's (USDA) Child and Adult Care Food Program (CACFP) serves millions of infants, children, and adults across the United States. The CACFP provides a great opportunity to introduce infants and children to healthy eating habits. This book reports on the importance of good nutrition at every age.

Hardcover ISBN: 978-1-53617-044-3
Retail Price: $160

Handbook of Chickpeas: Nutritional Value, Health Benefits and Management

Editors: Albert T. Lund and Noah D. Schultz

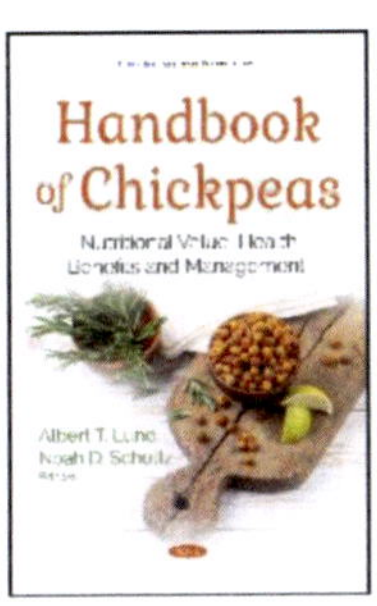

Series: Nutrition and Diet Research Progress

Book Description: Legumes are an important source of proteins, carbohydrates, vitamins, minerals, and dietary fiber. Chickpea is one of the most consumed legumes in the world. As such, *Handbook of Chickpeas: Nutritional Value, Health Benefits and Management* discusses the current information regarding the nutritional value of chickpea.

Hardcover ISBN: 978-1-53616-374-2
Retail Price: $230

To see a complete list of Nova publications, please visit our website at www.novapublishers.com